MATH for
CLINICAL
PRACTICE

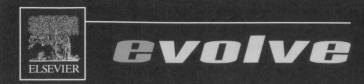

ELSEVIER

evolve

∴ *To access your Student Resources, visit:*
http://evolve.elsevier.com/Macklin/math/

Evolve® Student Resources for *Macklin: Math for Clinical Practice,*
second edition offers the following features:

- **Drug Calculations Companion, version 4:** A completely updated, interactive
  student tutorial that includes an extensive menu of various topic areas within drug
  calculations such as oral, parenteral, pediatric, and intravenous calculations to
  name a few. It contains over 600 practice problems covering ratio and proportion,
  formula, and dimensional analysis methods.

- **Student Practice Problems:** Provides additional practice and promotes active
  learning and application of content.

MATH for CLINICAL PRACTICE

Denise Macklin, BSN, RNC
Marietta, Georgia

Cynthia Chernecky, PhD, RN, CNS, AOCN
Professor
School of Nursing
Georgia Health Sciences University
Augusta, Georgia

Mother Helena Infortuna, MTS, BS
Saints Mary and Martha Orthodox Monastery
Wagener, South Carolina

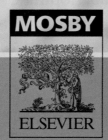

MOSBY

ELSEVIER

MOSBY
ELSEVIER

3251 Riverport Lane
Maryland Heights, Missouri 63043

Math for Clinical Practice, Second Edition   ISBN: 978-0-323-06499-6

NOTICE

Knowledge and best practice in this field are constantly changing. As new research and experience
broaden our knowledge, changes in practice, treatment and drug therapy may become necessary
or appropriate. Readers are advised to check the most current information provided (i) on procedures featured or (ii) by the manufacturer of each product to be administered, to verify the recommended dose or formula, the method and duration of administration, and contraindications. It is
the responsibility of the practitioner, relying on their own experience and knowledge of the patient,
to make diagnoses, to determine dosages and the best treatment for each individual patient, and
to take all appropriate safety precautions. To the fullest extent of the law, neither the Publisher nor
the Editors/Authors assumes any liability for any injury and/or damage to persons or property
arising out of or related to any use of the material contained in this book.

Library of Congress Cataloging-in-Publication Data
Macklin, Denise.
  Math for clinical practice / Denise Macklin, Cynthia Chernecky, Mother Helena Infortuna. — 2nd ed.
    p. ; cm.
  Includes index.
  ISBN 978-0-323-06499-6 (pbk. : alk. paper)
  1. Nursing—Mathematics. 2. Pharmaceutical arithmetic. I. Chernecky, Cynthia C. II. Helena
Infortuna, Mother. III. Title.
  [DNLM: 1. Drug Dosage Calculations—Problems and Exercises. 2. Mathematics—Problems and
Exercises. 3. Nursing Care—methods—Problems and Exercises. 4. Pharmaceutical Preparations—
administration & dosage—Problems and Exercises. QV 18.2 M158m 2010]
  RT68.M33 2010
  610.7301′5—dc22

     2009040476

Senior Editor: Yvonne Alexopoulos
Senior Developmental Editor: Danielle M. Frazier
Publishing Services Manager: Jeff Patterson
Project Manager: Tracey Schriefer
Book Designer: Paula Catalano

Printed in China

Last digit is the print number: 9   8   7   6   5   4   3   2

About the Authors

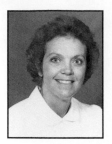

Denise Macklin is certified in adult/staff education. Denise has over 30 years of nursing experience, with 25 years in the specialty of IV therapy. She was included in *Who's Who in Media and Communications 1998*. She is the recipient of the Suzanne Herbst award for vascular access and a research grant related to vascular access education from the National Institute for Nursing Research. Denise has lectured around the United States on a wide variety of IV therapy topics. She has published articles in various publications, including *Journal of Intravenous Nursing, Journal of Vascular Access Devices, American Journal of Nursing*, and *Nursing Management and Dimensions of Critical Care*. She is a contributing author to *Saunders Manual of Medical-Surgical Nursing: A Guide to Clinical Decision Making*, co-author of *Real World Nursing Survival Guide: Fluids & Electrolytes*, and lead author of *Real World Nursing Survival Guide: IV Therapy*. Denise's work includes extensive experience in the production of training videos for vascular access and interactive programs for medical manufacturers and the Centers for Disease Control and Prevention.

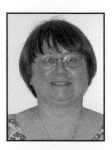

Dr. Cynthia Chernecky earned her degrees at the University of Connecticut (BSN), the University of Pittsburgh (MN), and Case Western Reserve University (PhD). She also earned an NIH fellowship at Yale University and was a postdoctoral visiting scholar at UCLA. She is also a recipient of the Oncology Nursing Society Mary Nowotny Excellence in Cancer Nursing Education Award and currently a nominee for the Oncology Nursing Society Excellence in Cancer Nursing Research Award. Her clinical area of expertise is critical care oncology, with publications including *Laboratory Tests and Diagnostic Procedures* (fourth edition), *Advanced and Critical Care Oncology Nursing: Managing Primary Complications*, and several titles from the *Real World Nursing Survival Guide Series*, including *ECGs & the Heart, Drug Calculations and Drug Administration, Fluids & Electrolytes, IV Therapy, Critical Care & Emergency Nursing*, and *Hemodynamic Monitoring*.

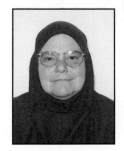

Mother Helena Infortuna was born of immigrant parents in Queens Village, New York. After working in Manhattan as a secretary, she entered the Sisters of Notre Dame de Namur, a teaching order, and was educated at Trinity College in Washington, D.C. While teaching high school mathematics in Pennsylvania, Maryland, New York, and Delaware, she earned her MTS degree from The Catholic University of America and other graduate mathematic credits from Villanova University, the University of Pennsylvania, and the University of Delaware, all through NSF grants. Mother Helena's 37 years in education have included administration as well as teaching. The first 28 years were in the Catholic school system, followed by 6 years at Newton High School in Elmhurst, a New York City public school. From there, she moved to Washington, D.C. and taught at both Northern Virginia Community College and Montgomery College. Settling into the Orthodox monastic community of Saints Mary and Martha in Wagener, South Carolina, she taught high school mathematics for 4 more years and is currently serving as a private mathematics instructor.

Contributors

Contributors for the Second Edition

Kathleen R. Wren, CRNA, PhD
Professor
Department of Nurse Anesthesia
Florida Hospital College of Health Sciences
Orlando, Florida

Contributors for the First Edition

Jean D. Balogh, RN, MSN, OCN
Assistant Professor
Department of Nursing
Augusta State University
Augusta, Georgia

Susan M. Buzhardt, RN, MSN, OCN
Nurse Instructor
Aiken Technical College
Graniteville, South Carolina

Corliss Grinstead Derrick, MSN
Instructor
School of Nursing
Georgia Health Sciences University
Augusta, Georgia

Rebecca K. Hodges, RN, MSN, CCRN
Critical Care Nurse Clinician
St. Joseph's Hospital
Augusta, Georgia

Barbara Kiernan, PhD, APRN
Assistant Professor, Parent-Child Nursing
School of Nursing
Georgia Health Sciences University
Augusta, Georgia

Patricia H. Revolinski, RN, MSN
Nurse Manager
Telemetry Unit
St. Joseph's Hospital
Augusta, Georgia

Rebecca Rule, MN, MPH
Assistant Professor
School of Nursing
Georgia Health Sciences University
Augusta, Georgia

Kathleen R. Wren, CRNA, PhD
Program Director, Nurse Anesthesia Program
School of Nursing
Louisiana State University Health Sciences Center
New Orleans, Louisiana

Timothy L. Wren, RN, MS
Assistant Professor, Clinical Nursing
School of Nursing
Louisiana State University Health Sciences Center
New Orleans, Louisiana

Content and Math Reviewers

Joyce Bedoian PhD(c), MSN, MBe, RN
Assistant Professor
Wilson School of Nursing
Midwestern State University
Wichita Falls, Texas

Billie E. Blake, EdD, MSN, BSN, RN
Associate Dean and Professor
St. Johns River Community College
Orange Park, Florida

Ruth A. Chaplen, MSN, RN, AOCN, APRN, BC
Clinical Instructor
College of Nursing
Wayne State University
Detroit, Michigan

Ruth Hansten, RN, MBA, PhD, FACHE
Principal
Hansten Healthcare PLLC
Port Ludlow, Washington

Pamela J. Schuler, RN, MSN
Nurse Educator
VA Sierra Nevada Health Care System
Reno, Nevada

Jill Scott, RN, MSN, CCRN
Nursing Professor
St. John's River Community College
Palatka, Florida

Tamara Shields, RN, MS, FNP-BC
Instructor of Nursing
St. Elizabeth School of Nursing
Lafayette, Indiana

Katherine Tate, RN, MN, PNP
Program Director
Professor of Pediatric Nursing
Ohlone College
Newark, California

Sharon Walker, MSN, RN
Nursing Instructor
Notre Dame College
South Euclid, Ohio

Ina E. Warboys, MS, RN
Clinical Assistant Professor
The University of Alabama
Huntsville, Alabama

Preface to the Instructor

Math for Clinical Practice presents a straightforward, real-life approach and focuses on mathematical calculations used in the clinical setting. The text focuses on linking mathematical principles to the prescription that is written and the medication sent to the nurse by the pharmacy. Only basic math skills that are required for calculations used in the clinical setting are included. Once these skills are reviewed, the text provides a comprehensive review. Without a firm foundation in the basics, calculation success is difficult. The text then proceeds to review the general calculation methods that are used in the clinical setting: percentage, ratio-proportion method, formula method, and body weight. This text focuses on the ratio-proportion method, but it does so because it lends itself easily to the clinical setting. The focus of the text is always on the use of math in the clinical setting. Rounding, for instance, is different in different chapters depending on the needs in the clinical setting. If a syringe is marked in tenths, then problems are rounded to the nearest tenth. If a whole number is clinically appropriate as with large volume infusions or non scored tablets, then the answer is rounded to the nearest whole number. The authors recognize that with calculators problems can be rounded to, for instance, the nearest thousand. However, the focus is on the real world and the connection of how math is used clinically. It is hoped that this approach will assist in a smooth transition from the classroom to the hospital.

Next, syringe usage, oral and parenteral medications, and medication reconstitution are reviewed. Common medications and methods of administration are used so that the student can feel confident that he or she will be prepared for what they encounter in practice. All common methods for administering medications are reviewed. In addition, examples are given for calculations that are unique to specific patient populations, such as insulin, intake and output, and heparin. Calculating insulin dosages based on dietary intake as well as sliding scale are reviewed in depth. Intake and output are discussed with examples from diverse clinical settings. Heparin is discussed based on the two major methods of calculation related to type of prescription and from two major clinical realities: premixed bags and pharmacy mixed bags. Intravenous therapy is reviewed, with the primary focus being infusion pumps. This approach more closely reflects the clinical setting where gravity infusions are becoming rare. Specialty units such as oncology, pediatrics, and intensive care are introduced. A math calculation specific to each area is discussed, such as body surface area for oncology, titration for intensive care, and body surface area for pediatrics.

In response to the importance of safety and quality care and current recommendations from The Joint Commission (TJC) and the Institute for Safe Medication Practices (ISMP), safety alerts, clinical alerts, human error alerts, and human error checks are integrated to minimize calculation errors. To support current TJC and ISMP recommendations, prescriptions are written out and abbreviations, acronyms, and symbols not recommended by TJC and ISMP are not used.

This reality-based book contains over 1200 clinically specific problems throughout the text, providing students the practice needed to master clinical calculations. Skills learned in early chapters are included in some of the review problems in later chapters. Once the use of syringes is reviewed, whenever a syringe is required for medication administration, an empty syringe is generally included with the problem to be marked appropriately. An oral syringe or medication cups are included when appropriate. The answer key includes syringes with plungers drawn back to the correct marking, as well as oral syringes and medicine cups. This feature enhances the real-life clinical experience in medication administration.

PEDAGOGICAL FEATURES

- **Clinical Connections** begin each chapter and explain why the chapter is important and how it relates to clinical practices enhancing the connection of the math calculation to the clinical setting.
- **Chapter Introductions** provide an overview of topics to be discussed in the chapter, focusing on what is relevant to the clinical setting. The introduction sets the foundation for the in-depth discussion and practice to follow and connects the calculation to the clinical setting.
- **Clinical Alert boxes** present information that, when applied in the clinical setting, creates the best practice care.
- **Safety Alert boxes** identify issues that may lead to medication errors. These alerts are based on the guidelines from the ISMP, as well as years of clinical practice by other health care professionals.
- **Human Error Alert boxes** identify common mistakes that can lead to incorrect drug calculations, enhancing the student's ability to troubleshoot calculations in the clinical setting.
- **Examples** include variations of the following **unique** step-by-step format:
  - **Prescription**—What is written on the patient's chart, incorporating current TJC and ISMP recommendations.

- **What You HAVE**—Pictures of what would be sent up from the pharmacy (labels) or a description of what will be on hand.
- **What You KNOW**—A breakdown of the prescription and information found in the patient's chart and on the drug insert or from the pharmacist, all of which is needed for the calculation.
- **What You WANT**—Identifies the missing information that must be found.
- **Critical Thinking**—The thought process that needs to occur to perform the calculation. A systematic approach is taken to help the student understand how to approach a calculation. The fill-in-the-blank questions require that the student identify information from the pharmacy label (What You HAVE) and from the prescription and patient chart (What You KNOW), all of which will be required to complete the calculation. This activity builds an organized approach to addressing clinical calculations.
- **Answer for Best Care**—A step-by-step calculation that follows the items outlined in Critical Thinking. This shows how to do the problem and does not just display the math calculation.
- **Human Error Check boxes**—Review how to check specific calculations to see if the calculation answer is correct, thus providing a systematic approach to checking drug calculations.
- **Does your answer fit the general guideline?**—Checks to see if the answer fits into acceptable clinical and scientific parameters. This is a step that should be carried out in the clinical setting.
- After the examples, there are **Practice Problems** that promote active learning and application of content. Answers worked out in ratio-proportion and formula methods are located in the answer key.
- At the end of the chapter is a **Chapter Review** that covers the entire chapter, enabling students to evaluate their understanding of chapter content. Answers only are listed in the answer key.

- At the end of the first four chapters, there is a **Comprehensive Review** for additional practice to promote a strong math foundation required for successful calculation activity.
- **Over 500 full-color illustrations** include full-color drug labels, parenteral and oral syringes, medicine cups, pumps, IV equipment, and much more.

ANCILLARIES

Evolve Resources for Math for Clinical Practice, second edition is available to enhance student instruction. This online resource is organized by chapter and includes the following:

- *New!* Lesson Plans
- *New!* Drug Label Glossary
- *New!* PowerPoint Slides
- Test Bank Questions
- Final Exam Questions
- Patient Scenarios based on disease groups (e.g., cardiac, renal, endocrine)
- Handouts

NEW VERSION! *Romans & Daugherty Dosages and Solutions CTB, version 3*. This generic test-bank, available on Evolve at evolve.elsevier.com/Macklin/math/, contains over 700 questions on general mathematics, converting within the same system of measurements, converting between different systems of measurement, oral dosages, parenteral dosages, flow rates, pediatric dosages, IV calculations, and more.

NEW VERSION! *Drug Calculations Companion, version 4*. This is a completely updated, interactive student tutorial that includes an extensive menu of various topic areas within drug calculations, such as oral, parenteral, pediatric, and intravenous calculations. It contains over 600 practice problems covering ratio and proportion, formula, and dimensional analysis methods. It is now available on Evolve at evolve.elsevier.com/Macklin/math/

This book focuses on clinical realities and the process of thinking so that best patient care can be accomplished.

Denise Macklin
Cynthia Chernecky
Mother Helena Infortuna

Preface to the Student

Math for Clinical Practice provides all the information, explanation, and practice needed to competently and confidently calculate drug dosages. It focuses on mathematical calculations used in the clinical setting. Take a look at the following features so that you can familiarize yourself with this text and maximize its value:

Clinical Connections explain why the chapter is important and how it relates to clinical practice.

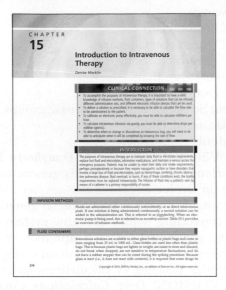

Safety Alert boxes identify issues that may lead to medication errors.

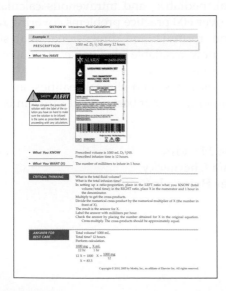

Human Error Alert boxes identify common mistakes that can lead to incorrect drug calculations, enhancing your ability to troubleshoot calculations in the clinical setting.

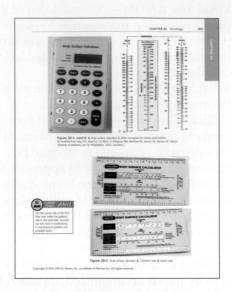

Clinical Alert boxes present information that, when applied in the clinical setting, creates the best practice care.

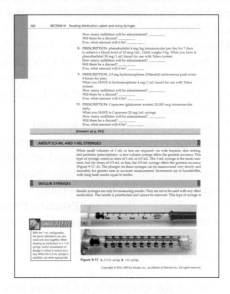

NEW VERSION! *Drug Calculations Companion, version 4.* This is a completely updated, interactive student tutorial that includes an extensive menu of various topic areas within drug calculations, such as oral, parenteral, pediatric, and intravenous calculations. It contains over 600 practice problems covering ratio and proportion, formula, and dimensional analysis methods. It is now available on Evolve at evolve.elsevier.com/Macklin/math/

evolve Look for this icon at the end of the chapters. It will refer you to the *Drug Calculations Companion, version 4* for additional practice problems and content information.

Acknowledgments

I would like to thank my colleague, mentor, and friend, Cynthia Chernecky, for her generosity of spirit and enthusiasm for life. Her support throughout our many professional activities has been invaluable to me. I would like to thank Mother Helena Infortuna for her contributions to this effort. It is truly a pleasure to work with her. I would also like to thank the contributing authors Jean Balogh, Sue Buzhardt, Pat Revolinski, Kathy and Timothy Wren, Barbara Kiernan, Rebecca Rule, Rebecca Hodges, and Corliss Derrick. Lending their special expertise to this book made it possible to complete a text that is current and will meet the needs of nursing students, and it truly demonstrates their devotion to enhancing nursing education.

I would like to thank Steve Nagy, PharmD; Cecily V. DiPiro, RPh, Medical College of Georgia Hospitals and Clinics; Kelly Farlow, RPh, Pharmaceutical Care Pharmacist for Oncology and Gastroenterology, Saint Joseph's Hospital Pharmacy; and Mark Stranz, RPh, for their significant input and assistance.

A special thanks for the never-ending encouragement, assistance, and friendship of my sister and partner Judith Carnahan. I would not have been able to complete the book or any of my many professional activities in research, authorship, and multimedia production without her. Also, a special thanks to my dear friend Nancy Willis. She has always provided me, without question, with whatever assistance I needed to complete a project. For this I will always be grateful.

I want to thank DeCapúa photography of Melbourne, Florida for the special assistance, flexibility, and creativity required to make my illustrative vision for this book a reality. Also, I would like to thank Dan Gunn of Gunn's Photo/Video of Atlanta for his efforts with the electronic pump photos.

I want to thank Yvonne Alexopoulos for her patience, suggestions, advice, and guidance. I want to thank Danielle Frazier, who kept me on track throughout a very complex development process. This book could not have become a reality without her attention to detail.

I would like to extend sincere thanks to Becton Dickinson & Company and Medicine-On-Time, who gave us permission to use photographs, illustrations, and other materials in the text.

Finally, I would like to thank my husband, Dana, who has believed in me and understood the long hours, missed meals, and trips that were required to complete this book.

Denise Macklin

This book has been a true delight from a clinical perspective. Many thanks to all the studnts who, through my many years of teaching, have made my career truly enlightening.

First, a special thanks to my Mother, Olga, for her endless proof reading, suggestions, understanding of the time commitment to this project, and hours of coffee and homemade cookies, perogies, and kulich. Special thanks to my co-editors and authors who shared their knowledge, expertise, time, effort, and words of encouragement, they are great role models. Many thanks to Yvonne Alexopoulos and Danielle Frazier, experts at Elsevier, who made this text a reality and very user friendly. My personal thanks to those who share time and knowledge with me, making me a better professional: Drs. Jean Brown, Mary Cooley, Linda Sarna, Denise Macklin, Ellie Fennell, May Wykle, and Ann Bavier. Special thanks to those with whom I share clinical: Pam Cushman, Christina Black, and the staff of 4-West MCGHI. I owe a great deal to the nuns of Saints Mary and Martha Orthodox Monastery in Wagener, South Carolina, who have a haven for rest and relaxation that I truly enjoy. Special thanks to Mother Thecla (Abbess), Mother Helena, and Sister Lubov. Finally, I thank my dog, who reminds me there is a need for breaks and walks.

Cynthia Chernecky

My thanks to Dr. Cynthia Chernecky for giving me yet another opportunity to help her with a most worthwhile task of helping nurses. I also thank the community of Saints Mary and Martha Orthodox Monastery for supporting me in this project, as well as our good God, who is so very good!

Mother Helena Infortuna

Contents

Renewing Math Skills

CHAPTER 1

Decimals: Relative Value, Addition, and Subtraction

Mother Helena Infortuna

CLINICAL CONNECTION

- Correct placement of decimal points in calculations is essential for error-free solutions and promotes quality patient care.
- Determining the relative value of decimals is necessary when comparing prescriptions with drug availability.
- Comparing the prescription relative value with the recommended dose range enhances appropriate dosage implementation.
- Addition and subtraction of decimals are common calculations in all clinical settings.
- Using relative value helps assist the practitioner in double-checking calculations to decrease human error.

INTRODUCTION

Since many medications involve dosages that contain decimals, it is essential to understand decimals, recognize the relative values of decimals, understand the importance of correct decimal placement, and be able to add and subtract decimal numbers. Identifying the relative value enables you to think about your answer to the drug calculation before you do the math. This will enable you to evaluate the math calculation that will affect patient care. For example, if you decide that you will need **less** than one tablet and your calculation results in an answer that you will need **more** than one tablet, you know that somewhere in your calculations there is a problem. Commonly the problem arises from improper decimal placement. Relative value is also important when evaluating how a number relates to a range of numbers such as recommended dose range or lab values (high and low).

WHAT ARE DECIMAL NUMBERS?

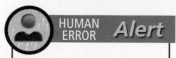

Improper decimal placement is a common error associated with medication administration.

Decimal numbers include both whole numbers and fractions. When written together, they are separated by a decimal point. Whole numbers are to the left of the decimal point and fraction numbers are to the right of the decimal point.

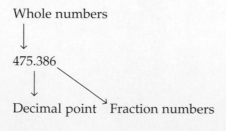

Whole numbers

475.386

Decimal point   Fraction numbers

The position of each digit (number) indicates its value:

Decimal point

Hundreds, tens, units (or ones) · Tenths, hundredths, thousandths

← Increasing value   Decreasing value →

To begin a review of decimal numbers, see Figure 1-1 for a series of digits with a value. (Only possible values for medications have been used.)

RELATIVE VALUE OF A DECIMAL NUMBER

Understanding the value of a decimal number, and recognizing the high and low values of each number, is the key to calculating and administering accurate dosages of medications. The relative value of a number is determined by the spaces to the left of the decimal point—the more spaces, the higher the value. (See Figure 1-1.) When comparing two or more numbers with the same quantity of spaces to the left of the decimal point, the first place from the left where they differ determines the relative value of each number. For example, if you have the numbers 34.5 and 32.6, the first place from the left where the two numbers differ is in the ones value, or the number 4 in 34.5 and the number 2 in 32.6. Since the number 4 is larger than the number 2, the larger of these two numbers is 34.5. If the numbers to the left of the decimal do not differ (are exactly the same), you begin comparing numbers to the right of the decimal point until you find a difference in the numbers. For example, if you have the numbers 29.82 and 29.61, the numbers to the left of the decimal point are the same; they both have the value 29. Therefore, you begin to look at the first space to the right of the decimal point to see if the numbers differ. In this case, they do differ—with one having a value of 8, in 29.82, and the other having a value of 6, in 29.61. Since 8 is a larger number than 6, the number with the highest value is 29.82.

Lining up the decimals vertically to each other enables you to more easily compare their values. In lining up the decimals, wherever there is an unequal number of spaces to the right and left of the decimal point you should add the value of zero (0) wherever there is a blank space; this decreases errors, especially when you begin to add and subtract values of numbers. These added zeros do not change the value of the number. For example, in comparing the values of the numbers 24.87 and 24.599, you would add a zero onto 24.87 when you line them up so that the number of spaces to the right and left of the decimal point is equal.

Line decimal points vertically:

24.870 ← Zero added
24.599

SAFETY ALERT

A zero is **always** placed to the left of the decimal point when there is no whole number. This zero highlights the decimal point and that the value of the number is less than one.

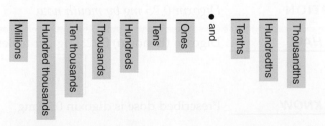

Figure 1-1 Decimal place values.

Example 1

Which is the higher value dexamethasone (Decadron), a 1.5-mg tablet or a 0.25-mg tablet?

CRITICAL THINKING

The decimal points must be lined up vertically when writing the numbers.
Do the numbers have the same number of spaces to the left of the decimal? Yes.
Do the numbers have the same number of spaces to the right of the decimal? No.
Do you need to add zeros anywhere? Yes.
Where is the first place from the left that is different?

ANSWER FOR BEST CARE

Line decimals up vertically and add zeros. Add a zero to the second space to the right of the decimal point in 1.5 to make it 1.50, so all numbers have the same number of spaces to the right and the left of the decimal point.

1.50 ← Add zero
0.25

The first place they differ is the first digit to the left of the decimal point.
Since 1 is greater than 0, 1.5 has the higher value.
Answer is 1.5.

Example 2

Which is the higher value, 0.225 or 0.25?

CRITICAL THINKING

The decimal points must be lined up vertically when writing the numbers.
Do the numbers have the same number of spaces to the left of the decimal? Yes.
Do the numbers have the same number of spaces to the right of the decimal? No.
Do you need to add zeros anywhere? Yes.
Where is the first place that the numbers differ?

ANSWER FOR BEST CARE

Line decimals up vertically.

0.225
0.250 ← Add zero

Add a zero to the third space to the right of the decimal point in 0.25 to make it 0.250, so all numbers have the same number of spaces.
These numbers have the same number of places to the left of the decimal and the same value (zero).
The first place they differ is the second place to the right of the decimal point.
Since 5 is greater than 2, 0.25 is the higher value.
Answer is 0.25.

   Understanding relative value enables you to determine if the prescription dose is higher or lower than the dose that you have on hand. Let's look at an example.

Example 3

PRESCRIPTION

Digoxin 0.25 mg by mouth now.

• What You HAVE

Digoxin (Lanoxin) 0.125 mg per tablet.

• What You KNOW

Prescribed dose is digoxin 0.25 mg.

• What You WANT

Is the prescribed dose higher than the dose that you have on hand?
Will you need less than one tablet, exactly one tablet, or more than one tablet?

CRITICAL THINKING	The decimal points must be lined up vertically when writing the numbers. Do the numbers have the same number of spaces to the left of the decimal? Yes. Do the numbers have the same number of spaces to the right of the decimal? No. Do you need to add zeros anywhere? Yes. What is the first place from the left that is different?
ANSWER FOR BEST CARE	Line decimals up vertically and add necessary zeros. 0.250 ← Add zero 0.125 Add a zero to the third space to the right of the decimal point in 0.25 so all numbers have the same number of digits. The first place the numbers differ is the first space to the right of the decimal point; since 2 is greater (bigger) than 1, 0.25 (0.250) has the higher value. The prescribed dose is larger (higher) than the dose you have on hand, so you will have to give more than one tablet. Answer is more than one tablet.

Example 4

PRESCRIPTION	*Lanoxin 0.125 mg by mouth daily.*
• **What You HAVE**	Lanoxin (digoxin) 0.125 mg per tablet.
• **What You KNOW**	The recommended dose range is 0.02 mg to 0.2 mg. Prescribed dose is Lanoxin 0.125 mg.
• **What You WANT**	Is the prescribed dose within the recommended dose range?
CRITICAL THINKING	The decimal points must be lined up vertically when writing the numbers. Do the numbers have the same number of spaces to the left of the decimal? Yes. Do the numbers have the same number of spaces to the right of the decimal? No. Do you need to add zeros anywhere? Yes. What is the first place from the left that is different?
ANSWER FOR BEST CARE	Line decimals up vertically and add necessary zeros. 0.125 0.020 ← Add zero 0.200 ← Add zeros Add a zero to the third space to the right of the decimal point in 0.02 and two zeros to 0.2 so all three numbers have the same number of spaces. The first place the numbers differ is the first space to the right of the decimal point. Since 2 is greater (bigger) than 1, 0.2 has a higher value than 0.125; since 1 is greater than 0, 0.125 has a greater value than 0.020 (0.02). The prescribed dose is within the recommended dose range.

PRACTICE PROBLEMS	**Directions:** *In problems 1 through 3, circle the number with the highest value.* **1.** (a) 2.5 (b) 3.55 (c) 3.75 **2.** (a) 1.25 (b) 1.5 (c) 1.35 **3.** (a) 0.175 (b) 0.125 (c) 0.15

4. PRESCRIPTION: nitroglycerin (Nitrostat) 0.4 mg by mouth now.
   You HAVE: 0.4-mg–strength tablets.

Will you NEED: less than one tablet, one tablet exactly, or more than one tablet?

5. PRESCRIPTION: warfarin sodium (Coumadin) 1.25 mg by mouth daily.
   You HAVE: 2.5-mg–strength tablets.

Will you NEED: less than one tablet, one tablet exactly, or more than one tablet?

6. PRESCRIPTION: levothyroxine (Synthroid) 0.05 mg by mouth today.
   You HAVE: 0.025-mg–strength tablets.

Will you NEED: less than one tablet, one tablet exactly, or more than one tablet?

7. PRESCRIPTION: glyburide (DiaBeta) 1.25 mg by mouth at breakfast.
   You HAVE: 2.5-mg–strength tablets.

Will you NEED: less than one tablet, one tablet exactly, or more than one tablet?

8. PRESCRIPTION: alprazolam (Xanax) 0.5 mg by mouth three times a day.
   You HAVE: 0.25-mg–strength tablets.

Will you NEED: less than one tablet, one tablet exactly, or more than one tablet?

9. PRESCRIPTION: lorazepam (Ativan) 1 mg by mouth now.
   You HAVE: 0.5-mg–strength tablets.

Will you NEED: less than one tablet, one tablet exactly, or more than one tablet?

10. PRESCRIPTION: prednisone (Deltasone) 7.5 mg by mouth now.
    You HAVE: 2.5-mg–strength tablets.

Will you NEED: less than one tablet, one tablet exactly, or more than one tablet?

(Answers on p. 437)

ADDITION OF DECIMAL NUMBERS

Addition is used in the clinical setting—for example, when adding doses, intake of fluids, hourly outputs, and in restricted diets (fluid, electrolyte, carbohydrate). Addition is the mathematical operation of combining numbers to determine their accumulative (total) value. The result is called the sum. To find the sum of decimal numbers, it is critical that the decimals are aligned vertically. Once the decimals are aligned, zeros are added to each number so that all numbers have the same number of numerical places. Add the numbers beginning from the farthest right column and continuing by moving left one column at a time. If the sum of the numbers in a column is 10 or greater, add the tens digit to the next column to the left. For example, if the sum of the numbers equaled a number that was between 10 and 19, you would add the number 1 to the next left column. If the sum of the numbers were 20 to 29, you would add a 2 to the next left column. If the sum were 30 to 39, you would add a 3 to the next left column. For sums of 40 to 49, add a 4; 50 to 59, add a 5; 60 to 69, add a 6; 70 to 79, add a 7; 80 to 89, add an 8; 90 to 99, add a 9; 100 to 109, add a 10; 110 to 119, add an 11; and so forth. Place the decimal point in the answer directly under the other decimal points. Once the sum is determined, if the last digit(s) on the right of the decimal point is zero, it does not change the value of the number and is eliminated.

> ✓**Human Error Check**
>
> To double-check your calculation, an easy method is to increase each decimal number to the nearest higher whole number. Add all whole numbers together and your actual answer should be less than or equal to this sum of the whole numbers.

Example 1

Add 12.5 and 0.25, knowing they have the same units of measurement.

CRITICAL THINKING

Write the numbers one under the other, aligning the decimal points.
Add zeros to numbers so that all columns have the same number of spaces.
Begin with the farthest right column and, moving one column to the left at a time, add each column.
Add the tens digit to the next column to the left when the column sum is 10 or greater.
Place the decimal point in the answer directly under the other decimal points.

ANSWER FOR BEST CARE

Align decimals vertically and add a zero after the 5 in the number 12.5 and before the 0 in 0.25.

$$\downarrow$$
$$12.50 \leftarrow \text{Add zero after } 5$$
$$\text{Add zero before } + 00.25$$

SAFETY *Alert*

A decimal point placed incorrectly is a major cause of medication error. It is important to place the decimal clearly and correctly.

$$\begin{array}{r}12.50 \\ + 00.25 \\ \hline 5 \end{array}$$ 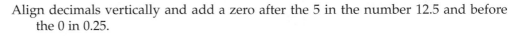 ← Begin with farthest right column of $0 + 5$. This equals 5, and since 5 is less than 10, there is no number to carry over to the next column.

Move left one column and add $5 + 2$, which equals 7. Since 7 is less than 10, there is no number to carry over to the next column.

$$\downarrow$$
$$\begin{array}{r}12.50 \\ + 00.25 \\ \hline .75 \end{array}$$

Move left to next column of $2 + 0$, which equals 2. Since 2 is less than 10, there is no number to carry over to the next column.

$$\downarrow$$
$$\begin{array}{r}12.50 \\ + 00.25 \\ \hline 2.75 \end{array}$$

Move left to the next column of $1 + 0$, which equals 1. Since 1 is less than 10, there is no number to carry over to the next column.

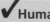
```
   ↓
  12.50
+ 00.25
  12.75
   ↑
```

Align the decimal point in the answer with the decimal points above.
The sum is 12.75 of the same units of measurement.

✔ **Human Error Check**

Round 12.5 up to 13.
Round 0.25 up to 1.
Add $13 + 1 = 14$.
Your answer should be less than or equal to 14.
The answer is 12.75. This is less than 14.

Example 2

Add 2.5 and 1.75, knowing that they have the same units of measurement.

CRITICAL THINKING

Write numbers one under the other, aligning the decimal points.
Add zeros to numbers so that all columns have the same number of spaces.
Begin with the farthest right column and moving one column to the left at a time add each column.
Add the tens digit to the next column to the left when the column sum is 10 or greater.
Place the decimal point in the answer directly under the other decimal points.

ANSWER FOR BEST CARE

Align decimals vertically.

```
  ↓
 2.5
+ 1.75
```

Add a zero after the 5 in the number 2.5.

```
 2.50 ←
+ 1.75
```

Begin adding the farthest right column of $0 + 5$. This equals 5, and since 5 is less than 10, there is no number to carry over to the next column.

```
   ↓
 2.50
+ 1.75
    5
```

Move left to the next column of $5 + 7$, which equals 12. Since 12 is more than 10, you carry over the **"one"** (because the number is between 10 and 19) to the next column.
Carry over → ①

```
    ↓
 2.50
+ 1.75
   25
```

Move left to the next column of $2 + 1 + 1$ (carry over), which equals 4. Since 4 is less than 10, there is no number to carry over to the next column.

$\downarrow$

Carry over → ①

$$\begin{array}{r} 2.50 \\ + \ 1.75 \\ \hline 4\,25 \end{array}$$

Align the decimal point in the answer with the decimal points above.

Carry over → ①

$$\begin{array}{r} 2.50 \\ + \ 1.75 \\ \hline 4.25 \end{array}$$

$\uparrow$

The sum is 4.25 of the same units of measurement.

✔ **Human Error Check**

Round 2.5 up to 3.
Round 1.75 up to 2.
Add $3 + 2 = 5$.
Your answer should be less than or equal to 5.
The answer is 4.25. This is less than 5.

Example 3

Using addition in the clinical setting.

ASSESSMENT

A patient has hourly urine outputs of 60 mL, 45.5 mL, 34.75 mL, and 20 mL.

• **What You WANT**

What is the total output in these 4 hours?

CRITICAL THINKING

Write numbers one under the other, aligning the decimal points.
Add zeros to numbers so that all columns have the same number of spaces.
Begin with the farthest right column and, moving one column to the left at a time, add each column.
Add the tens digit to the next column to the left when the column sum is 10 or greater.
Place the decimal point in the answer directly under the other decimal points.
Add the unit of measure—such as mg, g, or mL—to your answer.

ANSWER FOR BEST CARE

Align decimals vertically.

$\downarrow$

$$\begin{array}{r} 60 \\ 45.5 \\ 34.75 \\ + \ 20 \\ \hline \end{array}$$

Add a decimal point and two zeros after 60, add a zero after the 5 in 45.5, and add the decimal point and two zeros after the 0 in 20.

$$\begin{array}{r} 60.00 \\ 45.50 \\ 34.75 \\ + \ 20.00 \\ \hline \end{array}$$ ← Add decimal point and two zeros
← Add zero

← Add decimal point and two zeros

Begin adding the farthest right column of $0 + 0 + 5 + 0$. This equals 5, and since 5 is less than 10, there is no number to carry over to the next column.

$$
\begin{array}{r}
\downarrow \\
60.00 \\
45.50 \\
34.75 \\
+\ 20.00 \\
\hline
5
\end{array}
$$

Move left to next column: $0 + 5 + 7 + 0$. This equals 12 and, since 12 is larger than 10, the 1 is carried over to the next column.

$$
\begin{array}{r}
\downarrow \\
① \\
60.00 \\
45.50 \\
34.75 \\
+\ 20.00 \\
\hline
.25
\end{array}
$$

Move left to the next column of $1 + 0 + 5 + 4 + 0$, which equals 10. Since 10 is the same as 10, the 1 is carried over to the next column.

$$
\begin{array}{r}
\downarrow \\
①① \\
60.00 \\
45.50 \\
34.75 \\
+\ 20.00 \\
\hline
0.25
\end{array}
$$

Move left to the next column of $1 + 6 + 4 + 3 + 2$, which equals 16. Since 16 is more than 10, the 1 is carried over to the next column.

$$
\begin{array}{r}
\downarrow \\
①①① \\
60.00 \\
45.50 \\
34.75 \\
+\ 20.00 \\
\hline
60.25
\end{array}
$$

Move left to the next column. The only number here is the 1 you carried over. Place a 1 to the left of the 6.

$$
\begin{array}{r}
\downarrow \\
①①① \\
60.00 \\
45.50 \\
34.75 \\
+\ 20.00 \\
\hline
160.25
\end{array}
$$

Align the decimal point in the answer with the decimal points above.

$$
\begin{array}{r}
60.00 \\
45.50 \\
34.75 \\
+\ 20.00 \\
\hline
160.25
\end{array}
$$

The output sum is 160.25 mL.

✓**Human Error Check**

60 remains 60 (whole number).
Round 45.5 up to 46.
Round 34.75 up to 35.
20 remains 20.
Add 60 + 46 + 35 + 20 = 161.
Your answer should be less than or equal to 161.
The answer is 160.25. This is less than 161.

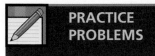

PRACTICE PROBLEMS

Directions: Find the sum (add the following) of the different strengths of the same medication or the sum of the combined strengths of different medications as named. Do a check to see if your answer is correct.

1. 1.5 + 1.25 = _____ Human error check _____

2. 0.35 + 1.275 = _____ Human error check _____

3. Meperidine (Demerol) 12.5 mg + hydroxyzine (Vistaril) 0.4 mg = _____ Human error check _____

4. One tablet labeled 0.5 mg and one tablet labeled 0.25 mg = _____ Human error check _____

5. One tablet labeled 1.5 mg and two tablets labeled 0.125 mg = _____ Human error check _____

6. One tablet labeled 30 mg, one tablet labeled 0.05 mg, and one tablet labeled 0.4 mg = _____ Human error check _____

7. One tablet labeled 1 mg, one tablet labeled 0.375 mg, and one tablet labeled 0.75 mg = _____ Human error check _____

8. One tablet labeled 2.5 mg and two tablets labeled 5 mg _____ Human error check _____

9. One tablet labeled 2.25 mg and two tablets labeled 0.75 mg _____ Human error check _____

10. Three tablets labeled 1 g and two tablets labeled 0.25 g _____ Human error check _____

(Answers on pp. 437–438)

SUBTRACTION OF DECIMAL NUMBERS

Subtraction is the opposite mathematical operation of addition. In subtraction the numbers are combined to determine the decreased value. The result is called the difference.

To find the difference of decimal numbers, write each number so that their decimal points are aligned. If there is a different number of digits to the right and/or the left of the decimal point, it will be helpful to add zeros to the shorter number to make the numbers have the same number of spaces, just as we did in addition. Subtract the numbers, beginning with the column farthest to the right of the decimal point, and move left, subtracting each column one column at a time. When the digit being subtracted is greater than the digit above it, the digit above it must be changed by placing a one in front of it and decreasing the digit in the column to the left of it by one (1). For example, in 1.7 subtracted from 5.3 (5.3 − 1.7) the 3 of 5.3 is changed to 13 (adding 10 + 3) and the 5 of 5.3 is changed to a 4 (5 − 1).

$$\begin{array}{r}
4\;13 \\
\cancel{5}.\cancel{3} \\
-1.7 \\
\hline
\end{array}$$

Subtract each column, starting with the farthest right column and moving left (first 13 − 7 and then 4 − 1), and place the decimal point in the answer directly under the other decimal points.

$$\begin{array}{r}
4\;13 \\
\cancel{5}.\cancel{3} \\
-1.7 \\
\hline
3.6 \\
\end{array}$$

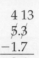

✓ **Human Error Check**

To double-check your calculation, an easy method is to **increase** higher value decimal number to nearest **higher** whole number and **decrease** the lower value decimal number to the nearest **lower** whole number. Subtract whole numbers and your actual answer should be less than or equal to this difference of the whole numbers.

Example 1

Subtract 0.5 mg from 2.5 mg.

CRITICAL THINKING

Write numbers one under the other, aligning the decimal points.

Add zeros to the left and the right of the decimal point so that all columns have the same number of spaces.

Begin subtraction with the farthest right column.

Is the digit being subtracted larger than the digit above it? If yes, then you must place "1" in front of it and decrease the digit in the next column to the left of it by the value of 1.

Subtract each column, moving left one column at a time.

Place the decimal point in the answer directly under the other decimal points.

Add the unit of measure—such as mg, g, or mL—to your answer.

ANSWER FOR BEST CARE

Align decimals.

$$\begin{array}{r}
\downarrow \\
2.5 \\
-0.5 \\
\hline
\end{array}$$

Begin subtracting with the farthest right column and subtract the bottom number from the top number (subtract 5 from 5 and then 0 from 2).

$$\begin{array}{r}
2.5 \\
-0.5 \\
\hline
0
\end{array} \leftarrow \text{Begin with right column}$$

Is the digit being subtracted larger than the digit above it? No.

$$\begin{array}{r}
2.5 \\
-0.5 \\
\hline
0
\end{array} \quad \text{5 is equal to 5 below}$$

Move one column left. 0 is less than 2.

$$\begin{array}{r}
\downarrow \\
2.5 \\
-0.5 \\
\hline
2\;0
\end{array}$$

Place the decimal point in the answer directly under the other decimal points.

$$\begin{array}{r} 2.5 \\ -\ 0.5 \\ \hline 2.0 \end{array}$$

The answer is 2 mg.

 Human Error Check

Increase 2.5 to 3.
Decrease 0.5 to 0.
3 − 0 = 3 (Answer is less than or equal to 3.)

Example 2

1.5 mg − 0.25 mg.

CRITICAL THINKING

Write numbers one under the other, aligning the decimal points.
Add zeros to numbers so that all columns have the same number of spaces.
Begin subtraction with the farthest right column.
Is the digit being subtracted larger than the digit above it? If yes, then you must add "1" in front of it and decrease the digit in the next column to the left of it by the value of 1.
Subtract each column, moving left one column at a time.
Place the decimal point in the answer directly under the other decimal points.
Add the unit of measure—such as mg, g, or mL—to your answer.

ANSWER FOR BEST CARE

Align decimals, since both numbers have milligrams as units of measure.

$$\begin{array}{r} \downarrow\ \ \ \\ 1.5 \\ -\ 0.25 \end{array}$$

Add zeros to even out digits to the right of the decimal point.

$$\begin{array}{r} 1.50 \leftarrow \\ -\ 0.25 \end{array}$$

Begin subtracting with the farthest right column and subtract the bottom number from the top number (subtract 5 from 0).

$$\begin{array}{r} \downarrow \\ 1.50 \\ -\ 0.25 \end{array}$$

5 is greater than 0. Put 1 in front of the 0. The 0 becomes 10. Decrease the 5 by 1. It becomes 4. Subtract 5 from 10.

$$\begin{array}{r} 4\,10 \\ 1.5\cancel{0} \\ -\ 0.25 \\ \hline 5 \end{array}$$

Move one column to the left. 2 is less than 4. Subtract 2 from 4.
Subtract second column

$$\begin{array}{r} \downarrow\ \ \ \\ 4\,10 \\ 1.5\cancel{0} \\ -\ 0.25 \\ \hline 25 \end{array}$$

Move one column to the left. 0 is less than 1. Subtract 0 from 1.

↓ Subtract third column

$$
\begin{array}{r}
4\,10 \\
1.\cancel{5}\cancel{0} \\
-\,0.25 \\
\hline
1\ 25
\end{array}
$$

Place the decimal point in the answer directly under the other decimal points.

$$
\begin{array}{r}
4\,10 \\
1.\cancel{5}\cancel{0} \\
-\,0.25 \\
\hline
1.25 \\
\uparrow
\end{array}
$$

The answer is 1.25 mg.

✔ **Human Error Check**

Increase 1.5 to 2.
Decrease 0.25 to 0.
2 − 0 = 2 (Answer is less than or equal to 2.)

Example 3

Using subtraction in the clinical setting.

PRESCRIPTION	*2.5-mg dose of medicine.*

• **What You HAVE** — One 0.75-mg tablet.

• **What You KNOW** — Prescribed dose is 2.5 mg.

• **What You WANT** — How many more milligrams must be ordered from the pharmacy?

CRITICAL THINKING

Is the prescribed dose larger or smaller than the dose on hand? Larger.
What you HAVE dose will be subtracted from the prescribed dose.
Write numbers one under the other, aligning the decimal points.
Add zeros to numbers so that all columns have the same number of spaces.
Begin subtraction with the farthest right column.
Is the digit being subtracted larger than the digit above it? If yes, then you must add "1" in front of it and decrease the digit in the column to the left of it by the value of 1.
Subtract each column, moving left one column at a time.
Place the decimal point in the answer directly under the other decimal points.
Add the unit of measure—such as mg, g, or mL—to your answer.

ANSWER FOR BEST CARE

Align decimals, since both numbers have milligrams as units of measure.

$$
\begin{array}{l}
2.5\ \ \text{mg (what is prescribed)} \\
-\,0.75\ \text{mg (what you HAVE)} \\
\hline
\end{array}
$$

Add zeros to even out digits to the right of the decimal point.

$$
\begin{array}{l}
2.50 \leftarrow \text{Add zero} \\
-\,0.75 \\
\hline
\end{array}
$$

Begin subtracting with the farthest right column and subtract the bottom number from the top number (subtract 5 from 0).

$$\downarrow$$
$$2.50$$
$$-\,0.75$$

5 is greater than 0. Put 1 in front of the 0. The 0 becomes 10. Decrease the 5 by 1. It becomes 4. Subtract 5 from 10.

$$4\,10$$
$$2.5\cancel{0}$$
$$-\,0.75$$
$$\overline{5}$$

Move one column to the left. 7 is larger than 4. Put 1 in front of the 4. The 4 becomes 14. Decrease the 2 by 1. It becomes 1. 7 from 14 is 7.

$$\downarrow$$
$$1\,14\,10$$
$$2.\cancel{5}\cancel{0}$$
$$-\,0.75$$
$$\overline{75}$$

Move one column to the left. 0 is smaller than 1. Subtract.

$$\downarrow$$
$$1\,14\,10$$
$$2.\cancel{5}\cancel{0}$$
$$-\,0.75$$
$$\overline{1\,75}$$

Place the decimal point in the answer directly under the other decimal points.

$$1\,14\,10$$
$$2.\cancel{5}\cancel{0}$$
$$-\,0.75$$
$$\overline{1.75}$$

The answer is 1.75 mg.

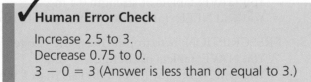

> **✔ Human Error Check**
>
> Increase 2.5 to 3.
> Decrease 0.75 to 0.
> 3 − 0 = 3 (Answer is less than or equal to 3.)

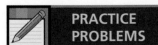

PRACTICE PROBLEMS

Directions: *Answer the following questions and do a check to see if your answer is correct.*

1. PRESCRIPTION: 2.5 mg by mouth. You HAVE: 1-mg tablets.
   How many more milligrams must you get from the pharmacy? _____
   Human error check _____

2. PRESCRIPTION: 20 mg. You HAVE: one 10-mg tablet.
   How many more milligrams must you get from the pharmacy? _____
   Human error check _____

3. PRESCRIPTION: 10 mg by mouth. You HAVE: one 7.5-mg tablet.
   How many more milligrams must you get from the pharmacy? _____
   Human error check _____

4. PRESCRIPTION: 30 mg. You HAVE: 22.5 mg.
   How many more milligrams must you get from the pharmacy? _____
   Human error check _____

5. PRESCRIPTION: 10 mg. You HAVE: 7.25 mg.
   How many more milligrams must you get from the pharmacy? _____
   Human error check _____

6. PRESCRIPTION: 0.25 mg. You HAVE: 0.125 mg.
   How many more milligrams must you get from the pharmacy? _____
   Human error check _____

7. PRESCRIPTION: 5 g by mouth. You HAVE: one tablet of strength 2.25 g.
   How many more grams must you get from the pharmacy? _____
   Human error check _____

8. PRESCRIPTION: 2.25 mg. You HAVE: 1.75 mg.
   How many more milligrams must you get from the pharmacy? _____
   Human error check _____

9. PRESCRIPTION: 3 mg. You HAVE: 2.25 mg.
   How many more milligrams must you get from the pharmacy? _____
   Human error check _____

10. PRESCRIPTION: 1 mg. You HAVE: 0.75 mg.
    How many more milligrams must you get from the pharmacy? _____
    Human error check _____

(Answers on pp. 438–439)

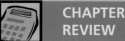

CHAPTER REVIEW

Answer each question as indicated for problems 1 through 7.

1. PRESCRIPTION: warfarin sodium (Coumadin) 1.25 mg by mouth.
   You HAVE: tablets of strength 2.5 mg.
   You will NEED: (a) 1 tablet (b) less than 1 tablet (c) more than 1 tablet ____

2. PRESCRIPTION: nitroglycerin (Nitrostat) 0.4 mg sublingual.
   You HAVE: tablets of strength 0.4 mg.
   You will NEED: (a) 1 tablet (b) less than 1 tablet (c) more than 1 tablet ____

3. PRESCRIPTION: benztropine mesylate (Cogentin) 2 mg by mouth.
   You HAVE: tablets of strength 0.5 mg.
   You will NEED: (a) 1 tablet (b) less than 1 tablet (c) more than 1 tablet ____

4. PRESCRIPTION: amlodipine (Norvasc) 7.5 mg by mouth.
   You HAVE: tablets of strength 2.5 mg.
   You will NEED: (a) 1 tablet (b) less than 1 tablet (c) more than 1 tablet ____

5. PRESCRIPTION: loratadine (Claritin) 10 mg by mouth.
   You HAVE: tablets of strength 10 mg.
   You will NEED: (a) 1 tablet (b) less than 1 tablet (c) more than 1 tablet ____

6. PRESCRIPTION: lisinopril (Prinivil) 2.5 mg by mouth.
   You HAVE: tablets of strength 5 mg.
   You will NEED: (a) 1 tablet (b) less than 1 tablet (c) more than 1 tablet ____

7. PRESCRIPTION: pentazocine (Talwin) 50 mg by mouth.
   You HAVE: tablets of strength 12.5 mg.
   You will NEED: (a) 1 tablet (b) less than 1 tablet (c) more than 1 tablet ____

Find the total doses for problems 8 through 14 (all tablets are the same drug).

8. One 0.5-mg tablet and one 0.25-mg tablet. Total dose is _____.

9. One 1.5-mg tablet and two 0.125-mg tablets. Total dose is _____.

10. One 30-mg tablet, one 0.05-mg tablet, and one 0.4-mg tablet.
    Total dose is _____ .

11. Two 0.5-mg tablets and one 1.5-mg tablet. Total dose is _____.

12. One 0.125-mg tablet and one 0.1-mg tablet. Total dose is _____.

13. Three 0.05-mg tablets and one 0.1-mg tablet. Total dose is _____.

14. One 0.4-mg tablet and one 2.5-mg tablet. Total dose is _____.

Answer the following questions for problems 15 through 21.

15. The patient needs 2.5 mg. You HAVE: one 1-mg tablet.
    How many more milligrams must you get from the pharmacy? _____

16. PRESCRIPTION: 20 mg. You HAVE: one 2.5-mg tablet.
    How many more milligrams must you get from the pharmacy? _____

17. PRESCRIPTION: 10 mg. You HAVE: one 2.5-mg tablet and one 5-mg tablet.
    How many more milligrams must you get from the pharmacy? _____

18. PRESCRIPTION: 30 mg. You HAVE: one tablet of strength 7.5 mg and one
    tablet of strength 15 mg.
    How many more milligrams must you get from the pharmacy? _____

19. PRESCRIPTION: 50 mg. You HAVE: two tablets of strength 12.5 mg.
    How many more milligrams must you get from the pharmacy? _____

20. PRESCRIPTION: 0.5 mg. You HAVE: three tablets of strength 0.125 mg.
    How many more milligrams must you get from the pharmacy? _____

21. The total dosage range for cefoperazone sodium (Cefobid) is 2 to 4 g/day
    in divided doses every 12 hours for moderate infections. The prescription is
    1.5 g every 12 hours. Is this within dosage recommendations? _____

22. Review the following math problem to determine whether it has been written
    correctly. Add 1.25, 100, 0.001, and 0.33.

$$
\begin{array}{r}
1.25 \\
100 \\
.001 \\
+\ 0.33 \\
\hline
2.59
\end{array}
$$

Add the medication doses for problems 23 through 30.

23. Demerol 75 mg + atropine 0.4 mg + Vistaril 1.5 mg. Total dose _____

24. Methocarbamol (Robaxin) 500 mg + 250 mg + 500 mg + 250 mg + 500 mg.
    Total dose _____

25. Add the following medications to make Phospho-Soda oral solution as a
    laxative for precolonoscopy: 18 g phosphate + 48 g biphosphate.
    Total dose _____

26. Valproate (Depakene) 750 mg + 500 mg + 250 mg + 750 mg.
    Total dose _____

27. 300 mg + 325 mg + 195 mg. Total dose _____

28. Demerol 50 mg + atropine 0.2 mg + Vistaril 25 mg. Total dose _____

29. Compute 24-hour dose: aspirin 325 mg + Motrin 400 mg + Tylenol 650 mg.
    Total dose _____

30. Prednisone 50 mg today and decrease the dose by 10 mg every day for the
    next 4 days. What is the total milligram dose for over 5 days? _____

(Answers on p. 439)

⊖volve **For additional practice problems, refer to the Mathematics Review section
of Drug Calculations Companion, version 4 on Evolve.**

Decimals: Multiplication and Division

Mother Helena Infortuna

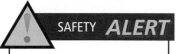

SAFETY **ALERT**

If a calculator is used, be sure to enter the numbers with their decimal points very accurately.

CLINICAL CONNECTION

- Either multiplication or division, or both, are commonly required in drug calculation.
- Understanding decimal placement in multiplication and division problems is crucial to error-free calculations.

INTRODUCTION

Calculating medication dosages often requires multiplying and dividing decimal numbers. The calculation can be done without a calculator and is a good way to double-check calculations done with a calculator. You will learn in Chapter 5 how to convert numbers with different units of measure to the same units of measure. In order to do calculations, all numbers must use the same unit of measure. In this chapter, all numbers in all problems use the same unit of measure.

MULTIPLICATION OF DECIMAL NUMBERS

Multiplication is the mathematical operation of repeated addition. The result is called the *product*. To find the product of decimal numbers, the placement of the decimal point in the answer is crucial. The number of decimal places in the product is the sum of the decimal places in each of the numbers of the multiplication problem.

To multiply decimal numbers:

1. Multiply as if they were whole numbers; don't worry about the decimal point yet!
2. In multiplication, place the last digit of each additional product to the left of the previous product's last digit.
3. Add products.
4. Count the number of decimal places to the **right** of the decimal point in each number.
5. Place the decimal point in the answer by counting from right to left, the total of the number of decimal places counted in the multiplication numbers. For example, if you multiply 2.3 × 4.5, there is one decimal place to the right of the decimal in 2.3 and one decimal place to the right of the decimal point in 4.5, so your answer will have 1 + 1 (or 2) decimal places. If you multiply 2.3 × 5.74, your answer will have 1 + 2 (or 3) decimal places.
6. If there are fewer digits in the answer than the total number of decimal places needed, add zeros to the left of the digits (as you are moving from right to left in counting the number of places). Also add one zero to the left of the decimal point if no whole number exists. For example, 0.31 × 0.12 = 372 in whole numbers. To count 4 decimal places (2 + 2), you need to add a zero to the left of the digits and a zero to the left of the decimal point to highlight decimal point location, so the answer is 0.0372.

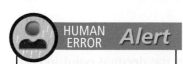

HUMAN ERROR *Alert*

In medication administration, all units of meausre must be the same or patient harm can occur.

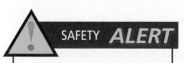

SAFETY **ALERT**

It is crucial that the total number of decimal places to the **right** of the decimal point are determined correctly. Carefully check your calculations.

Example 1

Multiply 3.5 × 0.25

CRITICAL THINKING

Multiply numbers as whole numbers.

Determine the number of decimal places to the right of the decimal point in each number.

Add the numbers together to determine the sum of decimal places.

Counting from the far right of your answer and, moving toward the left, count the sum of the decimal places.

Place the decimal point in your answer.

If you do not have enough spaces, add zeros after you have moved as far left as you can.

Add a zero to the left of the decimal point ONLY when no number exists there to highlight decimal point location.

ANSWER FOR BEST CARE

Multiply as whole numbers.

$$
\begin{array}{r}
35 \\
\underline{25} \\
175 \\
\underline{70} \quad \leftarrow \text{Product moved one space to the left} \\
875 \quad \leftarrow \text{Sum of both products}
\end{array}
$$

Count the number of decimal places to the right of the decimal point in each number.

3.5 × 0.25   There are three places.
 ↑   ↑↑

Place decimal point in answer the number of places starting from the right and moving left.

.875 ← Start counting from right to left
3,2,1

Add a zero to the left of the decimal point ONLY when no number exists there. This highlights decimal placement to prevent error.

↓

Answer = 0.875

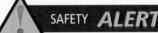

SAFETY ALERT

Place a zero to the left of the decimal point if no whole number exists there to highlight the decimal point location. This helps avoid the mistake of not seeing the decimal point and considering the answer as a whole number.

Example 2

Multiply 0.32 × 0.14

CRITICAL THINKING

Multiply numbers as whole numbers.

Determine the number of decimal places to the right of the decimal point in each number.

Add the numbers together to determine the sum of decimal places.

Counting from the far right of your answer and, moving toward the left, count the sum of the decimal places.

Place the decimal point in your answer.

If you do not have enough spaces, add zeros after you have moved as far left as you can.

Add a zero to the left of the decimal point ONLY when no number exists there.

ANSWER FOR BEST CARE

$$
\begin{array}{r}
32 \\
\times \ 14 \\
\hline
128 \\
\underline{32} \quad \leftarrow \text{Move product one space to the left} \\
448 \quad \leftarrow \text{Sum of both products}
\end{array}
$$

What is the number of decimal places to the right of the decimal point in each number?

$\downarrow\downarrow \quad \downarrow\downarrow$
0.32 × 0.14

There are two decimal places to the right in each number. Four decimal places are needed in the product. Place the decimal point in your answer by counting four places from the far right of your answer the sum of the decimal places.

Count four places to the left. Since there are only three whole numbers, a zero is added to the left of the last whole number and then the decimal point.

$\downarrow$ Add zero

Decimal placement → .0448
⁀⁀
4,3,2,1

To highlight the decimal point, add a zero to the left of the decimal point ONLY when no number exists there.

0.0448
↑

Example 3

You are to administer 3 tablets of 1.5 mg dexamethasone (Decadron).

• **What You WANT**

The total dose, in milligrams, you are to administer now.

CRITICAL THINKING

Multiply as if they are whole numbers.
What is the number of decimal places to the right of the decimal point in each number? What is the sum of these numbers of decimal places?
Place the decimal point in your answer by counting the number of places from the far right of your answer and, moving toward the left, the sum of the decimal places.
If you do not have enough spaces, add zeros after you have moved as far left as you can.
Add a zero to the left of the decimal point ONLY when no number exists there to highlight decimal point placement.
Answer should include the unit of measure.

ANSWER FOR BEST CARE

$$\begin{array}{r} 15 \\ \times\ 3 \\ \hline 45 \end{array}$$

Count the number of decimal places to the right of the decimal point in each number.

3 × 1.5
↑

The sum of these numbers of decimal places is 1.
Place the decimal point in your answer by counting the number of places from the far right of your answer the sum of the decimal places.

4.5
⁀

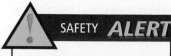

SAFETY **ALERT**

To avoid medication error, place decimal point correctly by counting decimal places accurately.

Add a zero to the left of the decimal point ONLY when no number exists there. (This is not necessary here.)
The total dose is 4.5 mg.

PRACTICE PROBLEMS

Directions: *Find the product by multiplying the following:*

1. $4 \times 0.5 =$ _____

2. $1.5 \times 0.1 =$ _____

3. $12.5 \times 3.5 =$ _____

4. $2.5 \times 5 =$ _____

5. $0.225 \times 2 =$ _____

6. $3 \times 1.5 =$ _____

7. $3.75 \times 1.5 =$ _____

8. $12.5 \times 0.5 =$ _____

9. $6.5 \times 1.5 =$ _____

10. $3 \times 12.25 =$ _____

(Answers on pp. 439–440)

DIVISION OF DECIMAL NUMBERS

SAFETY **ALERT**

When dividing without a calculator, the division symbol $\overline{)}$ is more useful than the other division symbol, ÷.

CLINICAL **ALERT**

As with all decimal number operations, the placement of the decimal point is crucial for correct dosages.

HUMAN ERROR **Alert**

Always place a zero to the left of the decimal point if there is no other number there; for example, always write 0.6 rather than .6.

Division is the opposite mathematical operation of multiplication. Division is repeated subtraction. The answer to a division problem is called the *quotient*.

Several symbols may be used to indicate division. It may be expressed as follows:

1.   (Dividend) $3 \div 2$ (Divisor) = Quotient

2.   (Divisor) $2\overline{)3}$ $\overset{\text{Quotient}}{}$ (Dividend)

3.   A fraction, as in 3 (Dividend)/2 (Divisor); 3/2 or $\frac{3}{2}$

In nursing, a formula that is often used is "Prescription" (Dividend)/divided by "Have" (Divisor), or $\dfrac{\text{Prescription}}{\text{Have}}$

For example, if you have 30 mg of prednisone prescribed and you have 10-mg tablets available, to determine how many tablets you give the patient, you divide 30 by 10 and get the answer, 3 tablets.

To find the quotient of decimal numbers, the divisor (the number performing the division, also called the denominator or "bottom number") must be a whole number (a number with no visible decimal point). When a number is being divided by a decimal number, the decimal point in the divisor must be moved to the right as many places as needed to make the divisor a whole number. For example, in $6.0 \div 0.5$ the decimal point in the 0.5 needs to be moved one place to the right to make the 0.5 the whole number 5. The decimal point in the dividend must be moved the same number of places to the right as was the divisor's; therefore, the decimal point in the 6.0 needs to be moved one place to the right, making the 6.0 become 60. The decimal point in the quotient is placed directly above the new position of the decimal point in the dividend. For example in $6.0 \div 0.5$, which becomes $5\overline{)60}$ or $5\overline{)60.0}$, the decimal point in the quotient is placed directly above the new position of the decimal point in the dividend, between the two zeros in this example. When a decimal number is being divided by a whole number, the decimal point in the quotient is placed directly above the decimal point in the dividend (number being divided).

Example 1

$4.25 \div 0.5$

CRITICAL THINKING

The dividend (prescription) is to the left of the ÷ symbol.
The divisor (HAVE) is to the right of the ÷ symbol.

The divisor must be converted to a whole number by moving the decimal point to the right. How many places to the right did you move the decimal point?

The decimal point in the dividend must be moved the same number of places to the right as the divisor's was moved.

The decimal point in the quotient is placed directly above the new position of the decimal point in the dividend (prescription).

Your answer may need to be rounded if there is a remainder in your division.

To check calculation, multiply quotient by the divisor. Answer should be equal or approximately equal (if rounding occurs).

ANSWER FOR BEST CARE	0.5 is the divisor (to the right of the ÷ symbol). Make divisor a whole number by moving the decimal point to the right one place.

$$0.\underset{\smile}{5} = 5$$

Move one place to the right in the dividend.

$$4.25 = 4\underset{\smile}{2}.5$$

Perform the calculation.

 SAFETY ALERT

When using a calculator to perform division, be sure the dividend number (numerator, top number, "prescription") is inputted first, then the division sign, ÷, followed by the divisor (denominator, bottom number, "have"). Be careful to place decimal points in the proper place when inputting the numbers.

$$
\begin{array}{r}
8.5 \\
5\overline{)42.5} \\
40 \\
\hline
2\,5 \\
2\,5 \\
\hline
\end{array}
$$

The decimal point in the quotient is placed directly above the new position of the decimal point in the dividend.

The quotient is 8.5.

✓ **Human Error Check**

8.5 × 5 = 42.5; therefore, calculation is correct.

Example 2

0.35 ÷ 0.24

CRITICAL THINKING	The dividend (prescription) is to the left of the ÷ symbol. The divisor (HAVE) is to the right of the ÷ symbol. The divisor must be converted to a whole number by moving the decimal point to the right. How many places to the right did you move the decimal point? The decimal point in the dividend must be moved the same number of places to the right as the divisor's was moved. The decimal point in the quotient is placed directly above the new position of the decimal point in the dividend (prescription). Your answer may need to be rounded if there is a remainder in your division. To check calculation, multiply quotient by the divisor. Answer should be equal or approximately equal (if rounding occurs).

ANSWER FOR BEST CARE	0.24 is the divisor (to the right of the ÷ symbol). Make divisor a whole number by moving the decimal point to the right two places.

$$0.\underset{\smile}{24} = 24$$

Move two places to the right in the dividend.

$$\underset{\smile}{.35} = 35$$

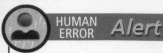

Perform the calculation.

$$24\overline{)35.00}$$ ← Zeros added to right of decimal

The decimal point in the quotient is placed directly above the position of the decimal point in the dividend.

11 is smaller → than 24; add a 0 to right of decimal and bring down

```
        1.45
   24)35.00
      24↓
      110←
       96↓
       140←
       120
        20 ← Remainder
```

Performing the calculation above by using four specific steps would include the following:

1. Setting up the division: $24\overline{)35.00}$
2. Beginning the division:

```
        1.
   24)35.00
      24
      11        Remainder
```

3. Continuing the division:

```
        1.4
   24)35.00
      24
      11 0
       9 6
       1 4        Remainder
```

4. Continuing the division so the answer is brought to two decimal points to the right of the decimal point:

```
        1.45
   24)35.00
      24
      11 0
       9 6
       1 40
       1 20
         20   Remainder
```

There may be times when you need to round the quotient. To round a number to an indicated decimal place, look at the digit to the right of it. If it is 5 or greater, increase the digit by 1. If the digit to the right of it is less than 5, leave the indicated digit as is. Since the 5 in 1.45 is 5 or greater, round the digit 4 up by 1 and make it a 5.

The quotient (answer) is 1.5

> ✔ **Human Error Check**
>
> $1.5 \times 24 = 36$

Example 3

PRESCRIPTION   *Give 7.5 mg of a medication in tablet form.*

- ***What You HAVE***   1.25-mg scored tablets.

- ***What You KNOW***   Prescribed dose is 7.5 mg.

- ***What You WANT***   How many tablets do you need to administer 7.5 mg?

CRITICAL THINKING

The dividend is what is prescribed.

The divisor is what you have.

The divisor must be converted to a whole number by moving the decimal point to the right. How many places to the right did you move the decimal point?

The decimal point in the dividend must be moved the same number of places to the right as the divisor's was moved.

The decimal point in the quotient is placed directly above the new position of the decimal point in the dividend.

Your answer may need to be rounded if there is a remainder in your division.

Unit of measure is number of tablets.

To check calculation, multiply quotient by the divisor. Answer should be equal or approximately equal (if rounding occurs).

ANSWER FOR BEST CARE

1.25 is the divisor.

Make divisor a whole number by moving the decimal point to the right two places.

1.25 = 125

7.5 is the dividend.

Move two places to the right in the dividend.

7.50 = 750

Perform the calculation.

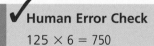

Since you have no remainder in your division, there is no need to round.

Your answer should be in units of measure, which in this case is number of tablets, NOT number of milligrams. When whole numbers only, not decimals, are used in prescribing, there is no decimal point used to avoid potential errors of reading the prescription/answer.

Answer is 6 tablets.

✓ **Human Error Check**

125 × 6 = 750

PRACTICE PROBLEMS

Directions: *Answer the following questions.*

1. Your patient is to receive a dose of 5.25 mg. The tablets available are labeled 1.5 mg. What is the dividend? _____ What is the divisor? _____ How many tablet(s) should you administer? _____

2. Your patient is to receive a dose of 0.75 mg. The tablets available are labeled 0.25 mg. What is the dividend? _____ What is the divisor? _____ How many tablet(s) will you administer? _____

3. Your patient is to receive a total dose of 4.5 mg. There are three tablets labeled 1.5 mg in his medicine drawer. Is this a correct dosage? _____

4. You are to give 125 mg. Scored tablets labeled 50 mg are available. What is the dividend? _____ What is the divisor? _____ How many tablet(s) will you administer? _____

5. A dose of 1.25 mg is needed. Tablets available are labeled 0.125 mg. What is the dividend? _____ What is the divisor? _____ How many tablet(s) are needed? _____

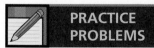

6. Your patient is to receive 1.25 mg. The scored tablets have strength 0.5 mg. How many tablet(s) should be in the drawer? _____

7. Your patient is to receive a total dose of 1.2 mg. The available tablets have strength 0.4 mg. What is the dividend? _____ What is the divisor? _____ How many tablet(s) should you administer? _____

8. You are to administer 8.75 mg. The tablets have strength 2.5 mg. What is the dividend? _____ What is the divisor? _____ How many tablet(s) should you administer? _____

9. Prescribed 0.625 mg of dexamethasone (Decadron). Tablets available have strength 0.25 mg. What is the dividend? _____ What is the divisor? _____ How many tablet(s) are needed? _____

10. The patient is to receive a total dose of 3.75 mg. There are three scored tablets labeled 2.5 mg in his medicine drawer. Is this a correct dosage? _____ If not, what should be in his medicine drawer? _____

(Answers on p. 440)

CHAPTER REVIEW

Find the product by multiplying the following.

1. $6 \times 0.5 =$ _____

2. $1.8 \times 0.1 =$ _____

3. $12.5 \times 4.5 =$ _____

4. $2.5 \times 7 =$ _____

5. $0.225 \times 4 =$ _____

6. $5 \times 1.5 =$ _____

7. $3.45 \times 1.5 =$ _____

8. $18.5 \times 0.5 =$ _____

9. $7.5 \times 1.5 =$ _____

10. $3 \times 12.15 =$ _____

Find the total dose for each patient situation for problems 11 through 20.

11. You are to administer two 0.75-mg tablets. _____

12. You are to administer 3½ (3.5) 1.5-mg tablets. _____

13. You are to administer 1½ (1.5) 0.1-mg tablets. _____

14. Your patient is to receive two 0.05-mg tablets and 1½ 1.5-mg tablets. _____

15. You are to give ½ of a 0.5-mg tablet and 1½ 2.5-mg tablets. _____

16. You are to give three 0.5-g tablets of sulfisoxazole. _____

17. 30-mcg thyroid tablets. There are 1½ tablets. _____

18. 0.4-mg nitroglycerin tablets. There are two tablets. _____

19. There are 2½ (2.5) 0.05-mg tablets. _____

20. Digoxin 0.125-mg tablets. There are 1½ tablets. _____

Answer the following questions for each patient situation in problems 21 through 30.

21. PRESCRIPTION: repaglinide (Prandin) 3.5 mg.
    HAVE: 0.5-mg tablets available.
    How many tablet(s) do you give? _____

22. PRESCRIPTION: prednisone 10 mg.
    HAVE: 2.5-mg tablets.
    How many tablet(s) do you give the patient? _____

23. PRESCRIPTION: pergolide (Permax) 0.15 mg.
    HAVE: Each tablet's strength is 0.05 mg.
    How many tablet(s) are needed? _____

24. PRESCRIPTION: 15 mg of olanzapine (Zyprexa) are prescribed. Tablets of strength 7.5 mg are available. How many tablet(s) are needed? _____

25. PRESCRIPTION: naratriptan (Amerge) 2.5 mg.
    HAVE: Tablets of 1 mg.
    How many tablet(s) do you give the patient? _____

26. PRESCRIPTION: moexipril (Univasc) 22.5 mg.
    HAVE: Tablets of strength 7.5 mg.
    How many tablet(s) do you give the patient? _____

27. PRESCRIPTION: metolazone (Mykrox) 1 mg.
    HAVE: There are three tablets each of strength 0.5 mg in the patient's medicine drawer.
    Is this a correct dosage? _____
    If not the correct dosage, what should be the exact number of tablets in the drawer? _____

28. PRESCRIPTION: meclizine (Antivert) 50 mg.
    HAVE: Tablets labeled 12.5 mg.
    How many tablet(s) are needed? _____

29. PRESCRIPTION: lorazepam (Ativan) 2.5 mg.
    HAVE: The tablets available are each labeled 0.5 mg.
    How many tablet(s) should you take from the automated medication dispensing machine? _____

30. PRESCRIPTION: digoxin (Lanoxin) 0.5 mg.
    HAVE: Tablets of strength 0.125 mg are available.
    How many tablet(s) do you need to give? _____

Answer the following questions for these nondrug calculations in problems 31 through 34.

31. An infant drinks 4 ounces of formula every 4 hours and 2.5 ounces of water twice a day. How much fluid in ounces will the infant drink in 1 day? _____

32. You know that 2 pounds of edema equals 1 L of fluid. A fluid overload patient has lost 15.25 pounds. How many liters of fluid have been removed? _____

33. A patient is supposed to have 1500 mL of fluid every 24 hours. You know that the patient is to have three-quarters of the fluid between breakfast (8 AM) and dinner (6 PM). How much fluid should be ingested between 8 AM and 6 PM? _____

34. The hematocrit of a patient is raised 2 g with each unit of packed cells that is administered. The patient has received 3 units of blood. The hematocrit prior

to blood administration was 7.5 g. What would you anticipate the new hematocrit would be? _____

Fill in the blanks for problem 35.

35. When multiplying, the decimal point in the answer is placed by counting the appropriate number of spaces, starting on the far _____ and moving to the _____.

(Answers on pp. 440–441)

⊝volve For additional practice problems, refer to the Mathematics Review section of Drug Calculations Companion, version 4 on Evolve.

Fractions: Reduction and Equations

Mother Helena Infortuna

CLINICAL CONNECTION

- In order to give medications safely, it is important to be able to determine the relative value of fractions, reduce fractions, and multiply and divide fractions.
- Understanding fractions is important in determining medication doses to be given at dosage intervals (i.e., 6 hours, 8 hours) over a 24-hour period, and in dietary planning.

INTRODUCTION

A fraction is a mathematical expression comparing two numbers by division. The top number is called the *numerator* (known as the *dividend* in division) and the bottom number is called the *denominator* (known as the *divisor* in division). Consider, for example, the following fraction:

$$\frac{3}{4} \quad \frac{\text{Numerator}}{\text{Denominator}}$$

Fractions are used in both the household and the apothecary measurement system. These systems are discussed in Chapters 4 and 5.

RELATIVE VALUE OF FRACTIONS

The relative value of two or more fractions may be determined in one of the following ways:

1. If the denominators are the same, the fraction with the **highest** numerator has the highest value. For example, the fractions $\frac{3}{8}$ and $\frac{5}{8}$ both have the denominator 8. Comparing numerators, a 5 is higher than a 3, so the fraction $\frac{5}{8}$ is larger.
2. If the numerators are the same, the fraction with the **lowest** denominator has the highest value. For example, the fractions $\frac{3}{5}$ and $\frac{3}{8}$ both have the numerator 3. Comparing denominators, a 5 is lower than an 8, so the fraction $\frac{3}{5}$ has the higher value.
3. When there is not a common numerator or denominator, each fraction is written as its decimal equivalent (by performing the indicated division); the fraction with the highest decimal number has the higher value. For example, in decimal form, $\frac{2}{5} = 0.4$ and $\frac{1}{8} = 0.125$. The higher decimal number is 0.4 (see Chapter 1 for decimal review), so $\frac{2}{5}$ has the higher value.

Example 1

$$\frac{1}{9}, \frac{4}{9}, \frac{7}{9}$$

| CRITICAL THINKING | Are the numerators the same?
Are the denominators the same?
Do I need to write each fraction as a decimal? |

| ANSWER FOR
BEST CARE | Since the denominators are the same (9), $\frac{7}{9}$ is the highest value because 7 is the highest numerator number. |

Example 2

$$\frac{3}{5}, \frac{3}{7}, \frac{3}{8}$$

| CRITICAL THINKING | Are the numerators the same?
Are the denominators the same?
Do I need to write each fraction as a decimal? |

| ANSWER FOR
BEST CARE | Since the numerators are the same, the fraction with the lowest denominator has the highest value. Therefore, $\frac{3}{5}$ has the highest value because 5, being lower than 7 and 8, is the lowest denominator. |

PRACTICE PROBLEMS

Directions: Identify the fraction with the highest value for problems 1 through 10.

1. (a) $\frac{1}{9}$ (b) $\frac{1}{2}$ (c) $\frac{1}{4}$

2. (a) $\frac{1}{7}$ (b) $\frac{4}{7}$ (c) $\frac{5}{7}$

3. (a) $\frac{2}{3}$ (b) $\frac{5}{6}$ (c) $\frac{3}{4}$

4. (a) $\frac{3}{2}$ (b) $\frac{3}{4}$ (c) $\frac{3}{8}$

5. (a) $\frac{5}{6}$ (b) $\frac{7}{6}$ (c) $\frac{9}{6}$

6. (a) $\frac{1}{4}$ (b) $\frac{1}{2}$ (c) $\frac{7}{8}$

7. (a) $\frac{1}{5}$ (b) $\frac{5}{7}$ (c) $\frac{5}{8}$

8. (a) $\frac{1}{2}$ (b) $\frac{1}{3}$ (c) $\frac{1}{5}$

9. (a) $\frac{3}{4}$ (b) $\frac{7}{8}$ (c) $\frac{9}{10}$

10. (a) $\frac{8}{3}$ (b) $\frac{5}{2}$ (c) $\frac{6}{5}$

11. Mr. Smith is to reduce his total caloric intake as much as possible. He is given the choice of decreasing his calories by $\frac{2}{3}, \frac{3}{4},$ or $\frac{5}{6}$. Which should he choose to get the greatest decrease in calories? _____

12. Ms. Smith is to decrease her total carbohydrate intake by the smallest amount prescribed by the dietitian. The dietitian gives her choices of $\frac{3}{8}, \frac{1}{4},$ or $\frac{3}{5}$. Which value is the lowest that Ms. Smith should choose? _____

(Answers on p. 441)

MULTIPLYING AND REDUCING FRACTIONS

Reducing fractions helps in dose calculations because it reduces errors. To reduce a fraction you divide both the numerator and the denominator by the same largest whole number that will divide both numbers. For example: $\frac{9}{24} = \frac{3}{8}$ because both the numerator, 9, and denominator, 24, can be divided by the same whole number, in this case 3.

$$\frac{9 \div 3}{24 \div 3} = \frac{3}{8}$$

Another example: $\frac{25}{125}$. The largest number that can be divided into both numbers is 25.

$$\frac{25 \div 25}{125 \div 25} = \frac{1}{5}$$

After you have reduced the fractions, you need to multiply the fractions. For example, $\frac{3}{8} \times \frac{1}{5}$. You do this by multiplying all the numerator numbers ($3 \times 1 = 3$) and then multiplying all the denominator numbers ($8 \times 5 = 40$). For medication dosage purposes, the resulting fraction, $\frac{3}{40}$, is then converted into a decimal by division. Remember to round your answer.

$$40\overline{)3.000} \quad 0.075$$

The rounded answer is 0.08.

Example 1

Multiply the following fractions: $\frac{2}{8} \times \frac{3}{6}$.

CRITICAL THINKING

To help avoid medication errors, reduce fractions when possible.
Reduce by dividing the numerators and denominators by the same number.
Multiply all the numerators first, then multiply all the denominators.
Convert the fraction answer to a decimal by dividing its numerator by its denominator ($\frac{numerator}{denominator}$).
Round the answer to the nearest tenth (one position to the right of the decimal point).
Include units of measure in the answer if applicable.

ANSWER FOR BEST CARE

The same largest number to divide both the numerator and denominator of the first fraction is 2. $\frac{2}{8} = \frac{1}{4}$.
The same largest number to divide both the numerator and denominator of the second fraction is 3. $\frac{3}{6} = \frac{1}{2}$.
Reduced problem becomes $\frac{1}{4} \times \frac{1}{2}$.
Multiplication of numerators is $1 \times 1 = 1$.
Multiplication of denominators is $4 \times 2 = 8$.
The resulting fraction from multiplication is $\frac{1}{8}$.
Express the final answer as a decimal to the nearest tenth.

$$8\overline{)1.00} \quad 0.12$$
$$\underline{8}$$
$$20$$
$$\underline{16}$$
$$4$$

 SAFETY **ALERT**

Failure to reduce fractions immediately and completely can lead to multiplication errors more easily and, hence, incorrect medication administration.

Does the decimal need to be rounded? Yes; the answer is 0.1. (There are alternative methods of obtaining the answer. If you do not reduce, you can arrive at the same answer: $\frac{2}{8} \times \frac{3}{6} = \frac{6}{48}$, which reduces by dividing the numerator and denominator by 6, equaling $\frac{1}{8}$, or just divide 6 by 48.)

Example 2

Multiply the following fractions: $\frac{5}{9} \times \frac{6}{7}$.

CRITICAL THINKING

To help avoid medication errors, reduce fractions when possible.
Reduce by dividing the numerators and denominators by the same number.
Multiply all the numerators first; then multiply all the denominators.
Convert the fraction answer to a decimal by dividing its numerator by its denominator.

Round the answer to the nearest tenth (one position to the right of the decimal point).

Include units of measure in the answer if applicable.

ANSWER FOR BEST CARE

The same largest number to divide both the numerator and denominator is 3.
The reduced fractions are $\frac{5}{3}$ and $\frac{2}{7}$.
Multiplication of numerators is $5 \times 2 = 10$.
Multiplication of denominators is $3 \times 7 = 21$.
The resulting fraction from multiplication is $\frac{10}{21}$.
Express the final answer as a decimal to the nearest tenth.

$$
\begin{array}{r}
0.47 \\
21\overline{)10.00} \\
\underline{8\ 4} \\
1\ 60 \\
\underline{1\ 47} \\
13
\end{array}
$$

Does the decimal need to be rounded? Yes; the answer is 0.5. (Using an alternative method: $\frac{5}{9} \times \frac{6}{7} = \frac{30}{63}$, which reduces by 3 to $\frac{10}{21}$.)

Example 3

Mr. Watts is currently taking 7 phenytoin sodium (Dilantin) capsules. He is supposed to reduce his capsule intake by $\frac{1}{6}$. How many capsules should he take?

    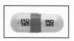 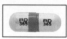 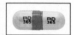

CRITICAL THINKING

To help avoid medication errors, reduce fractions when possible.
A whole number as a fraction is the whole number divided by one, so 7 is $\frac{7}{1}$.
Reduce by dividing the numerators and denominators by the same number.
Multiply all the numerators first; then multiply all the denominators.
Convert the fraction answer to a decimal by dividing its numerator by its denominator.
Round the answer to the nearest tenth (one position to the right of the decimal point).
Include units of measure in the answer if applicable.

ANSWER FOR BEST CARE

There is no same largest number to divide both the numerator and denominator.
The fractions are $\frac{1}{6}$ and $\frac{7}{1}$.
Multiplication of numerators is $1 \times 7 = 7$.
Multiplication of denominators is $6 \times 1 = 6$.
The resulting fraction from multiplication is $\frac{7}{6}$.
The fraction as a decimal is as follows:

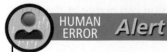

HUMAN ERROR *Alert*

Failure to make whole numbers into fractions by placing the whole number over 1 ($\frac{\text{whole number}}{1}$) can lead to multiplication errors more easily and lead to incorrect medication administration.

$$
\begin{array}{r}
1.16 \\
6\overline{)7.00} \\
\underline{6} \\
1\ 0 \\
\underline{6} \\
40 \\
\underline{36} \\
4
\end{array}
$$

Does the decimal need to be rounded? Yes; the answer is 1.2, clinically rounded to 1 capsule per day. He is to take 6 capsules a day.

PRACTICE PROBLEMS

Directions: Multiply the following fractions and give your answer as a fraction and as a decimal to the nearest tenth (one digit to the right of the decimal point).

1. $\frac{1}{2} \times \frac{1}{4}$

2. $\frac{1}{10} \times \frac{100}{1}$

3. $\frac{7}{8} \times \frac{4}{21}$

4. $\frac{8}{3} \times \frac{1}{5}$

5. $\frac{3}{4} \times \frac{14}{15}$

6. $\frac{150}{4} \times \frac{2}{5}$

7. $\frac{1000}{1} \times \frac{1}{1000}$

8. $\frac{2}{5} \times \frac{7}{9}$

9. $\frac{1}{5} \times \frac{3}{2}$

10. $\frac{2500}{3} \times \frac{1}{100}$

11. Mr. Johnson has essential hypertension and is to decrease his sodium intake by $\frac{1}{5} \times \frac{1}{2}$ daily. Write answer in both fraction and decimal form. _____

12. The nursing home protocol for weening patients off of tube feedings includes daily decreases of $\frac{1}{6} \times$ the mathematical fraction of $\frac{3}{2}$. What is the amount of decrease daily as a fraction and a decimal for the tube feeding? _____

(Answers on pp. 441–442)

DIVIDING FRACTIONS

The division of fractions is performed by multiplying by the reciprocal of the divisor (second fraction). To find the reciprocal of a fraction, replace the numerator (top) with the denominator (bottom) of the fraction and the denominator with the numerator. This is also referred to as "inverting the fraction." For example, the reciprocal of $\frac{2}{3}$ is $\frac{3}{2}$ and the reciprocal of $\frac{9}{4}$ is $\frac{4}{9}$.

When doing dose calculations, division of two fractions is usually indicated by a fraction line rather than the division symbol, $\div$.

To divide fractions:

1. Keep the first (numerator) fraction as written.
2. Write the reciprocal of the second (denominator) fraction.
3. Multiply the first fraction by the reciprocal of the second fraction or "invert the second fraction and then multiply."

Example 1

Divide the following fractions: $\dfrac{1/2}{3/4}$ or $\dfrac{1}{2} \div \dfrac{3}{4}$.

CRITICAL THINKING

Find the numerator fraction, the one on top, and keep it as is.

Find the denominator fraction, the one on the bottom.

Write the reciprocal of the denominator (second) fraction (the one on the bottom).

Multiply the numerator fraction by the reciprocal of the denominator fraction.

Reduce the fractions if possible.

Convert the fraction answer to a decimal by dividing its numerator by its denominator.

Round the answer to the nearest tenth (one position to the right of the decimal point).

Include units of measure in the answer if applicable.

ANSWER FOR BEST CARE

The numerator fraction is $\frac{1}{2}$ and is left as is.
The denominator fraction is $\frac{3}{4}$.
Determine the reciprocal of the denominator fraction, $\frac{4}{3}$.
Multiply the two fractions.

$$\frac{1}{2} \times \frac{4}{3}$$

Reduce by 2.

$$\frac{1}{1} \times \frac{2}{3} = \frac{2}{3}$$

Convert $\frac{2}{3}$ to a decimal = 0.66.
Round the answer = 0.7.

Example 2

Divide the following fractions: $\frac{1/25}{1/150}$ or $\frac{1}{25} \div \frac{1}{150}$.

CRITICAL THINKING

Find the numerator fraction, the one on top, and keep it as is.
Find the denominator fraction, the one on the bottom.
Write the reciprocal of the denominator (second) fraction (the one on the bottom).
Multiply the numerator fraction by the reciprocal of the denominator fraction.
Reduce the fractions if possible.
Convert the fraction answer to a decimal by dividing its numerator by its denominator.
Round the answer to the nearest tenth (one position to the right of the decimal point).

ANSWER FOR BEST CARE

The numerator fraction is $\frac{1}{25}$ and is left as is.
The denominator fraction is $\frac{1}{150}$.
Determine the reciprocal of the denominator fraction, $\frac{150}{1}$.

$$\frac{1}{25} \times \frac{150}{1}$$

Reduce by 25.

$$\frac{1}{1} \times \frac{6}{1} = \frac{6}{1}$$

Convert $\frac{6}{1}$ to a decimal = 6
Rounding the answer and placing units of measure are not necessary.

Example 3

Decrease the amount of wound-packing solution in milliliters per day by the standard wound reduction of the following mathematical fraction: $\frac{1/6}{1/9}$ or $\frac{1}{6} \div \frac{1}{9}$.

CRITICAL THINKING

Find the numerator fraction, the one on top, and keep it as is.
Find the denominator fraction, the one on the bottom.
Write the reciprocal of the denominator (second) fraction (the one on the bottom).
Multiply the numerator fraction by the reciprocal of the denominator fraction.
Reduce the fractions if possible.
Convert the fraction answer to a decimal by dividing its numerator by its denominator.
Round the answer to the nearest tenth (one position to the right of the decimal point).
Include units of measure in the answer if applicable.

ANSWER FOR BEST CARE

The numerator fraction is $\frac{1}{6}$ and is left as is.
The denominator fraction is $\frac{1}{9}$.

Determine the reciprocal of the denominator fraction, $\frac{9}{1}$.

$$\frac{1}{6} \times \frac{9}{1}$$

Reduce by 3.

$$\frac{1}{2} \times \frac{3}{1} = \frac{3}{2}$$

Convert $\frac{3}{2}$ to a decimal = 1.5 mL.
Rounding the answer is not necessary.

PRACTICE PROBLEMS

Directions: For problems 1 through 10, divide the following fractions and give your answers as fractions and as decimals rounded to the nearest tenth.

1. $\frac{1}{200} \div \frac{1}{75}$

2. $\frac{1}{6} \div \frac{1}{10}$

3. $\frac{1}{3} \div \frac{1}{6}$

4. $\frac{3}{4} \div \frac{7}{8}$

5. $\frac{1000}{1} \div \frac{250}{3}$

6. $\frac{3}{2} \div \frac{2}{5}$

7. $\frac{2}{15} \div \frac{3}{5}$

8. $\frac{125}{3} \div \frac{100}{1}$

9. $\frac{15}{1} \div \frac{3}{2}$

10. $\frac{225}{2} \div \frac{15}{4}$

11. The patient is on a reduced-calorie diet, with diet reduced by 1000 calories per day. This reduction is equal to $\frac{1}{3} \div \frac{1}{6}$ for your answer in pounds-per-week loss. How many pounds should the patient be losing? _____

12. Mr. Brown is to reduce his oral potassium supplement by a certain number of milliliters per day. This is based on the formula of $\frac{1}{2} \div \frac{1}{4}$. How many milliliters per day should he reduce his potassium supplement intake? _____

(Answers on p. 442)

EQUATIONS

An equation is a mathematical sentence that contains an equal sign (=) and a letter or an unknown entry known as a *variable*. The solution to an equation is a value that makes the sentence true. In calculating doses, you need to determine the value of an unknown (X). The unknown is what you WANT.

To determine the value of the X variable:
- Reduce the number when possible.
- Multiply the remaining numerators.
- Multiply the remaining denominators.
- Divide the numerator by the denominator ($\frac{numerator}{denominator}$).
- Round the answer to the nearest tenth.

Example 1

Determine the value of X if $X = 200 \times \frac{1}{50}$.

CRITICAL THINKING

What are the numerators?
What are the denominators?

Can the numbers be reduced?
Multiply the remaining numerators.
Multiply the remaining denominators.
Divide the numerator by the denominator ($\frac{numerator}{denominator}$).
Round the answer to the nearest tenth.

| **ANSWER FOR BEST CARE** | $\dfrac{\text{Numerators}}{\text{Denominators}}$ $\dfrac{200}{1} \times \dfrac{1}{50}$ |

Reduce by 50.

$$\frac{4}{1} \times \frac{1}{1} = \frac{4}{1}$$

Answer is X = 4.

Example 2

Determine the value of X if $X = \dfrac{125}{50} \times 4$.

| **CRITICAL THINKING** | What are the numerators?
What are the denominators?
Can the numbers be reduced?
Multiply the remaining numerators.
Multiply the remaining denominators.
Divide the numerator by the denominator ($\frac{numerator}{denominator}$).
Round the answer to the nearest tenth. |

| **ANSWER FOR BEST CARE** | $\dfrac{\text{Numerators}}{\text{Denominators}}$ $\dfrac{125}{50} \times \dfrac{4}{1}$ |

Reduce by 25.

$$\frac{5}{2} \times \frac{4}{1}$$

Reduce by 2.

$$\frac{5}{1} \times \frac{2}{1} = \frac{10}{1} = 10$$

Answer is X = 10.

Example 3

Determine the value of X if $X = \dfrac{0.5}{1.35} \times 1.5$.

| **CRITICAL THINKING** | What are the numerators?
What are the denominators?
Can the numbers be reduced?
Multiply the remaining numerators.
Multiply the remaining denominators.
Divide the numerator by the denominator ($\frac{numerator}{denominator}$).
Round the answer to the nearest tenth. |

| **ANSWER FOR BEST CARE** | $\dfrac{\text{Numerators}}{\text{Denominators}}$ $\dfrac{0.5}{1.35} \times \dfrac{1.5}{1}$ |

Decimal points may be eliminated from a single fraction by moving the decimal point an equal number of places to the right in both the numerator and the denominator. In the fraction on the left, move the decimal points two places to the

CHAPTER 3

right (both numerator and denominator will be whole numbers). The fraction on the right requires only moving the decimal points one place.

Move decimal points in each fraction.

$$\frac{\overset{\frown}{50}}{\underset{\smile}{135}} \times \frac{\overset{\frown}{15}}{10}$$

Reduce by 10.

$$\frac{5}{135} \times \frac{15}{1}$$

Reduce by 15.

$$\frac{5}{9} \times \frac{1}{1} = \frac{5}{9}$$

$\frac{5}{9}$ as a decimal $= 0.55$.

Round the answer, so the answer is X = 0.6.

Example 4

Determine the value of X if $X = \frac{2/150}{1/120} \times 3$.

CRITICAL THINKING

What are the numerators?
What are the denominators?
Can the numbers be reduced?
Multiply the remaining numerators.
Multiply the remaining denominators.
Divide the numerator by the denominator ($\frac{\text{numerator}}{\text{denominator}}$).
Round the answer to the nearest tenth.

ANSWER FOR BEST CARE

$\frac{\text{Numerators}}{\text{Denominators}} \frac{2/150}{1/120} \times \frac{3}{1}$

When dividing by a fraction, remember to invert it and then multiply.

$$\frac{2}{150} \times \frac{120}{1} \times \frac{3}{1}$$

Reduce by 10.

$$\frac{2}{15} \times \frac{12}{1} \times \frac{3}{1}$$

Reduce by 3.

$$\frac{2}{5} \times \frac{12}{1} \times \frac{1}{1} = \frac{24}{5} \text{ or } \frac{2}{5} \times \frac{4}{1} \times \frac{3}{1} = \frac{24}{5}$$

Convert to decimal: $5\overline{)24.0}$ (4.8)

No rounding is necessary, so the answer is X = 4.8.

PRACTICE PROBLEMS

Directions: Determine the value of X and give the answer as a decimal to the nearest tenth.

1. $X = \frac{20}{50} \times 2$

2. $X = \frac{250}{1000} \times 1.3$

3. $X = \frac{0.25}{1.25} \times 1.2$

4. $X = \frac{1/60}{1/150} \times 2.1$

5. $X = \frac{2}{7} \times 3.5$

6. $X = \frac{3/5}{6/25} \times 3$

7. $X = \frac{125/1}{75/1} \times 6$

8. $X = \frac{1.5}{2} \times \frac{3.5}{3}$

9. $X = \frac{1000/1}{100/1} \times 2.25$

10. $X = \frac{1/100}{1/1000} \times \frac{3.75}{2}$

(Answers on p. 443)

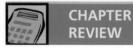

CHAPTER REVIEW

Determine the quantity of medication for each prescription.

1. PRESCRIPTION: morphine sulfate 30 mg.
   HAVE: morphine sulfate tablets labeled 15 mg.
   How many tablet(s) will you use? _____

2. PRESCRIPTION: 0.5 mg.
   HAVE: 0.25-mg tablets.
   How many tablet(s) do you give the patient? _____

3. PRESCRIPTION: atropine sulfate 0.6 mg.
   HAVE: 0.4 mg/mL.
   How many milliliters do you need? _____

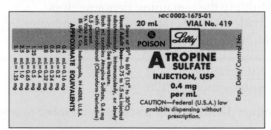

4. PRESCRIPTION: meperidine hydrochloride 100 mg.
   HAVE: 50-mg tablets.
   How many tablet(s) will you use? _____

5. PRESCRIPTION: 0.125 mg.
   HAVE: 0.5 mg scored tablets.
   How many tablet(s) are needed? _____

6. PRESCRIPTION: digoxin (Lanoxin) elixir 0.125 mg.
   HAVE: digoxin (Lanoxin) elixir 0.05 mg/mL.
   How many milliliters are needed? _____

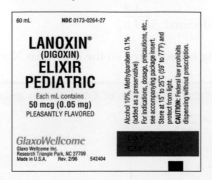

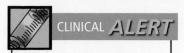

7. PRESCRIPTION: oral medication gr 6½.
   HAVE: The drug is available in gr 2 per ounce.
   How many ounces will be needed? _____

8. PRESCRIPTION: 0.5 g.
   HAVE: 1 g/0.5 mL.
   How many milliliters are needed? _____

9. PRESCRIPTION: docusate sodium (Colace) elixir 30 mg.
   HAVE: elixir of strength 20 mg/5 mL.

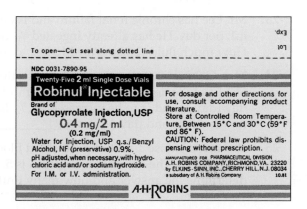

   How many milliliters are needed? _____

10. PRESCRIPTION: glycopyrrolate (Robinul) 1 mg.
    HAVE: glycopyrrolate (Robinul) of strength 0.2 mg/mL.

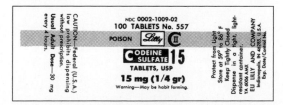

   How many milliliters are needed? _____

11. PRESCRIPTION: gr 1/100.
    HAVE: gr 1/150 tablets.
    How many tablet(s) are needed? _____

12. PRESCRIPTION: codeine sulfate gr ½.
    HAVE: Your supply of codeine sulfate tablets is labeled gr ¼.

   How many tablet(s) will you give? _____

13. PRESCRIPTION: 4 mg of liquid medication.
    HAVE: liquid available 1 mg/5 mL.
    How many milliliters do you need? _____

14.   PRESCRIPTION: lithium citrate (Eskalith) 300 mg.
      HAVE: lithium syrup 300 mg/5 mL.
      How many milliliters do you need? _____

15.   PRESCRIPTION: intravenous levofloxacin (Levaquin) 500 mg.
      HAVE: premixed 250 mg/50 mL.
      How many milliliters do you need? _____

Determine the value of X and give the answer as a decimal to the nearest tenth for problems 16 through 20.

16. $X = \dfrac{1/4}{1/6}$ _____

17. $X = \dfrac{1/6}{1/3} \times 2$ _____

18. $X = \dfrac{650}{325/10.15}$ _____

19. $X = \dfrac{250/5}{125/5}$ _____

20. $X = \dfrac{700}{100/15}$ _____

Answer the following questions for these nondrug calculations in problems 21 through 25.

21.   The patient is to receive ⅔ of 300 mL tube feeding for breakfast and lunch and is to receive ½ of 200 mL Ensure for dinner and bedtime feeding. How much tube feeding will the patient receive? _____

22.   Mr. Hall is on a 2400-calorie diet. He is to decrease his caloric intake by ⅓. What should be his total caloric daily intake? _____

23.   Mr. Lee has chronic renal failure and is on a total fluid restriction diet of 800 mL per day. He has already ingested ⁶⁄₁₀ of his total daily amount by 3 PM. How much fluid remains for Mr. Lee to ingest for the rest of the day? _____

24.   Mrs. Gardner is 3 days post colon resection and has positive bowel sounds. She has tolerated ice chips well. Her fluid intake is changed to 200 mL twice a day (day 1) and is to be increased by ½ daily for 3 days. What is the total for day 2, day 3, and day 4? Day 2 _____ Day 3 _____ Day 4 _____

25.   You are to infuse 1 unit of packed red blood cells for every gram of hemoglobin below 8. The current hemoglobin is 5. What equation would you use to determine the answer and how many units of packed red blood cells would you infuse? _____

(Answers on pp. 443–444)

⊘volve   **For additional practice problems, refer to the Mathematics Review section of Drug Calculations Companion, version 4 on Evolve.**

Systems of Measurement

Units of Measure

Mother Helena Infortuna

CLINICAL CONNECTION

- Recognize metric units used in the clinical setting.
- Recognize metric abbreviations used in the clinical setting.
- Convert from one metric unit to another to acquaint yourself with relationships of metric units to each other.
- Become familiar with units of measure for household measurement systems and understand the safety impact their continued use has on interpretation of medication prescription.
- Become familiar with milliequivalents and international units.

INTRODUCTION

The most common, most accurate, and safest system of measurement in the clinical setting all over the world is the metric system. The metric system is a decimal system of weights and measures that was originally proposed and accepted by an international committee that convened in France. The units used in the metric system are often denoted as SI units; SI comes from the system's French name, *Systeme International*. The SI units are common units seen in laboratory results, patient's height, fundal height in obstetrics, wounds, and intradermal skin reactions. It is the most common system of measurement for medications worldwide.

BASIC UNITS

The metric system uses the meter (m) as the unit of length, the gram (g) as the unit of weight, and the liter (L) as the unit of volume. Clinically, length is commonly used to measure size of induration for the Mantoux tuberculosis skin test in millimeters and length of walking is described in meters. Clinically it is common to see weight being used to determine medication doses based in kilograms and volume being used to denote total urinary output.

Prefixes are used to indicate basic units with each prefix being a power of ten. Table 4-1 provides a full set of metric system prefixes. Prefixes to these basic units common to the clinical setting are kilo (one thousand), centi (one hundredth), milli (one thousandth), and micro (one millionth). The relationships between the prefixes are as follows:

Weight

1 kilogram (kg) = 1000 g
1 gram (g) = 1000 mg
1 milligram (mg) = 1/1000 g or 0.001 g or 1000 mcg
1 microgram (mcg) = 1/1000 mg or 0.001 mg or 0.000001 g

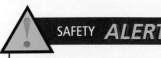

SAFETY ALERT

The abbreviation μg for microgram may be seen on drug labels; this abbreviation can be confused with mg. **Always** use the abbreviation **mcg** or preferably write out the word microgram instead of μg when transcribing medication prescriptions. Since μg is 1000 times smaller than mg, using the abbreviation μg creates a possibility for error in nursing care.

Table 4-1	Metric Units		
Prefix (Symbol)	**Power Times Standard Unit**	**Weight (Symbol)**	**Volume (Symbol)**
Kilo (k)	10^3	Kilogram (kg)	
Hecto (h)	10^2	Hectogram (hg)	
Deka (dk)	10^1	Dekagram (dkg)	
Standard Unit	**10^0**	**Gram (g)**	**Liter (L)**
Deci (d)	10^{-1}	Decigram (dg)	Deciliter (dL)
Centi (c)	10^{-2}	Centigram (cg)	Centiliter (cL)
Milli (m)	10^{-3}	Milligram (mg)	Milliliter (mL)
Micro (mc)	10^{-6}	Microgram (mcg)	Microliter (mcL)
Nano (n)	10^{-9}	Nanogram (ng)	Nanoliter (nL)
Pico (p)	10^{-12}	Picogram (pg)	Picoliter (pL)

Length

1 meter (m) = 100 cm or 1000 mm
1 centimeter (cm) = 1/100 m or 0.01 m or 10 mm
1 millimeter (mm) = 0.001 m or 0.1 cm

Volume

1 liter (L) = 1000 mL
1 milliliter (mL) = 1/1000 L or 0.001 L

Directions: *Write the abbreviations for each unit of measure and identify if it is by weight, length, or volume.*

1. Ten grams. _____
2. Two milliliters. _____
3. Six and three-tenths kilograms. _____
4. Seventy-five hundredths of a milligram. _____
5. One hundred micrograms. _____
6. Two hundredths of a liter. _____
7. Four and two-tenths micrograms. _____
8. Four liters. _____
9. One thousand milliliters. _____
10. Three and seven-tenths kilograms. _____
11. Two centimeters. _____
12. Thirty milliliters. _____
13. Three meters. _____
14. Seventy-four kilograms. _____
15. Four millimeters. _____

16. Three and one-half liters. _____

17. Twenty-five meters. _____

18. Sixty micrograms. _____

19. Two and one-half centimeters. _____

20. Two grams. _____

(Answers on p. 444)

CONVERSION OF METRIC UNITS

Calculating medication doses requires being able to convert kilo, standard, milli, and micro units of measure. To go from a larger unit to a smaller unit, you multiply by 1000. To go from a smaller unit to a larger unit you divide by 1000. Because of the decimal nature of the system, the multiplication can be done by moving the decimal point three places to the right and the division by moving the decimal point three places to the left. This is also a good check for your math.

Example 1

Convert the following metric measurement: 1.2 L = _____ mL.

- **What You HAVE**   1.2 L.

- **What You KNOW**   Conversion is necessary from liters to milliliters.

- **What You WANT**   Answer in equivalent milliliters.

CRITICAL THINKING

Decide whether you are converting from smaller unit to larger unit or vice versa.
If going from a larger unit to a smaller unit, you multiply by 1000 or move the decimal point three places to the right.
If going from a smaller unit to a larger unit, you divide by 1000 or move the decimal point three places to the left.
Label your answer with the correct unit of measure.

ANSWER FOR BEST CARE

In this case, from liters to milliliters is going from a larger unit to a smaller unit.
Multiply by 1000. So 1.2 becomes 1200.
Or you can move the decimal point three places to the right:

1200

Answer is 1.2 L = 1200 mL.

Example 2

Convert the following metric measurement: 0.2 mg = _____ g.

CRITICAL THINKING

Decide whether you are converting from smaller unit to larger unit or vice versa.
If going from a larger unit to a smaller unit, you multiply by 1000 or move the decimal point three places to the right.
If going from a smaller unit to a larger unit, you divide by 1000 or move the decimal point three places to the left.
Label your answer with the correct unit of measure.

ANSWER FOR BEST CARE

In this case, from milligrams to grams is going from a smaller unit to a larger unit.
Divide by 1000. So 0.2 becomes 0.0002.

Or you can move the decimal point three places to the left:

0.0002

Answer is 0.2 mg = 0.0002 g.

Example 3

Convert the following metric measurement: 100 mcg = _0.1 mg_ mg.

CRITICAL THINKING

Decide whether you are converting from smaller unit to larger unit or vice versa.
If going from a larger unit to a smaller unit, you multiply by 1000 or move the decimal point three places to the right.
If going from a smaller unit to a larger unit, you divide by 1000 or move the decimal point three places to the left.
Label your answer with the correct unit of measure.

ANSWER FOR BEST CARE

In this case, from micrograms to milligrams is going from a smaller unit to a larger unit.
Divide by 1000. So 100 (100.0) becomes 0.1.
Or you can move the decimal point three places to the left:

0.100 ← Drop the two zeros to the right of the 1

Answer is 100 mcg = 0.1 mg.

Example 4

Convert the following metric measurement: 150 mL = _____ L.

CRITICAL THINKING

Decide whether you are converting from smaller unit to larger unit or vice versa.
If going from a larger unit to a smaller unit, you multiply by 1000 or move the decimal point three places to the right.
If going from a smaller unit to a larger unit, you divide by 1000 or move the decimal point three places to the left.
Label your answer with the correct unit of measure.

ANSWER FOR BEST CARE

In this case, from milliliters to liters is going from a smaller unit to a larger unit.
Divide by 1000. So 150 (150.0) becomes 0.15.
Or you can move the decimal point three places to the left:
Add zero to highlight decimal → 0.150 ← Drop the zero to the right of the 5
Answer is 150 mL = 0.15 L.

 PRACTICE PROBLEMS

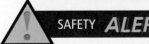 SAFETY **ALERT**

To avoid the possibility of inaccurate dosages, eliminate unnecessary trailing zeros at the end of decimal number. For example, 5.50 would become 5.5. Trailing zeros after a decimal point may be misread. For example, 3.0 may be misread as 30, which is a ten-fold increase and likely an overdose!

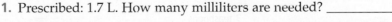

Directions: *Convert the following metric measurements.*

1. Prescribed: 1.7 L. How many milliliters are needed? _____

2. Prescribed: amikacin sulfate 0.5 g. What is the equivalent dose in milligrams? _____

3. Prescribed: 0.5 mL. How many milliliters are needed? _____

4. Prescribed: cefonicid 100 mg. What is the equivalent dose in grams? _____

5. Prescribed: 400 mcg. How many milligrams are needed? _____

6. There are 100 mL of penicillin V potassium solution. How many liters are there? _____

7. Prescribed: digoxin injection of 0.5 mg. What is the equivalent injection in micrograms? _____

8. Prescribed: cyanocobalamin 1 mg. What is the microgram equivalent? _____

9. Prescribed: naloxone HCL 0.4 mg/mL. You have naloxone HCL 400 mcg/mL. Are they equivalent? _____

10. You have 0.04 g furosemide and 4 mg was prescribed. Do you have enough? _____

(Answers on p. 444)

OTHER TYPES OF MEASUREMENTS

Although the metric system is the predominant and preferred measure in the clinical setting, other types of measurements are used in nursing. Among them are the household system, and the drug measurements known as *international units* and *milliequivalents*.

Household Measure

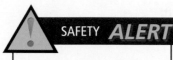

Household measurement is also referred to as *U.S. Customary Measurement* and is the least accurate of the systems because of the differences among the measuring devices. Household measurement is familiar because it is used in cookbooks and in recipes. To communicate with patients and to provide good home health care, it is necessary to be knowledgeable about this system. The household units that are most commonly used when working with medication doses are as follows:
- Drop, abbreviated gtt
- Teaspoon, abbreviated tsp or t = 60 gtt = 5 mL
- Tablespoon, abbreviated tbs, tbsp, or T = 15 mL
- Pound, abbreviated lb
- Fluid ounce, abbreviated oz = 30 mL

Less frequently used household units include cups (abbreviated c), quarts (abbreviated qt), and gallons (abbreviated gal). The U.S. Customary System of Volume Measurement, Table 4-2, gives additional unit equivalents.

Table 4-2	U.S. Customary System of Volume Measurement	
4 quarts (qt)	=	1 gallon (gal)
2 pints (pt)	=	1 quart (qt)
2 measuring cups (c)	=	1 pint (pt)
8 fluid ounces	=	1 measuring cup
2 tablespoons (T, tbs, or tbsp)	=	1 fluid ounce (fl oz)
3 teaspoons	=	1 tablespoon (tbsp)
1 teaspoon (t or tsp)	=	1 fluid dram (fl dr)
1 drop (gtt)	=	1 minim (m)
4 microdrops (mcgtt)	=	1 drop (gtt)

International Units

Heparin, insulin, penicillin, and epoetin alfa recombinant (Epogen, Procrit) are examples of medications that are measured in international units. To minimize misinterpretation, today the common abbreviation *U* is no longer used but the whole

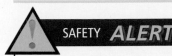

word *units* is written out. An international unit measures a medication in terms of its action or ability to produce a given result. It does not measure a medication in terms of its physical weight or volume. Therefore, to prepare dosages, the volume and dose strength listed on the medication labels must be recognized.

Milliequivalent Measures

Pharmacists and chemists define milliequivalent measure as an expression of the number of grams of equivalent weight of a drug contained in 1 mL of a normal solution. Milliequivalents (mEq) are specific to the medication used, and there is no mathematical conversion required to another system.

The common drugs using milliequivalents are sodium bicarbonate, sodium chloride, and potassium chloride. Since the dosage is individualized, there are no calculations involved. However, as with all medication to be administered, it is crucial that the labels are read accurately. With these vials you always want to note the total volume and the dose strength expressed in mEq/mL or more often noted in mEq/L.

PRACTICE PROBLEMS

Directions: *Express the amounts in correct notation for problems 1 through 5.*

1. One million units. _____

2. Twenty thousand units. _____

3. Seventeen units. _____

4. Seven thousand two hundred units. _____

5. Five hundred thousand units. _____

CLINICAL ALERT

Common medications that use milliequivalents come in both liquid and tablet form.

Directions: *Express the amounts in correct notation for problems 6 through 10.*

6. Twenty milliequivalents. _____

7. Thirty milliequivalents. _____

8. Fifteen milliequivalents. _____

9. Forty milliequivalents. _____

10. Ten milliequivalents. _____

(Answers on p. 444)

CHAPTER REVIEW

HUMAN ERROR Alert

Medications that come in milliequivalents also have on the box the number of milligrams contained in the tablet. Beware, it is the milliequivalent of electrolyte activity that is important, NOT the number of milligrams contained in the tablet or liquid. Do NOT confuse mEq with mg for strength or dose of medication.

For problems 1 through 5, write the abbreviation for each unit of measure and identify whether it is by weight or volume.

1. Five milliliters. _____

2. One and five-tenths milligrams. _____

3. Twenty-five hundredths of a milligram. _____

4. Two and five-tenths milliliters. _____

5. Five grams. _____
   Convert the following metric measurement for problems 6 through 20.

6. PRESCRIPTION: Gantrisin 500 mg. You have Gantrisin 0.5 g. Do you have enough? _____

7. PRESCRIPTION: injection of 5 g. How many milligrams are there? _____

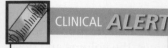

When total volume and dose strength are confused, dangerous results may occur to the patient.

! SAFETY **ALERT**

Do not confuse mEq with mg or mcg, since these abbreviations often look alike with poor handwriting.

8. PRESCRIPTION: digoxin elixir 50 mcg. What is the equivalent dose in milligrams? _____

9. PRESCRIPTION: Robinul 2 mL. You have 0.002 L. Do you have enough? _____

10. PRESCRIPTION: Nafcil injection of 2 g. What is the milligram equivalent? _____

11. There are 60 mL of digoxin elixir. How many liters are there? _____

12. If you have 2.5 L of a solution; how many milliliters do you have? _____

13. PRESCRIPTION: Aldomet 125 mg. What is the equivalent dose in grams? _____

14. There are 120 mL of Prozac liquid. How many liters are there? _____

15. PRESCRIPTION: phenobarbital 30 mg. What is the equivalent dose in micrograms? _____

16. PRESCRIPTION: Gantrisin 0.5 g. What is the equivalent dose in milligrams? _____

17. The size of an ulcer on a patient's foot is 10 mm. What is the size in centimeters? _____

18. PRESCRIPTION: Coumadin 2.5 mg. What is the equivalent dose in micrograms? _____

19. PRESCRIPTION: Vancocin 500 mg. What is the equivalent dose in grams? _____

20. PRESCRIPTION: Decadron 0.25 mg. What is the equivalent dose in micrograms? _____
    Express the amounts in correct notation for problems 21 through 25.

21. Twenty milliequivalents. _____

22. Thirty milliequivalents. _____

23. Fifteen milliequivalents. _____

24. Forty milliequivalents. _____

25. Ten milliequivalents. _____

(Answers on p. 444)

⊖volve **For additional information, refer to the Introducing Drug Measures section on the Drug Calculations Companion, version 4 on Evolve.**

Comprehensive Review

Cynthia Chernecky

Chapter 1

Directions: *For problems 1 through 3, circle the number with the highest value.*

1. (a) 1.9 (b) 3.75 (c) 4.5

2. (a) 1.65 (b) 1.6 (c) 1.42

3. (a) 0.166 (b) 0.125 (c) 0.13

Directions: *For problems 4 through 10, circle the correct needed dosage.*

4. PRESCRIPTION: nitroglycerin (Nitrostat) 0.6 mg buccal controlled-release STAT.
   You HAVE: 0.3-mg strength tablets.

   Will you NEED: less than one tablet, one tablet exactly, or more than one tablet?

5. PRESCRIPTION: warfarin sodium (Coumadin) 7.5 mg by mouth daily.
   You HAVE: 5-mg strength tablets.

   Will you NEED: less than one tablet, one tablet exactly, or more than one tablet?

6. PRESCRIPTION: valsartan (Diovan) 80 mg by mouth today.
   You HAVE: 80-mg strength tablets.
   Will you NEED: less than one tablet, one tablet exactly, or more than one tablet?

7. PRESCRIPTION: glyburide (DiaBeta) 2.5 mg by mouth at breakfast.
   You HAVE: 5-mg strength tablets.

   Will you NEED: less than one tablet, one tablet exactly, or more than one tablet?

8. PRESCRIPTION: telmisartan (Micardis) 40 mg by mouth three times a day.
   You HAVE: 80-mg strength tablets.
   Will you NEED: less than one tablet, one tablet exactly, or more than one tablet?

9. PRESCRIPTION: rifapentine (Priftin) 600 mg by mouth weekly.
   You HAVE: 150-mg tablet.
   Will you NEED: less than one tablet, one tablet exactly, or more than one tablet?

10. PRESCRIPTION: montelukast (Singulair) 10 mg by mouth daily.
    You HAVE: 10-mg strength tablets.
    Will you NEED: less than one tablet, one tablet exactly, or more than one tablet?

Directions: *Find the sum (add the following) of the different strengths of the same medication or the sum of the combined strengths of different medications as named for problems 11 through 20. Do a check to see if your answer is correct.*

11. 2.5 + 5 = _____ Human error check _____

12. 0.125 + 0.25 = _____ Human error check _____

13. 50 mg meperidine (Demerol) + 0.6 mg hydroxyzine (Vistaril) = _____ Human error check _____

14. One tablet labeled 0.2 mg and one tablet labeled 0.4 mg = _____ Human error check _____

15. One tablet labeled 0.25 mg and two tablets labeled 0.125 mg = _____ Human error check _____

16. One tablet labeled 10 mg, one tablet labeled 0.05 mg, and one tablet labeled 0.4 mg = _____ Human error check _____

17. One tablet labeled 2 mg, one tablet labeled 0.375 mg, and one tablet labeled 0.5 mg = _____ Human error check _____

18. Two tablets labeled 2.5 mg and two tablets labeled 5 mg = _____ Human error check _____

19. One tablet labeled 2.25 mg and two tablets labeled 0.5 mg = _____ Human error check _____

20. Three tablets labeled 0.5 g and two tablets labeled 0.25 g = _____ Human error check _____

Directions: *Answer the following questions for problems 21 through 30 and do a check to see if your answer is correct.*

21. PRESCRIPTION: 3 mg. You have 1-mg tablets.
    How many more milligrams must you obtain from the pharmacy? _____
    Human error check _____

22. PRESCRIPTION: 15 mg. You have one 10-mg tablet.
    How many more milligrams must you get from the pharmacy? _____
    Human error check _____

23. PRESCRIPTION: 7.5 mg. You have one 5-mg tablet.
    How many more milligrams must you get from the pharmacy? _____
    Human error check _____

24. PRESCRIPTION: 60 mg. You have 45 mg.
    How many more milligrams must you get from the pharmacy? _____
    Human error check _____

25. PRESCRIPTION: 9 mg. You have 2.5 mg.
    How many more milligrams must you get from the pharmacy? _____
    Human error check _____

26. PRESCRIPTION: 2.625 mg. You have 1.125 mg.
How many more milligrams must you get from the pharmacy? _____
Human error check _____

27. PRESCRIPTION: 4.5 g. You have one tablet of strength 2.25 g.
How many more grams must you get from the pharmacy? _____ Human error check _____

28. PRESCRIPTION: 2.65 mg. You have 1.75 mg.
How many more milligrams must you get from the pharmacy? _____
Human error check _____

29. PRESCRIPTION: 6.75 mg. You have 2.25 mg.
How many more milligrams must you get from the pharmacy? _____
Human error check _____

30. PRESCRIPTION: 3 mg. You have 0.75 mg.
How many more milligrams must you get from the pharmacy? _____
Human error check _____

(Answers on p. 445)

Chapter 2

Directions: *Calculate the answer by multiplying for problems 1 through 10.*

1. $2 \times 2.5 =$ _____
2. $2 \times 0.125 =$ _____
3. $325 \times 3 =$ _____
4. $250 \times 4 =$ _____
5. $250 \times 69.4 =$ _____
6. $0.5 \times 24.7 =$ _____
7. $0.025 \times 4 =$ _____
8. $0.075 \times 1 =$ _____
9. $2.6 \times 72.6 =$ _____
10. $20 \times 82.3 =$ _____

Directions: *Answer the following questions and do a check to see if your answer is correct for problems 11 through 20.*

11. Your patient is to receive a dose of 7.5 mg. The tablets available are labeled 1.5 mg.
What is the dividend? _____ What is the divisor? _____
How many tablet(s) should you administer? _____

12. Your patient is to receive a dose of 1 mg. The tablets available are labeled 0.25 mg.
What is the dividend? _____ What is the divisor? _____
How many tablet(s) will you administer? _____

13. Your patient is to receive a total dose of 3 mg. There are three tablets labeled 1.5 mg in his medicine drawer. Is this a correct dosage? _____

14. You are to give 62.5 mg. Scored tablets labeled 25 mg are available.
What is the dividend? _____ What is the divisor? _____
What is the total number of tablets? _____

15. A dose of 0.125 mg is needed. Tablets available are labeled 0.125 mg.
What is the dividend? _____ What is the divisor? _____
How many tablet(s) are needed? _____

16. Your patient is to receive 0.5 mg. The tablets have strength of 0.2 mg.
    What is the dividend? _____ What is the divisor? _____
    What will be the total number of tablets? _____

17. Your patient is to receive a total dose of 1.8 mg. The available tablets have
    strength of 0.6 mg.
    What is the dividend? _____ What is the divisor? _____
    How many tablet(s) should you administer? _____

18. You are to administer 7.5 mg. The tablets have strength of 2.5 mg.
    What is the dividend? _____ What is the divisor? _____
    How many tablet(s) should you administer? _____

19. PRESCRIPTION: 2.25 mg of dexamethasone (Decadron). Tablets available have
    strength of 0.75 mg.
    What is the dividend? _____ What is the divisor? _____
    How many tablet(s) are needed? _____

20. The patient is to receive a total dose of 6.25 mg. There are three tablets labeled
    2.5 mg in his medicine drawer. Is this a correct dosage? _____
    If not, what should be in his medicine drawer? _____

Directions: *Find the total dose for each patient situation for problems 21 through 30.*

21. You are to administer two 0.6-mg tablets. _____

22. You are to administer 2½ 1.5-mg tablets. _____

23. You are to administer 2½ 0.2-mg tablets. _____

24. Your patient is to receive two 0.25-mg tablets and 1½ 2.5-mg tablets. _____

25. You are to give ½ 0.8-mg tablet and 1½ 3.5-mg tablets. _____

26. You are to give 2½ 0.5-g tablets of sulfisoxazole. _____

27. You have 30-mcg thyroid tablets. There are 2½ tablets. _____

28. You have 0.4-mg nitroglycerin tablets. There are three tablets. _____

29. There are 1½ 0.05-mg tablets. _____

30. Digoxin 0.125-mg tablets. There are two tablets. _____

Directions: *Answer the following questions for each patient situation for problems 31
through 40.*

31. PRESCRIPTION: prednisolone (Delta-Cortef) 10 mg.
    HAVE: The tablets available are each labeled 5 mg.
    How many tablet(s) do you give? _____

32. PRESCRIPTION: 480 mg docusate sodium (Colace).
    HAVE: 240-mg capsules are available.
    How many capsule(s) do you give the patient? _____

33. PRESCRIPTION: acetaminophen 640 mg.
    HAVE: Each tablet available is of strength 160 mg.
    How many tablet(s) are needed? _____

34. PRESCRIPTION: baclofen (Lioresal) 30 mg.
    HAVE: 20-mg tablets.
    How many tablet(s) are needed? _____

35. PRESCRIPTION: buspirone hydrochloride (BuSpar) 25 mg.
    HAVE: 10-mg tablets.
    How many tablet(s) do you give the patient? _____

36. PRESCRIPTION: 180 mg diltiazem hydrochloride sustained-release capsules (Cardizem).
    HAVE: Capsules of strength 60 mg are available.
    How many capsule(s) do you give the patient? _____

37. PRESCRIPTION: cimetidine (Tagamet) 200 mg at bedtime.
    HAVE: There are three tablets, each of strength 400 mg, in the patient's medicine drawer.
    Is this a correct dosage? _____
    If not the correct dosage, what should be the exact number of tablets in the drawer? _____

38. PRESCRIPTION: warfarin sodium (Coumadin) 5 mg.
    HAVE: Tablets are labeled 2.5 mg.
    How many tablet(s) are needed? _____

39. PRESCRIPTION: hydrochlorothiazide (HydroDIURIL) 25 mg daily.
    HAVE: The tablets available are each labeled 12.5 mg.
    How many tablet(s) should you take from the automated medication dispensing machine? _____

40. PRESCRIPTION: 1.5 mg lorazepam (Ativan).
    HAVE: Tablets of strength 0.5 mg are available.
    How many tablet(s) do you need to give? _____

Directions: *Answer the following questions for these nondrug calculations in problems 41 through 50.*

41. An infant drinks 3 ounces of formula every 3 hours and 4 ounces of water three times a day. How much fluid in ounces will the infant drink in 1 day? _____

42. An infant drinks 5 ounces of formula every 4 hours and 2.5 ounces of water three times a day. How much fluid in ounces will the infant drink in 1 day? _____

43. You know that 2 pounds of edema equals 1 L of fluid. A fluid overload patient has lost 11 pounds. How many liters of fluid have been removed? _____

44. You know that 2 pounds of edema equals 1 L of fluid. A fluid overload patient has lost 8 pounds. How many liters of fluid have been removed? _____

45. A patient is supposed to have 1800 mL of fluid every 24 hours. You know that the patient is to have three-fourths of the fluid between breakfast (8 AM) and dinner (6 PM). How much fluid should be ingested between 8 AM and 6 PM? _____

46. A patient is supposed to have 800 mL of fluid every 24 hours. You know that the patient is to have three-fourths of the fluid between breakfast (8 AM) and dinner (6 PM). How much fluid should be ingested between 8 AM and 6 PM? _____

47. The hematocrit of a patient is raised 2 g with each unit of packed red blood cells that is administered. The patient has received 2 units of blood. The hematocrit before blood administration was 6.2 g. What would you anticipate the new hematocrit to be? _____

48. The hematocrit of a patient is raised 2 g with each unit of packed red blood cells that is administered. The patient has received 4 units of blood. The hematocrit before blood administration was 5.8 g. What would you anticipate the post transfusion hematocrit to be? _____

49. Your renal patient is restricted to 40 mL of fluid every 2 hours. How many milliliters of fluid can your patient have per day? _____

50. Your renal patient can have half of his 24-hour oral fluid total with breakfast. His 24-hour oral fluid total is 540 mL. How many milliliters of fluid can he have with breakfast? _____

(Answers on p. 445)

Chapter 3

Directions: *Identify the fraction with the highest value for problems 1 through 10 and answer the questions in problems 11 and 12.*

1. (a) $\frac{1}{8}$ (b) $\frac{1}{6}$ (c) $\frac{1}{4}$ _____

2. (a) $\frac{1}{6}$ (b) $\frac{4}{16}$ (c) $\frac{5}{16}$ _____

3. (a) $\frac{2}{3}$ (b) $\frac{3}{6}$ (c) $\frac{3}{4}$ _____

4. (a) $\frac{4}{9}$ (b) $\frac{4}{11}$ (c) $\frac{5}{4}$ _____

5. (a) $\frac{3}{4}$ (b) $\frac{2}{4}$ (c) $\frac{1}{4}$ _____

6. (a) $\frac{3}{4}$ (b) $\frac{1}{2}$ (c) $\frac{3}{5}$ _____

7. (a) $\frac{2}{5}$ (b) $\frac{3}{4}$ (c) $\frac{3}{8}$ _____

8. (a) $\frac{1}{4}$ (b) $\frac{1}{3}$ (c) $\frac{1}{5}$ _____

9. (a) $\frac{1}{2}$ (b) $\frac{1}{5}$ (c) $\frac{1}{4}$ _____

10. (a) $\frac{8}{4}$ (b) $\frac{6}{5}$ (c) $\frac{9}{8}$ _____

11. Mr. Lewis is to reduce his total caloric intake as much as possible. He is given the choice of decreasing his calories by one-half, three-fourths, or two-thirds. Which should he choose to get the greatest decrease in calories? _____

12. Ms. Forest is to decrease her total carbohydrate intake by the smallest amount prescribed by the dietitian. The dietitian gives her choices of three-eighths, one-sixth, or two-thirds. Which value is the lowest that Ms. Forest could choose? _____

Directions: *Multiply the following fractions and give your answer as a fraction and as a decimal to the nearest tenth (one digit to the right of the decimal) for problems 13 through 24.*

13. $\frac{1}{2} \times \frac{1}{8} =$ _____ _____

14. $\frac{1}{5} \times \frac{100}{1} =$ _____ _____

15. $\frac{8}{10} \times \frac{6}{8} =$ _____ _____

16. $\frac{7}{2} \times \frac{1}{3} =$ _____ _____

17. $\frac{3}{4} \times \frac{8}{16} =$ _____ _____

18. $\frac{160}{4} \times \frac{2}{5} =$ _____ _____

19. $\frac{4000}{1} \times \frac{4}{4000} =$ _____ _____

20. $\frac{3}{5} \times \frac{6}{7} =$ _____ _____

21. $\frac{2}{5} \times \frac{7}{2} =$ _____ _____

22. $\frac{2400}{5} \times \frac{1}{100} =$ _____ _____

23. Mr. Jefferson has essential hypertension and is to decrease his sodium intake by $\frac{1}{4} \times \frac{1}{2}$ daily. Write answer in both fraction and decimal form. _____ _____

24. The nursing home protocol for weening patients off of tube feedings includes daily decreases of $\frac{1}{4}$ times the mathematical fraction of $\frac{3}{2}$. What is the amount of decrease daily as a fraction and a decimal for the tube feeding? _____

Directions: *For problems 25 through 36, divide the fractions and give your answers as fractions and as decimals rounded to the nearest tenths.*

25. $\frac{1}{200} \div \frac{1}{90} =$ _____ _____

26. $\frac{1}{8} \div \frac{1}{10} =$ _____ _____

27. $\frac{1}{2} \div \frac{1}{8} =$ _____ _____

28. $\frac{1}{4} \div \frac{5}{8} =$ _____ _____

29. $\frac{1000}{1} \div \frac{200}{3} =$ _____ _____

30. $\frac{5}{2} \div \frac{3}{5} =$ _____ _____

31. $\frac{4}{15} \div \frac{3}{5} =$ _____ _____

32. $\frac{125}{7} \div \frac{100}{1} =$ _____ _____

33. $\frac{18}{1} \div \frac{3}{2} =$ _____ _____

34. $\frac{225}{2} \div \frac{15}{4} =$ _____ _____

35. The patient is on a reduced-calorie diet that is reduced by 1000 calories per day. This reduction is equal to $\frac{1}{4} \div \frac{1}{3}$ for your answer in pounds-per-week loss. How many pounds should the patient be losing? _____

36. Mr. Sands is to reduce his oral potassium supplement by a certain number of milliliters per day. This is based on the formula of $\frac{1}{3} \div \frac{1}{12}$. How many milliliters per day should he reduce his potassium supplement intake? _____

Directions: *For problems 37 through 46, determine the value of X, giving the answer as a decimal to the nearest tenth.*

37. $X = \frac{10}{45} \times 2$ _____

38. $X = \frac{750}{1000} \times 1.4$ _____

39. $X = \frac{0.5}{1.25} \times 1.3$ _____

40. $X = \frac{1/20}{1/140} \times 2.6$ _____

41. $X = \frac{3}{7} \times 4.8$ _____

42. $X = \frac{2/5}{7/25} \times 5$ _____

43. $X = \frac{150/1}{75/1} \times 3$ _____

44. $X = \frac{1.2}{2} \times \frac{3.5}{6}$ _____

45. $X = \frac{700/1}{100/1} \times 3.25$ _____

46. $X = \frac{1/100}{3/1000} \times \frac{2.5}{3}$ _____

Directions: *Answer the following questions for these nondrug calculations in problems 47 through 50.*

47. The patient is to receive one-fourth of the 600 mL (the total amount daily) for breakfast. How much tube feeding will the patient receive for breakfast? _____

48. Your patient is on a 2800-calorie diet. He needs to decrease his daily caloric intake by one-fifth. What amount should he decrease daily and what is his new daily diet in number of total calories? _____ _____

49. You are to increase fluid intake by 100 mL for every 250 mL the patient has in output in the next 2 hours. At the end of 2 hours, the patient's output is 750 mL. How much should you increase the patient's intake? _____

50. You are to infuse 2 units of platelets for every 25,000 decrease in platelet count. The patient's previous platelet count was 280,000 and now the platelet count is 205,000. How many units of platelets should you infuse? _____

(Answers on pp. 445–446)

Chapter 4

Directions: *For problems 1 through 10, write the abbreviations for each unit of measure and identify whether it is by weight, length, or volume.*

1. Four grams. _____

2. Five milliliters. _____

3. Sixty-nine and three-tenths kilograms. _____

4. Twenty-five hundredths of a milligram. _____

5. Ten meters. _____

6. Five hundredths of a liter. _____

7. One hundred sixty micrograms. _____

8. Three liters. _____

9. Thirty-one centimeters. _____

10. Thirteen millimeters. _____

Directions: *For problems 11 through 20, convert the metric measurements as necessary and answer the questions.*

11. PRESCRIPTION: 1.5 L. How many milliliters are needed? _____

12. PRESCRIPTION: amikacin sulfate 0.4 g. What is the equivalent dose in milligrams? _____

13. PRESCRIPTION: 0.8 L. How many milliliters are needed? _____

14. PRESCRIPTION: cefonicid 200 mg. What is the equivalent dose in grams? _____

15. PRESCRIPTION: 600 mcg. How many milligrams are needed? _____

16. There are 200 mL of penicillin V potassium solution. How many liters are there? _____

17. PRESCRIPTION: digoxin injection of 0.5 mg. What is the equivalent injection in micrograms? _____

18. PRESCRIPTION: cyanocobalamin 0.5 mg. What is the microgram equivalent? _____

19. PRESCRIPTION: naloxone HCL 0.2 mg/mL. You have naloxone HCL 200 mcg/mL. Are they equivalent? _____

20. You have 0.08 g furosemide (Lasix), and 8 mg was prescribed. Do you have enough? _____

(Answers on p. 446)

Conversion

Mother Helena Infortuna, Susan Buzhardt, and Jean Balogh

INTRODUCTION

In order to calculate medication dosages accurately, the nurse must know how to convert between the systems of measurement: metric and household. The importance of knowing how to convert between systems may arise when a physician's or advanced practice nurse's medication prescription is not written in the same measurement system as the medication that is supplied. *Conversion* means changing a measure to its equivalent within the same system—for example, grams to milligrams—or changing a measure from one system to another system, such as ounces (household) to milliliters. When you convert from a larger unit of measure to a smaller unit of measure, you will multiply. When you convert from a smaller unit of measure to a larger unit of measure, you will divide.

It is important for the nurse to have a working knowledge of measurement system equivalents. Table 5-1 lists commonly used metric equivalents. Table 5-2 lists commonly used equivalents for weight, volume, and length in the metric and household systems of measurement.

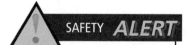

SAFETY ALERT

It is essential to know that when changing from one system to another, the conversions are not exact. Approximate equivalents are used from one system to another.

CONVERTING WITHIN THE METRIC SYSTEM

The metric system is a decimal system. Decimals are based on powers of 10 (e.g., 10^2 [hundreds], 10^3 [thousands]). Since it is a decimal system, conversion between units of measure in the metric system can be accomplished by moving the decimal point. When converting from a larger unit of measure to a smaller unit of measure, the decimal point is moved to the right. The number of places to move the decimal point equals the power of 10.

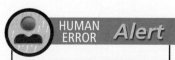

HUMAN ERROR Alert

When computing medication dosages, the approximate equivalent should not differ by more than 10% from the prescribed dose.

Table 5-1	Equivalents within the Metric System
1 kg	=	1000 g
1 g	=	1000 mg
1 mg	=	1000 mcg
1 L	=	1000 mL

Table 5-2	Equivalents for Units of Measure	
Metric	**Apothecary**	**Household**
60 mg	gr 1	
1 g	gr 15	
1 kg		2.2 lb
0.45 kg		1 lb
5 mL		1 tsp
15 mL	oz ½	1 tbsp
30 mL	oz 1	2 tbsp
500 mL		16 oz
		1 pint
1000 mL		1 quart
		32 oz
1 cm		0.4 inches
2.5 cm		1 inch

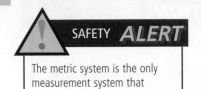

SAFETY **ALERT**

The metric system is the only measurement system that can use the movement of the decimal points.

Example 1

Convert 0.4 g to milligrams.

Larger → Smaller
0.4 g = ? mg

Conversion factor is 1000. Move the decimal point three spaces to the right.

0.4 = 400 mg

Or multiply by 1000.

0.4 g × 1000 = 400.0

The movement of the decimal point to the right is the same as multiplying by the conversion factor.

 When converting from a smaller unit of measure to a larger unit of measure, move the decimal point to the left. The number of places to move the decimal point equals the power of 10.

Example 2

Convert 400 mg to grams.

Smaller → Larger
400 mg = ? g

Conversion factor is 1000. Move the decimal point three spaces to the left.

400 mg = 0.400 = 0.4 g

Or divide by 1000.

$$\frac{400 \text{ mg}}{1000} = 0.4 \text{ g}$$

The movement of the decimal point to the left is the same as dividing by the conversion factor.

Example 3

Convert 3 mcg to milligrams.

Smaller → Larger
3 mcg = ? mg

Conversion factor is 1000. Move the decimal point three spaces to the left.

3 mcg = 0.003 = 0.003 mg

Or divide by 1000.

$$\frac{3 \text{ mcg}}{1000} = 0.003 \text{ mg}$$

PRACTICE PROBLEMS

Directions: *Convert the following.*

1. 0.05 mg to mcg _____
2. 0.6 mg to g _____
3. 2.5 g to mg _____
4. 75 mg to mcg _____
5. 0.006 mcg to mg _____
6. 35 g to mg _____
7. 50 mg to g _____
8. 13 mcg to mg _____
9. 0.055 mg to mcg _____
10. 0.0006 mg to mcg _____

(Answers on p. 446)

⚠ SAFETY *ALERT*

Before a drug calculation can be computed, the prescribed medication and the medication on hand must be in the same unit of measure.

Example 1

PRESCRIPTION   *Metoprolol tartrate 0.025 g by mouth every morning.*

• **What You HAVE**   Lopressor 50 mg.

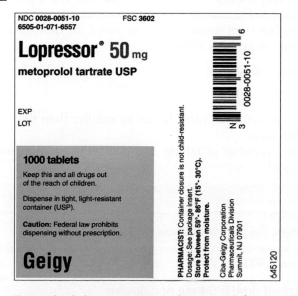

• **What You KNOW**   Prescribed dose is 0.025 g of metoprolol.

1000 mg = 1 g.

Conversion is from larger to smaller.

• **What You WANT**   To convert grams to milligrams.

CRITICAL THINKING	Do the ordered metoprolol tartrate units of measure match the available metoprolol tartrate units of measure? No. What measurement system is being used? The metric system. Can decimals be moved to make the conversion? Yes. Which way should the decimal be moved? Three places to the right.
ANSWER FOR BEST CARE	Converting from larger to smaller. Decimal is moved right. 0.025 g = ? mg 0.025 g = 25 mg 1000 × 0.025 = 25 mg Is the amount prescribed larger or smaller than the amount on hand? Smaller. Will the number of tablets to be administered be more than one tablet or less? Less.

Example 2

PRESCRIPTION	*Lanoxin 125 mcg by mouth every day.*
• **What You HAVE**	Lanoxin 0.125-mg tablets.
• **What You KNOW**	Prescribed dose is 125 mcg of Lanoxin. 1000 mcg = 1 mg. Conversion is from smaller to larger.
• **What You WANT**	To convert micrograms to milligrams.
CRITICAL THINKING	Do the ordered Lanoxin units of measure match the available units of measure? No. What measurement system is being used? The metric system. Can decimals be moved to make the conversion? Yes. Which way should the decimal be moved? Three places to the left.
ANSWER FOR BEST CARE	Converting from smaller to larger, move the decimal to the left. Conversion factor is 1000. 125 mcg = 0.125 mg 125 ÷ 1000 = 0.125 Is the amount prescribed larger or smaller than the amount on hand? Neither: it's the same. Will the number of tablets to be administered be more than one tablet or less? Equal.

Example 3

PRESCRIPTION	*Naloxone 0.4 mg intravenous now.*
• **What You HAVE**	Naloxone 400 mcg/mL.
• **What You KNOW**	Prescribed dose is 0.4 mg of naloxone. 1000 mg = 1 mcg. Conversion is from larger to smaller.
• **What You WANT**	To convert milligrams to micrograms.

CRITICAL THINKING	Do the ordered naloxone units of measure match the available units of measure? No. What measurement system is being used? The metric system. Can decimals be moved to make the conversion? Yes.

ANSWER FOR BEST CARE	Which way should the decimal be moved? Three places to the right. 0.4 mg = ? mcg 0.4 mg = 400 mcg Is the amount prescribed larger or smaller than the amount on hand? Neither: it's the same. Will the quantity to be administered be more than 1 mL or less? Equal. Does your answer fit the general guideline? Yes, the desired dose is equal to the dose on hand.

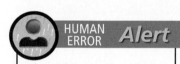

PRACTICE PROBLEMS

Directions: *Solve the following conversion problems. Be sure to label and check your answers.*

1. PRESCRIPTION: The patient is to receive cyproheptadine hydrochloride (Periactin) 6000 mcg by mouth twice a day.
   HAVE: 4-mg scored tablet.
   Convert micrograms to milligrams. _____

2. The patient is to receive 0.4 L of GoLytely by mouth the day before a colonoscopy.
   Convert liters to milliliters. _____

3. PRESCRIPTION: Zyloprim 0.6 g by mouth every day.
   HAVE: allopurinol (Zyloprim) 300-mg scored tablets.
   Convert grams to milligrams. _____

4. 1 g of a drug is equal to how many kilograms? _____

5. The advanced practice nurse has prescribed cyanocobalamin (vitamin B$_{12}$) 500 mcg by mouth.
   How many milligrams will the nurse give? _____

6. PRESCRIPTION: cephalexin monohydrate (Keflex) 0.5 g orally every 12 hours.
   HAVE: Keflex 250-mg tablets.
   Convert grams to milligrams. _____

7. PRESCRIPTION: Premarin 1.25 mg by mouth daily.
   HAVE: 625-mcg tablets.
   Convert milligrams to micrograms. _____

8. PRESCRIPTION: 0.8 g of Megace by mouth each day.
   HAVE: 40 mg/mL.
   Convert grams to milligrams. _____

9. PRESCRIPTION: theophylline elixir 0.2 g.
   HAVE: 80 mg per 15 mL.
   Convert grams to milligrams. _____

10. 0.1 kg of a drug is equivalent to how many grams? _____

HUMAN ERROR *Alert*

When utilizing numbers that divide evenly in half, always set up a math equation to double-check the math, since doing the math in your head can easily lead to a double dose or a half dose of medication.

(Answers on pp. 446–447)

CONVERTING BETWEEN SYSTEMS OF MEASUREMENT

Conversion between the household units of measure and the metric system may occur because patients are accustomed to using the household units of measure.

Example 1

A child weighs 20 kg. The mother asks, "How many pounds does the baby weigh?"

• **What You KNOW**	Changing larger to smaller.
• **What You WANT**	Convert kilograms to pounds.
CRITICAL THINKING	What systems of measurement are being used? The metric and household measurement systems.
	How can an equivalent be found between the two units of measure? Through memorization of equivalents or by referring to an equivalents table, an equivalent conversion can be identified.
	1 kg = 2.2 lb
ANSWER FOR BEST CARE	Multiply numbers when changing from larger to smaller.
	20 × 2.2 = 44 lb

Example 2

The patient reports to you that she has drunk half a cup of juice, 2 cups of coffee, and $\frac{3}{4}$ cup of water with her breakfast. What is her intake in milliliters?

• **What You KNOW**	A cup is equal to 8 ounces.
	Converting from larger to smaller.
• **What You WANT**	Total intake in milliliters.
CRITICAL THINKING	What systems are being used? The household and metric systems.
	How can an equivalent be found between the two units of measure? Through memorization of equivalents or by referring to an equivalents table, an equivalent conversion can be identified.
	1 ounce = 30 mL

ANSWER FOR BEST CARE

8 ounces × 30 mL = 240 mL × 2 (coffee) = 480 mL

$$\frac{1}{2} \text{ (juice)} \times \frac{8 \text{ ounces}}{1} = \frac{8}{2} = 4 \text{ ounces} \times 30 \text{ mL} = 120 \text{ mL}$$

$$\frac{3}{4} \text{ (water)} \times \frac{8 \text{ ounces}}{1} = \frac{24}{4} = 6 \text{ ounces} \times 30 \text{ mL} = 180 \text{ mL}$$

480 + 120 + 180 = 780 mL

Example 3

PRESCRIPTION	*Amoxicillin 25 mg/kg by mouth every 12 hours. The patient weighs 18 pounds.*
• **What You HAVE**	Amoxil 125 mg/5 mL.
• **What You KNOW**	The physician's prescription utilizes the metric system of measurement for amoxicillin. This system of measurement indicates that for each kilogram of body weight,

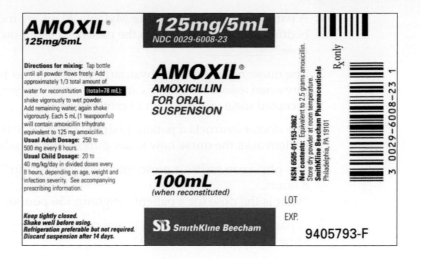

25 mg of amoxicillin needs to be administered. The patient's weight is in pounds, not kilograms.

• **What You WANT**

The amount of milliliters needed to deliver a 25 mg/kg dose of amoxicillin to a patient weighing 18 pounds.

CRITICAL THINKING

Do the prescribed units of measure match the available units of measure? No.
What systems are being used? One system is household and one is metric.
How can an equivalent be found between the two units of measure? Through memorization of equivalents or by referring to an equivalents table, an equivalent conversion can be identified.

ANSWER FOR BEST CARE

2.2 lb = 1 kg

$$\frac{18 \text{ lb}}{2.2 \text{ lb}} = 8.2 \text{ kg (rounded from 8.18)}$$

How many milligrams of amoxicillin must be administered for each kilogram of body weight?
25 mg of amoxicillin must be administered for each kilogram of body weight (25 mg/kg).
25 mg × 8.2 kg = 205 mg of amoxicillin per dose.

PRACTICE PROBLEMS

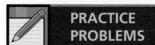

Directions: *Solve the following conversion problems. Be sure to label and check your answers.*

1. PRESCRIPTION: Phenobarbital 60 mg.
   HAVE: Phenobarbital 60 mg.

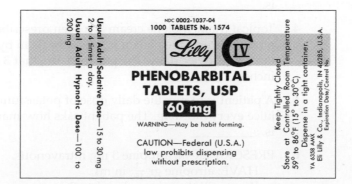

How many tablet(s) equal the prescribed dose? _____

2. A patient is prescribed to take Mylanta 20 mL by mouth after each meal and at bedtime. The nurse instructs the patient to take how many teaspoons for each dose? _____

3. The nurse reports to the physician that the wound is 6 inches by 8 inches; the physician asks the nurse to convert those measurements into the hospital's accepted measuring system of centimeters. _____

4. The doctor instructs a patient to drink 2 L of clear fluids in 24 hours. The patient asks the nurse how many ounces that equals. _____

5. The physician writes a prescription for gentamicin 2 mg/kg intravenous every 8 hours.
   What is the dose for a patient weighing 156 pounds? _____

6. A patient with heart disease is prescribed aspirin gr 5 by mouth each morning. How many mg is each tablet? _____

7. PRESCRIPTION: guaifenesin syrup 2 teaspoons by mouth every 4 hours as needed for cough.
   HAVE: guaifenesin syrup unit dose cups 100 mg/5 mL.
   How many milliliters should be given for each ordered dose? _____

8. A patient received 1.5 L of intravenous fluid in the emergency room. The patient asks how many quarts this is equivalent to. _____

9. A patient experiencing pain is prescribed morphine sulfate gr $\frac{1}{4}$ by mouth every 4 hours as needed. The pharmacy has 15-mg immediate-release morphine tablets available. What should the patient receive per dose? _____

10. The advanced practice nurse prescribes atropine gr $\frac{1}{200}$ intramuscular preoperatively. The vial available reads atropine 0.4 mg/mL. Calculate the correct dose. _____

(Answers on p. 447)

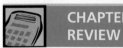

CHAPTER REVIEW

Solve the following conversion problems. Be sure to label and check your answers.

1. Prepare a gr $\frac{1}{6}$ intramuscular injection of morphine sulfate from a vial labeled gr $\frac{1}{8}$ grs/mL. _____

2. PRESCRIPTION: citalopram (Celexa) oral solution 30 mg by mouth every day. This dose requires 15 mL.
   How many tablespoons will the patient take per dose? _____

3. A newborn is 55 cm long. The mother asks how many inches this is. _____

4. Topical triamcinolone cream has been prescribed for a skin rash. The nurse instructs the patient to cover the 3 cm by 4 cm rash on the arm with the cream twice daily. The patient asks what 3 cm by 4 cm is equal to in inches. _____

5. A patient is to mix the daily dose of potassium in 180 mL of orange juice every morning. The patient asks how many ounces this is. _____

6. PRESCRIPTION: atropine 3 mg intravenous.
   HAVE: atropine gr $\frac{1}{150}$ in mL.
   What will the nurse administer? _____ mL.

7. A patient with end-stage lung cancer has been taking 20 mg of concentrated oral morphine every 3 hours for the past 48 hours. How many grams of morphine has the patient had in the last 48 hours? _____

8. A patient is prescribed to drink one 300 mL bottle of magnesium citrate. The patient asks how many ounces there are in the bottle of magnesium citrate. _____

9. The physician has prescribed epoetin alfa 50 units per kg of body weight. The patient weighs 165 pounds. How many units of drug will the patient receive? _____

10. A postoperative patient has returned to the surgical unit after receiving a total of 6.4 L of intravenous fluid during the operative procedure. How many milliliters of fluid did the patient receive? _____

11. The physician instructs a patient to force fluids to at least 3000 mL per day. The patient asks how many 8-ounce glasses this equals. _____

12. The advanced practice nurse prescribes gabapentin 1.8 g per day in three divided doses. Available capsules are 300 mg. How many milligrams will the patient receive per dose? _____

13. A patient is prescribed to take Maalox 1 ounce by mouth 1 hour after meals and at bedtime. The patient asks what 1 ounce is equivalent to in table-spoons. _____

14. Convert ciprofloxacin 500 mg to a dose in grains. _____

15. Prepare a 1500-mcg dose of risperidone. Risperidone tablets available equal 3 mg. _____

16. Prepare a 15-mg dose of morphine sulfate intramuscular from a vial labeled gr $\frac{1}{6}$ /mL. _____

17. The physician prescribes 0.8 g streptomycin intramuscular. The pharmacy dispenses streptomycin vials of 400 mg/mL. What will the nurse give? _____ mL.

18. A child who weighs 35 pounds is to receive amoxicillin 30 mg/kg. What amoxicillin dose will the child receive? _____

19. A patient is to receive 9 mcg of interferon alfacon–1 subcutaneous three times a week for the next 6 months. How many milligrams will the patient receive weekly? _____

20. The nurse practitioner prescribes 325 mg of aspirin daily. How many grains would this be? _____

21. The nurse is to administer KCL mixed in 30 mL by mouth daily. The patient is to be discharged on this medication and only has a tablespoon at home. How many tablespoons should the patient take daily? _____

22. Your patient is prescribed upon discharge to receive Robitussin cough syrup 0.5 ounces now and every 4 hours. How many tablespoons should the patient receive now? _____

23. Your nursing home patient has signs of mild heart failure and is prescribed furosemide (Lasix) 20 mg orally now. You have available Lasix 40 mg/5 mL. How many milliliters should you administer now? _____

24. Your 8-year-old patient is to receive amoxicillin and potassium clavanate (Augmentin) 500 mg orally every 8 hours for an ear infection. The oral solution comes in 125 mg/5 mL. How many teaspoons should the mother give the child every 8 hours after discharge? _____

25. Your intensive care patient receives codeine gr 2 as an oral elixir for pain now. How many milligrams should you administer? _____

(Answers on p. 447)

⊖volve   **For additional information, refer to the Introducing Drug Measures section of the Drug Calculations Companion, version 4 on Evolve.**

Calculations for the Clinical Setting

CHAPTER 6

Percentages

Mother Helena Infortuna

CLINICAL CONNECTION

- Understanding percentages is essential for effective implementation of nursing care in all clinical settings.
- Converting percentages to decimals or fractions is a necessary skill to help determine correct dosages of medications.

INTRODUCTION

Since intravenous solutions and parenteral medications involve percentages, an understanding of percentages is necessary to give excellent patient care. This is particularly true in acute care settings and home care settings.

PERCENTAGES

HUMAN ERROR *Alert*

If using a calculator to determine the decimal, be sure to enter the percent number, then the division key, and then enter the number 100.

SAFETY *ALERT*

When converting clinical percentages to decimals, the conversion is always 1 or less than 1. For example 100% = 1 and 58% = 0.58.

A ratio (a divisional comparison of two quantities) that compares a number with 100 is called a *percentage*, or a percent (%). Percentages are used in writing medication prescriptions, such as magnesium sulfate 50%; in assessing the size of burns on the entire body (i.e., 15% of the body is burned); as an expression of the total body surface area in prescribing chemotherapy (see Chapter 22); with external medication solutions such as hydrocortisone cream, eye drops and eye ointments, ear drops and Dakin's solution (a very strong antiseptic wound-cleansing solution); and with internal solutions, such as intravenous fluids of 0.9% sodium chloride and 5% dextrose in water (D_5W) or peritoneal dialysate 1.5%, 2.5%, 4.25% dextrose or sorbitol concentrations.

Percentages can be written as fractions or decimals. For example, 5% would be $\frac{5}{100}$ as a fraction (reduced to $\frac{1}{20}$ as a fraction) or 0.05 as a decimal, and 10% would be $\frac{10}{100}$ ($\frac{1}{10}$ as a reduced fraction) or 0.1 as a decimal.

The decimal equivalent can be determined in one of the following ways: divide the percent number by 100; for example, 20% is:

$$100\overline{)20.0} \qquad 0.2$$

Or you can move the decimal point of the percent number two places to the left. If no decimal is visible, place the decimal point at the right of the number. For example, for 5%, the number is 5 and moving the decimal point of 5.0 two places to the left results in 0.050 or, properly written, 0.05.

Example 1

Write 9% as a fraction and as a decimal.

| **CRITICAL THINKING** | For fraction: put percent number over 100.
For decimal: move decimal point of the percent number two places to the left, or divide by 100. |

| **ANSWER FOR BEST CARE** | Fraction: $\frac{9}{100}$

Decimal: 09. or 0.09

Or divide: $\quad 0.09$
$\qquad 100\overline{)9.0}$ |

Example 2

Write 30% as a fraction and as a decimal.

| **CRITICAL THINKING** | For fraction: put percent number over 100.
For decimal: move decimal point of the percent number two places to the left, or divide by 100. |

| **ANSWER FOR BEST CARE** | Fraction: $\frac{30}{100} = \frac{3}{10}$

Decimal: 30. or 0.3

Or divide: $\quad 0.3$
$\qquad 100\overline{)30.0}$ |

Example 3

Write 0.5% as a fraction and as a decimal.

| **CRITICAL THINKING** | For fraction: put percent number over 100.
For decimal: move decimal point of the percent number two places to the left, or divide by 100. |

| **ANSWER FOR BEST CARE** | Fraction: $\frac{0.5}{100} = \frac{5}{1000}$

Decimal: 00.5 or 0.005

Or divide: $\quad 0.005$
$\qquad 100\overline{)0.500}$ |

| **PRACTICE PROBLEMS** | Directions: *Write each percentage as a fraction and then as a decimal.* |

1. 4% _____

2. 0.9% _____

HUMAN ERROR *Alert*

3. 0.45% _____

4. 50% _____

5. 10% _____

6. 25% _____

Remember: If decimal number ends in zero(s), the zero(s) are dropped. If the decimal has no number to the left of the decimal, a zero is placed there to help avoid medication errors.

7. 35% _____

8. 75% _____

HUMAN ERROR *Alert*

9. 0.6% _____

10. 43% _____

With fractions, use whole numbers rather than decimal numbers to avoid errors.

11. A patient's hematocrit increases 3% for every unit of packed red blood cells infused. Mrs. Smith has had 4 units of packed red blood cells infused. What percent of increase in hematocrit can you expect? _____

12. Your patient is prescribed an eye ointment in a 1:5 solution. The pharmacy has sent up the eye ointment labeled 20%. Is this the correct ointment? _____

(Answers on p. 447)

PERCENTAGES OF MEDICATIONS IN SOLUTIONS

To determine the grams of medication in a percent solution:
1. Change the percentage to its fraction or decimal equivalent.
2. Multiply the total number of milliliters of solution by the equivalent (fraction or decimal).
3. Write your answer containing the appropriate units and medication name.

Example 1

Determine the grams of medication in the prescribed percent solution.

PRESCRIPTION	*1000 mL of a 1% solution.*
• **What You HAVE**	1000-mL solution.
• **What You KNOW**	Prescribed is 1% solution.
• **What You WANT (X)**	Number of grams of medication contained in the solution.
CRITICAL THINKING	Change percentage to its equivalent as a fraction or decimal. For fraction, put number over 100; for decimal, move decimal point two places to the left. Multiply milliliters you HAVE by the equivalent. Write answer in appropriate units for each medication.
ANSWER FOR BEST CARE	$1\% = \frac{1}{100}$ or 0.01 $$1000 \times \frac{1}{100} = 10 \text{ or } 1000 \times 0.01 = 10$$ 10 g of the drug are in the solution.

Example 2

Determine the grams of medication in the prescribed percent solution.

PRESCRIPTION	*250 mL of a 5% solution.*
• **What You HAVE**	250-mL solution.
• **What You KNOW**	Prescribed is 5% solution.
• **What You WANT (X)**	Number of grams of medication contained in the solution.
CRITICAL THINKING	Change percentage to its equivalent as a fraction or decimal. For fraction, put number over 100; for decimal, move decimal point two places to the left. Multiply milliliters you HAVE by the equivalent. Write answer in appropriate units for each medication.
ANSWER FOR BEST CARE	$5\% = \frac{5}{100}$ or $\frac{1}{20} = 0.05$ $$250 \times 0.05 = 12.50 \text{ or } 250 \times \frac{1}{20} = \frac{250}{20} = \frac{25}{2} = 12.5$$ The intravenous dose contains 12.5 g of drug in the solution.

PRACTICE PROBLEMS

Directions: *In each of the following problems, determine the number of grams of drug the solution will contain.*

1. 1000 mL of a 0.3% solution. _____

2. 1000 mL of a 10% solution. _____

3. 500 mL of a 20% solution. _____

4. 500 mL of a 25% solution. _____

5. 500 mL of a 0.45% hydrocortisone solution. _____

6. 50 mL of a 0.1% solution. _____

7. 300 mL of a 10% multivitamin (MVI) solution. _____

8. 250 mL of a 20% dextrose solution. _____

9. 100 mL of a 5% sodium bicarbonate solution. _____

10. 750 mL of a 3% salt solution. _____

(Answers on p. 447)

CHAPTER REVIEW

Write each percentage as a fraction and as a decimal for problems 1 through 15.

1. 15% _____ _____

2. 40% _____ _____

3. 0.1% _____ _____

4. 1.25% _____ _____

5. 0.03% _____ _____

6. 8% _____ _____

7. 0.6% _____ _____

8. 0.25% _____ _____

9. 50% _____ _____

10. 10% _____ _____

11. 45% _____ _____

12. 33% _____ _____

13. 80% _____ _____

14. 0.7% _____ _____

15. 42% _____ _____

Answer each question for problems 16 through 25.

16. A patient's hematocrit increases 3% for every unit of packed red blood cells infused. Mrs. Smith has had 3 units of packed red blood cells infused. What percent of increase in hematocrit can you expect? _____

17. Your patient is prescribed an eye ointment in a 1:4 solution. The pharmacy has sent up the eye ointment labeled 20%. Is this the correct ointment? _____

18. Ms. Smith has a wound that needs to be irrigated with the strongest Dakin's solution that the pharmacy has on hand. The pharmacy states that they have

the following three solutions: (a) 5%, (b) 10%, and (c) 20%. Which solution do you obtain from the pharmacy? _____

19. The doctor prescribes an ophthalmic solution to decrease inflammation of the patient's right eye. He prescribes that you use the weakest solution first. The solutions the pharmacy has on hand are (a) 0.05%, (b) 1%, (c) 0.02%. Which solution should you use first? _____

20. FIO_2 is the percentage of supplemental oxygen a patient is receiving. To determine PaO_2, multiply the FIO_2 by 5. Mr. Henry's FIO_2 is 18%. What is his estimated PaO_2? _____

21. Spilled urine should be cleaned up with 1% bleach. How many milliliters of bleach are added to 100 mL of water? _____

22. Catheter-related infections occur in 7% of patients with central venous access. The ICU staff inserts 500 central lines annually. How many catheter-related infections might you expect? _____

23. To determine the fullness of an MDI inhaler, you float the inhaler in a bowl of water. If the inhaler is 70% full, it will lie on its side below the surface of the water. If it is less than 30% full, it will float at a 30-degree angle with half the inhaler above the surface of the water. Your patient's canister is lying on its side below the surface of the water. What percentage of medication is left in the MDI? _____

24. A sputum culture is 98% accurate when diagnosing tuberculosis. You have done sputum cultures on 500 jailed inmates. How many inmates could have active tuberculosis but test negative for their culture? _____

25. Without the use of anticoagulants, the risk of deep vein thrombosis (DVT) after joint arthroplasty is approximately 53%. Your hospital does 400 arthroplasties annually. How many patients are at risk for DVT if no anticoagulants are used? _____

(Answers on pp. 447–448)

ɘvolve   **For additional practice problems, refer to the Mathematics Review section of the Drug Calculations Companion, version 4 on Evolve.**

Ratio-Proportion Method

Mother Helena Infortuna, Denise Macklin, Susan Buzhardt, and Jean Balogh

CLINICAL CONNECTION

- Understanding the elements of a ratio-proportion will ensure the proper arrangement of information collected from the prescription and the medication supplied by the pharmacy, as well as accurate calculations.
- Using the ratio-proportion method offers a systematic approach to solving clinical math calculations, including medication and nonmedication problems.

INTRODUCTION

There are different methods to calculate medication dosages. Ratio-proportion is one method that provides a logical approach to solving dosage calculations. To understand the method, it is important to understand what a ratio is, what a proportion is, how to set up a ratio-proportion, how to solve for an unknown, and what are the potential issues that can result in calculation errors.

RATIO

HUMAN ERROR *Alert*

Strength and volumes for the same medications often differ, so be extra careful when using ratios.

SAFETY *ALERT*

Ratios are always written in their simplest (reduced) terms.

A ratio is a divisional comparison of two quantities using either a colon or a fraction line. With drug dosages, the relationship between the weight (strength) of a drug and the volume of medication (such as one tablet or capsule, or 1 mL of solution with liquid medications) is expressed as a ratio. This is often spoken of in nursing as the dose.

$$\frac{\text{Strength}}{\text{Volume}} \text{ or Strength: Volume}$$

When expressing a medication dose as a ratio, the unit of measure should be included with the numeric value:

$$\frac{\text{(Strength)}}{\text{(Volume)}} \frac{10 \text{ mg}}{5 \text{ mL}} \rangle \text{Unit of measure}$$

Ratios are also used in determining hourly infusion rates (see Chapter 15) and intake and output (I&O) for hydration purposes (see Chapter 19). This is common in the elderly and infants or anyone with tube feedings or those requiring monitoring of urinary output.

Throughout this chapter, compare What You HAVE, What You KNOW, and What You WANT and answer the questions in the Critical Thinking section.

Example 1

- **What You HAVE**   Ampicillin 250-mg capsule.

- **What You WANT**   To write a ratio for what you HAVE.

CRITICAL THINKING   What is the strength? _250 _g_
What is the volume? _1 cap_

Write the ratio as $\dfrac{\text{strength}}{\text{volume}}$ and as strength : volume.

ANSWER FOR BEST CARE   The strength is 250 mg.
The volume is 1 capsule.

As a ratio: $\dfrac{250 \text{ mg ampicillin}}{1 \text{ capsule}}$ or 250 mg : 1 capsule.

Example 2

- **What You HAVE**   Demerol 100 mg in 1 mL.

- **What You WANT**   To write a ratio for what you HAVE.

CRITICAL THINKING   What is the strength? _100mg_
What is the volume? _1ml_

Write the ratio as $\dfrac{\text{strength}}{\text{volume}}$ and as strength : volume.

ANSWER FOR BEST CARE   The strength is 100 mg.
The volume is 1 mL.

As a ratio: $\dfrac{100 \text{ mg Demerol}}{1 \text{ mL}}$ or 100 mg : 1 mL.

Example 3

- **What You HAVE**   Lanoxin 0.25-mg tablet.

- **What You WANT**   To write a ratio for what you HAVE.

CRITICAL THINKING   What is the strength? _0.25 mg_
What is the volume? _1 tab_

Write the ratio as $\dfrac{\text{strength}}{\text{volume}}$ and as strength : volume.

ANSWER FOR BEST CARE   The strength is 0.25 mg.
The volume is 1 tablet.

As a ratio: $\dfrac{0.25 \text{ mg Lanoxin}}{1 \text{ tablet}}$ or 0.25 mg : 1 tablet.

PRACTICE PROBLEMS   Directions: *Write a ratio from the following medication information, using both a fraction line and a colon.*

1. Gentamicin 40 mg in 1 mL. _40mg/1ml   40mg : 1ml_

2. Keflex 125 mg in 5-mL solution. _125mg/5ml   125mg : 5ml_

3. Diabinese 250 mg in one tablet. _____ 250mg/1 tab

4. Docusate sodium 100 mg in 10-mL solution. _____ 100mg/10ml

5. Levothyroxine sodium (Synthroid) 0.05 mg in one tablet. _____ 0.05mg/1 tab

6. Aspirin 325 mg in one tablet. _____ 325mg/1 tab

7. Lorabid 200 mg in 5 mL. _____ 200mg/5ml

8. Demerol 50 mg in 5 mL. _____ 50mg/5ml

9. Phenobarbital 60 mg in one tablet. _____ 60mg/1 tab

10. Cimetidine HCL 250 mg in one tablet. _____ 250mg/1 tab

(Answers on p. 448)

RATIO MEASURES

Although ratio strengths are not readily seen in dosages, it is necessary to understand what they mean because of their use in the clinical setting, such as with dressing changes, eye drops, ear drops, and ointments. Ratio strength compares parts of a drug to parts of a solution.

Think of this as a stated number of drops of a medicine in a stated number of drops of water. So if you have 50 drops of red food coloring in 100 drops of water in one vial and in another vial have 2 drops of red food coloring in 100 drops of water, the vial with 50 drops of food coloring will be darker and have a greater strength, whereas the vial with 2 drops of red coloring will be lighter in color and have a lesser strength.

✔ **Human Error Check**

Comparison of ratio strengths can be double-checked by converting all ratio fractions using a common denominator, and the one fraction with the highest numerator is the stronger solution. For example, with $^1/_{10}$, $^2/_{10}$, and $^7/_{10}$, the $^7/_{10}$ solution is the stronger solution.

Example 1

PRESCRIPTION	*A 1:100 solution.*
• *What You HAVE*	You have a 1:100 solution.
• *What You KNOW*	Prescribed is 1:100 solution.
• *What You WANT*	A ratio measure.
CRITICAL THINKING	A ratio measure consists of parts of drug in parts of solution. What are the parts of drug? _____ 1 What are the parts of solution? _____ 100
ANSWER FOR BEST CARE	A 1:100 solution contains 1 part drug in 100 parts solution. Ratio measure: $\dfrac{1}{100}$ or 0.01.

Example 2

Epinephrine is a solution with a strength of 1:1000 when used subcutaneously for treating anaphylaxis.

• **What You HAVE**   Epinephrine 30 mL of 1:1000 solution.

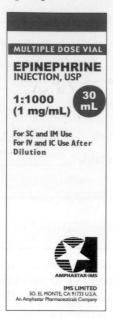

• **What You KNOW**   Prescribed is 1:1000 solution.

• **What You WANT**   A ratio measure.

CRITICAL THINKING

A ratio measure consists of parts of drug in parts of solution.
What are the parts of drug? _____
What are the parts of solution? _____1000_____

ANSWER FOR BEST CARE

A 1:1000 solution contains 1 part drug in 1000 parts solution.

Ratio measure: $\dfrac{1}{1000}$ or 0.001.

PRACTICE PROBLEMS

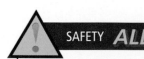

Directions: *In each of the following, which is the strongest solution?*

1. (a) 1:5 (b) 1:50 (c) 1:500

2. (a) 1:1000 (b) 1:500 (c) 1:300

3. (a) 1:10 (b) 1:20 (c) 1:100

4. (a) 1:3 (b) 1:2 (c) 1:5

5. (a) 1:1000 (b) 1:100 (c) 1:10

6. (a) 1:50 (b) 1:10 (c) 1:60

7. (a) 1:250 (b) 1:10,000 (c) 1:100

8. (a) 1:40 (b) 1:3 (c) 1:80

9. (a) 1:1 (b) 1:20 (c) 1:100

10. (a) 1:12 (b) 1:120 (c) 1:6

11. Ms. Smith has a wound that needs to be irrigated with the strongest Dakin's solution that the pharmacy has on hand. The pharmacy states that they have the following three solutions: (a) 1:20, (b) 1:10, and (c) 1:3. Which solution do you obtain from the pharmacy?

12. The doctor prescribes an ophthalmic solution to decrease inflammation of the patient's right eye. He prescribes that you use the weakest solution first. The

SAFETY ***ALERT***

Medications that use ratio strength also include metric measure and are usually prescribed by the number of milliliters.

solutions the pharmacy has on hand are as follows: (a) 1:8, (b) 3:5, and (c) 1:2. Which solution should you use first?

(Answers on p. 448)

PROPORTION

An equation of two ratios is a proportion: 100 mg/mL = 200 mg/2 mL. In a proportion the cross-products are equal. The cross-product is found by multiplying the numerator (top number) of one fraction (ratio) by the denominator (bottom number) of the other fraction (ratio). Consider the following example:

$$\frac{\text{Numerator}}{\text{Denominator}} \quad \frac{100 \text{ mg}}{1 \text{ mL}} \diagdown\diagup \frac{200 \text{ mg}}{2 \text{ mL}}$$

$100 \times 2 = 200 \times 1$, or $200 = 200$.

SOLVING FOR AN UNKNOWN (X) IN THE RATIO-PROPORTION METHOD

The ratio-proportion method can be used when only one ratio (two values) is complete and the second ratio is incomplete (one value known and one value unknown).

Using the fraction notation for ratios is the easiest and safest method when writing your calculations, because it makes the cross-multiplication process easy to visualize. The unknown value is always represented by the letter X.

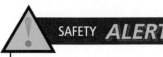

SAFETY *ALERT*

Using fraction notation for the ratios makes cross-multiplication easier.

✓ **Human Error Check**

Replacing the number obtained for X in the original equation and cross-multiplying is an easy way to double-check your calculation.

Example 1

$$\frac{3}{36} = \frac{4}{X}$$

Step 1: Cross-multiply to get the product.

$$\frac{3}{36} \diagdown\diagup \frac{4}{X}$$

$3X = 4 \times 36 \quad 3X = 144$

Step 2: Divide the numerical product by the number in front of X to get the value for X.

$$3\overline{)144}^{\,48} \quad \text{or} \quad \frac{144}{3} = \frac{48}{1}$$

$X = 48$

✓ **Human Error Check**

Replace the number obtained for X in the original equation. Cross-multiply. The cross-products should be equal.

$$\frac{3}{36} \diagdown\diagup \frac{4}{48} \text{ (number obtained for X)}$$

$3 \times 48 = 36 \times 4$
$144 = 144$

Example 2

$$\frac{20}{50} = \frac{X}{75}$$

Step 1: Cross-multiply to get the product.

$50X = 20 \times 75$ $50X = 1500$

Step 2: Divide the numerical product by the number in front of X to get the value for X.

$50\overline{)1500}^{\,30}$ or $\dfrac{1500}{50} = \dfrac{30}{1}$

$X = 30$

> ✔ **Human Error Check**
>
> Replace the number obtained for X in the original equation. Cross-multiply. The cross-products should be equal.
>
> $\dfrac{20}{50} = \dfrac{30}{75}$ (number obtained for X)
>
> $20 \times 75 = 50 \times 30$
> $1500 = 1500$

Example 3

$$\frac{1/4}{3} = \frac{2}{X}$$

Step 1: Cross-multiply to get the products.

$\frac{1}{4}X = 3 \times 2$ $\frac{1}{4}X = 6$

Step 2: Divide the numerical product by the number in front of X to get the value for X.

$6 \div \frac{1}{4}$

Since the divisor is a fraction, multiply by the reciprocal.

$X = 6 \times \frac{4}{1} = 24$

> ✔ **Human Error Check**
>
> Replace X with 24 in the original equation. The cross-products should be equal.
>
> $\dfrac{1/4}{3} = \dfrac{2}{24}$
>
> $\frac{1}{4} \times 24 = 3 \times 2$
>
> $6 = 6$

PRACTICE PROBLEMS

Directions: *Solve the following problems for X.*

1. $\frac{9}{27} = \frac{300}{X}$ _900_

2. $\frac{34}{2} = \frac{X}{3}$ _51_

3. $\frac{1.3}{X} = \frac{0.65}{23}$ _46_

4. $\frac{1000}{2.3} = \frac{1200}{X}$ _2.76_

5. $\frac{1/8}{10} = \frac{2}{X}$ _160_

6. $\frac{75}{1} = \frac{30}{X}$ 0.4

7. $\frac{3000}{2.2} = \frac{1800}{X}$ 1.32

8. $\frac{X}{54} = \frac{9}{81}$ 6

9. $\frac{2}{9} = \frac{1/3}{X}$ 1.5

10. $\frac{125}{5} = \frac{X}{30}$ 750

(Answers on pp. 448–449)

Calculating Medication Doses

In the clinical setting, the medication dose that you HAVE (strength/volume), which is supplied by the pharmacy, is the complete ratio; the dose prescribed is the incomplete ratio because you KNOW the dose strength written in the prescription, but you need to determine what volume of medication you WANT to administer to the patient (X). Since a proportion must have two equal ratios, the units of measure for both dose strength (mg, mcg, g, etc.) and volume in both ratios must be the same.

For example, the prescription is to give 60 mg of a medication by mouth. What you HAVE is 40 mg per tablet. What you WANT is the number of tablets (X) that equal 60 mg:

Complete Ratio   **Incomplete Ratio**
(HAVE)

$$\frac{40 \text{ mg}}{1 \text{ tablet}} = \frac{60 \text{ mg (KNOW)}}{X \text{ tablet (WANT)}}$$

Unit of measure Strength the same   Unit of measure Volume the same

Before setting up a ratio-proportion, the medication you HAVE and the prescription must be compared. First, they must be the same medication (as discussed in Chapter 11), must use the same system of measurement (as discussed in Chapter 4), and must use the same unit of measure (as discussed in Chapter 5).

If the prescribed dose and the dose you HAVE use a different systems of measurement and/or different units of measure than the prescribed dose, the prescribed dose must be converted to match the dose you HAVE before the ratio-proportion can be set up. For example:

The prescription is to give two teaspoons of cough syrup by mouth. What you have is 15 mg/5 mL. You will need to convert teaspoons to the metric system.

The prescription is to give 125 mcg by mouth. What you HAVE is 0.125 mg/tablet. You will need to convert 125 mcg to milligrams (0.125 mg) before proceeding with the calculation.

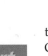

HUMAN ERROR *Alert*

Most prescriptions use the metric system. However, always compare the prescription with the medication you HAVE to avoid medication errors.

✓ Human Error Check

Before performing a calculation, it is important to take a moment and compare the relative value of the prescribed medication and that of the medication you have. Ask the question: Is the dose prescribed larger or smaller than what you have on hand? If the prescribed dose is smaller than the dose you HAVE, the final volume will be less than the volume you HAVE on hand. If the prescribed dose is larger, the final volume will be more than the volume you HAVE on hand. When you complete the calculation, compare your answer with this mental calculation. For example, the prescribed dose of 60 mg is larger than the 40-mg tablet you HAVE on hand. Thus, the calculation answer will require more than one tablet. If your answer is for less than one tablet, you know that a problem exists with the calculation and you should repeat the process.

HUMAN ERROR *Alert*

Be sure the units of measure are in the same position in each ratio of the proportion.

HUMAN ERROR *Alert*

Labeling the problem and the answer with the proper units of measure will enable you to identify errors in setting up the proportion before any calculation error occurs.

To perform a medication dose calculation, you must:

1. Determine if the prescribed medication and what you HAVE are the same medication.
2. Compare system of measurement and the units of measure of the prescribed medication and the medication you HAVE.
3. Compare the relative value of the prescribed medication and the medication you HAVE.
4. Set up a ratio-proportion: the complete ratio on the LEFT is the medication dose strength per volume you HAVE; the RIGHT incomplete ratio contains what you KNOW (prescribed dose) in the numerator, with X (what you WANT) placed in the denominator to represent the unknown volume to be administered.
5. Multiply to get the cross-products.
6. Divide the numerical cross-product by the numerical multiplier of X (the number in front of X).
7. The result is the answer for X.
8. Label the answer properly in units (i.e., number of tablets, number of milliliters).

In the following examples, the prescribed medication and what you HAVE are the same.

> ✓ **Human Error Check**
>
> Check calculation by placing the number obtained for X in the original equation. Cross-multiply. The cross-products should be equal or approximately equal.

Example 1

| **PRESCRIPTION** | *Lorazepam 3 mg IV every 6 hours as needed.* |

- **What You HAVE** — Lorazepam 4 mg/mL.

- **What You KNOW** — Prescribed dose is 3 mg.

- **What You WANT (X)** — The milliliters (dose volume) needed to deliver a 3-mg dose of lorazepam.

CRITICAL THINKING

Do the prescribed dose and the dose you HAVE use the same unit of measure? _____

Is prescribed dose larger or smaller than the dose you HAVE? _____

Will the final volume be more or less than the medication volume you HAVE? _____

In setting up a ratio-proportion, place in the LEFT ratio the medication dose strength per volume you HAVE on hand; in the RIGHT ratio, make what you KNOW the numerator and place X in the denominator.

Multiply to get the cross-products.

Divide the numerical cross-product by the number multiplier of X (the number in front of X).

The result is the answer for X.

Label answer properly in units (i.e., number of tablets, number of milliliters).

Check answer by placing the number obtained for X in the original equation. Cross-multiply. The cross-products should be approximately equal.

ANSWER FOR BEST CARE

Unit of measurement comparison? Yes; milligrams.
Dose larger or smaller? Smaller.
The final volume will be less than 1 mL.

$$\frac{\text{Strength}}{\text{Volume}} \quad \frac{\overset{\text{HAVE}}{4 \text{ mg}}}{1 \text{ mL}} = \frac{3 \text{ mg}}{\text{X mL}} \quad \frac{\text{(KNOW)}}{\text{(WANT)}}$$

Cross-multiply to solve for X.

4X = 3

$$X = 4\overline{)3.00} \atop \begin{array}{r} 0.75 \\ \underline{28} \\ 20 \\ \underline{20} \end{array}$$

Label with the unit of measure.

X = 0.75 mL

> ✔ **Human Error Check**
>
> Replace X with 0.75.
>
> $\dfrac{4}{1} = \dfrac{3}{0.75}$ 4 × 0.75 = 3 × 1   3 = 3
>
> 0.75 mL is less than 1 mL

Example 2

PRESCRIPTION	*Phenytoin sodium 300 mg by mouth at hour of sleep.*
• **What You HAVE**	Phenytoin sodium 125 mg/5 mL.
• **What You KNOW**	Prescribed dose is 300 mg.
• **What You WANT (X)**	The milliliters (dose volume) needed to administer 300 mg of phenytoin.

CRITICAL THINKING

Do the prescribed dose and the dose you HAVE use the same unit of measure? _____

Is prescribed dose larger or smaller than the dose you HAVE? _____

Will the final volume be more or less than the medication volume you HAVE? _____

In setting up a ratio-proportion, place in the LEFT ratio the medication dose strength per volume you HAVE on hand; in the RIGHT ratio, make what you KNOW the numerator and place X in the denominator.

Multiply to get the cross-products.

Divide the numerical cross-product by the number multiplier of X (the number in front of X).

The result is the answer for X.

Label answer properly in units (i.e., number of tablets, number of milliliters).

Check answer by placing the number obtained for X in the original equation. Cross-multiply. The cross-products should be approximately equal.

ANSWER FOR BEST CARE

Unit of measurement comparison? Yes; milliliters.

Dose larger or smaller? Larger.

The final volume will be more than 5 mL (the supplied volume).

HAVE

$\dfrac{125 \text{ mg}}{5 \text{ mL}} = \dfrac{300 \text{ mg}}{X \text{ mL}}$ (KNOW) (WANT)

Cross-multiply to solve for X.

125X = 5 × 300

125X = 1500

$$X = \frac{1500}{25}$$

$$125\overline{)1500}$$
$$\underline{125}$$
$$250$$
$$\underline{250}$$

Label with the unit of measure.

X = 12 mL

> ✔ **Human Error Check**
>
> Replace X with 12.
>
> $\dfrac{125}{5} = \dfrac{300}{12}$ 125 × 12 = 300 × 5   1500 = 1500
>
> 12 mL is larger than 5 mL.

Example 3

PRESCRIPTION	*Captopril 12.5 mg by mouth twice a day.*
• **What You HAVE**	25-mg tablets.

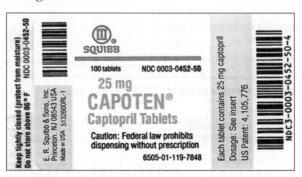

• **What You KNOW**	Prescribed dose is 12.5 mg.
• **What You WANT (X)**	The number of tablets (dose volume) required to administer 12.5 mg of captopril.

CRITICAL THINKING

Do the prescribed dose and the dose you HAVE use the same unit of measure? _____

Is prescribed dose larger or smaller than the dose you HAVE? _____
Will the final volume be more or less than medication volume you HAVE? _____
In setting up a ratio-proportion, place the medication dose strength per volume you
    HAVE on hand in the LEFT ratio; in the RIGHT ratio, make what you KNOW
    the numerator and place X in the denominator.
Multiply to get the cross-products.
Divide the numerical cross-product by the numerical multiplier of X (the number in
    front of X).
The result is the answer for X.
Label the answer properly in units (i.e., number of tablets, number of milliliters).
Check answer by placing the number obtained for X in the original equation. Cross-
    multiply. The cross-products should be approximately equal.

ANSWER FOR BEST CARE

Unit of measurement comparison? Yes; milligrams.
Dose larger or smaller? Smaller.

The final volume will be less than one tablet (the supplied volume).

HAVE

$$\frac{25 \text{ mg}}{1 \text{ tablet}} = \frac{12.5 \text{ mg}}{X \text{ tablet}} \quad \frac{(KNOW)}{(WANT)}$$

Cross-multiply to solve for X.

$$25X = 12.5$$

$$X = \frac{12.5}{25}$$

$$25\overline{)12.5}^{\,0.5}$$
$$125$$

Label with the unit of measure.

X = 0.5 tablet

✓ **Human Error Check**

Replace X with 0.5.

$$\frac{25}{1} = \frac{12.5}{0.5} \quad 25 \times 0.5 = 12.5 \times 1 \quad 12.5 = 12.5$$

0.5 tablet is less than 1 tablet.

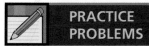 **PRACTICE PROBLEMS**

Directions: *Solve the following problems using the ratio-proportion method. Be sure to label and check your answers.*

1. Prepare a 20-mEq dose of potassium chloride (Kaon) by mouth.
   HAVE: 40 mEq/15 mL.

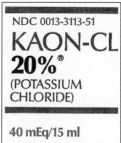

NDC 0013-3113-51

KAON-CL
20%®
(POTASSIUM CHLORIDE)

40 mEq/15 ml

CHERRY
Sugar-Free
Each 15 ml (tablespoonful) supplies 40 mEq each of potassium and chloride (as potassium chloride, 3 g), with saccharin and alcohol 5%.

CAUTION: Federal law prohibits dispensing without prescription.

ONE PINT

《*Adria*》®

$$\frac{40}{15} = \frac{20}{x} \quad 7.5 \text{ ml}$$

How many milliliters will be administered? ___7.5 ml___

2. PRESCRIPTION: The physician has prescribed warfarin sodium (Coumadin) 7.5 mg by mouth now.
   HAVE: The pharmacy sends scored tablets of 2.5 mg.

$$\frac{2.5 \text{ mg}}{1} \quad \frac{7.5 \text{ mg}}{x}$$

COUMADIN® 2½ mg
(Warfarin Sodium Tablets, USP)
Crystalline
DuPont Pharma
Wilmington, Delaware 19880
LOT
EXP

How many tablet(s) will be administered? ___3 tab___

3. PRESCRIPTION: diphenhydramine HCL (Benadryl) 50 mg by mouth at bedtime.
   HAVE: elixir 12.5 mg/5 mL

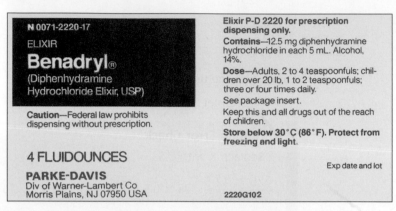

$$\frac{12.5 mg}{5 ml} = \frac{50 mg}{x}$$

How many milliliters will you administer? ___20 ml___

4. Prepare a 150-mg dose of ranitidine hydrochloride (Zantac) syrup by mouth.
   HAVE: 15 mg/1 mL.

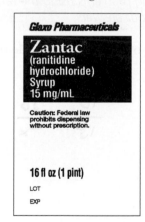

$$\frac{15 mg}{1 ml} = \frac{150 mg}{x}$$

How many milliliters will be administered? ___10 ml___

5. PRESCRIPTION: benztropine mesylate (Cogentin) 2 mg by mouth every day.
   HAVE: 0.5-mg tablets.

NDC 0006-0021-68
100 TABLETS
COGENTIN® 0.5 mg
(BENZTROPINE MESYLATE)
Dist. by:
MERCK & CO., INC.
West Point, PA 19486, USA

$$\frac{0.5 mg}{1} = \frac{2}{x}$$

How many tablet(s) will be administered? ___4 tab___

6. A patient is to receive acetaminophen 650 mg by mouth.
   HAVE: acetaminophen oral solution 500 mg/15 mL.
   How many milliliters will be administered? ___19.5 ml___

   $$\frac{500 mg}{15 ml} = \frac{650 mg}{x}$$

7. PRESCRIPTION: dexamethasone (Decadron) 2 mg by mouth.
   HAVE: 0.25-mg tablets.

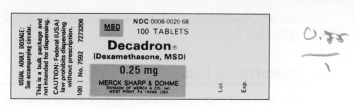

$$\frac{0.25}{1} = \frac{2-g}{1}$$

How many tablet(s) will be administered? ___8 tab___

8. PRESCRIPTION: Levothyroxine sodium tablets 0.2 mg by mouth.
   HAVE: 50-mcg tablets.

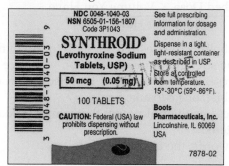

$$\frac{.05\,mg}{1} = \frac{.2-g}{r}$$

Prepare a 0.2-mg dose. ___4 tab___

9. PRESCRIPTION: digoxin 0.25 mg by mouth daily.
   HAVE: 0.125-mg tablets.

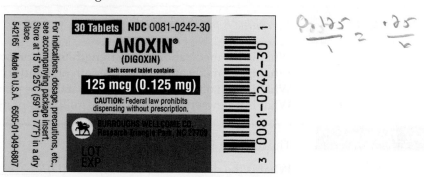

$$\frac{0.125}{1} = \frac{.25}{r}$$

How many tablet(s) will be administered? ___2 tab___

10. Prepare a 2500-unit injection of heparin sodium.
    HAVE: 10,000 units/mL.

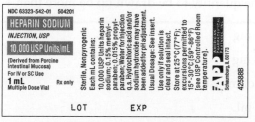

$$\frac{10,000}{1\,ml} = \frac{2500}{r}$$

How many milliliters will be administered? 0.25 ml

(Answers on p. 449)

FORMULA METHOD

The formula method is a variation of the ratio-proportion method. It consists of knowing what it is you desire (the prescription) and what you have on hand (what you received from the pharmacy). From these two known entities, you can accurately calculate the desired dosage to be administered by setting up an equation (Chapter 3).

Calculations Using Similar Units

As in ratio-proportion calculation, the nurse using the formula method solves for an unknown quantity or "X." The variables that the nurse must remember can be written in a mathematical format:

when solving a proportion once, you cross-multiply

$$X = \frac{\text{Prescribed Dose} \times \text{Volume You Have}}{\text{Dose You Have}}$$

"D" symbolizes the **desired** strength (dose) in the prescription (e.g., 1 mg, 1 g).
"H" is the strength of the medication you **have** on hand (e.g., 5 mg, 5 g).
"V" represents the **volume** of the medication on hand, whether solid or liquid (e.g., one tablet, one capsule, 5 mL).
"X" represents the **unknown**: the volume, equal to the dose prescribed, that will be administered.
In other words, the formula is as follows:

$$\frac{\text{Desired (Prescription)}}{\text{Have}} \times \textbf{Volume} = \textbf{X} \text{ (Unknown) or } \frac{D}{H} \times V = X$$

Example 1

PRESCRIPTION	*Morphine 3 mg intravenous push.*

What is the medication dose strength in the prescription (D = desired)? 3 mg.
What is the medication dose strength on hand (H = have)? Morphine 4 mg.
What is the volume of the dose on hand (V = volume)? 1 mL.
What is unknown (X)? How many milliliters of morphine to be administered.

CRITICAL THINKING

The formula is $\frac{D}{H} \times V = X$.

What is the desired dose of morphine (D)? _____
What is the strength of the morphine on hand (H)? _____
Are the units of measure the same? _____
What is the volume of the morphine on hand (V)? _____
Is the dose prescribed larger or smaller than that of the medication on hand? _____
Will the quantity to be drawn up be more than 1 mL or less? _____

ANSWER FOR BEST CARE

D = 3 mg

H = 4 mg

Units of measure same.

V = 1 mL

Quantity less.

$$\frac{3 \text{ mg (D)}}{4 \text{ mg (H)}} \times 1 \text{ mL (V)} = X$$

$$3 \div 4 \times 1 \text{ mL} = X$$

$$0.75 \times 1 \text{ mL} = X$$

$$0.75 \text{ mL} = X$$

0.75 mL is less than 1 mL.

Does your answer fit the general guidelines? Yes; the desired dose is smaller than the dose on hand; therefore, the unknown quantity should be smaller.

Converting Units

In the previous examples, the desired doses and doses on hand were equivalent in units of measure. This may not be the case in all medication orders. The nurse may need to convert the prescribed medication units of measure to the same units of measure on the medication label supplied by the pharmacy before applying the formula method.

Example 2

PRESCRIPTION	*Levothyroxine (Synthroid) 0.125 mg intravenous push.*

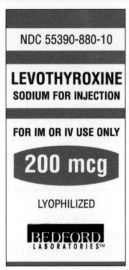

What is the medication dose in the prescription (D = desired)? 0.125 mg.
What is the medication strength on hand (H = have)? 200 mcg.
What is the volume of the dose on hand (V = volume)? 1 mL.
What is unknown (X)? How many mL of levothyroxine to be administered.

CRITICAL THINKING	The formula is $\dfrac{D}{H} \times V = X$.

What is the desired dose of levothyroxine (D)? _____
What is the strength of the levothyroxine on hand (H)? _____
Are the units of measure the same? _____
Convert prescription unit of measure to medication-on-hand unit of measure.
What is the volume of the levothyroxine on hand (V)? _____
Is the dose prescribed larger or smaller than that of the medication on hand? _____
Will the quantity be more or less than 1 mL? _____

ANSWER FOR BEST CARE	D = 0.125 mg

H = 200 mcg

Units of measure are not the same; the prescription is in milligrams, and the medication on hand is in micrograms.

V = 1 mL

Dose smaller.
Quantity less.

Convert milligrams to micrograms by moving the decimal three places to the right (larger to smaller) or multiply by 1000 (1 mg = 1000 mcg; see Chapter 5).

0.125 = 125 mcg   or   0.125 mg × 1000 = 125 mcg

125 mcg is smaller than 200 mcg.

$$\frac{125 \text{ mcg (D)}}{200 \text{ mcg (H)}} \times 1 \text{ mL (V)} = X$$

125 ÷ 200 = 0.625

0.625 × 1 mL = X

0.625 mL = X. Rounded to the nearest hundredth is 0.63 mL.

0.63 mL is less than 1 mL.

Does your answer fit the general guidelines? Yes; the desired dose is smaller than the dose on hand; therefore, the unknown quantity should be smaller.

Example 3

PRESCRIPTION   *Cefuroxime (Zinacef) 1.5 g intravenous.*

What is the medication dose in the prescription (D = desired)? 1.5 g.
What is the medication strength on hand (H = have)? 750 mg.
What is the volume of the dose on hand (V = volume)? 8 mL.
What is unknown (X)? How many milliliters of cefuroxime to be administered.

CRITICAL THINKING

$$\frac{D}{H} \times V = X.$$

What is the desired dose of cefuroxime (D)? _____
What is the strength of the cefuroxime on hand (H)? _____
Are the units of measurement the same? _____
Convert prescription unit of measure to medication-on-hand unit of measure.
What is the volume of the cefuroxime on hand (V)? _____
Is the dose prescribed larger or smaller than that of the medication on hand? _____
Will the quantity be more or less than 8 mL? _____

ANSWER FOR BEST CARE

D = 1.5 g

H = 750 mg

Units of measure are not the same; the prescription is in grams, and the drug on hand is in milligrams.

V = 8 mL

Dose larger.
Quantity more.
Convert grams to milligrams by moving the decimal point three places to the right (larger to smaller) or by multiplying by 1000 (1 g = 1000 mg; see Chapter 5).

1.500 = 1500 mg or 1.5 g × 1000 = 1500 mg

1500 mg is larger than 750 mg.

$$\frac{1500 \text{ mg (D)}}{750 \text{ mg (H)}} \times 8 \text{ mL} = X$$

1500 ÷ 750 = 2

$2 \times 8 \text{ mL} = X$

$16 \text{ mL} = X$

16 mL is larger than 8 mL.

Does your answer fit the general guidelines? Yes; the desired dose is larger than the dose on hand; therefore, the unknown quantity should be larger.

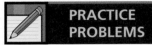

PRACTICE PROBLEMS

Directions: *Solve each problem for the exact unknown mathematical quantity using the formula $\frac{D}{H} \times V = X$.*

1. You will administer furosemide (Lasix) 60 mg intravenous push twice a day. The medication-dispensing system contains vials with furosemide 10 mg/mL.

   > **4 mL** Single-dose   25 Units/**NDC 0074-6102-04**   **EXP**
   > **LOT**
   > **FUROSEMIDE** Injection, USP
   > **40 mg (10 mg/mL)**
   > For I.V. or I.M. use. Protect from light.   ℞ only
   > ABBOTT LABORATORIES, NORTH CHICAGO, IL 60064, USA   **82**

   What is D? _____
   What is H? _____
   What is V? _____
   Is the amount prescribed larger or smaller than the amount on hand? _____
   Will the quantity be more or less than or the same as 1 mL? _____
   The nurse will administer _____ for one dose.

2. You will administer dexamethasone (Decadron) 15 mg intravenous push now. The medication-dispensing system contains vials with dexamethasone 20 mg/mL.
   What is D? _____
   What is H? _____
   What is V? _____
   Is the amount prescribed larger or smaller than the amount on hand? _____
   Will the quantity be more or less than 1 mL? _____
   The nurse prepares a syringe that contains _____.

3. Administer naloxone (Narcan) 0.2 mg intravenous push now. The medication cabinet contains vials with 0.4 mg/mL of naloxone.

   > **1 mL** 10 Single-dose Ampuls   **NDC 0074-1212-01**
   > **NALOXONE HYDROCHLORIDE** Injection, USP
   > **0.4 mg/mL**   **Protect from light.**
   > For I.M., I.V. or S.C. use.   **Keep ampuls in tray until time of use.**
   > Each mL contains naloxone hydrochloride 0.4 mg; sodium chloride added to adjust tonicity. pH adjusted with hydrochloric acid. 0.31 mOsmol/mL (calc.). pH 4.0 (3.0 to 6.5). Usual dosage: See insert. Store at 15° to 30°C (59° to 86°F).   ℞ only
   > ©Abbott 1996, 2002   Printed in USA
   > ABBOTT LABORATORIES, NORTH CHICAGO, IL 60064, USA   58-2852-2/R8-11/01   EXP
   > LOT

   What is D? _____
   What is H? _____
   What is V? _____
   Is the amount prescribed larger or smaller than the amount on hand? _____
   Will the quantity be more or less than or the same as 1 mL? _____
   The nurse administers _____.

4. The physician prescribes morphine 5 mg intravenous push now.

NDC 10019-178-44

Morphine
Sulfate Injection, USP

10 mg/mL   ℞ only
FOR SC, IM OR SLOW IV USE
NOT FOR EPIDURAL OR
INTRATHECAL USE
25 x 1 mL DOSETTE® Vials

Baxter   **ESI LEDERLE™**
Mfd. for an affiliate of **Baxter Healthcare Corporation**
Deerfield, IL 60015 USA
by: Elkins-Sinn, Cherry Hill, NJ 08003   400-830-01

Each mL contains morphine sulfate 10 mg, monobasic sodium phosphate, monohydrate 10 mg, dibasic sodium phosphate, anhydrous 2.8 mg, sodium formaldehyde sulfoxylate 3 mg and phenol 2.5 mg in Water for Injection. pH 2.5-6.5; sulfuric acid added, if needed, for pH adjustment. Sealed under nitrogen.
Usual Dosage: See package insert.
PROTECT FROM LIGHT.
Store at 15°-30°C (59°-86°F).
Avoid freezing.
NOTE: Do not use if color is darker than pale yellow, if it is discolored in any other way or if it contains a precipitate.
DOSETTE® is a registered trademark of A.H. Robins Company.

The medication-dispensing system contains syringes with 10 mg/mL.
What is D? _____
What is H? _____
What is V? _____
Is the amount prescribed larger or smaller than the amount on hand? _____
Will the quantity be more or less than or the same as 1 mL? _____
The nurse will administer _____.

5. The patient is to receive diphenhydramine (Benadryl) 12.5 mg intravenous push prior to a blood transfusion. The patient's medication drawer contains diphenhydramine vials with 25 mg/mL.
What is D? _____
What is H? _____
What is V? _____
Is the amount prescribed larger or smaller than the amount on hand? _____
Will the quantity be more or less than or the same as 1 mL? _____
The patient will receive _____.

6. The nurse is to give filgrastim (Neupogen) 0.63 mg subcutaneous. The pharmacy has sent vials that contain filgrastim 300 mcg/mL.

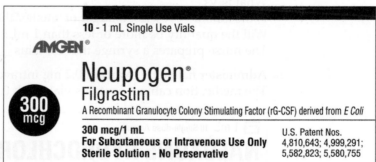

10 - 1 mL Single Use Vials

AMGEN®

Neupogen®
Filgrastim
A Recombinant Granulocyte Colony Stimulating Factor (rG-CSF) derived from *E Coli*

300 mcg/1 mL
For Subcutaneous or Intravenous Use Only
Sterile Solution - No Preservative

U.S. Patent Nos.
4,810,643; 4,999,291;
5,582,823; 5,580,755

Is the amount prescribed larger or smaller than the amount on hand? _____
Will the quantity be more or less than or the same as 1 mL? _____
The nurse prepares a syringe with how many milliliters? _____

7. The nurse is to administer levothyroxine (Synthroid) 0.25 mg intravenous push.
The pharmacy delivers vials containing Synthroid 200 mcg/mL.
Is the amount prescribed larger or smaller than the amount on hand? _____

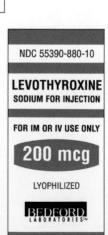

NDC 55390-880-10

LEVOTHYROXINE
SODIUM FOR INJECTION

FOR IM OR IV USE ONLY

200 mcg

LYOPHILIZED

BEDFORD
LABORATORIES™

Will the quantity be more or less than or the same as 1 mL? _____
The nurse prepares a syringe that contains _____.

8. The physician prescribes atropine sulfate (Atropine) 600 mcg intravenous every 6 hours.
The pharmacy dispenses Atropine 400 mcg/mL.

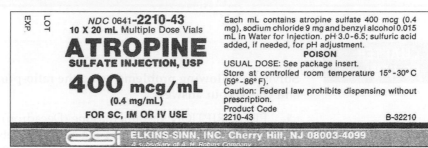

Is the amount prescribed larger or smaller than the amount on hand? _____
Will the quantity be more or less than or the same as 1 mL? _____
The patient receives _____ mL.

9. The nurse practitioner prescribes cefoxitin (Mefoxin) 400 mg intravenous every 6 hours.

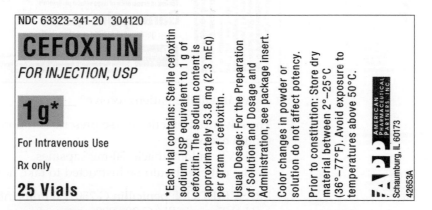

When reconstituted, a vial of cefoxitin contains 1 g/10 mL.
Is the amount prescribed larger or smaller than the amount on hand? _____
Will the quantity be more or less than or the same as 10 mL? _____
One dose contains _____.

10. A patient is to receive a loading dose of levothyroxine (Synthroid) 0.05 mg intravenous push.

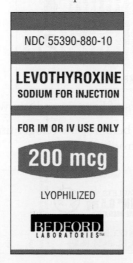

The pharmacy dispenses a vial that contains Synthroid 200 mcg/mL.
Is the amount prescribed larger or smaller than the amount on hand? _____
Will the quantity be more or less than or the same as 1 mL? _____
The nurse prepares a syringe that contains _____.

(Answers on pp. 449–450)

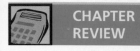

CHAPTER REVIEW

Solve the following problems using the ratio-proportion method. Be sure to label and check your answers.

1.   PRESCRIPTION: dexamethasone (Decadron) 6 mg by mouth every morning.
     HAVE: dexamethasone 4-mg scored tablets.
     How many tablet(s) will be administered? _____

2.   The nurse is to administer gentamicin (Garamycin) 50 mg intramuscular.
     HAVE: gentamicin 80 mg/2 mL vial.

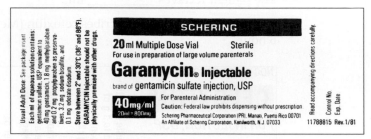

     What will the patient receive? _____

3.   The advanced practice nurse prescribes indomethacin (Indocin) 100 mg by mouth every day.
     HAVE: indomethacin 50-mg capsules.
     The patient should be instructed to take how many capsules? _____

4.   PRESCRIPTION: penicillin G 250,000 units intramuscular.
     HAVE: penicillin G 300,000 units/mL.
     How many milliliters will be administered? _____

5.   Prepare 7000 units heparin sodium injection for subcutaneous administration.
     HAVE: heparin sodium available in 10,000 units/mL.

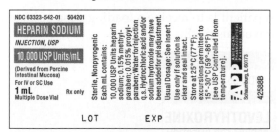

     How many milliliters of heparin sodium will be administered? _____

6.   PRESCRIPTION: 1 mg benztropine (Cogentin) by mouth every day.
     HAVE: 0.5 mg benztropine tablets.

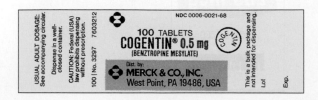

How many tablet(s) will the patient receive per dose? _____

7. Prepare an 80-mg dose of Solu-Cortef.
   HAVE: hydrocortisone sodium succinate (Solu-Cortef) 100 mg/2 mL.

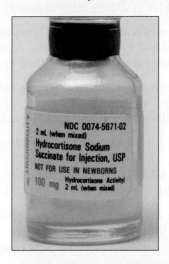

How many milliliters will be administered? _____

8. PRESCRIPTION: venlafaxine hydrochloride (Effexor) 75 mg by mouth daily.
   HAVE: Effexor scored tablets labeled 37.5 mg.
   How many tablet(s) will be administered? _____

9. PRESCRIPTION: chlordiazepoxide (Librium) 0.5 mL intramuscular every 6 hours as needed.
   HAVE: 5 mL ampule containing 100 mg Librium.
   How many milliliters will be administered? _____

10. PRESCRIPTION: phenytoin sodium (Dilantin) suspension 100 mg by mouth three times a day.
    HAVE: dosage strength of 125 mg/5 mL.
    How many milliliters will the patient receive per dose? _____

11. PRESCRIPTION: carvedilol (Coreg) 3.125 mg by mouth twice daily.
    HAVE: carvedilol 6.25 mg per tablet.
    How many tablet(s) will be administered? _____

12. PRESCRIPTION: thioridazine hydrochloride (Mellaril) 75 mg by mouth three times a day.
    HAVE: Mellaril oral solution 30 mg/mL.

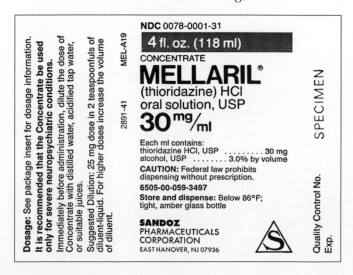

How many milliliters will be administered? _____

13. PRESCRIPTION: verapamil hydrochloride (Isoptin) 120 mg by mouth now.
    HAVE: verapamil hydrochloride (Isoptin) tablets at 80 mg.
    How many tablet(s) will be administered? _____

14. A patient will be receiving filgrastim (Neupogen) 480 mcg subcutaneous injec-
    tion daily for 10 days. The filgrastim vial contains 300 mcg/mL. The patient
    asks what volume of the filgrastim will be given in each injection? _____

15. PRESCRIPTION: diazepam (Valium) 8 mg intramuscularly every 4 hours.
    HAVE: Valium 5 mg/mL.
    How many milliliters will be administered? _____

16. PRESCRIPTION: fexofenadine (Allegra) 120 mg by mouth in two divided
    doses daily.
    HAVE: 30-mg tablets sent by the pharmacy.
    How many tablet(s) per dose will the patient be instructed to take? _____

17. PRESCRIPTION: thiethylperazine (Torecan) 10 mg intramuscularly every 8
    hours as needed for pain.
    HAVE: thiethylperazine 2-mL ampule containing 5 mg/mL.
    What will the patient receive per dose? _____

18. The infectious disease advanced practice nurse prescribes lamivudine (Epivir)
    oral solution 150 mg by mouth twice a day.
    HAVE: lamivudine labeled 5 mg/mL.
    What will the patient receive per dose? _____

19. PRESCRIPTION: valsartan (Diovan) 320 mg by mouth daily.
    HAVE: valsartan 160-mg capsules.
    How many capsule(s) will be administered? _____

20. A patient who receives all food, fluids, and medications via a gastrostomy
    tube is prescribed 100 mg of furosemide (Lasix). The pharmacy provides furo-
    semide (Lasix) oral solution 40 mg/5 mL. What volume will the nurse admin-
    ister? _____

(Answers on p. 450)

⊖volve **For additional practice problems, refer to the Methods of Calculating
Dosages section of the Drug Calculations Companion, version 4 on Evolve.**

Body Weight

Cynthia Chernecky and Denise Macklin

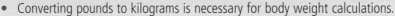

CLINICAL CONNECTION

- Converting pounds to kilograms is necessary for body weight calculations.
- Recognizing the relationship between dose strength and weight is necessary in developing the ratios required to utilize the ratio-proportion method.
- Understanding how to round to the nearest hundredth is necessary for successful calculation.

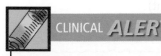

CLINICAL *ALERT*

Conversion calculators exist on-line or by handheld devices.

HUMAN ERROR *Alert*

Be aware that your weight in kilograms is smaller than your equivalent weight in pounds by at least 50%. For example, 100 lb is about 50 kg.

INTRODUCTION

Determining a medication dosage based on body weight is relevant to medical-surgical, oncology, pediatric, and critical care nursing. Unlike common medication prescriptions that are written in dose strength/volume, prescriptions based on body weight are written in dose strength (e.g., milligrams, micrograms, units) per weight in kilograms. When using weight in body weight computations, weight is expressed in kilograms (kg), not pounds (lb). Thus, it may often be necessary to convert pounds to kilograms to successfully complete a body weight calculation. The conversion factor is easiest to use quickly in the clinical setting when it is committed to memory. With practice (combined with memorization of the conversion factor), mastery of this process is assured.

CONVERTING POUNDS TO KILOGRAMS

To convert pounds to kilograms, divide the number of pounds by 2.2 (pounds/2.2). Remember that the divisor must be converted to a whole number by moving the decimal point to the right; the decimal point must be moved the same number of places to the right in the dividend. The decimal point in the quotient is placed directly above the new position of the decimal point in the dividend. In the chemical setting, it is best not to round, but for practice purposes you may round to the nearest tenth. However, in the clinical setting rounding to the tenth is acceptable.

PRACTICE PROBLEMS

Directions: *Convert pounds to kilograms. Round answers to nearest hundredth.*

1. 135 ÷ 2.2 = ___62.36___
2. 247 ÷ 2.2 = ___112.27___
3. 185 ÷ 2.2 = ___84.09___
4. 124 ÷ 2.2 = ___56.36___
5. 146 ÷ 2.2 = ___66.36___
6. 222 ÷ 2.2 = ___100.91___
7. 201 ÷ 2.2 = ___91.36___
8. 175 ÷ 2.2 = ___79.50___

9. $156 \div 2.2 =$ _70.91_

10. $168 \div 2.2 =$ _76.36_

(Answers on p. 451)

CALCULATING BODY WEIGHT

SAFETY *ALERT*

Always double- or triple-check your calculations with other professionals such as nurses, pharmacists, and physicians.

When using the ratio-proportion method to calculate body weight, the ratios are set up with strength (mg or mcg) in the numerator and weight (kg) in the denominator. The complete ratio on the right is written using dose strength per 1 kg, as found in the prescription that you KNOW. What you WANT is the total strength of medication for the patient's weight in kilograms (total weight) that will be administered. Therefore, X is placed in the numerator of the incomplete ratio on the left; the patient's weight you KNOW is placed in the denominator.

$$\underset{\text{KNOW}}{\frac{\text{Dose strength}}{1 \text{ kilogram}}} = \underset{\text{WANT}}{\frac{\text{X (unknown total strength)}}{\text{Patient's weight in kilograms (total weight)}}}$$

Example 1

PRESCRIPTION

Tacrolimus (FK506, Prograf) 0.05 mg/kg/day in 1000 mL D_5W by continuous intravenous infusion daily for prophylaxis of organ transplant rejection. Weight = 246 lb.

- **What You HAVE**   1000 mL D_5W.

- **What You KNOW**   Prescribed dose strength is tacrolimus 0.05 mg/kg/day.
Weight is 246 lb.

- **What You WANT (X)** Total strength of tacrolimus to be added to the intravenous solution.

CRITICAL THINKING

Convert weight to kilograms by dividing pounds by 2.2.
In setting up a ratio-proportion, place in the LEFT ratio the medication dose strength per 1 kg; in the RIGHT ratio, place an X in the numerator and the patient's weight in kilograms in the denominator. So you have $\frac{\text{mg}}{\text{kg}} \times \frac{\text{mg}}{\text{kg}}$.
Cross-multiply to solve for X.
Check answer by placing the number obtained for X in the original equation. Cross-multiply. The cross-products should be equal.
Label the problem and the answer with the proper units of measure.

ANSWER FOR BEST CARE

Convert pounds to kilograms.

$$
\begin{array}{r}
111.81 \quad \text{(round to the nearest hundredth)} \\
22\overline{)2460.00} \\
\underline{22} \\
26 \\
\underline{22} \\
40 \\
\underline{22} \\
180 \\
\underline{176} \\
40
\end{array}
$$

$$\underset{\text{(dose strength)}}{\frac{0.05 \text{ mg}}{1 \text{ kg}}} \times \underset{\overset{\text{WANT}}{\text{X (total mg)}}}{\frac{\text{X (total mg)}}{111.81 \text{ kg (patient's weight)}}}$$

$1X = 0.05 \times 111.81$

$X = 5.59$

✔ **Human Error Check**

Replace X with 5.59 and cross-multiply.

$$\frac{0.05}{1} = \frac{5.59}{111.8}$$

$$5.59 = 5.59$$

Answer: 5.59 mg of Tacrolimus to be added into the 1000 mL D₅W.

Example 2

PRESCRIPTION   *Filgrastim (Neupogen) 5 mcg/kg/day intravenous over 30 minutes daily x 5 days. Weight = 174 lb.*

• **What You HAVE**   50-mL minibag of D₅W with filgrastim.

• **What You KNOW**   Prescribed dose strength is filgrastim (Neupogen) 5 mcg/kg/day.
Weight in pounds is 174 lb.

• **What You WANT (X)**   Weight in kilograms.
Total strength of filgrastim to be added to the intravenous solution.

CRITICAL THINKING

Convert pounds to kilograms by dividing the pounds by 2.2.
In setting up a ratio-proportion, place in the LEFT ratio the medication dose strength per 1 kg; in the RIGHT ratio, place an X in the numerator and the patient's weight in kilograms in the denominator. So you have $\frac{mcg}{kg} \times \frac{mcg}{kg}$.
Cross-multiply to solve for X.
Check answer by placing the number obtained for X in the original equation. Cross-multiply. The cross-products should be equal.
Label the problem and the answer with the proper units of measure.

ANSWER FOR BEST CARE

Convert pounds to kilograms.

```
      79.09
 22)1740
      154
      200
      198
      200
      198
```

HAVE   WANT

(dose strength) $\frac{5\ mcg}{1\ kg} \times \frac{X\ (total\ mcg)}{79.09\ kg\ (patient's\ weight)}$

$1X = 5 \times 79$

$X = 395.45$

✔ **Human Error Check**

Replace X with 395 and cross-multiply.

$$\frac{5}{1} = \frac{395.45}{79.09}$$

$$395.45 = 395.45$$

Answer: 395 mcg/day of filgrastim to be added into the 50 mL D₅W.

Example 3

PRESCRIPTION   *Phenobarbital 20 mg/kg intravenous push over 10 minutes for status epilepticus. Weight = 160 lb.*

- **What You HAVE**   Phenobarbital 130 mg/mL.

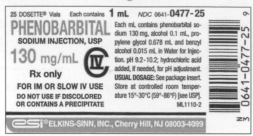

- **What You KNOW**   Prescribed dose strength is phenobarbital 20 mg/kg.
                       Weight is 160 lb.

- **What You WANT (X)**   Weight in kilograms.
                           Total strength of phenobarbital to be administered.

CRITICAL THINKING   Convert pounds to kilograms by dividing the pounds by 2.2.
In setting up a ratio-proportion, place in the LEFT ratio the medication dose strength per 1 kilogram; in the RIGHT ratio, place an X in the numerator and the patient's weight in kilograms in the denominator. So you have $\frac{mg}{kg} \times \frac{mg}{kg}$.
Cross-multiply to solve for X.
Check answer by placing the number obtained for X in the original equation. Cross-multiply. The cross-products should be equal.
Label the problem and the answer with the proper units of measure.

ANSWER FOR BEST CARE   Convert pounds to kilograms.

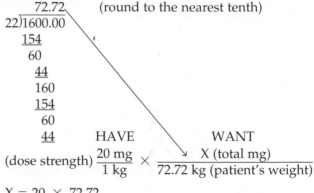

$X = 20 \times 72.72$

$X = 1454.4$

> ✓ **Human Error Check**
>
> Replace X with 1454 and cross-multiply.
>
> $$\frac{20}{1} = \frac{1454}{72.72}$$
>
> $1454.4 = 1454.4$

Answer: Total strength of phenobarbital to be administered is 1454 mg.

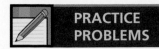

PRACTICE PROBLEMS

Directions: *Determine the total strength of medication for each problem, round your answers to the nearest whole number, and label your answer with the appropriate unit of measure.*

1. PRESCRIPTION: rocuronium bromide (Zemuron) 0.6 mg/kg intravenous push prior to tracheal intubation. Weight = 210 lb.
   Weight in kilograms ___95.5 kg___
   Dose strength ___0.6/kg___
   Total strength ___57 mg___

2. PRESCRIPTION: epoetin alfa recombinant (Epogen) 150 units/kg weekly intravenous over 30 minutes. Weight = 140 lb.
   Weight in kilograms ___63.64 kg___
   Dose strength ___150/kg___
   Total strength ___9546 units___

3. PRESCRIPTION: vancomycin hydrochloride (Vancocin) 15 mg/kg intravenous over 60 minutes. Weight = 220 lb.
   Weight in kilograms ___100 kg___
   Dose strength ___15 mg/kg___
   Total strength ___1500 mg___

4. PRESCRIPTION: metoclopramide (Reglan) 0.8 mg/kg intravenous every 4 hours over 15 minutes × 3 doses. Weight = 132 lb.
   Weight in kilograms ___60 kg___
   Dose strength ___0.8 mg/kg___
   Total strength ___48 mg___

5. PRESCRIPTION: granisetron hydrochloride (Kytril) 10 mcg/kg intravenous over 15 minutes 1 hour prior to chemotherapy.
   Weight = 73 kg.
   Weight in kilograms ___73 kg___
   Dose strength ___10 mcg/kg___
   Total strength ___730 mcg___

6. PRESCRIPTION: diltiazem hydrochloride (Cardizem) intravenous bolus 0.25 mg/kg over 2 minutes STAT. Weight = 82 kg.
   Weight in kilograms ___82 kg___
   Dose strength ___0.25 mg/kg___
   Total strength ___20.5 = 21 mg___

7. PRESCRIPTION: amphotericin B (Fungizone) 0.4 mg/kg/day intravenous × 8 weeks. Weight 140 lb.
   Weight in kilograms ___63.63 kg___
   Dose strength ___0.4 mg/kg___
   Total strength ___25 mg___

8. PRESCRIPTION: trimethoprim and sulfamethoxazole (Septra) 8 mg/kg/day every 6 hours over 60 minutes × 8 doses. Weight = 122 lb.
   Weight in kilograms ___55.45 kg___
   Dose strength ___8 mg/kg___
   Total strength ___443 mg___

9. PRESCRIPTION: netilmicin sulfate (Netromycin) 2.2 mg/kg intravenous piggyback every 8 hours, in 50 mL normal saline over 30 minutes. Give first dose now. Weight = 60 kg.
   Weight in kilograms ___60 kg___
   Dose strength ___2.2 mg/kg___
   Total strength ___132 mg___

10. PRESCRIPTION: hydroxyurea (Hydrea) 15 mg/kg/day.
    Weight = 158 lb.
    Weight in kilograms __71.9__
    Dose strength __15 mg/kg__
    Total strength __1077 mg__

(Answers on p. 451)

CHAPTER REVIEW

Determine the total strength of medication for each problem, round your answers to the nearest tenth, and label your answer with the appropriate unit of measure.

1. PRESCRIPTION: rocuronium bromide (Zemuron) 0.4 mg/kg intravenous push prior to tracheal intubation. Weight = 254 lb. __46.2 mg__

2. PRESCRIPTION: epoetin alfa recombinant (Epogen) 100 units/kg weekly subcutaneous. Weight = 186 lb. __8454 units__

3. PRESCRIPTION: vancomycin hydrochloride (Vancocin) 10 mg/kg intravenous over 60 minutes. Weight = 166 lb. _____

4. PRESCRIPTION: metoclopramide (Reglan) 0.6 mg/kg intravenous every 4 hours over 15 minutes × 3 doses. Weight = 118 lb. _____

5. PRESCRIPTION: granisetron hydrochloride (Kytril) 10 mcg/kg intravenous over 15 minutes 1 hour prior to chemotherapy. Weight = 82 kg. _____

6. PRESCRIPTION: diltiazem hydrochloride (Cardizem) intravenous bolus 0.25 mg/kg over 2 minutes STAT. Weight = 94 kg. _____

7. PRESCRIPTION: amphotericin B (Fungizone) 0.4 mg/kg/day intravenous × 8 weeks. Weight = 206 lb. _____

8. PRESCRIPTION: trimethoprim and sulfamethoxazole (Septra) 4 mg/kg/day every 6 hours over 60 minutes × 8 doses. Weight = 94 lb. _____

9. PRESCRIPTION: netilmicin sulfate (Netromycin) 2.2 mg/kg intravenous piggyback every 8 hours, in 50 mL normal saline over 30 minutes. Give first dose now. Weight = 74 kg. _____

10. PRESCRIPTION: hydroxyurea (Hydrea) 10 mg/kg/day. Weight = 188 lb. _____

11. PRESCRIPTION: rocuronium bromide (Zemuron) 0.6 mg/kg intravenous push prior to tracheal intubation. Weight = 158 lb. _____

12. PRESCRIPTION: epoetin alfa recombinant (Epogen) 150 units/kg subcutaneous. Weight = 124 lb. _____

13. PRESCRIPTION: vancomycin hydrochloride (Vancocin) 15 mg/kg intravenous over 60 minutes. Weight = 170 lb. _____

14. PRESCRIPTION: metoclopramide (Reglan) 0.8 mg/kg intravenous every 4 hours over 15 minutes × 3 doses. Weight = 102 lb. _____

15. PRESCRIPTION: granisetron hydrochloride (Kytril) 5 mcg/kg intravenous over 15 minutes 1 hour prior to chemotherapy. Weight = 73 kg. _____

16. PRESCRIPTION: diltiazem hydrochloride (Cardizem) intravenous bolus 0.25 mg/kg over 2 minutes STAT. Weight = 96 kg. _____

17. PRESCRIPTION: amphotericin B (Fungizone) 0.2 mg/kg/day intravenous × 8 weeks. Weight = 140 lb. _____

18. PRESCRIPTION: trimethoprim and sulfamethoxazole (Septra) 8 mg/kg/day every 6 hours over 60 minutes × 8 doses. Weight = 142 lb. _____

19. PRESCRIPTION: tobramycin (Nebcin) 0.75 mg/kg intravenous piggyback every 8 hours, in 50 mL normal saline over 30 minutes. Give first dose now. Weight = 60 kg. _____

20. PRESCRIPTION: kanamycin (Kantrex) 15 mg/kg/day. Weight = 140 lb. _____

(Answers on pp. 451–452)

ⓔvolve **For additional practice problems, refer to the Pediatric Calculations section of the Drug Calculations Companion, version 4 on Evolve.**

Reading Medication Labels and Using Syringes

Using Syringes

Denise Macklin

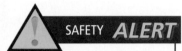

SAFETY ALERT

The unmarked calibration marks between numbered markings are commonly four. But the volume represented by these calibration markings is different depending on the size of the syringe.

INTRODUCTION

Syringes are widely used in clinical practice. Hypodermic syringes come in a variety of sizes, with varying capacity from 0.5 mL to 60 mL. Insulin syringes have either a 0.3-mL, 0.5-mL, or 1-mL capacity. Syringes that are 5 mL or larger are commonly used with intravenous administration. Oral syringes come in 10-mL and 60-mL capacities, have large tips to which you cannot attach a needle, and are used to draw up liquids such as tube feeding and oral medications (Figure 9-1).

SYRINGES

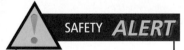

SAFETY ALERT

Understanding the calibration marks on the outside of the barrel is critical to being successful in drawing up the correct amount of medicine.

All syringes have three main parts: barrel, plunger, and tip. The barrel is the hollow tube that holds the medication. It comes in a variety of lengths and diameters. On the outside of the barrel are black calibration markings that identify a specific solution volume. Calibrations use the metric system (Figure 9-2). The first marking on the calibration nearest the tip is a zero followed by four short interim markings and then a longer, numbered marking; this arrangement (four short interim markings and one longer, numbered marking) continues for the length of the barrel.

Syringes of 1 mL and 0.5 mL are calibrated in hundredths (Figure 9-3).

Calibration markings in tenths include those for syringes of 2 mL, 2.5 mL, and 3 mL (Figure 9-4).

Larger syringes such as 5 mL, 6 mL, and 10 mL are calibrated in two-tenth increments (Figure 9-5).

Syringes 20 mL and larger are calibrated in 1-mL increments (Figure 9-6).

The plunger is the mechanism that withdraws medication from the medication container and then is pushed by your thumb to administer the medication. The inner tip of the plunger looks like a dome with a tip followed below by an upper ring that touches the barrel, followed by a lower ring that is attached to the plunger and seals the barrel to prevent leaking. The upper ring (nearest the dome) is used to measure the correct volume (Figure 9-7).

Finally, there is the tip. Some syringes come with straight slip tips (Figure 9-8, A); however, the safest tip is the Luer-Lok tip, which allows needles to be twisted on and locked in place (Figure 9-8, B). Oral syringe tips are large (Figure 9-9). A needle cannot be attached to an oral syringe tip.

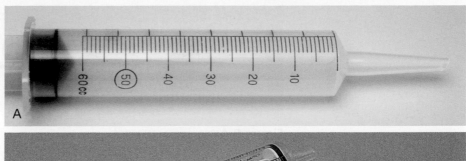

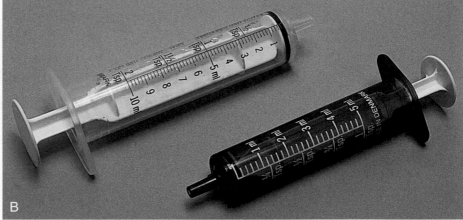

Figure 9-1 A, 60-mL oral syringe. **B,** 5-mL and 10-mL oral syringes. (**B** from Clayton BD, Stock YN, Harroun, RD: Basic pharmacology for nurses, ed 14, St Louis, 2007, Mosby.)

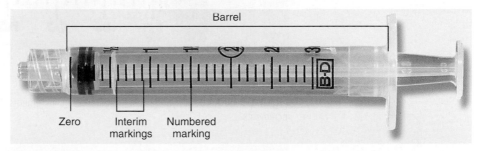

Figure 9-2 Barrel of the syringe with calibration markings. (Used with permission from Becton, Dickinson, and Company.)

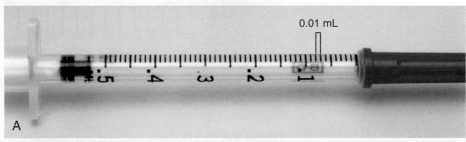

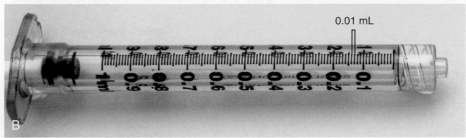

Figure 9-3 A, 0.5-mL syringe calibrated in 0.01-mL increments. **B,** 1-mL syringe calibrated in 0.01-mL increments.

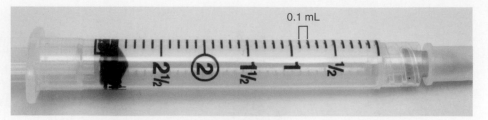

Figure 9-4 3-mL syringe calibrated in 0.1-mL increments.

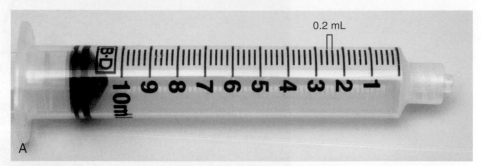

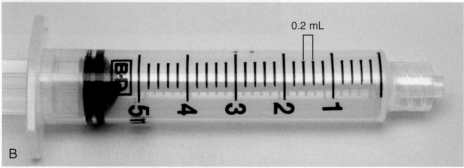

Figure 9-5 A, 10-mL syringe calibrated in 0.2-mL increments. **B,** 5-mL syringe calibrated in 0.2-mL increments.

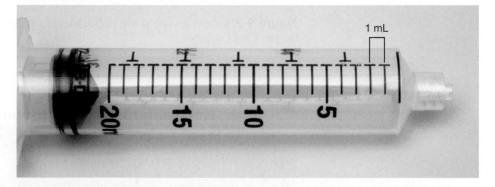

Figure 9-6 20-mL syringe calibrated in 1-mL increments.

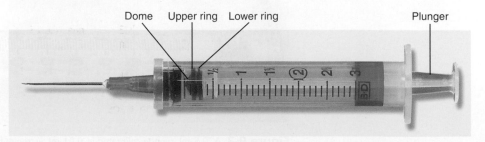

Figure 9-7 Parts of the plunger.

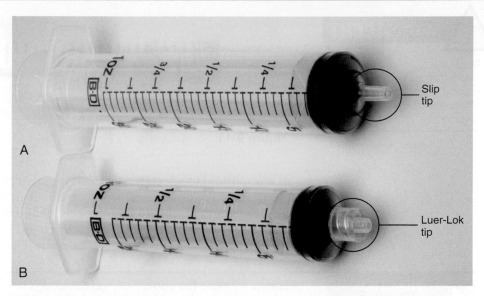

Figure 9-8 A, Slip tip. **B,** Luer-Lok tip.

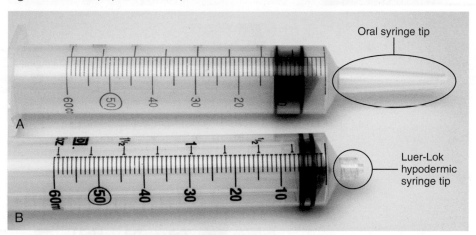

Figure 9-9 A, Oral syringe tip. **B,** Luer-Lok hypodermic syringe tip.

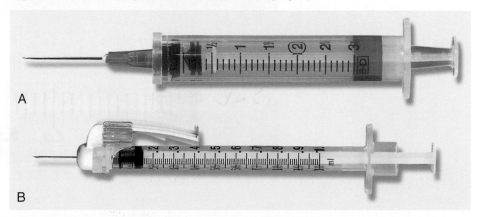

Figure 9-10 A, BD Safety-Lok™ 3-mL syringe. **B,** BD SafetyGlide™ tuberculin syringe. (Used with permission from Becton, Dickinson, and Company.)

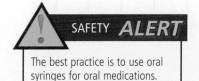

SAFETY **ALERT**

The best practice is to use oral syringes for oral medications.

Safety systems that protect the needle after medication is drawn up and after patient usage are required with syringes (Figure 9-10).

Some syringes come with a needle attached and some allow the needle to be added. Needles vary in size, gauge (circumference), inner diameter, and length. Needle selection is dependent on patient size, route of administration (intramuscular, intradermal, or subcutaneous), and the viscosity (thickness) of the solution being administered.

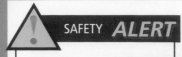

SAFETY **ALERT**

Needle protection guidelines require that needles are never recapped and always disposed of in needle-stick prevention containers.

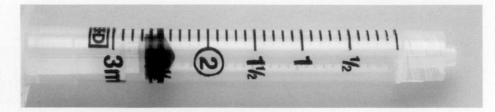

Figure 9-11 2.5 mL drawn up in a 3-mL syringe.

It is important to select the size of syringe that best allows for accurate calibration of medication. For example, drawing up 2.5 mL in a 5-mL syringe would be very difficult. You would be able to find the 2-mL marking, but since the increments are in two-tenths, finding the exact 0.5 marking would be difficult. A better choice would be a 3-mL syringe with one-tenth calibrations (Figure 9-11).

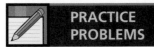

PRACTICE PROBLEMS

Directions: *Choose the correct syringe size based on the prescription and place the correct letter in the space.*

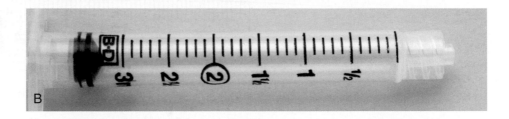

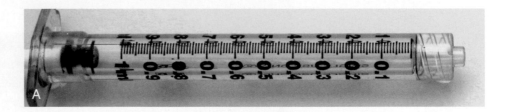

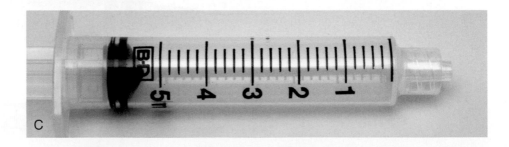

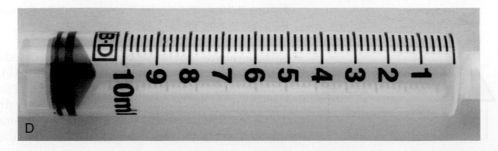

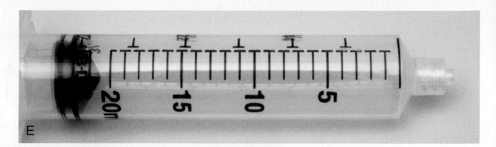

E

1. 1.3 mL ___B___
2. 0.52 mL ___A___
3. 8.5 mL ___D___
4. 0.25 mL ___A___
5. 2.8 mL ___C___
6. 7.6 mL ___D___
7. 16 mL ___E___
8. 4.5 mL ___C___
9. 0.8 mL ___A___
10. 18 mL ___E___
11. 1.5 mL ___B___

Directions: *Read the following syringes and write the amount in milliliters.*

12. ___12 mL___

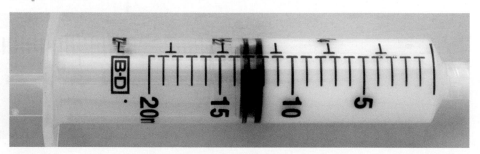

13. ___.3 mL___

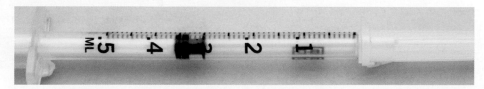

14. ___.25 mL___

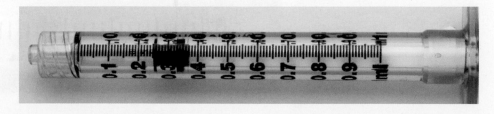

15. _16 ml_

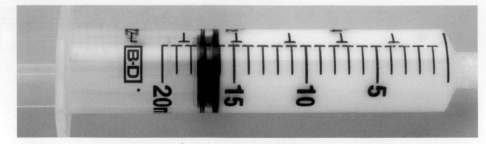

16. _2.7 ml_

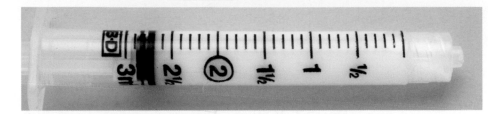

17. _2.3 ml_

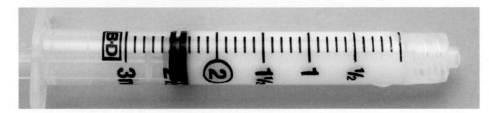

18. _8 ml_

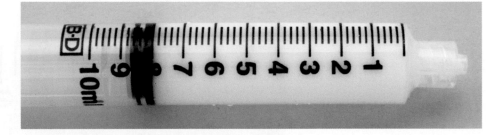

19. _3 ml_

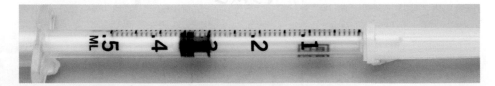

20. _1.2 ml_

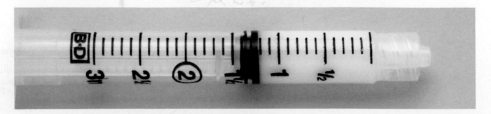

21. _1.6 mL_

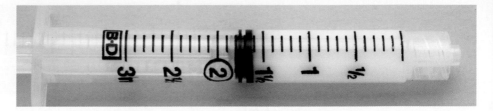

Directions: _Draw a line through the syringe where you would pull the plunger back for the prescribed volume._

22. 1.3 mL

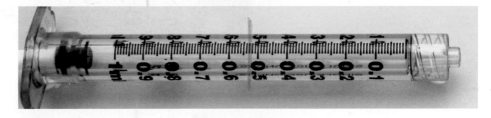

23. 0.53 mL

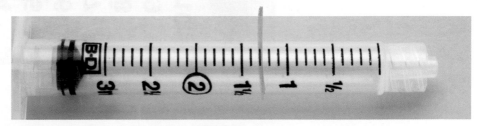

24. 8 mL

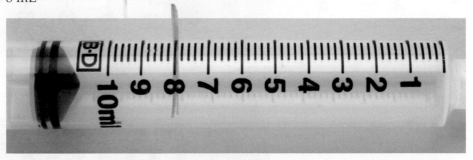

25. 0.25 mL

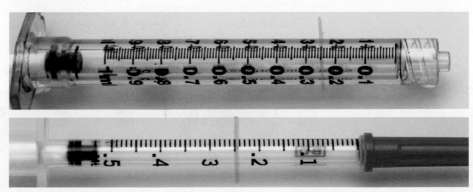

26. 2.8 mL

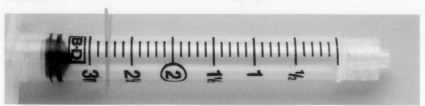

27. 7.6 mL

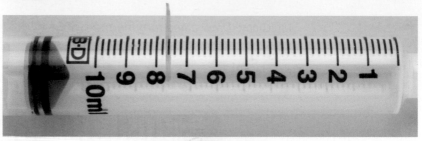

28. 16 mL

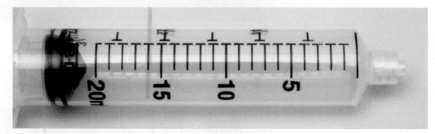

29. 4.4 mL

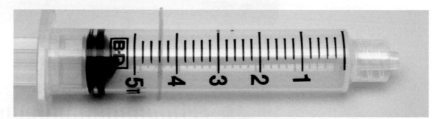

30. 0.87 mL

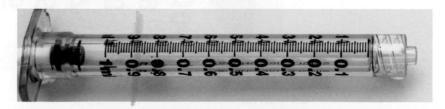

31. 18 mL

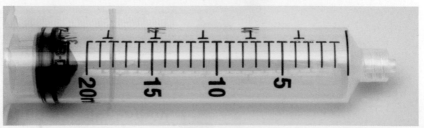

(Answers on p. 452)

PREFILLED SYRINGES

Prefilled syringes are single-dose syringes that come filled with sterile drug and are designed to be used only once. Some prefilled syringes come complete, including total dose prescribed, and either with a needle already attached or one that can be attached (Figure 9-12). In certain syringes the medication container is the plunger (Figure 9-13), whereas others use a cartridge system and require a plunger extension system be used to activate the syringe (Figure 9-14).

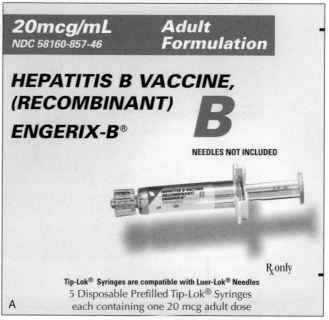

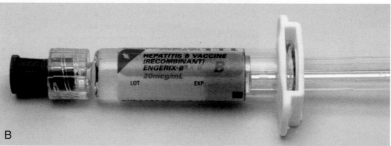

Figure 9-12 Complete prefilled syringes.

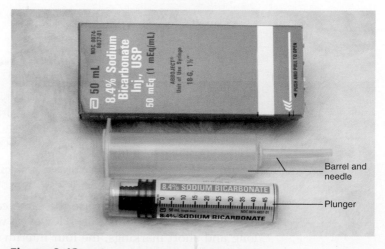

Figure 9-13 Medication container is a plunger.

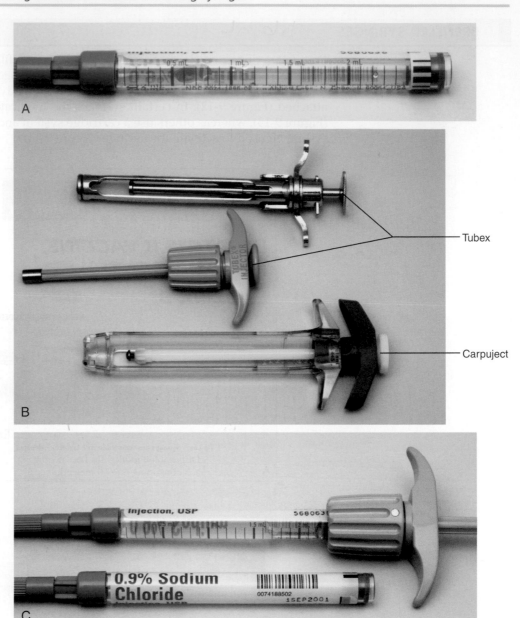

Figure 9-14 **A,** Cartridge system. **B,** Tubex and Carpuject systems. **C,** Cartridge and Tubex system assembled.

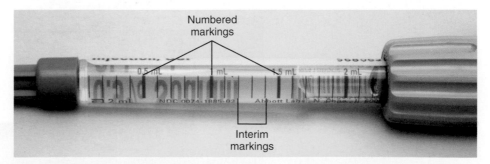

Figure 9-15 Prefilled syringe with calibration markings.

Many prefilled syringes use the same calibration marking system as found on their hypodermic counterpart. However, with some prefilled syringes, instead of long and short markings, the four interim markings are thin bands followed by a fifth bold wider numbered marking (Figure 9-15).

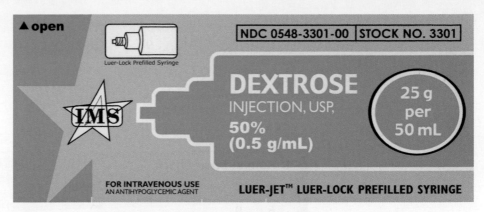

Figure 9-16 Single-dose prefilled syringe.

With some prefilled syringes, the entire dose of medication is to be administered as a single dose (Figure 9-16).

When the entire syringe volume is not required, you will need to discard (waste) in the sink (in the presence of another nurse when the drug is a narcotic) the amount of drug that is in excess of the amount prescribed prior to medication administration. This enables you to safely administer the prescribed amount.

Example 1

PRESCRIPTION	*Benzathine penicillin G (Bicillin) 900,000 units intramuscular STAT.*

- **What You HAVE** — Prefilled syringe.
Total dose strength is 1,200,000 units.
Total dose volume is 2 mL Bicillin.

- **What You KNOW** — Prescribed dose strength is 900,000 units.

- **What You WANT (X)** — Dose volume to be administered.
Appropriate plunger system for administration.

CRITICAL THINKING

Is the prescribed dose larger or smaller than the available dose? _____
Will the final volume be more or less than 2 mL? _____
Will you need more than one syringe or will you need to discard excess? _____
In setting up a ratio-proportion, place in the LEFT ratio the medication dose strength per volume you HAVE on hand; in the RIGHT ratio, place what is prescribed in the numerator and place X in the denominator.
Cross-multiply to solve for X.
Divide by the number in front of X to get the value for X.
Label the problem and the answer with the proper units of measure.
Check answer by placing the number obtained for X in the original equation. Cross-multiply. The cross-products should be equal.
Determine discard by subtracting prescribed volume from total volume.

ANSWER FOR BEST CARE

Prescribed dose? Smaller.
Final dose? It will be less.
Discard? Necessary.
Perform calculation.

$$\frac{\text{HAVE}}{}$$
$$\frac{1,200,000 \text{ units}}{2 \text{ mL}} = \frac{900,000 \text{ units (prescribed)}}{X}$$

Reduce.

$$\frac{6}{1 \text{ mL}} = \frac{9}{X} \quad 6X = 9 \quad X = \frac{9}{6}$$

$$6\overline{)9}^{\,1.5}$$

$$X = 1.5 \text{ mL}$$

✓ **Human Error Check**

Replace X with 1.5 and cross-multiply.

$$\frac{6}{1} = \frac{9}{1.5}$$

$$9 = 9$$

Determine discard.

2.0 mL	(total volume)
− 1.5 mL	(prescribed volume)
0.5 mL	(discard)

Example 2

PRESCRIPTION	*Morphine sulfate 3 mg intravenous push every 4 hours for pain.*

- **What You HAVE**

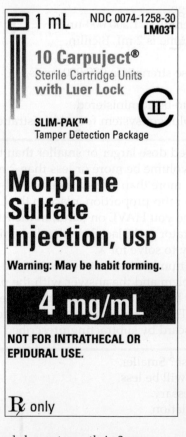

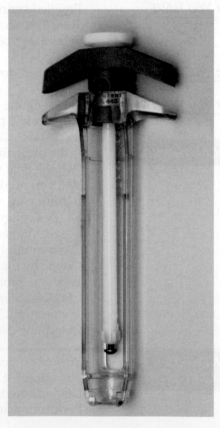

- **What You KNOW**   Prescribed dose strength is 3 mg.

- **What You WANT (X)**   Dose volume to be administered.

CRITICAL THINKING	Are the prescribed medication and the supplied medication the same drug? _____
	What is the medication dose strength/volume you HAVE? _____
	Is the prescribed dose larger or smaller than the available dose? _____
	Will you need more than one syringe or will you need to discard excess? _____
	In setting up a ratio-proportion, place in the LEFT ratio the medication dose strength per volume you HAVE on hand; in the RIGHT ratio, place what is prescribed in the numerator and place X in the denominator.
	Cross-multiply to solve for X.
	Divide by the number in front of X to get the value for X.
	Label the problem and the answer with the proper units of measure.
	Check answer by placing the number obtained for X in the original equation. Cross-multiply. The cross-products should be equal.
	Determine discard by subtracting prescribed volume from total volume.

ANSWER FOR BEST CARE	Prescribed medication and supplied medication? Same.
	Medication dose strength per volume? 4 mg/mL.
	Prescribed dose? Smaller.
	Discard? Necessary.
	Perform calculation

$$\frac{4 \text{ mg}}{1 \text{ mL}} = \frac{3 \text{ mg}}{X \text{ mL}} =$$

$$4X = 3 \quad X = \frac{3}{4}$$

$$\begin{array}{r} 0.75 \\ 4\overline{)3.0} \end{array}$$

$$X = 0.75 \text{ mL}$$

> ✔ **Human Error Check**
>
> Replace X with 0.75 and cross-multiply.
>
> $$\frac{4}{1} = \frac{3}{0.75}$$
>
> $$3 = 3$$

Determine discard.

$$\begin{array}{r} 0910 \\ \cancel{1}.\cancel{0}0 \text{ mL (total volume)} \\ -0.75 \text{ mL (prescribed volume)} \\ \hline 0.25 \text{ mL (discard)} \end{array}$$

When the prescription identifies the volume to be administered, the calculation consists of subtracting the prescribed volume from the supplied volume.

Example 3

PRESCRIPTION	*Flush central line with 6 mL 0.9% saline after each usage.*

• **What You HAVE**

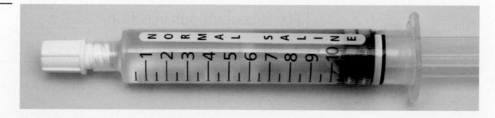

- **What You KNOW**

Prescribed dose volume is 6 mL.

- **What You WANT (X)**

Syringe volume to be discarded.
Appropriate plunger system for administration.

CRITICAL THINKING

Are the prescribed medication and the supplied medication the same drug? _____
What is the total volume? _____
Is the prescribed dose larger or smaller than the available dose? _____
Determine discard by subtracting prescribed volume from total volume.

ANSWER FOR BEST CARE

Prescribed medication and supplied medication? Same.
Total volume? 10 mL.
Prescribed dose? Smaller.
Perform calculation.

$$\begin{array}{r} 10 \text{ mL (total volume)} \\ - \quad 6 \text{ mL (prescribed volume)} \\ \hline 4 \text{ mL (discard)} \end{array}$$

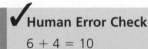

✓ Human Error Check

6 + 4 = 10

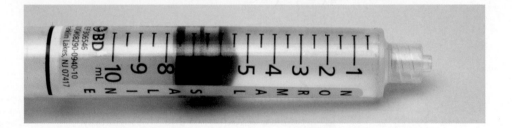

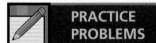 **PRACTICE PROBLEMS**

Directions: *Fill in the blanks.*

1. PRESCRIPTION: dalteparin sodium (Fragmin) 2500 units 2 hours before surgery.

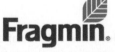

10 x 0.2 mL single dose syringes, preassembled with needle guards
NDC 0013-2426-91

Fragmin®

dalteparin sodium injection

5000 IU (anti-Xa) per 0.2 mL

For subcutaneous injection

How many milliliters will be administered? _____
Will there be a discard? _____
If so, what amount will it be? _____

2. PRESCRIPTION: filgrastim (Neupogen) injection 5 mcg/kg subcutaneous daily for 2 weeks. Patient weighs 60 kg. What you have is filgrastim (Neupogen) injection 300 mcg/0.5 mL prefilled syringe.
How many milliliters will be administered? _____
Will there be a discard? _____
If so, what amount will it be? _____

3. PRESCRIPTION: interferon beta-1B (Rebif) 25 mcg subcutaneous every other day.
What you HAVE is interferon beta-1B (Rebif) 44 mcg/0.5 mL prefilled syringes.
How many milliliters will be administered? _____
Will there be a discard? _____
If so, what amount will it be? _____

4. PRESCRIPTION: Humira (adalimumab) 0.04 g subcutaneous weekly.
What you HAVE is adalimumab 40 mg/0.8 mL syringe.
How many milliliters will be administered? _____
Will there be a discard? _____
If so, what amount will it be? _____

5. PRESCRIPTION: 2,400,000 units penicillin G procaine using multiple sites now.
What you HAVE is penicillin G procaine 600,000 units/mL Tubex®.
How many milliliters will be administered? _____
Will there be a discard? _____
If so, what amount will it be? _____

6. PRESCRIPTION: meperidine (Demerol) 25 mg intravenous push now.
What you HAVE is meperidine 50 mg/mL prefilled syringe.
How many milliliters will be administered? _____
Will there be a discard? _____
If so, what amount will it be? _____

7. PRESCRIPTION: morphine sulfate 3 mg intravenous now.

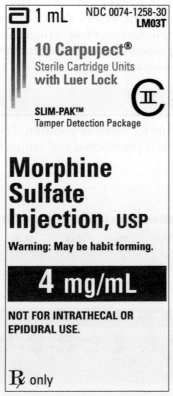

1 mL   NDC 0074-1258-30
                    LM03T

10 Carpuject®
Sterile Cartridge Units
with Luer Lock

SLIM-PAK™
Tamper Detection Package

Morphine Sulfate Injection, USP

Warning: May be habit forming.

4 mg/mL

NOT FOR INTRATHECAL OR EPIDURAL USE.

℞ only

How many milliliters will be administered? _____
Will there be a discard? _____
If so, what amount will it be? _____

8. PRESCRIPTION: phenobarbital 4 mg/kg intramuscular per day for 7 days to achieve a blood level of 10 mcg/mL. Child weighs 9 kg. What you have is phenobarbital 30 mg/1 mL barrel for use with Tubex system.
   How many milliliters will be administered? _____
   Will there be a discard? _____
   If so, what amount will it be? _____

9. PRESCRIPTION: 2.5 mg hydromorphone (Dilaudid) intravenous push every 4 hours for pain.
   What you HAVE is hydromorphone 4 mg/1 mL barrel for use with Tubex system.
   How many milliliters will be administered? _____
   Will there be a discard? _____
   If so, what amount will it be? _____

10. PRESCRIPTION: Copaxone (glatiramer acetate) 20,000 mcg intramuscular daily.
    What you HAVE is Copaxone 20 mg/mL syringe.
    How many milliliters will be administered? _____
    Will there be a discard? _____
    If so, what amount will it be? _____

(Answers on p. 453)

ABOUT 0.5-ML AND 1-ML SYRINGES

When small volumes of 1 mL or less are required—as with heparin, skin testing, and pediatric prescriptions—a low-volume syringe offers the greatest accuracy. This type of syringe comes in sizes of 1 mL or 0.5 mL. The 1-mL syringe is the most common, but for doses of 0.5 mL or less, the 0.5-mL syringe offers the greatest accuracy (Figure 9-17, A). The plunger on these syringes can be maneuvered very slowly and smoothly for greater ease in accurate measurement. Increments are in hundredths, with long hash marks equal to tenths.

INSULIN SYRINGES

Insulin syringes are only for measuring insulin. They are not to be used with any other medication. The needle is preattached and cannot be removed. This type of syringe is

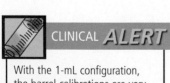

CLINICAL ALERT

With the 1-mL configuration, the barrel calibrations are very small and close together. When drawing up medication in a 1-mL syringe, careful visualization of dosage is critical to ensure accuracy. When the 0.5-mL syringe is available, use when appropriate.

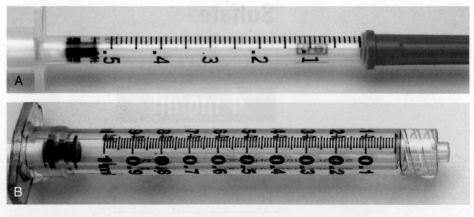

Figure 9-17 **A,** 0.5-mL syringe. **B,** 1-mL syringe.

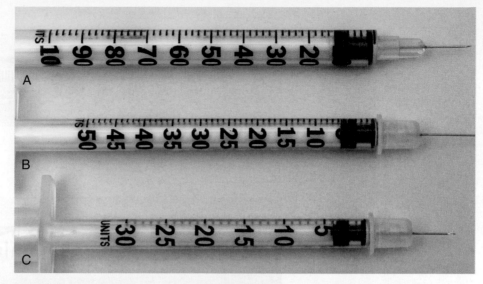

Figure 9-18 Insulin syringes. **A,** 1 mL (100 units). **B,** 0.5 mL (50 units). **C,** 0.3 mL (30 units).

calibrated in units. Insulin is standardized to 100 units per milliliter. A 1-mL syringe is calibrated for 100 units and each increment equals 2 units with numbered markings every 10 units. Low-dose insulin syringes of 0.5 mL (50 units) and 0.3 mL (30 units) are calibrated in 1-unit increments and are numbered every 5 units (Figure 9-18).

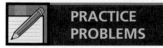 **PRACTICE PROBLEMS**

Directions: *Read the following syringes and write the amount in the blank in milliliters.*

1. _____

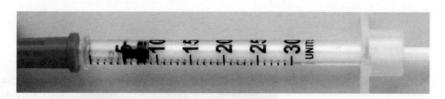

2. _____

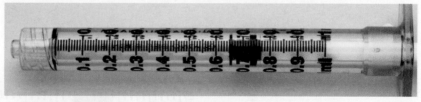

3. _____

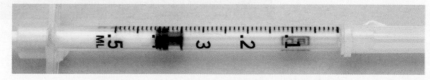

4. _____

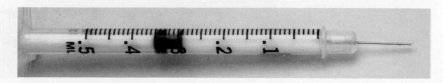

5. _____

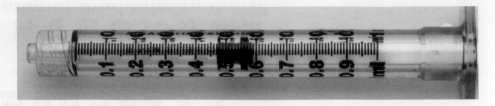

6. _____

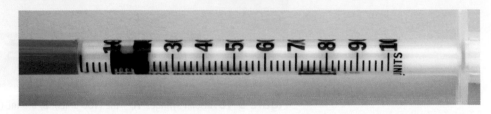

7. _____

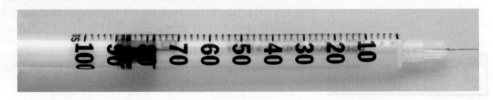

8. _____

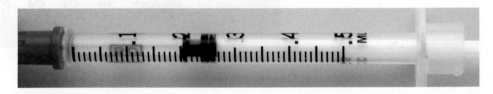

9. _____

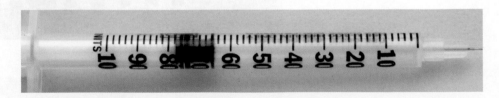

10. _____

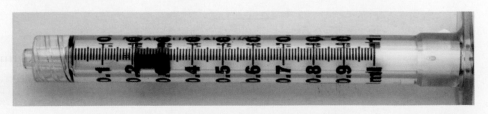

Directions: *Mark the following syringes with the correct amount.*

11. 0.8 mL

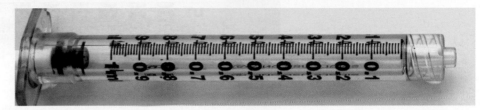

12. 8 units

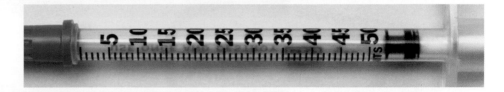

13. 0.74 mL

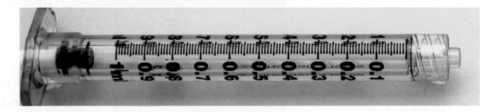

14. 58 units

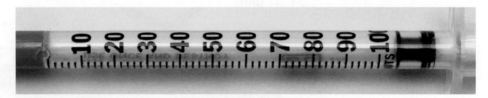

15. 0.25 mL

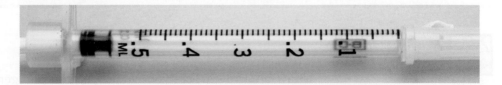

16. 0.25 mL

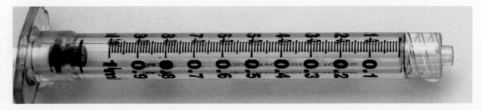

17. 10 units

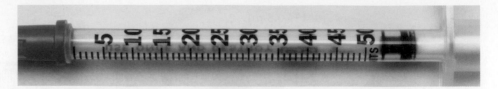

18. 0.38 mL

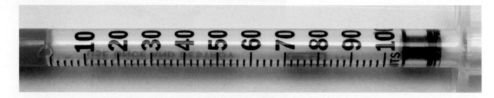

19. 10 units

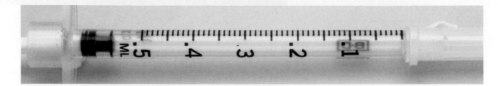

20. 0.47 mL

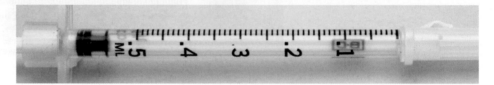

21. 47 units

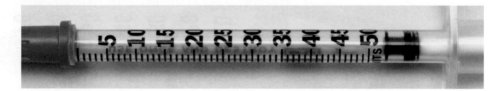

(Answers on pp. 453–454)

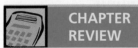

CHAPTER REVIEW

Draw an arrow where you would pull the plunger back to in order to obtain the correct volume.

1. 2.3 mL

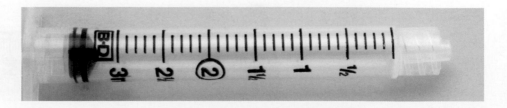

2. 1.5 mL

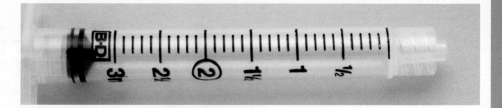

3. 15 mL

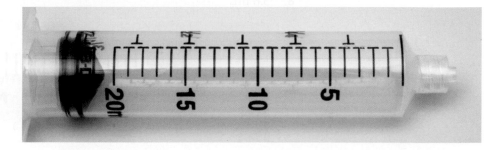

4. 7.2 mL

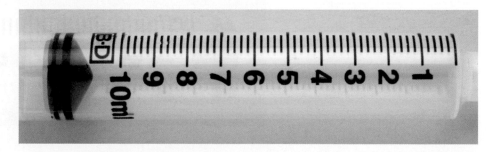

5. 2.8 mL

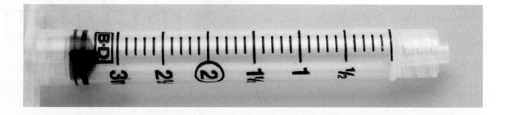

6. 4.4 mL

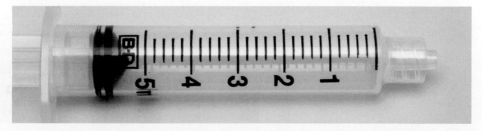

7. 12 mL

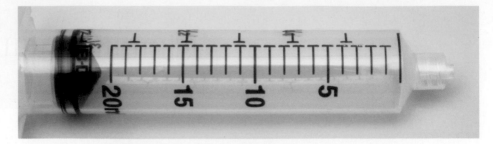

8. 3.6 mL

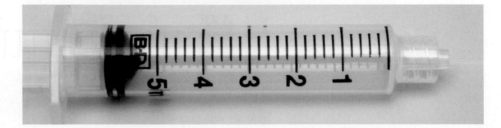

9. 10 mL

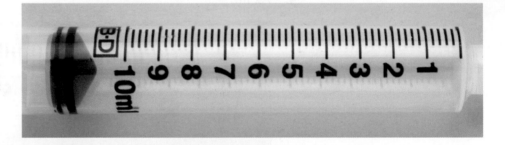

10. 18 mL

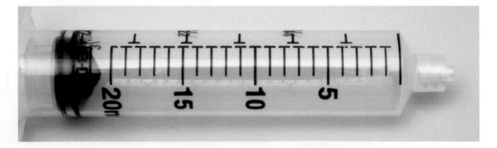

Read the following 1-mL, 0.5-mL, and insulin syringes and enter the volume amount in the blank space provided.

11.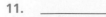

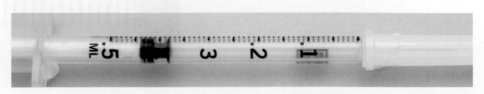

CHAPTER 9

12. _____

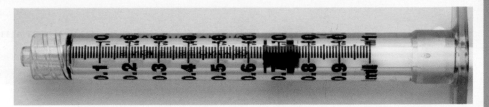

13. _____

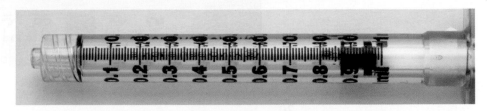

14. _____

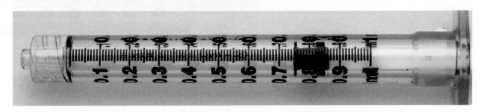

15. _____

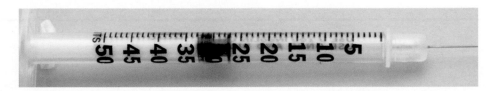

16. _____

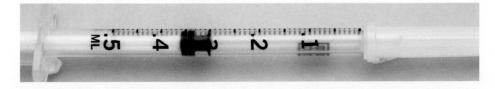

17. _____

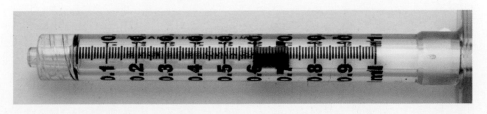

18. _____

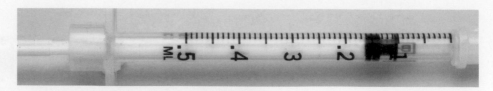

19. _____

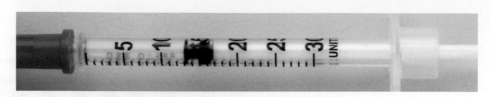

20. _____

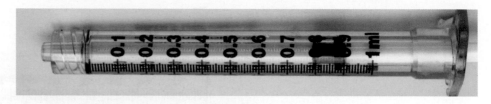

(Answers on p. 454)

evolve   **For additional practice problems, refer to the Safety in Medication Administration section of the Drug Calculations Companion, version 4 on Evolve.**

Oral Medications

Denise Macklin

CLINICAL CONNECTION

- To complete medication calculations, you must be able to read the drug label to locate necessary computation information for clinical implementation.
- The drug label must be compared to the prescription correctly to determine whether a calculation is necessary prior to preparing the medication for each patient.

INTRODUCTION

Oral medications are the most common type of prescription. Oral medications come prepared as solids (tablets, scored tablets, chewable sublingual tablets, enteric-coated tablets [dissolved in the intestine], timed-release tablets, capsules, timed-release capsules, gelatin capsules, powders) and as liquids (Figure 10-1).

Oral medications come in different dose strengths. Scored tablets can be divided, but nonscored tablets, enteric-coated tablets, extended- or delayed-release tablets, and capsules cannot be divided and must be given whole. In the clinical setting you will most commonly see unit dose labels.

MEDICATION LABELS

SAFETY ALERT

Altering oral medications that must be given whole may result in an alteration of the drug's action (increase absorption speed, alter the absorption rate, cause the drug to be inactivated) and cause unintended outcomes. Always consult a drug reference book or your pharmacist if you are uncertain.

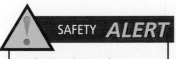

SAFETY ALERT

Medications have only one generic name but may have more than one trade name.

Starting at the top of the label, the first line (usually in large bold print) is the trade (brand) name of the drug, which is the registered name given by the manufacturer. The prescription may use this name (Figure 10-2).

Under (or near) the trade name is the generic name of the drug. By law the generic name must be on a drug label. There are some medications whose generic name is so common that it is the only name appearing on the label. One example is phenobarbital. Generic medications only have the generic name on the label.

Moving down the label, next is the dose strength of the medication (see Figure 10-2). This refers to the amount of drug that is available in the detailed unit of measure listed. This is the dose that you will compare with the prescription to determine whether you need to perform a calculation before administration.

Some labels will list the medication strength using different but comparable units of measure (see Figure 10-2). The label identifies the composition of the drug. Examples are tablet, capsule, liquid suspensions, or solution (Figure 10-3).

The route of administration is identified on labels. With tablets and capsules, the route of administration is assumed to be oral; however, because all tablets, capsules, and liquids are not always given orally, any variation from oral administration is listed on the label (Figure 10-4).

If the drug requires reconstitution, the instructions will be outlined on the label (see Chapter 13) (Figure 10-5).

Sometimes a drug requires special handling, such as protection from light or specific storage requirements. These directions will appear on the drug label (Figure 10-7).

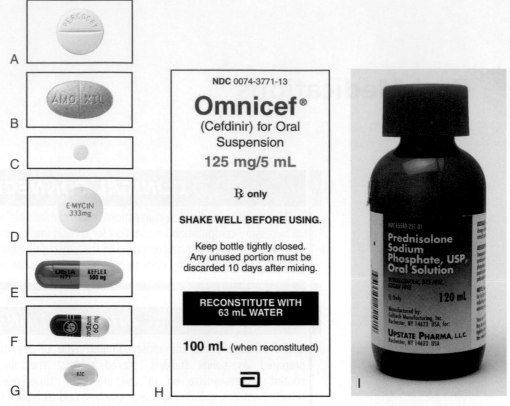

Figure 10-1 Types of oral medications. **A,** Scored tablet. **B,** Chewable tablet. **C,** Sublingual. **D,** Timed-release tablet. **E,** Capsule. **F,** Timed-release capsule. **G,** Gelatin capsule. **H,** Powder. **I,** Solution. (**A** through **G** from Mosby's drug consult 2007, St Louis, 2007, Mosby.)

HUMAN ERROR *Alert*

If a prescription uses the trade name and a generic drug is dispensed without a trade name on the label it is safest to confirm the drug with the pharmacist or the *Physicians' Desk Reference* (PDR) or other drug reference prior to administration.

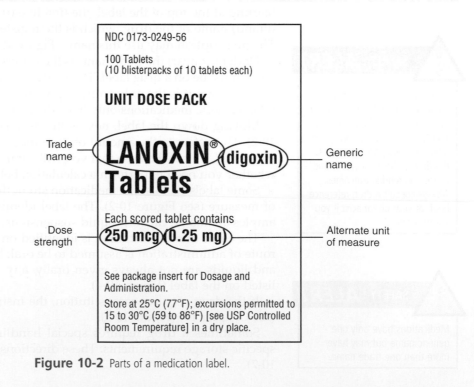

Figure 10-2 Parts of a medication label.

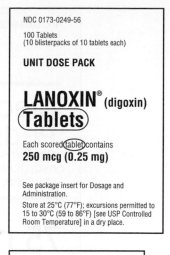

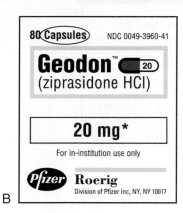

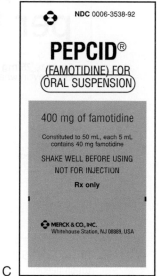

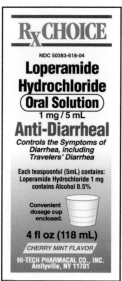

Figure 10-3 Composition of drugs. **A,** Tablets. **B,** Capsules. **C,** Oral suspension. **D,** Oral solution.

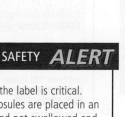

SAFETY *ALERT*

Reading the label is critical. Some capsules are placed in an inhaler and not swallowed and some medications are taken by the sublingual or buccal routes. An oral dose is often different than an intravenous dose. ALWAYS double-check the dose and route of administration.

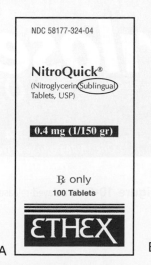

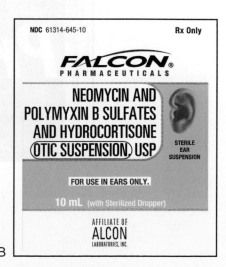

Figure 10-4 A, Sublingual tablets. **B,** Otic suspension.

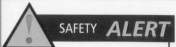

Be sure to take note if the product is labeled as a slow- or extended-release medication. This may be denoted with the letters XL, ES, or, SR after the medication's name (Figure 10-6). Many medications come in the same strength, but in both immediate- and slow-release forms.

NDC 0009-0760-04

Cleocin Pediatric®
clindamycin palmitate hydrochloride for oral solution, USP

75 mg
per 5 mL

Equiv. to **75 mg per 5 mL** clindamycin when (reconstituted)

— 100 mL
   (when mixed)

Pharmacia &Upjohn

LOT: K C 0 8 0 3
EXP.:   0 3 / 2 0 1 4

Figure 10-5 Label showing reconstitution needed.

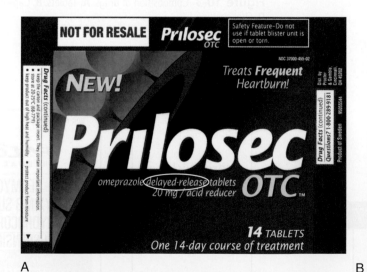

NOT FOR RESALE   Prilosec OTC

Safety Feature–Do not use if tablet blister unit is open or torn.

NDC 37000-455-02

NEW!

Treats **Frequent** Heartburn!

Dist. by Procter & Gamble, Cincinnati, OH 45202

Product of Sweden   96905544

Drug Facts (continued) Questions? 1-800-289-9181

Drug Facts (continued)
• keep the carton and package insert. They contain important information.
• store at 20-25°C (68-77°F)
• keep product out of high heat and humidity
• protect product from moisture

Prilosec OTC™
omeprazole (delayed-release) tablets
20 mg / acid reducer

14 TABLETS
One 14-day course of treatment

A

NDC 0245-0041-01
Klor-Con® 10
Potassium Chloride
(Extended-release) Tablets, USP

10 mEq (750 mg)

Unit Dose, 100 Tablets   **Rx only**

UPSHER-SMITH

B

Figure 10-6 **A,** Delayed-release tablets. **B,** Extended-release tablets.

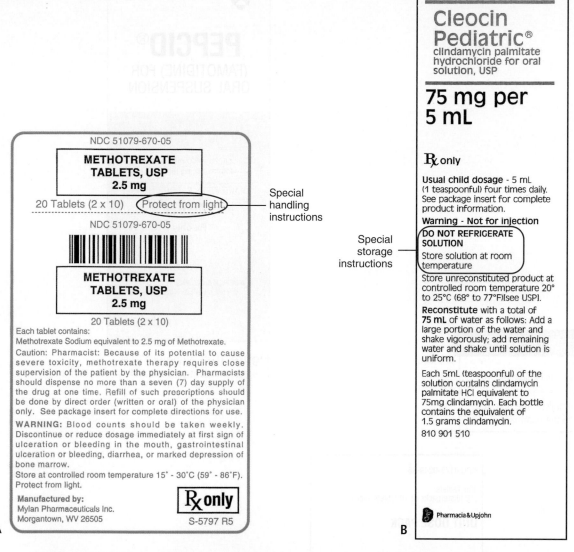

NDC 51079-670-05

**METHOTREXATE
TABLETS, USP
2.5 mg**

20 Tablets (2 x 10)   Protect from light   —— Special handling instructions

NDC 51079-670-05

**METHOTREXATE
TABLETS, USP
2.5 mg**

20 Tablets (2 x 10)

Each tablet contains:
Methotrexate Sodium equivalent to 2.5 mg of Methotrexate.

Caution: Pharmacist: Because of its potential to cause severe toxicity, methotrexate therapy requires close supervision of the patient by the physician. Pharmacists should dispense no more than a seven (7) day supply of the drug at one time. Refill of such prescriptions should be done by direct order (written or oral) of the physician only. See package insert for complete directions for use.

WARNING: Blood counts should be taken weekly. Discontinue or reduce dosage immediately at first sign of ulceration or bleeding in the mouth, gastrointestinal ulceration or bleeding, diarrhea, or marked depression of bone marrow.
Store at controlled room temperature 15˚ - 30˚C (59˚ - 86˚F).
Protect from light.

Manufactured by:
Mylan Pharmaceuticals Inc.
Morgantown, WV 26505

R͟x only

S-5797 R5

A

NDC 0009-0760-04

**Cleocin
Pediatric®**
clindamycin palmitate
hydrochloride for oral
solution, USP

**75 mg per
5 mL**

R͟x only

Usual child dosage - 5 mL
(1 teaspoonful) four times daily.
See package insert for complete
product information.

Warning - Not for injection

**DO NOT REFRIGERATE
SOLUTION**
Store solution at room
temperature   —— Special storage instructions
Store unreconstituted product at
controlled room temperature 20°
to 25°C (68° to 77°F)(see USP).

Reconstitute with a total of
75 mL of water as follows: Add a
large portion of the water and
shake vigorously; add remaining
water and shake until solution is
uniform.

Each 5mL (teaspoonful) of the
solution contains clindamycin
palmitate HCl equivalent to
75mg clindamycin. Each bottle
contains the equivalent of
1.5 grams clindamycin.

810 901 510

Pharmacia & Upjohn

B

Figure 10-7 A, Label showing special handling instructions. **B,** Label showing specific storage requirements.

Suspensions always include directions to shake well before each administration (Figure 10-8).

The drug manufacturer's name is commonly located at the bottom of the label but can appear in different areas on the label; the expiration date (drug is to be administered before this date) can be found by finding the abbreviation **exp** (Figure 10-9).

All medication labels (which are required by U.S. federal law and the laws of most other countries) include a lot number. This number, which refers to a batch of drugs that were manufactured at a specific time, is needed if a medication recall is required. The lot number is always placed on paperwork associated with vaccinations. Also, the national drug code (NDC) is a drug-specific identifying number that is required by the federal government of the United States (Figure 10-10).

Bar coding is also seen on drug labels. Bar coding is an electronic system for identifying the drug. It can be used for ordering, tracking, charging, and in some settings for comparing the specific drug with a specific patient. This system is the same as the one used on products that you purchase in stores (Figure 10-11).

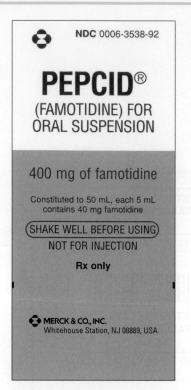

NDC 0006-3538-92

PEPCID®
(FAMOTIDINE) FOR ORAL SUSPENSION

400 mg of famotidine

Constituted to 50 mL, each 5 mL
contains 40 mg famotidine

(SHAKE WELL BEFORE USING)

NOT FOR INJECTION

Rx only

❖ MERCK & CO., INC.
Whitehouse Station, NJ 08889, USA

Figure 10-8 Suspension label includes directions to shake well.

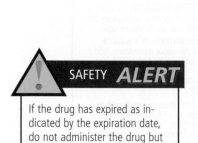

SAFETY **ALERT**

If the drug has expired as indicated by the expiration date, do not administer the drug but return it to the pharmacy.

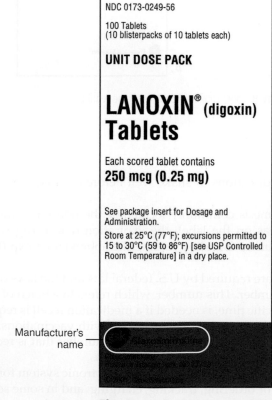

NDC 0173-0249-56

100 Tablets
(10 blisterpacks of 10 tablets each)

UNIT DOSE PACK

LANOXIN® (digoxin)
Tablets

Each scored tablet contains
250 mcg (0.25 mg)

See package insert for Dosage and
Administration.
Store at 25°C (77°F); excursions permitted to
15 to 30°C (59 to 86°F) [see USP Controlled
Room Temperature] in a dry place.

Manufacturer's
name —

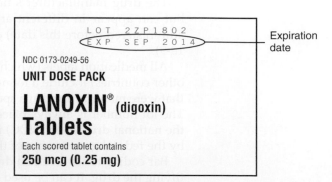

LOT 2ZP1802
(EXP SEP 2014)   — Expiration
                                       date

NDC 0173-0249-56

UNIT DOSE PACK

LANOXIN® (digoxin)
Tablets

Each scored tablet contains
250 mcg (0.25 mg)

Figure 10-9 Labels showing manufacturer name and expiration date, respectively.

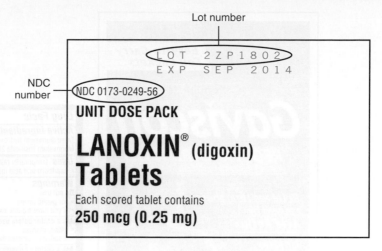

Figure 10-10 Label includes NDC and lot numbers.

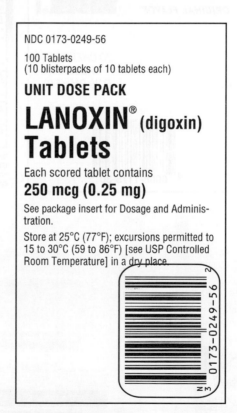

Figure 10-11 Bar code.

Medications may contain more than one drug (e.g., Vytorin, a new anticholesterol medication that contains both ezetimibe and simvastatin). All the different drugs and their strengths are listed on the medication label (Figure 10-12).

There may be some medications, such as acetylsalicylic acid (aspirin) and acetaminophen (Tylenol), that may be stored in some settings in bottles. Unlike the common unit dose system, the drug label will include the total volume in the container—for example, 250 tablets in the one bottle.

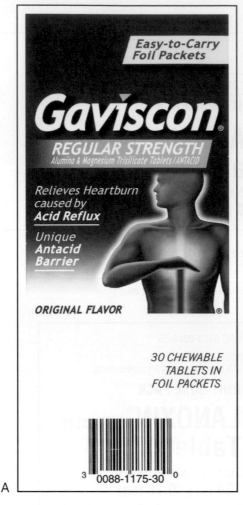

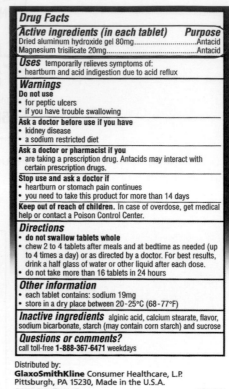

Drug Facts

Active ingredients (in each tablet)	Purpose
Dried aluminum hydroxide gel 80mg	Antacid
Magnesium trisilicate 20mg	Antacid

Uses temporarily relieves symptoms of:
• heartburn and acid indigestion due to acid reflux

Warnings
Do not use
• for peptic ulcers
• if you have trouble swallowing

Ask a doctor before use if you have
• kidney disease
• a sodium restricted diet

Ask a doctor or pharmacist if you
• are taking a prescription drug. Antacids may interact with certain prescription drugs.

Stop use and ask a doctor if
• heartburn or stomach pain continues
• you need to take this product for more than 14 days

Keep out of reach of children. In case of overdose, get medical help or contact a Poison Control Center.

Directions
• **do not swallow tablets whole**
• chew 2 to 4 tablets after meals and at bedtime as needed (up to 4 times a day) or as directed by a doctor. For best results, drink a half glass of water or other liquid after each dose.
• do not take more than 16 tablets in 24 hours

Other information
• each tablet contains: sodium 19mg
• store in a dry place between 20–25°C (68–77°F)

Inactive ingredients alginic acid, calcium stearate, flavor, sodium bicarbonate, starch (may contain corn starch) and sucrose

Questions or comments?
call toll-free 1-888-367-6471 weekdays

Distributed by:
GlaxoSmithKline Consumer Healthcare, L.P. Pittsburgh, PA 15230, Made in the U.S.A.
©2003 GlaxoSmithKline   50068004

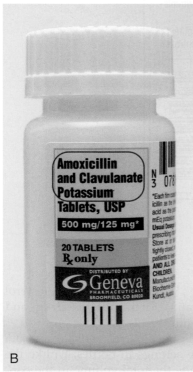

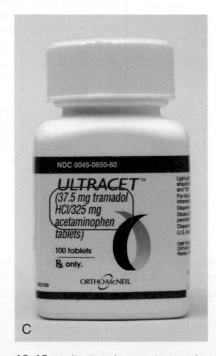

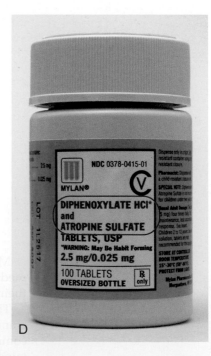

Figure 10-12 Medications that contain more than one drug.

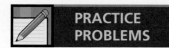
PRACTICE PROBLEMS

Directions: *Answer the questions for each medication label.*

1.

	NDC 0074-2415-12
Abbo Pac UNIT DOSE	100 Tablets Abbo-Pac®

Dilaudid® **2mg**
hydromorphone HCl

Each tablet contains:
hydromorphone HCl .... 2 mg

Tablet identification marking change adopted December, 2001.

℞ only

Tamper-Evident: Do not accept if sealed blister unit has been broken or opened.

See back panel for lot number and expiration date.

THIS PACKAGE FOR HOUSEHOLDS WITHOUT YOUNG CHILDREN.

13-2215-R1

What is the trade name? _____
What is the generic name? _____
What is the dose strength? _____
Measurement system is _____

2. What is the generic name? _____
What is the trade name? _____
What is the dose strength? _____
Measurement system is _____
Drug composition is _____

3.

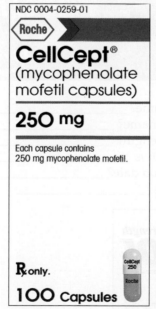
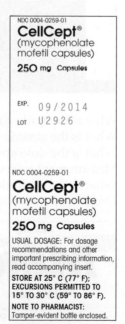

NDC 0004-0259-01

◇ **Roche** ▶

CellCept®
(mycophenolate
mofetil capsules)

250 mg

Each capsule contains
250 mg mycophenolate mofetil.

℞ only.

100 Capsules

NDC 0004-0259-01

CellCept®
(mycophenolate
mofetil capsules)

250 mg Capsules

EXP. 09/2014
LOT U2926

NDC 0004-0259-01

CellCept®
(mycophenolate
mofetil capsules)

250 mg Capsules

USUAL DOSAGE: For dosage recommendations and other important prescribing information, read accompanying insert.

STORE AT 25° C (77° F); EXCURSIONS PERMITTED TO 15° TO 30° C (59° TO 86° F).

NOTE TO PHARMACIST: Tamper-evident bottle enclosed.

What is the generic name? _____
What is the trade name? _____
What is the dose strength? _____
Measurement system is _____
Drug manufacturer is _____
What is the expiration date? _____
Drug composition is _____
Special handling is _____

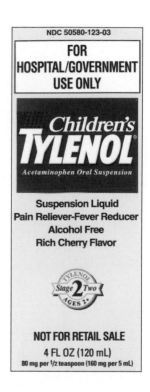
NDC 50580-123-03

FOR HOSPITAL/GOVERNMENT USE ONLY

Children's TYLENOL®
Acetaminophen Oral Suspension

Suspension Liquid
Pain Reliever-Fever Reducer
Alcohol Free
Rich Cherry Flavor

TYLENOL Stage 2 Two AGES 2+

NOT FOR RETAIL SALE
4 FL OZ (120 mL)
80 mg per ½ teaspoon (160 mg per 5 mL)

4.

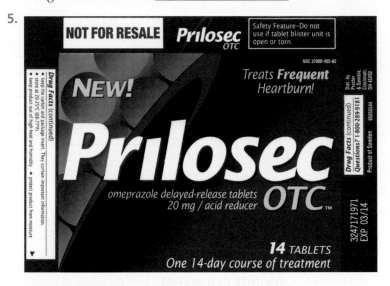

NDC 50580-451-03

Extra Strength

TYLENOL®

Pain Reliever - Fever Reducer   ACETAMINOPHEN

For Hospital and Government Use Only

UNIT DOSE PACK

McNeil

150 CAPLETS – 500 mg each

What is the trade name? _____

What is the generic name? _____

What is the dose strength? _____

Measurement system is _____

Drug composition is _____

Drug manufacturer is _____

5.

NOT FOR RESALE   *Prilosec* OTC

Safety Feature–Do not use if tablet blister unit is open or torn.

NDC 37000-455-02

*Treats **Frequent** Heartburn!*

Drug Facts (continued)
- keep the carton and package insert. They contain important information.
- store at 20-25°C (68-77°F)
- keep product out of high heat and humidity
- protect product from moisture

NEW!

Prilosec OTC™

omeprazole delayed-release tablets
20 mg / acid reducer

Dist. by Procter & Gamble, Cincinnati, OH 45202

Drug Facts (continued)
Questions? 1-800-289-9181

Product of Sweden   95855544

3247171971
EXP 03/14

14 TABLETS
One 14-day course of treatment

What is the trade name? _____

What is the generic name? _____

What is the dose strength? _____

Measurement system is _____

What is the expiration date? _____

Drug composition is _____

6.

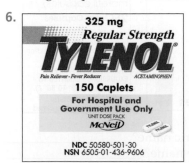

325 mg
Regular Strength

TYLENOL®

Pain Reliever - Fever Reducer   ACETAMINOPHEN

150 Caplets

For Hospital and Government Use Only

UNIT DOSE PACK

McNeil

NDC 50580-501-30
NSN 6505-01-436-9606

What is the trade name? _____

What is the generic name? _____

What is the dose strength? _____

Drug composition is _____

Measurement system is _____

7.

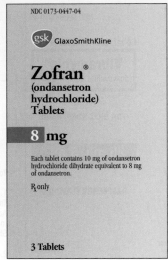

NDC 0173-0447-04

gsk GlaxoSmithKline

Zofran®
(ondansetron
hydrochloride)
Tablets

8 **mg**

Each tablet contains 10 mg of ondansetron
hydrochloride dihydrate equivalent to 8 mg
of ondansetron.

R̳ only

3 Tablets

What is the trade name? _____

What is the generic name? _____

What is the dose strength? _____

Measurement system is _____

Drug composition is _____

Drug manufacturer is _____

8.

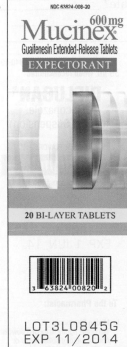

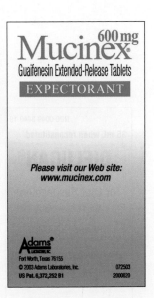

NDC 63824-008-20

Mucinex® 600 mg

Guaifenesin Extended-Release Tablets

EXPECTORANT

20 BI-LAYER TABLETS

3 63824 00820 2

LOT3L0845G
EXP 11/2014

Mucinex® 600 mg

Guaifenesin Extended-Release Tablets

EXPECTORANT

Please visit our Web site:
www.mucinex.com

Adams®
ADAMS LABORATORIES, INC.
Fort Worth, Texas 76155
© 2003 Adams Laboratories, Inc.   072503
US Pat. 6,372,252 B1   2000820

What is the trade name? _____

What is the generic name? _____

What is the dose strength? _____

Measurement system is _____

What is the expiration date? _____

Drug composition is _____

Drug manufacturer is _____

9.

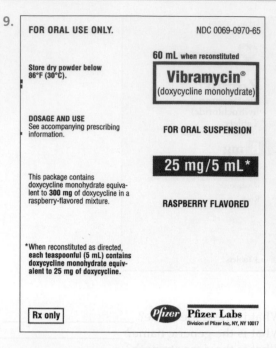

FOR ORAL USE ONLY.   NDC 0069-0970-65

60 mL when reconstituted

Vibramycin®
(doxycycline monohydrate)

FOR ORAL SUSPENSION

25 mg/5 mL*

RASPBERRY FLAVORED

Store dry powder below
86°F (30°C).

DOSAGE AND USE
See accompanying prescribing
information.

This package contains
doxycycline monohydrate equivalent to **300 mg** of doxycycline in a
raspberry-flavored mixture.

*When reconstituted as directed,
**each teaspoonful (5 mL) contains
doxycycline monohydrate equivalent to 25 mg of doxycycline.**

| Rx only |

Pfizer Pfizer Labs
Division of Pfizer Inc, NY, NY 10017

0630K03A
EXP 1JUL 14

To the Pharmacist:

1. Mixing Directions:
Tap bottle lightly to loosen powder.
Add 47.6 mL of water to the bottle
to make a total volume of 60 mL.
Shake well.

2. This prescription, when in suspension, will maintain its potency
for two weeks when kept at room
temperature.

**DISCARD UNUSED PORTION
AFTER TWO WEEKS.**

What is the trade name? _____

What is the generic name? _____

What is the dose strength? _____

Measurement system is _____

What is the expiration date? _____

Drug composition is _____

Drug manufacturer is _____

10.

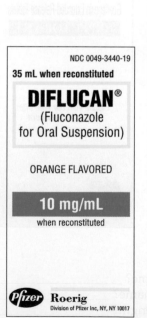

NDC 0049-3440-19
35 mL when reconstituted

DIFLUCAN®
(Fluconazole
for Oral Suspension)

ORANGE FLAVORED

10 mg/mL

when reconstituted

0400K03A
EXP 1 JUN 14

To the Pharmacist:

1. Mixing Directions:
Tap bottle lightly to loosen powder.
Add 24 mL of distilled water or
Purified Water (USP) to the bottle.
Shake well.

2. Store reconstituted suspension
between 41°F (5°C) and 86°F
(30°C). Protect from freezing.

Shake well before each use.
Discard unused portion after
2 weeks.

NDC 0049-3440-19
35 mL when reconstituted

DIFLUCAN®
(Fluconazole
for Oral Suspension)

ORANGE FLAVORED

10 mg/mL

when reconstituted

Pfizer Roerig
Division of Pfizer Inc, NY, NY 10017

What is the trade name? _____

What is the generic name? _____

What is the dose strength? _____

Measurement system is _____
What is the expiration date? _____
Drug composition is _____
Drug manufacturer is _____

(Answers on pp. 454–455)

CALCULATING SOLID MEDICATION DOSAGES

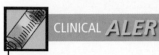

CLINICAL ALERT

If a tablet is not scored, it cannot be divided and must be administered whole.

Comparing the prescription with the drug you HAVE on hand to determine that you have the correct drug is the first step to medication administration. This step comes before any calculation can be started. Compare the prescribed dose with the inscribed dose on the medication label you HAVE to determine if they are the same drug. If they are the same drug, decide whether a drug calculation will be required. Commonly, one tablet or capsule will be required. When calculations are necessary, usually no more than three tablets or capsules will be required. There are some drugs—for example, HIV medications, steroids, and potassium—that exceed this rule. With scored tablets, the calculated dose may be in half-tablet increments. Compare the routes of administration. The medication you HAVE must include the same route of administration as the prescribed medication.

Example 1

PRESCRIPTION *Digoxin 0.374 mg orally daily.*

- **What You HAVE**

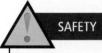

SAFETY ALERT

When possible it is safest for the prescribed dose to be the same as or simple multiples of the medication that is provided by the pharmacy.

NDC 0173-0249-56

100 Tablets
(10 blisterpacks of 10 tablets each)

UNIT DOSE PACK

LANOXIN® (digoxin)
Tablets

Each scored tablet contains
250 mcg (0.25 mg)

See package insert for Dosage and Administration.

Store at 25°C (77°F); excursions permitted to 15 to 30°C (59 to 86°F) [see USP Controlled Room Temperature] in a dry place.

- **What You KNOW** Prescribed dose is 0.374 mg.

- **What You WANT (X)** How many tablets needed to supply digoxin 0.374 mg.

CRITICAL THINKING

Are the prescribed medication and the medication you HAVE the same? _____
Does the prescribed dose use the same system of measurement as the medication you HAVE? _____
Does the prescribed dose use the same equivalent measurement within the same system? _____
Is the prescribed dose larger or smaller than the dose you HAVE? _____
In setting up a ratio-proportion, place in the LEFT ratio the medication dose strength per volume you HAVE on hand; in the RIGHT ratio place the prescribed dose in the numerator and place X (the unknown volume) in the denominator.

SAFETY **ALERT**

When computing medication doses, the approximate equivalent should not differ by more than 10% from the prescribed dose.

Multiply to get the cross-products.
Divide the numerical cross-product by the numerical multiplier of X (the number in front of X).
The result is the answer for X.
Label answer properly in units (i.e., number of tablets, number of milliliters).
Check answer by placing the number obtained for X in the original equation. Cross-multiply. The cross-products should be approximately equal.

ANSWER FOR BEST CARE

Medication comparison? Yes.
System of measurement? Yes; metric.
Unit of measure comparison? Yes; milligrams.
Dose larger.
Perform calculation.

HUMAN ERROR **Alert**

Except when administering special medications, calculation results that require more than three tablets or capsules being administered to a patient at one time should be repeated. The prescription should be reviewed, and a drug reference book and/or the pharmacist consulted.

$$\frac{0.25 \text{ mg}}{1 \text{ tablet}} = \frac{0.374 \text{ mg}}{X \text{ tablet}}$$

(HAVE)   (KNOW)
         (WANT)

$0.25X = 0.374$

$$\begin{array}{r} 1.49 \text{ (rounded to nearest tenth)} \\ 25\overline{)037.40} \\ \underline{25} \\ 124 \\ \underline{100} \\ 240 \\ 225 \end{array}$$

$X = 1.5$

Label with the unit of measure.
1.5 tablets

HUMAN ERROR **Alert**

Always anticipate the result of your computation by looking at the relative value of the dose prescribed and the dose you HAVE on hand, determining whether the dose prescribed is greater or less than the dose you HAVE. Compare this with the final calculation result. If calculation answer differs from the anticipated result, recalculate the problem.

✓ **Human Error Check**

Replace X with 1.5 and cross-multiply.

$$\frac{0.25}{1} = \frac{0.374}{1.5}$$

$1.25 \times 1.5 = 1 \times 0.374$
$375 \approx 374$

Guideline: Only scored tablets can be divided. Is the tablet scored? Yes.

NDC 0173-0249-56

100 Tablets
(10 blisterpacks of 10 tablets each)

UNIT DOSE PACK

LANOXIN® (digoxin)
Tablets

Each scored tablet contains
250 mcg (0.25 mg)

See package insert for Dosage and Administration.
Store at 25°C (77°F); excursions permitted to 15 to 30°C (59 to 86°F) [see USP Controlled Room Temperature] in a dry place.

Example 2

PRESCRIPTION	*Clarithromycin 1 g orally once daily for 7 days.*

• What You HAVE

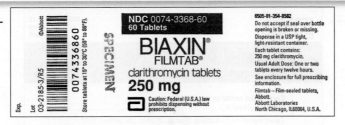

• What You KNOW   Prescribed dose is 1 g.

• What You WANT (X)   How many tablets required to administer clarithromycin 1 g.

CRITICAL THINKING

Are the prescribed medication and the medication you HAVE the same? _____

Does the prescribed dose use the same system of measurement as the medication you HAVE? _____

Does the prescribed dose use the same equivalent measurement within the same system? _____

Is the prescribed dose larger or smaller than the dose you HAVE? _____

In setting up a ratio-proportion, place in the LEFT ratio the medication dose strength per volume you HAVE on hand; in the RIGHT ratio place the prescribed dose in the numerator and place X (the unknown volume) in the denominator.

Multiply to get the cross-products.

Divide the numerical cross-product by the numerical multiplier of X (the number in front of X).

The result is the answer for X.

Label answer properly in units (i.e., number of tablets, number of milliliters).

Check answer by placing the number obtained for X in the original equation. Cross-multiply. The cross-products should be approximately equal.

ANSWER FOR BEST CARE

Medication comparison? Yes.

System of measurement? Yes; metric.

Unit of measure comparison? No; prescribed grams and supplied milligrams.

Dose larger.

Convert grams to milligrams.

1 g = 1000 mg

Perform calculation.

$$\frac{250 \text{ mg}}{1 \text{ tablet}} = \frac{1000 \text{ mg}}{X \text{ tablet}} \qquad 250X = 1000$$

$$\begin{array}{r} 4 \\ 250\overline{)1000} \\ \underline{1000} \end{array}$$

X = 4

Label with the unit of measure.

4 tablets

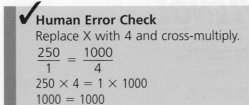

> **✓ Human Error Check**
> Replace X with 4 and cross-multiply.
> $$\frac{250}{1} = \frac{1000}{4}$$
> 250 × 4 = 1 × 1000
> 1000 = 1000

Example 3

PRESCRIPTION   *Morphine 4 mg orally every 4 hours for pain.*

- **What You HAVE**

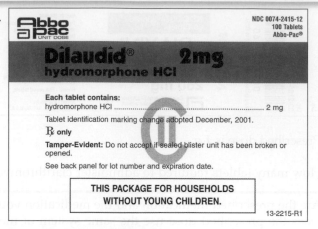

Abbo-Pac UNIT DOSE

NDC 0074-2415-12
100 Tablets
Abbo-Pac®

Dilaudid® 2mg
hydromorphone HCl

Each tablet contains:
hydromorphone HCl .... 2 mg

Tablet identification marking change adopted December, 2001.

℞ only

Tamper-Evident: Do not accept if sealed blister unit has been broken or opened.

See back panel for lot number and expiration date.

**THIS PACKAGE FOR HOUSEHOLDS
WITHOUT YOUNG CHILDREN.**

13-2215-R1

- **What You KNOW**   Prescribed dose is 4 mg.

- **What You WANT (X)** How many tablets required to administer morphine 4 mg.

CRITICAL THINKING

Are the prescribed medication and the medication you HAVE the same? _____

Does the prescribed dose use the same system of measurement as the medication you HAVE? _____

Does the prescribed dose use the same equivalent measurement within the same system? _____

Is the prescribed dose larger or smaller than the dose you HAVE? _____

In setting up a ratio-proportion, place in the LEFT ratio the medication dose strength per volume you HAVE on hand; in the RIGHT ratio place the prescribed dose in the numerator and place X (the unknown volume) in the denominator.

Multiply to get the cross-products.

Divide the numerical cross-product by the numerical multiplier of X (the number in front of X).

The result is the answer for X.

Label answer properly in units (i.e., number of tablets, number of milliliters).

Check answer by placing the number obtained for X in the original equation. Cross-multiply. The cross-products should be approximately equal.

ANSWER FOR BEST CARE

Medication comparison? No; the generic name of Dilaudid is hydromorphone, which is 7 to 10 times more potent than morphine. You have been supplied with the wrong drug.

Do not proceed with the calculation. Contact the pharmacy.

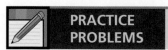

PRACTICE PROBLEMS

Directions: *Answer the questions under each problem related to the medication label provided.*

1. PRESCRIPTION: Tylenol 650 mg by mouth every 4 hours for pain.

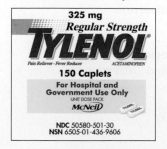

325 mg
Regular Strength
TYLENOL®
Pain Reliever · Fever Reducer   ACETAMINOPHEN
150 Caplets
**For Hospital and
Government Use Only**
UNIT DOSE PACK
McNeil

NDC 50580-501-30
NSN 6505-01-436-9606

Are the prescribed medication and the supplied medication the same drug?
_____

What is the generic name for Tylenol? _____

Does the prescribed dose use the same system of measurement? _____

Does the prescribed dose use the same equivalent measurement within the same system? _____

Is the prescribed dose the same as, larger, or smaller than the supplied dose?
_____

How many caplet(s) will be administered? _____

2. PRESCRIPTION: metformin 500 mg by mouth twice a day.

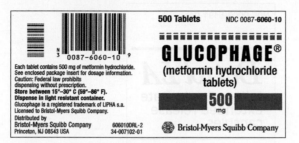

Are the prescribed medication and the supplied medication the same drug?
_____

What is the trade name for metformin? _____

Does the prescribed dose use the same system of measurement? _____

Is the prescribed dose the same as, larger, or smaller than the supplied dose?
_____

How many tablet(s) will be administered? _____

3. PRESCRIPTION: Capoten 25 mg by mouth twice a day.

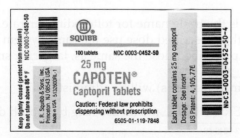

Are the prescribed medication and the supplied medication the same drug?
_____

What is the generic name for Capoten? _____

Does the prescribed dose use the same system of measurement? _____

Is the prescribed dose the same as, larger, or smaller than the supplied dose?
_____

How many tablet(s) will be administered? _____

4. PRESCRIPTION: Lasix 120 mg by mouth daily.

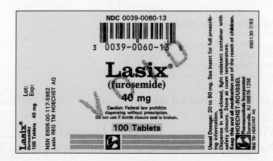

Are the prescribed medication and the supplied medication the same drug? _____

What is the generic name for Lasix? _____

Does the prescribed dose use the same system of measurement? _____

Does the prescribed dose use the same equivalent measurement within the same system? _____

Is the prescribed dose the same as, larger, or smaller than the supplied dose? _____

How many tablet(s) will be administered? _____

5. PRESCRIPTION: tolterodine tartrate extended-release 4 mg by mouth daily.

NDC 0009-5191-01

Detrol® LA
tolterodine tartrate
extended release
capsules

4 mg   ͭᴹ

30 Capsules   **PHARMACIA**

Are the prescribed medication and the supplied medication the same drug? _____

What is the trade name for tolterodine tartrate? _____

Does the prescribed dose use the same system of measurement? _____

Is the prescribed dose the same as, larger, or smaller than the supplied dose? _____

How many tablet(s) will be administered? _____

6. PRESCRIPTION: Lanoxin 250 mcg by mouth daily.

NDC 0173-0249-56

100 Tablets
(10 blisterpacks of 10 tablets each)

UNIT DOSE PACK

**LANOXIN® (digoxin)
Tablets**

Each scored tablet contains
250 mcg (0.25 mg)

See package insert for Dosage and
Administration.
Store at 25°C (77°F); excursions permitted to
15 to 30°C (59 to 86°F) [see USP Controlled
Room Temperature] in a dry place.

Are the prescribed medication and the supplied medication the same drug? _____

What is the generic name for Lanoxin? _____

Does the prescribed dose use the same system of measurement? _____

Does the prescribed dose use the same equivalent measurement within the same system? _____

Is the prescribed dose the same as, larger, or smaller than the supplied dose? _____

How many tablet(s) will be administered? _____

7. PRESCRIPTION: Ativan 2 mg by mouth twice a day.

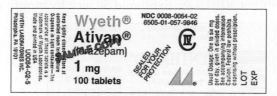

Are the prescribed medication and the supplied medication the same drug? _____

What is the generic name for Ativan? _____

Does the prescribed dose use the same system of measurement? _____

Does the prescribed dose use the same equivalent measurement within the same system? _____

Is the prescribed dose the same as, larger, or smaller than the supplied dose? _____

How many tablet(s) will be administered? _____

8. PRESCRIPTION: Nitrostat 1/150 gr sublingually 5 minutes apart for angina. Do not take more than three tablets in 15 minutes.

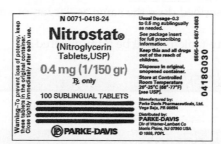

The patient reports that he has taken two tablets. How many milligrams has he taken? _____

9. PRESCRIPTION: Lopressor 100 mg by mouth daily.

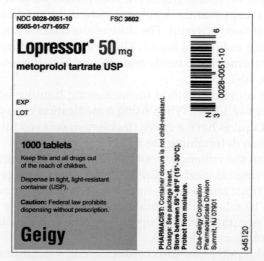

Are the prescribed medication and the supplied medication the same drug? _____

What is the generic name of Lopressor? _____

Does the prescribed dose use the same system of measurement? _____
Does the prescribed dose use the same equivalent measurement within the same system? _____
Is the prescribed dose the same as, larger, or smaller than the supplied dose? _____

How many tablet(s) will be administered? _____

10. PRESCRIPTION: Synthroid 50 mcg by mouth daily.

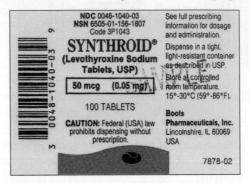

Are the prescribed medication and the supplied medication the same drug? _____

What is the generic name for Synthroid? _____
Does the prescribed dose use the same system of measurement? _____
Does the prescribed dose use the same equivalent measurement within the same system? _____
Is the prescribed dose the same as, larger, or smaller than the supplied dose? _____

How many tablet(s) will be administered? _____

(Answers on p. 455)

CALCULATING LIQUID MEDICATION DOSAGES

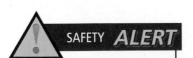

SAFETY ALERT

Be careful to identify the dose strength and the dose volume. Do not confuse **dose strength/dose volume** and **total strength/total volume** when performing calculations.

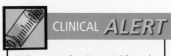

CLINICAL **ALERT**

Only use oral syringes with oral medications.

Oral medications also come in liquid form. These are used for patients who have difficulty swallowing; have a nasogastric, gastrostomy, or jejunostomy tube; or are an infant or young child. The medication label is similar to the tablet and capsule labels except that the label will state if the medication is an elixir, oral suspension, oral solution, or syrup. The dose of the medication will be listed as drug **strength** in a specific **volume** of liquid. This is the **dose/volume.** The label will also identify the **total volume** of the bottle and may include the total strength of the entire container (Figure 10-13).

One common method for measuring liquid medications is a calibrated medicine cup (Figure 10-14). When using a medication cup, you need to have the liquid at eye level. Liquids have a curve (meniscus); you read the lowest point of the curve (center) when determining the volume (Figure 10-15).

When the volume cannot be accurately determined by using a medication cup, an oral syringe is used (Figure 10-16). An oral syringe has a longer tip than a hypodermic syringe and is large enough that a needle cannot be applied. With small-volume doses, 10-mL and 5-mL oral syringes are available (Figure 10-17). Once the medication is accurately drawn up in the syringe, it may be easier to dispense by putting it back into a medicine cup.

Oral liquids may also be dispensed by a calibrated dropper. The dropper comes with a specific medication. This dropper is medication-specific and is not interchangeable with other medications (Figure 10-18).

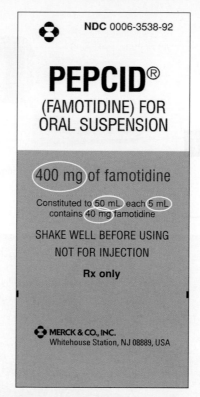

NDC 0006-3538-92

PEPCID®
(FAMOTIDINE) FOR ORAL SUSPENSION

400 mg of famotidine

Constituted to 50 mL, each 5 mL contains 40 mg famotidine

SHAKE WELL BEFORE USING

NOT FOR INJECTION

Rx only

MERCK & CO., INC.
Whitehouse Station, NJ 08889, USA

Figure 10-13 Medication label of a liquid drug.

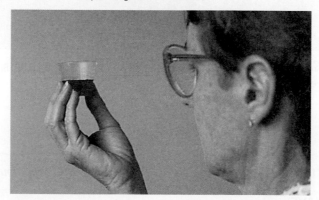

Figure 10-14 Calibrated medicine cup. (From Elkin MK, Perry AG, Potter PA: Nursing interventions and clinical skills, ed 3, St Louis, 2004, Mosby.)

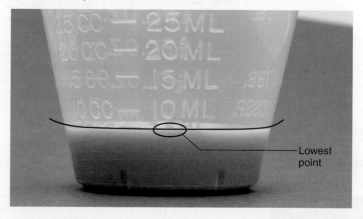

Lowest point

Figure 10-15 Medicine cup showing curve (meniscus).

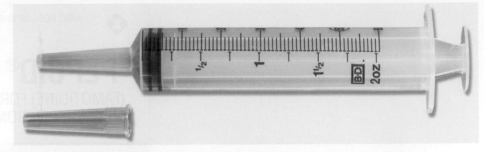

Figure 10-16 2-oz oral syringe. (Used with permission from Becton, Dickinson, and Company.)

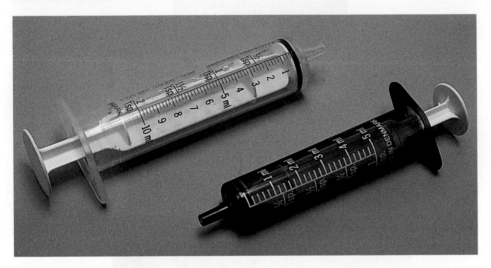

Figure 10-17 5-mL and 10-mL oral syringes. (From Clayton BD, Stock YN, Harroun RD: Basic pharmacology for nurses, ed 14, St Louis, 2007, Mosby.)

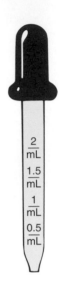

Figure 10-18 Medicine dropper. (From Clayton BD, Stock YN, Harroun RD: Basic pharmacology for nurses, ed 14, St Louis, 2007, Mosby.)

Example 1

PRESCRIPTION   *Docusate sodium elixir 120 mg by mouth daily.*

• What You HAVE

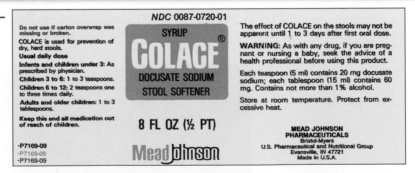

NDC 0087-0720-01

SYRUP

COLACE®

DOCUSATE SODIUM

STOOL SOFTENER

8 FL OZ (½ PT)

Mead Johnson

Do not use if carton overwrap was missing or broken.

COLACE is used for prevention of dry, hard stools.

Usual daily dose

Infants and children under 3: As prescribed by physician.

Children 3 to 6: 1 to 3 teaspoons.

Children 6 to 12: 2 teaspoons one to three times daily.

Adults and older children: 1 to 3 tablespoons.

Keep this and all medication out of reach of children.

·P7169-09
·P7169-09
·P7169-09

The effect of COLACE on the stools may not be apparent until 1 to 3 days after first oral dose.

WARNING: As with any drug, if you are pregnant or nursing a baby, seek the advice of a health professional before using this product.

Each teaspoon (5 ml) contains 20 mg docusate sodium; each tablespoon (15 ml) contains 60 mg. Contains not more than 1% alcohol.

Store at room temperature. Protect from excessive heat.

MEAD JOHNSON
PHARMACEUTICALS
Bristol-Myers
U.S. Pharmaceutical and Nutritional Group
Evansville, IN 47721
Made in U.S.A.

• What You KNOW   Prescribed dose is 120 mg.

• What You WANT (X)   How many milliliters required to administer docusate sodium 120 mg.

CRITICAL THINKING   Are the prescribed medication and the medication you HAVE the same? _____

Does the prescribed dose use the same system of measurement as the medication you HAVE? _____

CHAPTER 10

Does the prescribed dose use the same equivalent measurement within the same system? _____

Is the prescribed dose larger or smaller than the dose you HAVE? _____

In setting up a ratio-proportion, place in the LEFT ratio the medication dose strength per volume you HAVE on hand; in the RIGHT ratio place the prescribed dose in the numerator and place X (the unknown volume) in the denominator.

Multiply to get the cross-products.

Divide the numerical cross-product by the numerical multiplier of X (the number in front of X).

The result is the answer for X.

Label answer properly in units (i.e., number of tablets, number of milliliters).

Check answer by placing the number obtained for X in the original equation. Cross-multiply. The cross-products should be approximately equal.

ANSWER FOR BEST CARE

Medication comparison? Yes.

System of measurement? Yes; metric.

Unit of measure comparison? Yes; milliliters.

Dose larger.

Perform calculation.

$$\frac{20 \text{ mg}}{5 \text{ mL}} = \frac{120 \text{ mg}}{X \text{ mL}} \qquad 20X = 600$$

$$20\overline{)600} \quad \frac{30}{}$$
$$\underline{600}$$

X = 30

Label with the unit of measure.

30 mL

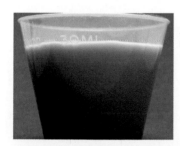

✓ **Human Error Check**
Replace X with 30 and cross-multiply.
$$\frac{20}{5} = \frac{120}{30}$$
$20 \times 30 = 120 \times 5$
$600 = 600$

Example 2

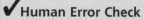

PRESCRIPTION *Nystatin (Mycostatin) oral suspension 500,000 units by mouth every 6 hours.*

• *What You HAVE*

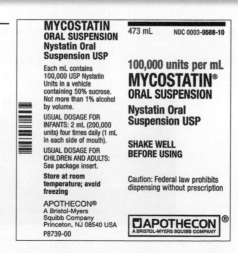

MYCOSTATIN
ORAL SUSPENSION
Nystatin Oral
Suspension USP

473 mL   NDC 0003-0588-10

Each mL contains
100,000 USP Nystatin
Units in a vehicle
containing 50% sucrose.
Not more than 1% alcohol
by volume.

USUAL DOSAGE FOR
INFANTS: 2 mL (200,000
units) four times daily (1 mL
in each side of mouth).

USUAL DOSAGE FOR
CHILDREN AND ADULTS:
See package insert.

Store at room
temperature; avoid
freezing

APOTHECON®
A Bristol-Myers
Squibb Company
Princeton, NJ 08540 USA

P8739-00

100,000 units per mL
MYCOSTATIN®
ORAL SUSPENSION
Nystatin Oral
Suspension USP

SHAKE WELL
BEFORE USING

Caution: Federal law prohibits
dispensing without prescription

□APOTHECON ®
A BRISTOL-MYERS SQUIBB COMPANY

- *What You KNOW* ———————— Prescribed dose is 500,000 units.

- *What You WANT (X)* ———————— How many milliliters required to administer nystatin 500,000 units.

<table>
<tr><td>CRITICAL THINKING</td><td>Are the prescribed medication and the medication you HAVE the same? _____
Does the prescribed dose use the same system of measurement as the medication you HAVE? _____
Does the prescribed dose use the same equivalent measurement within the same system? _____
Is the prescribed dose larger or smaller than the dose you HAVE? _____
In setting up a ratio-proportion, place in the LEFT ratio the medication dose strength per volume you HAVE on hand; in the RIGHT ratio, place the prescribed dose in the numerator and place X (the unknown volume) in the denominator.
Multiply to get the cross-products.
Divide the numerical cross-product by the numerical multiplier of X (the number in front of X).
The result is the answer for X.
Label answer properly in units (i.e., number of tablets, number of milliliters).
Check answer by placing the number obtained for X in the original equation. Cross-multiply. The cross-products should be approximately equal.</td></tr>
</table>

ANSWER FOR BEST CARE

Medication comparison? Yes.
System of measurement? Yes; metric.
Unit of measure comparison? Yes; milliliters.
Dose larger.
Perform calculation.

$$\frac{100,000 \text{ mg}}{1 \text{ mL}} = \frac{500,000 \text{ mg}}{X \text{ mL}}$$

Reduce.

$$\frac{1}{1} = \frac{5}{X}$$

$$X = 5$$

Label with the unit of measure.
5 mL

> ✔ **Human Error Check**
>
> Replace X with 5.
>
> $$\frac{1}{1} = \frac{5}{5}$$
>
> $1 \times 5 = 5 \times 1$
> $5 = 5$

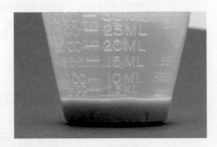

Example 3

PRESCRIPTION	*Fluoxetine hydrochloride oral solution 30 mg by mouth daily in the morning.*

- **What You HAVE**

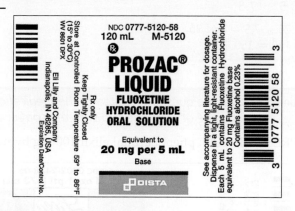

- **What You KNOW**   Prescribed dose is 30 mg.

- **What You WANT (X)**   How many milliliters required to administer fluoxetine hydrochloride 30 mg.

CRITICAL THINKING	Are the prescribed medication and the medication you HAVE same? _____
	Does the prescribed dose use the same system of measurement as the medication you HAVE? _____
	Does the prescribed dose use the same equivalent measurement within the same system? _____
	Is the prescribed dose larger or smaller than the dose you HAVE? _____
	In setting up a ratio-proportion, place in the LEFT ratio the medication dose strength per volume you HAVE on hand; in the RIGHT ratio, place the prescribed dose in the numerator and place X (the unknown volume) in the denominator.
	Multiply to get the cross-products.
	Divide the numerical cross-product by the numerical multiplier of X (the number in front of X).
	The result is the answer for X.
	Label answer properly in units (i.e., number of tablets, number of milliliters).
	Check answer by placing the number obtained for X in the original equation. Cross-multiply. The cross-products should be approximately equal.

ANSWER FOR BEST CARE	Medication comparison? Yes.
	System of measurement? Yes; metric.
	Unit of measure comparison? Yes; milliliters.
	Dose larger.
	Perform calculation.

$$\frac{20 \text{ mg}}{5 \text{ mL}} = \frac{30 \text{ mg}}{X \text{ mL}}$$

$$\begin{array}{r} 7.5 \\ 20\overline{)150.0} \\ \underline{140} \\ 100 \end{array}$$

X = 7.5

Label with the unit of measure.

7.5 mL

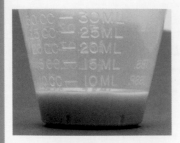

✓ **Human Error Check**

Replace X with 7.5 and cross-multiply.

$$\frac{20}{5} = \frac{30}{7.5}$$

$20 \times 7.5 = 5 \times 30$
$150 = 150$

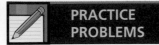

PRACTICE PROBLEMS

Directions: *Answer the questions related to the medication labels provided. Mark the oral syringe or medicine cup with the correct volume to be administered.*

1. PRESCRIPTION: phenobarbital elixir 100 mg by mouth at bedtime.

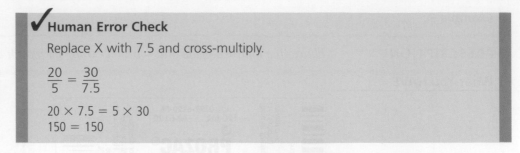

Dose/volume _____

Administer _____

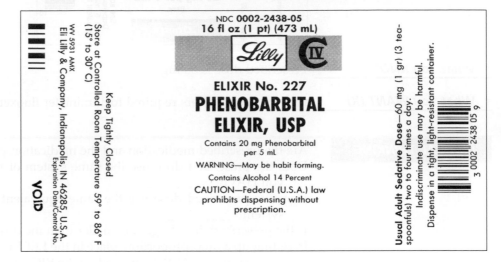

2. PRESCRIPTION: penicillin V potassium oral solution 500 mg by mouth every 8 hours.

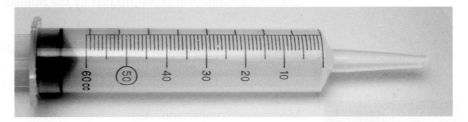

Trade name _____

Dose/volume _____
Administer _____

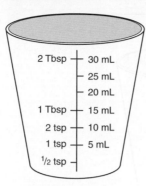

3. PRESCRIPTION: ranitidine syrup 300 mg by mouth at bedtime.

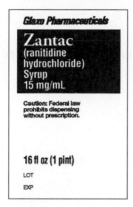

Trade name _____
Dose/volume _____
Administer _____

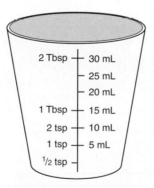

4. PRESCRIPTION: thioridazine HCl oral solution 300 mg by mouth three times a day.

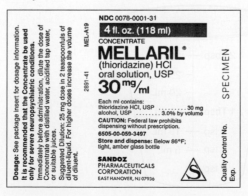

Trade name _____

Dose/volume _____

Administer _____

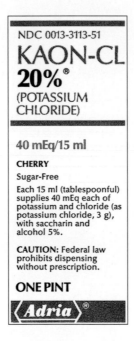

5. PRESCRIPTION: potassium chloride syrup 80 mEq by mouth daily.

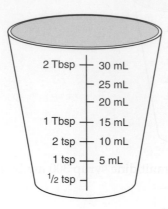

Trade name _____

Dose/volume _____

Administer _____

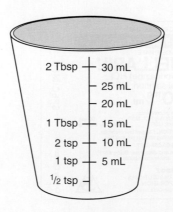

6. PRESCRIPTION: diphenhydramine hydrochloride elixir 40 mg by mouth three times a day.

N 0071-2220-17 ELIXIR **Benadryl**® (Diphenhydramine Hydrochloride Elixir, USP) **Caution**—Federal law prohibits dispensing without prescription. **4 FLUIDOUNCES** **PARKE-DAVIS** Div of Warner-Lambert Co Morris Plains, NJ 07950 USA	**Elixir P-D 2220 for prescription dispensing only.** **Contains**—12.5 mg diphenhydramine hydrochloride in each 5 mL. Alcohol, 14%. **Dose**—Adults, 2 to 4 teaspoonfuls; chil- dren over 20 lb, 1 to 2 teaspoonfuls; three or four times daily. See package insert. Keep this and all drugs out of the reach of children. **Store below 30°C (86°F). Protect from freezing and light.** Exp date and lot 2220G102

Trade name _____

Dose/volume _____

Administer _____

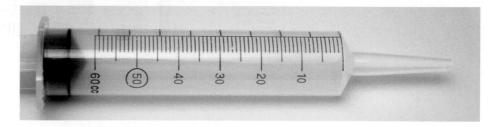

7. PRESCRIPTION: clindamycin oral solution 50 mg by mouth four times a day.

NDC 0009-0760-04

Cleocin Pediatric®
clindamycin palmitate
hydrochloride for oral
solution, USP

75 mg
per 5 mL

Equiv. to **75 mg per 5 mL**
clindamycin when reconstituted

**Pharmacia
&Upjohn**

100 mL
(when mixed)

Trade name _____

Dose/volume _____

Administer _____

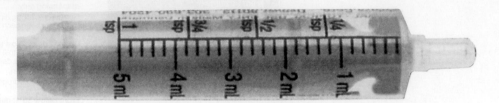

8. PRESCRIPTION: Suprax oral suspension 200 mg by mouth every 12 hours.

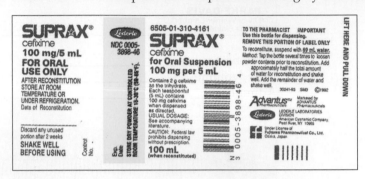

Generic name _____

Dose/volume _____

Administer _____

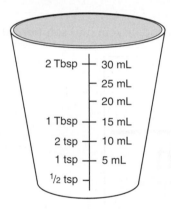

2 Tbsp	30 mL
	25 mL
	20 mL
1 Tbsp	15 mL
2 tsp	10 mL
1 tsp	5 mL
½ tsp	

9. PRESCRIPTION: Digoxin 150 mcg by mouth daily.

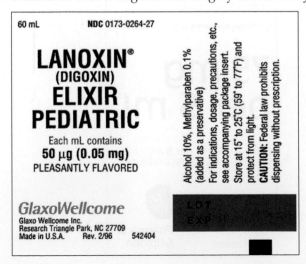

Trade name _____

Dose/volume _____

Administer _____

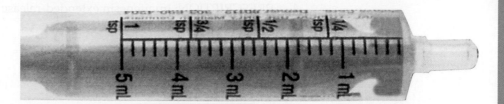

10. PRESCRIPTION: Amoxicillin 0.25 g by mouth every 6 hours.

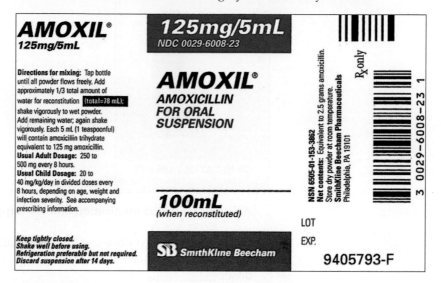

Trade name _____

Dose/volume _____

Administer _____

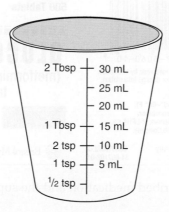

(Answers on pp. 455–456)

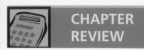

CHAPTER REVIEW

Answer the questions under each item using the medication label provided.

1. PRESCRIPTION: guaifenesin extended-release 1.2 g by mouth every 12 hours.

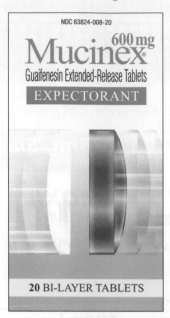

NDC 63824-008-20

Mucinex® 600 mg
Guaifenesin Extended-Release Tablets
EXPECTORANT

20 BI-LAYER TABLETS

Are the prescribed medication and the supplied medication the same drug? _____

Does the prescribed dose use the same unit of measurement? _____
Is the prescribed dose the same as, larger, or smaller than the supplied dose? _____
How many tablet(s) will be administered? _____

2. PRESCRIPTION: metformin (Glucophage) 1000 mg by mouth daily.

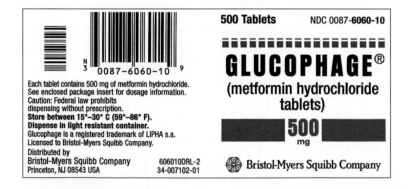

N 3 0087-6060-10 9

500 Tablets   NDC 0087-**6060-10**

GLUCOPHAGE®
(metformin hydrochloride tablets)
500 mg

Each tablet contains 500 mg of metformin hydrochloride.
See enclosed package insert for dosage information.
Caution: Federal law prohibits dispensing without prescription.
Store between 15°–30° C (59°–86° F).
Dispense in light resistant container.
Glucophage is a registered trademark of LIPHA s.a.
Licensed to Bristol-Myers Squibb Company.
Distributed by
Bristol-Myers Squibb Company
Princeton, NJ 08543 USA

606010DRL-2
34-007102-01

✿ Bristol-Myers Squibb Company

Are the prescribed medication and the supplied medication the same drug? _____

Does the prescribed dose use the same system of measurement? _____
Does the prescribed dose use the same equivalent measurement within the same system? _____
Is the prescribed dose the same as, larger, or smaller than the supplied dose? _____
How many tablet(s) will be administered? _____

3. PRESCRIPTION: lorazepam (Ativan) 2 mg by mouth at bedtime.
Are the prescribed medication and the supplied medication the same drug? _____

Does the prescribed dose use the same system of measurement? _____

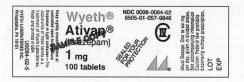

Is the prescribed dose the same as, larger, or smaller than the supplied dose? _____

How many tablet(s) will be administered? _____

4. PRESCRIPTION: codeine sulfate 30 mg by mouth every 6 hours for pain.

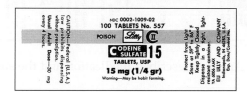

Are the prescribed medication and the supplied medication the same drug? _____

Does the prescribed dose use the same system of measurement? _____

Is the prescribed dose the same as, larger, or smaller than the supplied dose? _____

How many tablet(s) will be administered? _____

5. PRESCRIPTION: potassium chloride syrup 27 mEq by mouth daily.

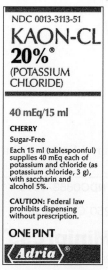

Are the prescribed medication and the supplied medication the same drug? _____

Does the prescribed dose use the same system of measurement? _____

How many milliliters will be administered? _____

Mark the medicine cup with the volume to be administered.

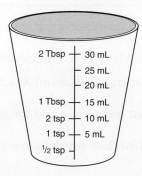

6. PRESCRIPTION: penicillin VK oral solution 250 mg by mouth twice a day.

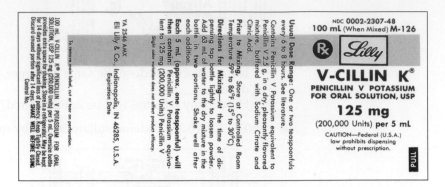

Are the prescribed medication and the supplied medication the same drug?

_____

Does the prescribed dose use the same system of measurement? _____
How many milliliters will be administered? _____
Mark the medicine cup with the volume to be administered.

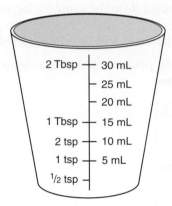

7. PRESCRIPTION: prazosin (Minipress) 3 mg by mouth twice a day.

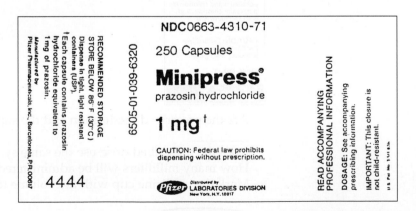

Are the prescribed medication and the supplied medication the same drug?

_____

How many capsule(s) will be administered? _____

8. PRESCRIPTION: glipizide (Glucotrol XL) 5 mg by mouth 30 minutes before breakfast.
Are the prescribed medication and the supplied medication the same drug?

_____

Does the prescribed dose use the same system of measurement? _____

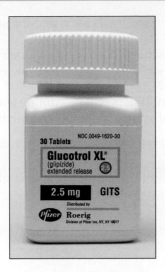

Is the prescribed dose the same as, larger, or smaller than the supplied
dose? _____
How many tablet(s) will be administered? _____

9. PRESCRIPTION: levofloxacin (Levaquin) 500 mg by mouth once daily for
10 days.

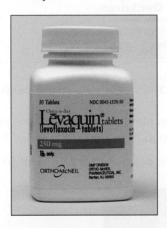

Are the prescribed medication and the supplied medication the same drug?
_____
Does the prescribed dose use the same system of measurement? _____
Is the prescribed dose the same as, larger, or smaller than the supplied
dose? _____
How many tablet(s) will be administered? _____

10. PRESCRIPTION: fluoxetine oral solution 40 mg by mouth daily.

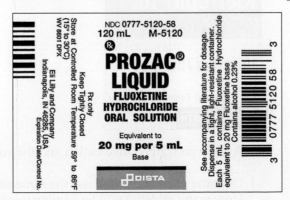

Are the prescribed medication and the supplied medication the same drug?
_____

Does the prescribed dose use the same system of measurement? _____
Does the prescribed dose use the same equivalent measurement within the same system? _____
How many milliliters will be administered? _____
Mark the oral syringe with the volume to be administered.

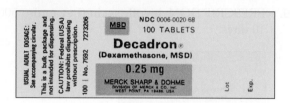

11. PRESCRIPTION: dexamethasone 1.5 mg by mouth with breakfast and dinner for 2 days, then 0.75 mg by mouth with breakfast and dinner the third day, then 0.75 mg by mouth with breakfast for 2 days (the fourth and fifth days).

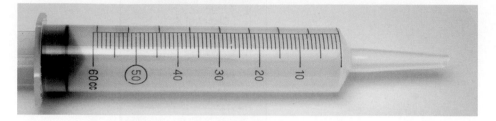

Are the prescribed medication and the supplied medication the same drug?
_____

Does the prescribed dose use the same system of measurement? _____
How many total tablets will be needed for the course of therapy? _____

12. PRESCRIPTION: potassium chloride ER 30 mEq by mouth daily.

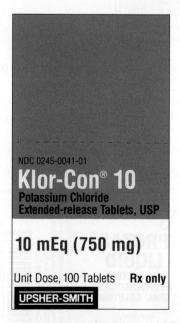

Are the prescribed medication and the supplied medication the same drug?
_____

Does the prescribed dose use the same unit of measurement? _____
How many tablet(s) will be administered? _____

13. PRESCRIPTION: methotrexate chemotherapy 10 mg by mouth daily.

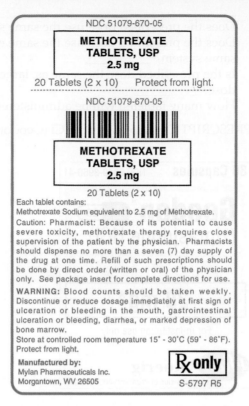

Are the prescribed medication and the supplied medication the same drug? _____

Does the prescribed dose use the same system of measurement? _____
Is the prescribed dose the same as, larger, or smaller than the supplied dose? _____
How many tablet(s) will be administered? _____

14. PRESCRIPTION: ondansetron hydrochloride (Zofran) 24 mg by mouth 30 minutes before chemotherapy administration.

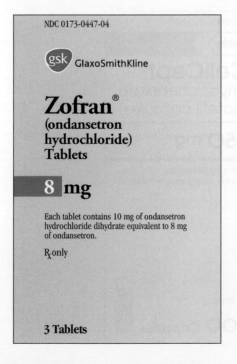

Are the prescribed medication and the supplied medication the same drug?
_____

Does the prescribed dose use the same system of measurement? _____

Does the prescribed dose use the same equivalent measurement within the same system? _____

Is the prescribed dose the same as, larger, or smaller than the supplied dose? _____

How many tablet(s) will be administered? _____

15. PRESCRIPTION: ziprasidone HCl (Geodon) 60 mg by mouth twice a day.

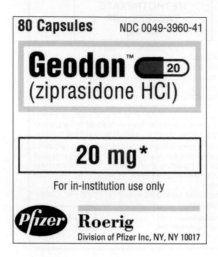

Are the prescribed medication and the supplied medication the same drug?
_____

Does the prescribed dose use the same system of measurement? _____

Is the prescribed dose the same as, larger, or smaller than the supplied dose? _____

How many capsule(s) will be administered? _____

16. PRESCRIPTION: mycophenolate mofetil (CellCept) 1.5 g by mouth twice a day.

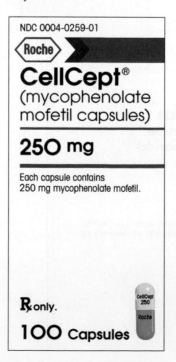

Are the prescribed medication and the supplied medication the same drug?
_____

Does the prescribed dose use the same unit of measurement? _____
How many capsule(s) will be administered? _____

17. PRESCRIPTION: loperamide hydrochloride solution (Imodium) 2 mg by mouth after each loose bowel movement.

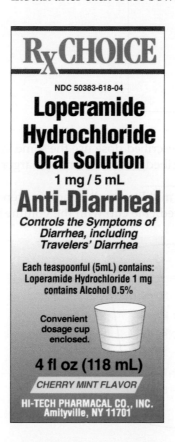

Are the prescribed medication and the supplied medication the same drug?
_____

Does the prescribed dose use the same system of measurement? _____
How many milliliters will be administered? _____
Mark the medicine cup with the volume to be administered.

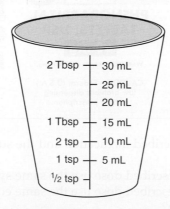

18. PRESCRIPTION: ranitidine hydrochloride (Zantac) syrup 150 mg by mouth at bedtime.

Are the prescribed medication and the supplied medication the same drug?
_____

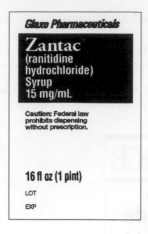

Does the prescribed dose use the same system of measurement? _____

Is the prescribed dose the same as, larger, or smaller than the supplied dose? _____

How many milliliters will be administered? _____

Mark the medicine cup with the volume to be administered.

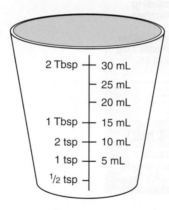

19.   PRESCRIPTION: phenobarbital 120 mg by mouth at bedtime.

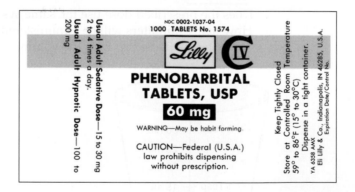

Are the prescribed medication and the supplied medication the same drug?

_____

Does the prescribed dose use the same system of measurement? _____

Does the prescribed dose use the same equivalent measurement within the same system? _____

Is the prescribed dose the same as, larger, or smaller than the supplied dose? _____

How many tablet(s) will be administered? _____

20. PRESCRIPTION: metformin (Glucophage) 1 g by mouth with morning and evening meal.

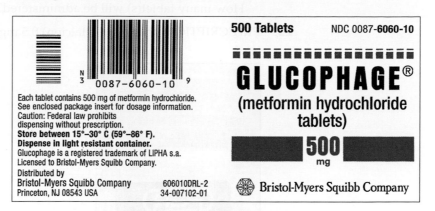

Are the prescribed medication and the supplied medication the same drug?

_____

Does the prescribed dose use the same unit of measurement? _____
Is the prescribed dose the same as, larger, or smaller than the supplied dose? _____
How many tablet(s) will be administered? _____

21. PRESCRIPTION: phenytoin sodium (Dilantin) extended-release 120 mg by mouth now.

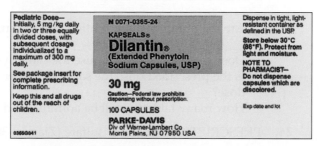

Are the prescribed medication and the supplied medication the same drug?

_____

Does the prescribed dose use the same system of measurement? _____
Is the prescribed dose the same as, larger, or smaller than the supplied dose? _____
How many capsule(s) will be administered? _____

22. PRESCRIPTION: ferrous sulfate (Feosol) 324 mg by mouth now.

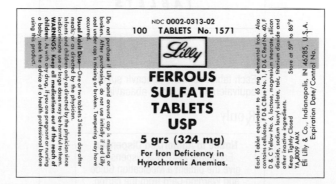

Are the prescribed medication and the supplied medication the same drug?

_____

Does the prescribed dose use the same system of measurement? _____

Is the prescribed dose the same as, larger, or smaller than the supplied dose? _____

How many tablet(s) will be administered? _____

23. PRESCRIPTION: triazolam (Halcion) 0.5 mg by mouth at bedtime.

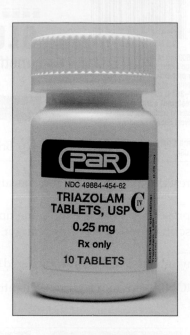

Are the prescribed medication and the supplied medication the same drug? _____

Does the prescribed dose use the same system of measurement? _____

Is the prescribed dose the same as, larger, or smaller than the supplied dose? _____

How many tablet(s) will be administered? _____

24. PRESCRIPTION: abacavir sulfate (Ziagen) 300 mg by mouth twice a day.

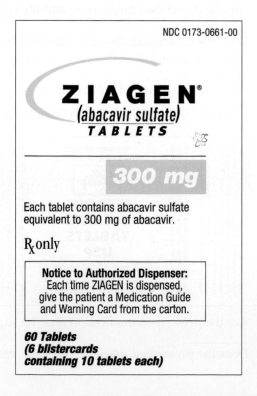

Are the prescribed medication and the supplied medication the same drug? _____

Does the prescribed dose use the same system of measurement? _____
Is the prescribed dose the same as, larger, or smaller than the supplied dose? _____
How many tablet(s) will be administered? _____

25. PRESCRIPTION: phenobarbital 60 mg by mouth at bedtime.

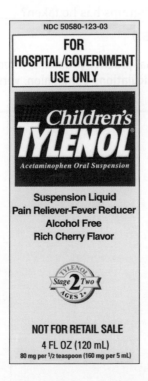

Are the prescribed medication and the supplied medication the same drug? _____

Does the prescribed dose use the same system of measurement? _____
Is the prescribed dose the same as, larger, or smaller than the supplied dose? _____
How many tablet(s) will be administered? _____

26. PRESCRIPTION: acetaminophen (Tylenol) elixir 80 mg by mouth now.

Are the prescribed medication and the supplied medication the same drug? _____

Does the prescribed dose use the same system of measurement? _____
Is the prescribed dose the same as, larger, or smaller than the supplied dose? _____

How many milliliters will be administered? _____

Mark the medicine cup with the volume to be administered.

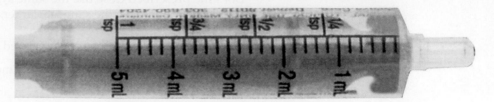

27. Mr. Tucker reports that he has taken three nitroglycerin tablets, each 5 minutes apart. He gives you the bottle.

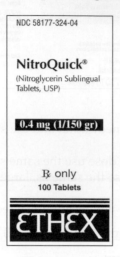

NDC 58177-324-04

NitroQuick®

(Nitroglycerin Sublingual Tablets, USP)

0.4 mg (1/150 gr)

℞ only
100 Tablets

ƎTHEX

How many milligrams has he taken? _____

(Answers on pp. 456–457)

ℰvolve   **For additional practice problems, refer to the Basic Calculations section of the Drug Calculations Companion, version 4 on Evolve.**

Parenteral Medications

Denise Macklin

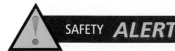

CLINICAL CONNECTION

- Understanding of the different routes of administration and common administration guidelines is important for correct administration of parenteral medications.
- It is very important to read labels carefully and determine the unit of measure and dose strength/volume. These factors will be used when performing drug calculations before administering the dose to the patient.

INTRODUCTION

Parenteral medications are medications that are administered through injection. The routes of administration include the following:

1. *Intramuscular (IM):* Into the muscle
2. *Intradermal (ID):* Into the dermis, as in a skin test
3. *Subcutaneous (Subcut):* Into the subcutaneous tissue, as with insulin and heparin
4. *Intravenous (IV):* Into a vein
5. *Intrathecal/epidural:* Into the spinal fluid
6. *Intraosseus (IO):* Into the bone
7. *Intraperitoneal (IP):* Into the peritoneal cavity

SAFETY ALERT

Any discrepancy between the medication administration record (MAR), current dose, and your calculations, should warrant assistance from another professional.

PARENTERAL MEDICATIONS

CLINICAL ALERT

Many antibiotics come in powder form and need to be mixed (see Chapter 12) before administration.

CLINICAL ALERT

Some intravenous push medications require dilution owing to their acidity. For example, dilute IV push morphine, phenergen, and versed.

Intramusuclar injections are less common today than in the past. The most common method of administering parenteral medications in the clinical setting is intravenous by either slow push, intermittent, piggyback, or continuous infusion. However, it is still important to be knowledgeable about all routes of administration. In this chapter prescriptions will use the intramuscular, subcutaneous, and intravenous push routes. The prescriptions that follow may not use the most common route of administration for a particular drug in the clinical setting (although it is acceptable) but have been chosen to offer the best opportunity for calculation and syringe practice. Except for intravenous push medications, intravenous prescriptions are prepared in the pharmacy. Parenteral medications commonly come prepared as a liquid in vials or in ampules, but they can also come as powders that require reconstitution (discussed in Chapter 12) or in prefilled syringes (discussed in Chapter 9) (Figure 11-1).

Solution containers are either single-dose or multidose (Figure 11-2). Single-dose is for single usage and multidose may be used more than once (Figure 11-3). Parenteral labels have many similarities to oral medication labels (discussed in Chapter 10). The labels include the trade name of the drug, which is the trademark of the drug manufacturer (may or may not be present); the generic name of the drug (always present); the lot number; an expiration date (drug is to be administered before this date); and a bar code (Figure 11-4).

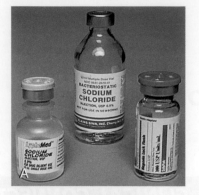

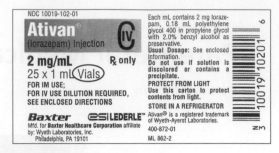

NDC 10019-102-01

Ativan®
(lorazepam) Injection

2 mg/mL

25 x 1 mL Vials

FOR IM USE;
FOR IV USE DILUTION REQUIRED,
SEE ENCLOSED DIRECTIONS

C IV

Rx only

Each mL contains 2 mg lorazepam, 0.18 mL polyethylene
glycol 400 in propylene glycol
with 2.0% benzyl alcohol as
preservative.
Usual Dosage: See enclosed
information.
Do not use if solution is
discolored or contains a
precipitate.
PROTECT FROM LIGHT
Use this carton to protect
contents from light.
STORE IN A REFRIGERATOR
Ativan® is a registered trademark
of Wyeth-Ayerst Laboratories.
400-872-01
ML 862-2

Baxter   **esiLEDERLE™**
Mfd. for **Baxter Healthcare Corporation** affiliate
by: Wyeth Laboratories, Inc.
Philadelphia, PA 19101

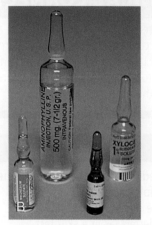

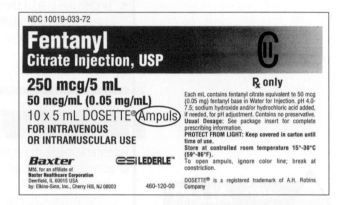

NDC 10019-033-72

Fentanyl
Citrate Injection, USP

250 mcg/5 mL
50 mcg/mL (0.05 mg/mL)

10 x 5 mL DOSETTE® Ampuls

FOR INTRAVENOUS
OR INTRAMUSCULAR USE

C II

Rx only

Each mL contains fentanyl citrate equivalent to 50 mcg
(0.05 mg) fentanyl base in Water for Injection. pH 4.0-
7.5; sodium hydroxide and/or hydrochloric acid added,
if needed, for pH adjustment. Contains no preservative.
Usual Dosage: See package insert for complete
prescribing information.
PROTECT FROM LIGHT: Keep covered in carton until
time of use.
Store at controlled room temperature 15°-30°C
(59°-86°F).
To open ampuls, ignore color line; break at
constriction.

DOSETTE® is a registered trademark of A.H. Robins
Company

Baxter   **esiLEDERLE™**
Mfd. for an affiliate of
Baxter Healthcare Corporation
Deerfield, IL 60015 USA
by: Elkins-Sinn, Inc., Cherry Hill, NJ 08003   460-120-00

---

a   Fliptop Vial   Sterile Powder   10 Units/**NDC 0074-6533-01**
                                                        6533

STERILE VANCOMYCIN HYDROCHLORIDE, USP
For Intravenous Use.   Rx only

Equivalent to **1 g** Vancomycin

MUST BE FURTHER DILUTED BEFORE USE. SEE INSERT.

ABBOTT LABORATORIES, NORTH CHICAGO, IL 60064, USA

(01) 1 030074 653301 3

C

---

1 gram/10 mL Vial   NDC 0004-1964-01

Roche

ROCEPHIN®
(ceftriaxone sodium) FOR INJECTION

1 gram   Single Use Vials

For Intramuscular or Intravenous Use.
Each vial contains ceftriaxone sodium powder
equivalent to 1 gram ceftriaxone.   Rx only.

10 VIALS (Not actual size)

D

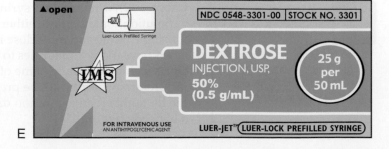

▲ open

Luer-Lock Prefilled Syringe

NDC 0548-3301-00   STOCK NO. 3301

IMS

DEXTROSE
INJECTION, USP,
50%
(0.5 g/mL)

25 g
per
50 mL

FOR INTRAVENOUS USE
AN ANTIHYPOGLYCEMIC AGENT

LUER-JET™ LUER-LOCK PREFILLED SYRINGE

E

Figure 11-1 Parenteral medications. **A,** Vials. **B,** Ampules. **C,**
Sterile powder. **D,** Powder. **E,** Luer-Lok prefilled syringe. (**A** and **B** from
Elkin MK, Perry AG, Potter PA: Nursing interventions and clinical skills,
ed 4, St Louis, 2008, Mosby.)

CHAPTER 11

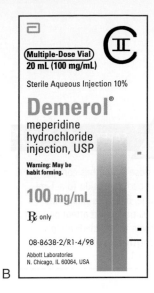

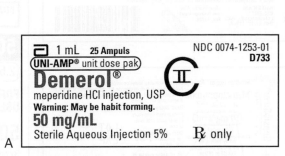

Figure 11-2 A, Unit dose pack. **B,** Multidose vial.

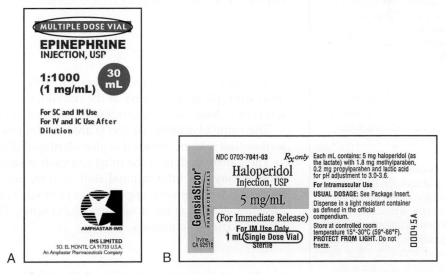

Figure 11-3 A, Multidose vial. **B,** Single-dose vial.

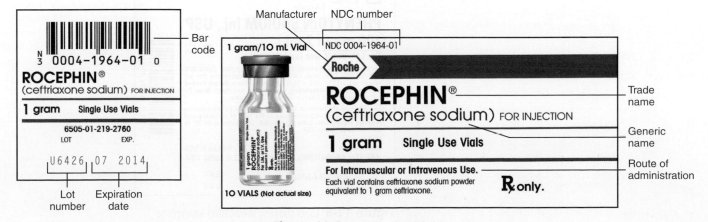

Figure 11-4 Parts of a drug label.

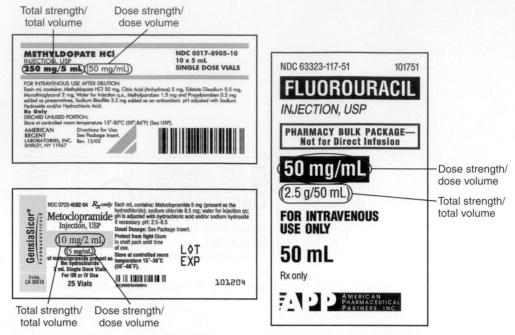

Total strength/total volume — Dose strength/dose volume

Dose strength/dose volume

Total strength/total volume

Total strength/total volume — Dose strength/dose volume

Figure 11-5 Labels showing dose strength/dose volume and total strength/total volume.

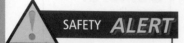
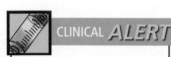
The difference between a parenteral label and an oral label is the inclusion of the **total strength/total volume** of the container, as well as a **dose strength** described in terms of a **dose volume,** commonly (but not always) mg/mL (Figure 11-5).

The route of administration is always identified. Sometimes the route of administration that is to be avoided is also identified (Figures 11-7 and 11-8).

The metric system is the most common system used with medications. But medications may use international unit system, percentages, ratios, or milliequivalents (Figure 11-9). It is very important to read labels carefully and to identify the unit of measure as well as the dose strength/volume. These factors will be used when performing drug calculations.

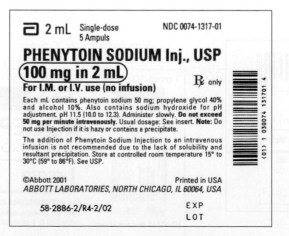

Figure 11-6 Label showing medication strength to volume.

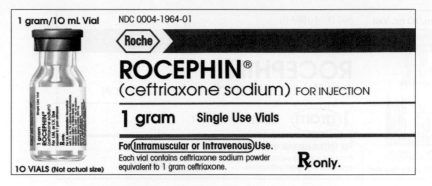

1 gram/10 mL Vial NDC 0004-1964-01

〈Roche〉

ROCEPHIN®
(ceftriaxone sodium) FOR INJECTION

1 gram **Single Use Vials**

For Intramuscular or Intravenous Use.
Each vial contains ceftriaxone sodium powder
equivalent to 1 gram ceftriaxone.

℞ only.

10 VIALS (Not actual size)

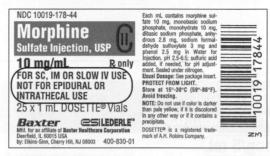

NDC 10019-178-44

Morphine Ⓒ
Sulfate Injection, USP
10 mg/mL ℞ only
FOR SC, IM OR SLOW IV USE
NOT FOR EPIDURAL OR
INTRATHECAL USE
25 x 1 mL DOSETTE® Vials

Baxter eSi LEDERLE™
Mfd. for an affiliate of **Baxter Healthcare Corporation**
Deerfield, IL 60015 USA
by: Elkins-Sinn, Cherry Hill, NJ 08003   400-830-01

Each mL contains morphine sulfate 10 mg, monobasic sodium
phosphate, monohydrate 10 mg,
dibasic sodium phosphate, anhydrous 2.8 mg, sodium formaldehyde sulfoxylate 3 mg and
phenol 2.5 mg in Water for
Injection. pH 2.5-6.5; sulfuric acid
added, if needed, for pH adjustment. Sealed under nitrogen.
Usual Dosage: See package insert.
PROTECT FROM LIGHT.
Store at 15°-30°C (59°-86°F).
Avoid freezing.
NOTE: Do not use if color is darker
than pale yellow, if it is discolored
in any other way or if it contains a
precipitate.
DOSETTE® is a registered trademark of A.H. Robins Company.

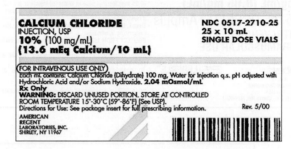

CALCIUM CHLORIDE
INJECTION, USP
10% (100 mg/mL)
(13.6 mEq Calcium/10 mL)

NDC 0517-2710-25
25 x 10 mL
SINGLE DOSE VIALS

FOR INTRAVENOUS USE ONLY
Each mL contains: Calcium Chloride (Dihydrate) 100 mg, Water for Injection q.s. pH adjusted with
Hydrochloric Acid and/or Sodium Hydroxide. 2.04 mOsmol/mL.
Rx Only
WARNING: DISCARD UNUSED PORTION. STORE AT CONTROLLED
ROOM TEMPERATURE 15°-30°C (59°-86°F) (See USP).
Directions for Use: See package insert for full prescribing information.

AMERICAN
REGENT
LABORATORIES, INC.
SHIRLEY, NY 11967

Rev. 5/00

Figure 11-7 Labels showing routes of administration.

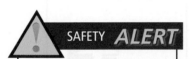

SAFETY *ALERT*

Never assume that if a medication can be given intravenously
it can also be given by other
routes.

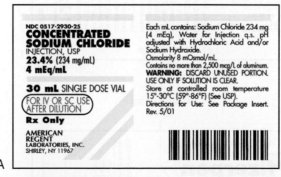

NDC 0517-2930-25
**CONCENTRATED
SODIUM CHLORIDE**
INJECTION, USP
23.4% (234 mg/mL)
4 mEq/mL

30 mL SINGLE DOSE VIAL
FOR IV OR SC USE
AFTER DILUTION
Rx Only

AMERICAN
REGENT
LABORATORIES, INC.
SHIRLEY, NY 11967

Each mL contains: Sodium Chloride 234 mg
(4 mEq), Water for Injection q.s. pH
adjusted with Hydrochloric Acid and/or
Sodium Hydroxide.
Osmolarity 8 mOsmol/mL.
Contains no more than 2,500 mcg/L of aluminum.
WARNING: DISCARD UNUSED PORTION.
USE ONLY IF SOLUTION IS CLEAR.
Store at controlled room temperature
15°-30°C (59°-86°F) (See USP).
Directions for Use: See Package Insert.
Rev. 5/01

A

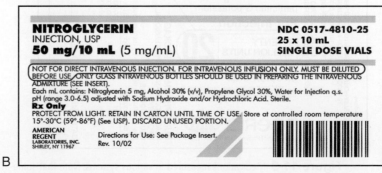

NITROGLYCERIN
INJECTION, USP
50 mg/10 mL (5 mg/mL)

NDC 0517-4810-25
25 x 10 mL
SINGLE DOSE VIALS

NOT FOR DIRECT INTRAVENOUS INJECTION. FOR INTRAVENOUS INFUSION ONLY. MUST BE DILUTED
BEFORE USE. ONLY GLASS INTRAVENOUS BOTTLES SHOULD BE USED IN PREPARING THE INTRAVENOUS
ADMIXTURE (SEE INSERT).
Each mL contains: Nitroglycerin 5 mg, Alcohol 30% (v/v), Propylene Glycol 30%, Water for Injection q.s.
pH (range 3.0-6.5) adjusted with Sodium Hydroxide and/or Hydrochloric Acid. Sterile.
Rx Only
PROTECT FROM LIGHT. RETAIN IN CARTON UNTIL TIME OF USE. Store at controlled room temperature
15°-30°C (59°-86°F) (See USP). DISCARD UNUSED PORTION.

AMERICAN
REGENT
LABORATORIES, INC.
SHIRLEY, NY 11967

Directions for Use: See Package Insert.
Rev. 10/02

B

Figure 11-8 A, Potassium chloride label. **B,** Nitroglycerin label.

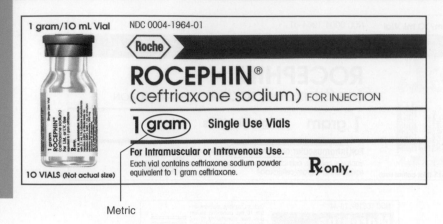

Metric

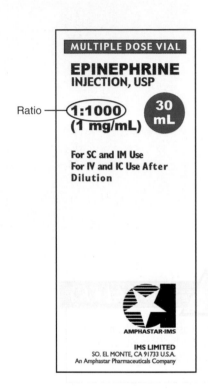

Ratio

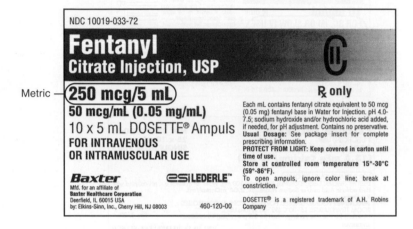

Metric

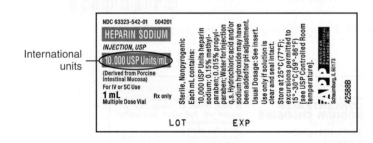

International units

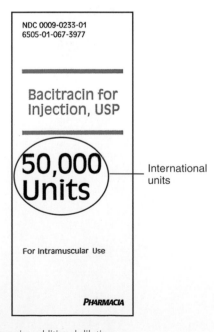

International units

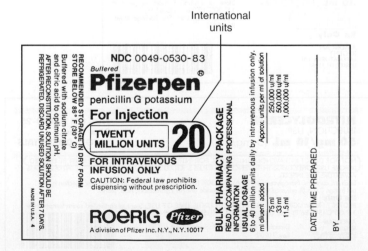

International units

Figure 11-9 Medications measured in various systems. Note that some drugs require additional dilution.

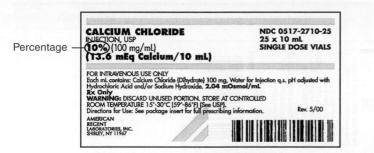

Percentage → **CALCIUM CHLORIDE**
INJECTION, USP
10% (100 mg/mL)
(13.6 mEq Calcium/10 mL)

NDC 0517-2710-25
25 x 10 mL
SINGLE DOSE VIALS

FOR INTRAVENOUS USE ONLY
Each mL contains: Calcium Chloride (Dihydrate) 100 mg, Water for Injection q.s. pH adjusted with Hydrochloric Acid and/or Sodium Hydroxide. **2.04 mOsmol/mL**
Rx Only
WARNING: DISCARD UNUSED PORTION. STORE AT CONTROLLED ROOM TEMPERATURE 15°-30°C (59°-86°F) (See USP).
Directions for Use: See package insert for full prescribing information.

AMERICAN
REGENT
LABORATORIES, INC.
SHIRLEY, NY 11967

Rev. 5/00

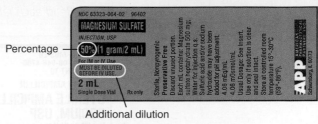

Percentage → **MAGNESIUM SULFATE**
50% (1 gram/2 mL)
For IM or IV Use
MUST BE DILUTED BEFORE IV USE. ← Additional dilution
2 mL
Single Dose Vial   Rx only

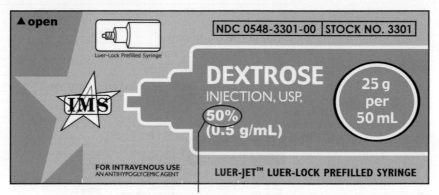

▲ open   Luer-Lock Prefilled Syringe

NDC 0548-3301-00 | STOCK NO. 3301

IMS

DEXTROSE
INJECTION, USP,
50%
(0.5 g/mL)

25 g per 50 mL

FOR INTRAVENOUS USE
AN ANTIHYPOGLYCEMIC AGENT

LUER-JET™ LUER-LOCK PREFILLED SYRINGE

Percentage

Milliequivalents

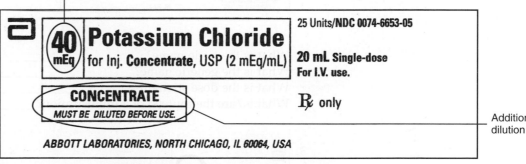

40 mEq **Potassium Chloride**
for Inj. **Concentrate**, USP (2 mEq/mL)

25 Units/NDC 0074-6653-05

20 mL Single-dose
For I.V. use.

CONCENTRATE
MUST BE DILUTED BEFORE USE.

℞ only

← Additional dilution

ABBOTT LABORATORIES, NORTH CHICAGO, IL 60064, USA

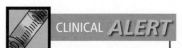

CLINICAL ALERT

Not all intravenous medications can or should be given as an intravenous push. Many require that they be diluted in some other solution and be infused over a longer period. With some intravenous push medications, once the correct dose volume has been calculated, further dilution is required before administration.

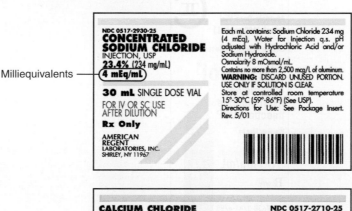

NDC 0517-2930-25
CONCENTRATED SODIUM CHLORIDE
INJECTION, USP
23.4% (234 mg/mL)
Milliequivalents → **4 mEq/mL**

30 mL SINGLE DOSE VIAL
FOR IV OR SC USE
AFTER DILUTION
Rx Only

AMERICAN
REGENT
LABORATORIES, INC.
SHIRLEY, NY 11967

Each mL contains: Sodium Chloride 234 mg (4 mEq), Water for Injection q.s. pH adjusted with Hydrochloric Acid and/or Sodium Hydroxide.
Osmolarity 8 mOsmol/mL.
Contains no more than 2,500 mcg/L of aluminum.
WARNING: DISCARD UNUSED PORTION. USE ONLY IF SOLUTION IS CLEAR.
Store at controlled room temperature 15°-30°C (59°-86°F) (See USP).
Directions for Use: See Package Insert.
Rev. 5/01

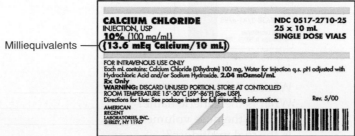

CALCIUM CHLORIDE
INJECTION, USP
10% (100 mg/mL)
Milliequivalents → **(13.6 mEq Calcium/10 mL)**

NDC 0517-2710-25
25 x 10 mL
SINGLE DOSE VIALS

FOR INTRAVENOUS USE ONLY
Each mL contains: Calcium Chloride (Dihydrate) 100 mg, Water for Injection q.s. pH adjusted with Hydrochloric Acid and/or Sodium Hydroxide. **2.04 mOsmol/mL**
Rx Only
WARNING: DISCARD UNUSED PORTION. STORE AT CONTROLLED ROOM TEMPERATURE 15°-30°C (59°-86°F) (See USP).
Directions for Use: See package insert for full prescribing information.

AMERICAN
REGENT
LABORATORIES, INC.
SHIRLEY, NY 11967

Rev. 5/00

Figure 11-9 cont'd Medications measured in various systems. Note that some drugs require additional dilution.

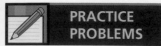

PRACTICE PROBLEMS

Directions: *Read each label and locate information necessary to fill in the blanks.*

1.

NDC 0015-7403-20
NSN 6505-00-946-4700
EQUIVALENT TO
500 mg AMPICILLIN
STERILE AMPICILLIN SODIUM, USP
For IM or IV Use
CAUTION: Federal law prohibits dispensing without prescription.

For IM use, add 1.8 mL diluent (read accompanying circular). Resulting solution contains 250 mg ampicillin per mL.
Use solution within 1 hour.
This vial contains ampicillin sodium equivalent to 500 mg ampicillin.
Usual Dosage: Adults—250 to 500 mg IM q. 6h.
READ ACCOMPANYING CIRCULAR for detailed indications, IM or IV dosage and precautions.
APOTHECON®
A Bristol-Myers Squibb Company
Princeton, NJ 08540 USA   7403200RL-2

Cont:
Exp. Date:

What is the trade name? _____
What is the generic name? _____
What is the dose strength? _____
What is/are the route(s) of administration? _____

2.

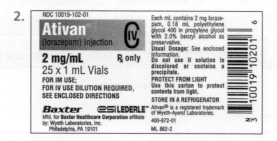

NDC 10019-102-01
Ativan®
(lorazepam) Injection
2 mg/mL
25 × 1 mL Vials
FOR IM USE;
FOR IV USE DILUTION REQUIRED, SEE ENCLOSED DIRECTIONS
Baxter **eSiLEDERLE™**
Mfd. for **Baxter Healthcare Corporation** affiliate by: Wyeth Laboratories, Inc.
Philadelphia, PA 19101

C IV
℞ only

Each mL contains 2 mg lorazepam, 0.18 mL polyethylene glycol 400 in propylene glycol with 2.0% benzyl alcohol as preservative.
Usual Dosage: See enclosed information.
Do not use if solution is discolored or contains a precipitate.
PROTECT FROM LIGHT
Use this carton to protect contents from light.
STORE IN A REFRIGERATOR
Ativan® is a registered trademark of Wyeth-Ayerst Laboratories.
400-872-01
ML 862-2

What is the trade name? _____
What is the generic name? _____
What is the dose strength? _____
What is/are the route(s) of administration? _____

3.

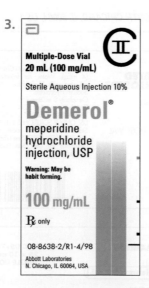

Multiple-Dose Vial
20 mL (100 mg/mL)

Sterile Aqueous Injection 10%

Demerol®
meperidine hydrochloride injection, USP

Warning: May be habit forming.

100 mg/mL

℞ only

08-8638-2/R1-4/98

Abbott Laboratories
N. Chicago, IL 60064, USA

C II

What is the trade name? _____
What is the generic name? _____
What is the dose volume? _____
Is the vial multidose? _____
Is the vial single-dose? _____

4.

NDC 10019-028-05

See opposite panel for additional
prescribing information.

Midazolam HCl Injection

5 mg/5 mL* (1 mg/mL*)

R̠ only   C̶I̶V̶

10 x 5 mL Vials
FOR INTRAMUSCULAR OR INTRAVENOUS USE
STERILE

Baxter
Mfd. for an affiliate of
Baxter Healthcare Corporation
Deerfield, IL 60015 USA
by: **MOVA** PHARMACEUTICAL CORPORATION
Caguas PR 00725 USA

460-015-03

What is the trade name? _____

What is the dose volume? _____

What is/are the route(s) of administration? _____

5.

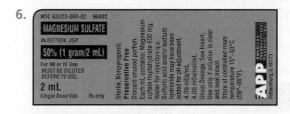

6 VIAFLEX PLUS Single Dose Containers

Diflucan®
(fluconazole) injection   **400 mg**

ISO-OSMOTIC **SODIUM CHLORIDE** DILUENT

Pfizer Roerig   **200 mL**
(2 mg/mL)*   NDC 0049-3436-26
2B3436
STERILE NONPYROGENIC

* Each 200 mL contains 400 mg of fluconazole and 1.8 g of Sodium Chloride (USP) in Water
for Injection (USP). Osmolarity 315 mOsmol/L (CALC).
DOSAGE: Intravenously as directed by a physician. See package insert.
CAUTIONS: Squeeze and inspect inner container which maintains product sterility.
Discard if leaks are found. Do not add supplementary medication. Must not be used in series
connections. Do not use unless solution is clear.
Rx only
STORAGE: STORE UNITS IN MOISTURE BARRIER OVERWRAP BETWEEN 77°F (25°C) AND
41°F (5°C) UNTIL READY TO USE. AVOID EXCESSIVE HEAT. **PROTECT FROM FREEZING.**

VIAFLEX PLUS   **SINGLE DOSE CONTAINER**   PL 146 PLASTIC
DIFLUCAN IS A REGISTERED TRADEMARK OF PFIZER INC.
VIAFLEX AND PL 146 ARE REGISTERED TRADEMARKS OF BAXTER INTERNATIONAL INC.
MANUFACTURED FOR **ROERIG, A DIV OF PFIZER INC,** NY, NY 10017 USA
BY BAXTER HEALTHCARE CORPORATION, DEERFIELD, IL 60015 USA
03-4585-00-4   6505-01-319-6652   7-4-1-431   1214

What is the trade name? _____

What is the generic name? _____

What is the dose volume? _____

What is/are the route(s) of administration? _____

Is the container multidose? _____

Is the container single-dose? _____

6.

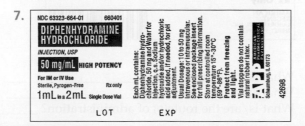

NDC 63323-064-02   96402

MAGNESIUM SULFATE
INJECTION, USP

50% (1 gram/2 mL)

For IM or IV Use
MUST BE DILUTED
BEFORE IV USE.

2 mL
Single Dose Vial   Rx only

Sterile, Nonpyrogenic
Preservative Free
Discard unused portion.
Each mL contains: Magnesium
sulfate heptahydrate 500 mg;
Water for Injection q.s.
Sulfuric acid and/or sodium
hydroxide may have been
added for pH adjustment.
4.06 mEq/mL
4.06 mOsmol/mL
Usual Dosage: See insert.
Use only if solution is clear
and seal intact.
Store at controlled room
temperature 15°-30°C
(59°-86°F).

APP AMERICAN
PHARMACEUTICAL
PARTNERS, INC.
Schaumburg, IL 60173

What is the generic name? _____

What is the dose volume? _____

What is/are the route(s) of administration? _____

7.

NDC 63323-664-01   660401

DIPHENHYDRAMINE
HYDROCHLORIDE

INJECTION, USP

50 mg/mL HIGH POTENCY

For IM or IV Use
Sterile, Pyrogen-Free   Rx only

1 mL in a **2 mL** Single Dose Vial

LOT   EXP

Each mL contains:
Diphenhydramine hydro-
chloride, 50 mg and Water for
Injection, q.s. Sodium
hydroxide and/or hydrochloric
acid added, if needed, for pH
adjustment.
Usual Dosage: 10 to 50 mg
Intravenous or intramuscular.
See enclosed package insert
for full prescribing information.
Store at controlled room
temperature 15°-30°C
(59°-86°F).
Protect from freezing
and light.
Vial stoppers do not contain
natural rubber latex.

APP AMERICAN
PHARMACEUTICAL
PARTNERS, INC.
Schaumburg, IL 60173

42698

What is the generic name? _____

What is the dose volume? _____

What is/are the route(s) of administration? _____

Is the vial multidose? _____

Is the vial single-dose? _____

8.

NITROGLYCERIN
INJECTION, USP
50 mg/10 mL (5 mg/mL)

NDC 0517-4810-25
25 x 10 mL
SINGLE DOSE VIALS

NOT FOR DIRECT INTRAVENOUS INJECTION. FOR INTRAVENOUS INFUSION ONLY. MUST BE DILUTED BEFORE USE. ONLY GLASS INTRAVENOUS BOTTLES SHOULD BE USED IN PREPARING THE INTRAVENOUS ADMIXTURE (SEE INSERT).
Each mL contains: Nitroglycerin 5 mg, Alcohol 30% (v/v), Propylene Glycol 30%, Water for Injection q.s. pH (range 3.0-6.5) adjusted with Sodium Hydroxide and/or Hydrochloric Acid. Sterile.
Rx Only
PROTECT FROM LIGHT. RETAIN IN CARTON UNTIL TIME OF USE. Store at controlled room temperature 15°-30°C (59°-86°F) (See USP). DISCARD UNUSED PORTION.

AMERICAN
REGENT
LABORATORIES, INC.
SHIRLEY, NY 11967

Directions for Use: See Package Insert.
Rev. 10/02

What is the generic name? _____

What is the dose volume? _____

What is/are the route(s) of administration? _____

What route of administration is not to be used? _____

Is the vial multidose? _____

Is the vial single-dose? _____

9.

10 - 1 mL Single Use Vials

AMGEN®

Neupogen®
Filgrastim

A Recombinant Granulocyte Colony Stimulating Factor (rG-CSF) derived from *E Coli*

**300
mcg**

300 mcg/1 mL
For Subcutaneous or Intravenous Use Only
Sterile Solution - No Preservative

U.S. Patent Nos.
4,810,643; 4,999,291;
5,582,823; 5,580,755

What is the trade name? _____

What is the generic name? _____

What is the dose volume? _____

What is/are the route(s) of administration? _____

Is the vial multidose? _____

Is the vial single-dose? _____

10.

NDC 0517-2930-25
**CONCENTRATED
SODIUM CHLORIDE**
INJECTION, USP
23.4% (234 mg/mL)
4 mEq/mL

30 mL SINGLE DOSE VIAL

FOR IV OR SC USE
AFTER DILUTION

Rx Only

AMERICAN
REGENT
LABORATORIES, INC.
SHIRLEY, NY 11967

Each mL contains: Sodium Chloride 234 mg (4 mEq), Water for Injection q.s. pH adjusted with Hydrochloric Acid and/or Sodium Hydroxide.
Osmolarity 8 mOsmol/mL.
Contains no more than 2,500 mcg/L of aluminum.
WARNING: DISCARD UNUSED PORTION. USE ONLY IF SOLUTION IS CLEAR.
Store at controlled room temperature 15°-30°C (59°-86°F) (See USP).
Directions for Use: See Package Insert.
Rev. 5/01

What is the generic name? _____

What is the dose volume? _____

What is/are the route(s) of administration? _____

(Answers on p. 457)

GUIDELINES FOR DOSE ADMINISTRATION

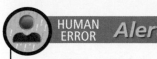

HUMAN ERROR *Alert*

Always verify the route of administration of all medications to avoid adverse patient reactions.

When administering parenteral medications, there are common guidelines for the volume that can be safely administered with one syringe.

Common guidelines for dose administration are as follows:

Subcutaneous: 0.5-1 mL for adult, <0.5 mL for child <0.1 mL for infant.

Intramuscular: <3 mL for adult, <2 mL for child, <1 mL for infant.

Intravenous push: The time over which a medication is administered is important. Each medication has its own guidelines for administration. For example, a particular medication may require administering at 10 mg over 1 minute, 80 mg over 5 minutes, and so forth.

Intrathecal: <3 mL bolus for adult, <2 mL for children, <0.5 mL for infant.

Intradermal: <0.5 mL for adult, <0.3 mL for child, <0.1 mL for infant.

CALCULATING PARENTERAL DOSAGES

CLINICAL *ALERT*

The patient's condition must be considered in conjunction with the guidelines when you are determining the number of syringes and injection sites.

With the ratio-proportion method, parenteral medication calculations utilize the dose strength/dose volume you HAVE as the left (complete) ratio. The right (incomplete) ratio has the prescribed dose in the numerator and X (the unknown volume) in the denominator. When a medication is given intravenous push, it may be necessary to determine how much volume is going to be pushed over a specific time period. What you want to know is the volume of medication that can be given in a specific time, such as 1 minute. What you HAVE is the intravenous push guideline in volume (mL)/time (minute). Note that in this ratio-proportion, the volume will be in the numerator. Rounding is determined by syringe calibration (p. 104) (i.e., 3 mL syringes round to the nearest tenth).

Example 1

| PRESCRIPTION | *Atropine sulfate 0.6 mg intravenous push now.* |

• **What You HAVE**

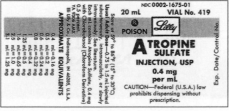

• **What You KNOW**   Prescribed dose is 0.6 mg.

• **What You WANT (X)**   The number of milliliters required to administer atropine sulfate 0.6 mg.

CRITICAL THINKING

Are the prescribed medication and the medication you HAVE the same? _____

Does the prescribed dose use the same system of measurement as the medication you HAVE? _____

Does the prescribed dose use the same equivalent measurement within the same system? _____

Is the prescribed dose larger or smaller than the dose you HAVE? _____

In setting up a ratio-proportion, place in the LEFT ratio the medication dose strength per volume you HAVE on hand; in the RIGHT ratio, place the prescribed dose in the numerator and place X (the unknown volume) in the denominator.

Multiply to get the cross-products.

Divide the numerical cross-product by the numerical multiplier of X (the number in front of X).

The result is the answer for X.

Label answer properly in units (i.e., number of tablets, number of milliliters).

Check answer by placing the number obtained for X in the original equation. Cross-multiply. The cross-products should be approximately equal.

ANSWER FOR BEST CARE

Medication comparison? Yes.
System of measurement? Yes; metric.
Unit of measure comparison? Yes; milliliters
Dose larger.
Perform calculation.

$$\frac{0.4 \text{ mg}}{1 \text{ mL}} = \frac{0.6 \text{ mg}}{X \text{ mL}} \qquad 0.4X = 0.6$$

$$0.6 \div 0.4 = 4\overline{\smash{)}6.0} \\ \underline{4} \\ 20$$

$$\begin{array}{r} 1.5 \end{array}$$

$$X = 1.5$$

Label with the unit of measure.
1.5 mL

✓ **Human Error Check**

Replace X with 1.5 and cross-multiply.

$$\frac{0.4}{1} = \frac{0.6}{1.5}$$

$0.4 \times 1.5 = 1 \times 0.6$
$0.6 = 0.6$

Guideline: The dose volume is less than the 3-mL maximum volume for intramuscular administration.

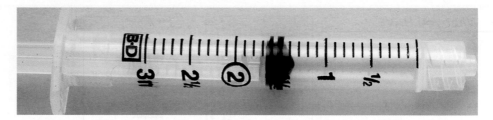

Example 2

PRESCRIPTION   *Midazolam hydrochloride (Versed) 4 mg intramuscular 1 hour before surgery.*

• **What You HAVE**

NDC 10019-028-05

See opposite panel for additional prescribing information.

Midazolam HCl Injection

5 mg/5 mL* (1 mg/mL*)

10 x 5 mL Vials
**FOR INTRAMUSCULAR OR INTRAVENOUS USE
STERILE**

℞ only

Baxter
Mfd. for an affiliate of
Baxter Healthcare Corporation
Deerfield, IL 60015 USA
by: **MOVA** PHARMACEUTICAL CORPORATION
Caguas PR 00725 USA

460-015-03

• **What You KNOW**   Prescribed dose is 4 mg.

• **What You WANT (X)**   The milliliters required to administer midazolam hydrochloride 4 mg.

CRITICAL THINKING	Are the prescribed medication and the medication you HAVE the same drug? _____

Does the prescribed dose use the same system of measurement as the medication you HAVE? _____

Does the prescribed dose use the same equivalent measurement within the same system? _____

Is the prescribed dose larger or smaller than the dose you HAVE? _____

In setting up a ratio-proportion, place in the LEFT ratio the medication dose strength per volume you HAVE on hand; in the RIGHT ratio, place the prescribed dose in the numerator and place X (the unknown volume) in the denominator.

Multiply to get the cross-products.

Divide the numerical cross-product by the numerical multiplier of X (the number in front of X).

The result is the answer for X.

Label answer properly in units (i.e., number of tablets, number of milliliters).

Check answer by placing the number obtained for X in the original equation. Cross-multiply. The cross-products should be approximately equal.

ANSWER FOR BEST CARE	Medication comparison? Yes.

System of measurement? Yes; metric.

Unit of measure comparison? Yes; milligrams.

Dose larger.

Perform calculation.

$$\frac{1\ mg}{X\ mL} = \frac{4\ mg}{X\ mL}$$

$$X = 4$$

Label with the unit of measure.

4 mL

> ✔ **Human Error Check**
>
> Replace X with 4 and cross-multiply.
>
> $$\frac{1}{1} = \frac{4}{4}$$
>
> $1 \times 4 = 1 \times 4$
> $4 = 4$

Guideline: Intramuscular: <3 mL for an adult, <2 mL for a child, and <1 mL for an infant. Because 4 mL is larger than the recommended maximum volume for intramuscular injections, the dose should be divided into two syringes.

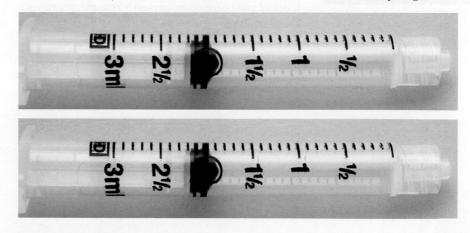

Example 3

PRESCRIPTION   *Digoxin (Lanoxin) 250 mcg intravenous push now.*

- **What You HAVE**

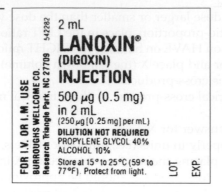

542282

2 mL
LANOXIN®
(DIGOXIN)
INJECTION
500 µg (0.5 mg)
in 2 mL
(250 µg [0.25 mg] per mL)
DILUTION NOT REQUIRED
PROPYLENE GLYCOL 40%
ALCOHOL 10%
Store at 15° to 25°C (59° to
77°F). Protect from light.

FOR I.V. OR I.M. USE
BURROUGHS WELLCOME CO.
Research Triangle Park, NC 27709

LOT
EXP.

- **What You KNOW**   Prescribed dose is 250 mcg.

- **What You WANT (X)**   The milliliters required to administer digoxin 200 mcg.

CRITICAL THINKING   Are the prescribed medication and the medication you HAVE the same? _____
Does the prescribed dose use the same system of measurement as the medication
    you HAVE? _____
Does the prescribed dose use the same equivalent measurement within the same
    system? _____
Is the prescribed dose larger or smaller than the dose you HAVE? _____
In setting up a ratio-proportion, place in the LEFT ratio the medication dose strength
    per volume you HAVE on hand; in the RIGHT ratio, place the prescribed dose in
    the numerator and place X (the unknown volume) in the denominator.
Multiply to get the cross-products.
Divide the numerical cross-product by the numerical multiplier of X (the number in
    front of X).
The result is the answer for X.
Label answer properly in units (i.e., number of tablets, number of milliliters).
Check answer by placing the number obtained for X in the original equation. Cross-
    multiply. The cross-products should be approximately equal.

**ANSWER FOR
BEST CARE**   Medication comparison? Yes.
System of measurement? Yes; metric.
Unit of measure comparison? Yes; micrograms.
Dose smaller.
Perform calculation.

$$\frac{500 \text{ mcg}}{2 \text{ mL}} = \frac{250 \text{ mcg}}{X \text{ mL}}$$

$$500X = 500$$

$$500\overline{)500}^{1}$$

$$X = 1$$

Label with the unit of measure.
1 mL

✓ **Human Error Check**

Replace X with 1 and cross-multiply.

$$\frac{500}{2} = \frac{250}{1}$$

$500 \times 1 = 250 \times 2$
$500 = 500$

Guideline: Administer intravenous digoxin injections over 5 minutes. Determine how many milliliters per minute to infuse.

$$\frac{\text{(volume)}}{\text{(time)}} \frac{1 \text{ mL}}{5 \text{ min}} = \frac{\text{X mL}}{1 \text{ min}} \frac{\text{(unknown volume)}}{\text{(time)}}$$

$5X = 1$

$$5\overline{)1.0}^{\,0.2}$$

$X = 0.2$

Label with the unit of measure.
0.2 mL/min
While digoxin can be given undiluted, it can also be diluted fourfold or greater with sterile water for injection. In the clinical setting, the dose volume might be further diluted to make the final volume 5 mL by adding 4 mL of sterile water. Then you would administer 1 mL/min. This enhances the ease and accuracy of the injection.

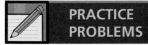
PRACTICE PROBLEMS

Directions: *Complete calculation using the medication label provided as what you HAVE on hand, and mark each syringe with appropriate volume.*

1.

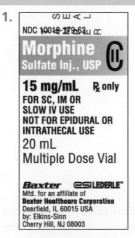

NDC 10019-179-63

Morphine **C**II
Sulfate Inj., USP

15 mg/mL   ℞ only
FOR SC, IM OR
SLOW IV USE
NOT FOR EPIDURAL OR
INTRATHECAL USE
20 mL
Multiple Dose Vial

Baxter ℮SILEDERLE™
Mfd. for an affiliate of
Baxter Healthcare Corporation
Deerfield, IL 60015 USA
by: Elkins-Sinn
Cherry Hill, NJ 08003

PRESCRIPTION: morphine sulfate 25 mg intramuscular every 3 hours for pain.
Is the prescribed dose larger or smaller than the dose you HAVE? _____
Administer _____

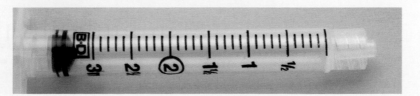

2.

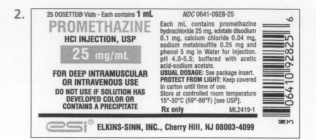

25 DOSETTE® Vials - Each contains **1 mL**

PROMETHAZINE
HCl INJECTION, USP

25 mg/mL

**FOR DEEP INTRAMUSCULAR
OR INTRAVENOUS USE**
**DO NOT USE IF SOLUTION HAS
DEVELOPED COLOR OR
CONTAINS A PRECIPITATE**

NDC 0641-0928-25

Each mL contains promethazine
hydrochloride 25 mg, edetate disodium
0.1 mg, calcium chloride 0.04 mg,
sodium metabisulfite 0.25 mg and
phenol 5 mg in Water for Injection.
pH 4.0-5.5; buffered with acetic
acid-sodium acetate.
USUAL DOSAGE: See package insert.
PROTECT FROM LIGHT: Keep covered
in carton until time of use.
Store at controlled room temperature
15°-30°C (59°-86°F) [see USP].

Rx only   ML2419-1

esi® ELKINS-SINN, INC., Cherry Hill, NJ 08003-4099

PRESCRIPTION: promethazine (Phenergan) 30 mg intramuscular now.
Is the prescribed dose larger or smaller than the dose you HAVE? _____
Administer _____

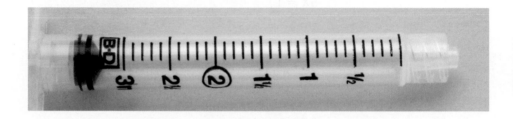

3.

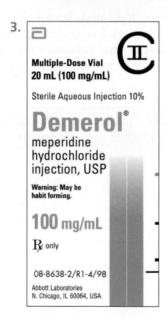

Λ

Multiple-Dose Vial
20 mL (100 mg/mL)

Sterile Aqueous Injection 10%

Demerol®
meperidine
hydrochloride
injection, USP

**Warning: May be
habit forming.**

100 mg/mL

R̶x only

08-8638-2/R1-4/98

Abbott Laboratories
N. Chicago, IL 60064, USA

Cⁱⁱ

PRESCRIPTION: meperidine (Demerol) 160 mg intramuscular pre-op on call.
Is the prescribed dose larger or smaller than the dose you HAVE? _____
Administer _____

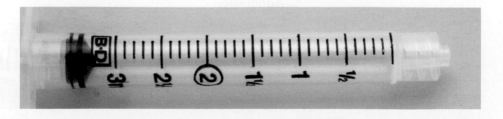

4.
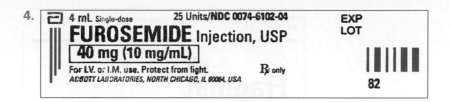

PRESCRIPTION: furosemide (Lasix) 40 mg intravenous push now over 2 minutes.
Is the prescribed dose larger or smaller than the dose you HAVE? _____
Administer _____
Volume/time _____

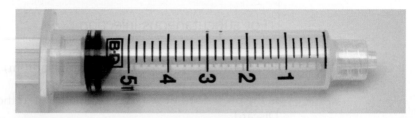

5.
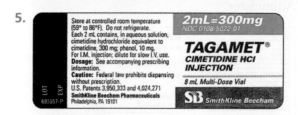

PRESCRIPTION: cimetidine (Tagamet) 300 mg intramuscular.
Is the prescribed dose larger or smaller than the dose you HAVE? _____
Administer _____

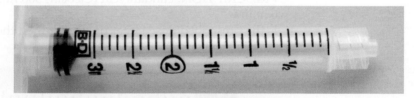

6.
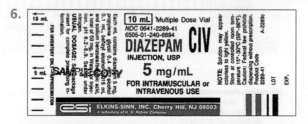

PRESCRIPTION: Valium (diazepam) 7.5 mg intramuscular every 4 hours for severe anxiety.
Is the prescribed dose larger or smaller than the dose you HAVE? _____
Administer _____

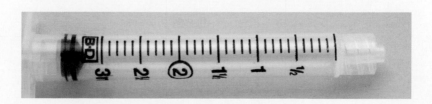

7.

10 x 0.2 mL single dose syringes, preassembled with needle guards
NDC 0013-2426-91

Fragmin.

dalteparin sodium injection

5000 IU (anti-Xa) per 0.2 mL

For subcutaneous injection

PRESCRIPTION: Fragmin (dalteparin sodium) 2500 units subcutaneous daily for 5 days.
Is the prescribed dose larger or smaller than the dose you HAVE? _____
Discard _____
Administer _____

8.

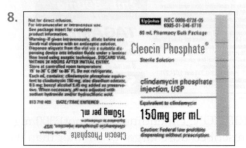

Upjohn NDC 0009-0728-05
6505-01-346-6718

80 mL Pharmacy Bulk Package

Cleocin Phosphate®
Sterile Solution

clindamycin phosphate
injection, USP

Equivalent to clindamycin

150mg per mL

Caution: Federal law prohibits
dispensing without prescription.

PRESCRIPTION: clindamycin (Cleocin) 300 mg intravenous piggyback every 6 hours.
Is the prescribed dose larger or smaller than the dose you HAVE? _____
Administer _____

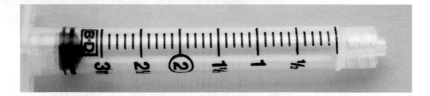

9.

5 mL   **MULTIPLE DOSE**
NDC 0003-0293-20
NSN 6505-01-210-4472

40 mg per mL

KENALOG®-40

**Triamcinolone
Acetonide Injectable
Suspension, USP**

Rx only

Read all sides

🔷 **Bristol-Myers
Squibb Company**

PRESCRIPTION: Kenalog (triamcinolone) 20 mg intramuscular daily.
Is the prescribed dose larger or smaller than the dose you HAVE? _____
Administer _____

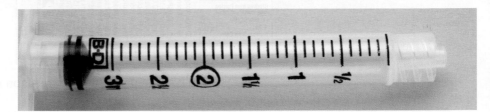

10.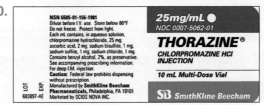

PRESCRIPTION: chlorpromazine (Thorazine) 50 mg intramuscular now.
Is the prescribed dose larger or smaller than the dose you HAVE? _____
Administer _____

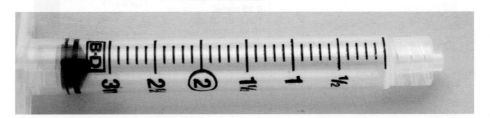

(Answers on pp. 457–458)

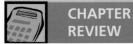

**CHAPTER
REVIEW**

Complete each calculation using the medication label provided as what you HAVE
on hand, and mark each syringe with the appropriate volume.

1.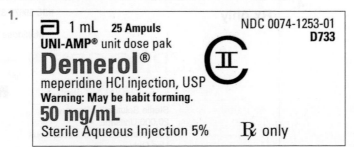

PRESCRIPTION: meperidine hydrochloride (Demerol) 75 mg intramuscular every 3 hours as needed for pain.
Administer _____

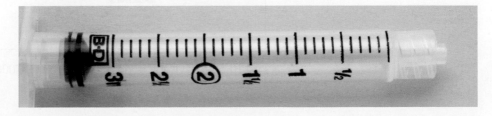

2.

NDC 63323-542-01   504201

HEPARIN SODIUM

INJECTION, USP

10,000 USP Units/mL

(Derived from Porcine
Intestinal Mucosa)
For IV or SC Use

1 mL   Rx only
Multiple Dose Vial

Sterile, Nonpyrogenic
Each mL contains:
10,000 USP Units heparin
sodium; 0.15% methyl-
paraben; 0.015% propyl-
paraben; Water for Injection
q.s.Hydrochloric acid and/or
sodium hydroxide may have
been added for pH adjustment.
Usual Dosage: See insert.
Use only if solution is
clear and seal intact.
Store at 25°C (77°F);
excursions permitted to
15°-30°C (59°-86°F)
[see USP Controlled Room
temperature].

APP PHARMACEUTICAL PARTNERS, INC.
Schaumburg, IL 60173

42588B

LOT   EXP

PRESCRIPTION: heparin sodium injection of 8700 units subcutaneous every 8 hours.

Administer _____

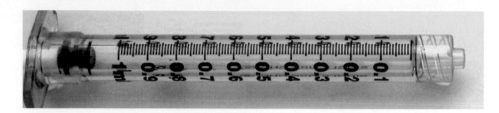

3.

NDC 10019-506-10

Bumetanide

Injection, USP

0.25 mg/mL   Rx only
FOR IV OR IM USE
10 mL Multiple Dose Vial

Baxter
Mfd. for **Baxter Healthcare Corporation** affiliate
by: Gensia Sicor Pharmaceuticals, Irvine, CA 92618

Each mL contains: Bumetanide 0.25 mg,
Sodium Chloride 8.5 mg, and Ammonium
Acetate 4.0 mg, as buffers, Disodium Edetate
0.1 mg, Benzyl Alcohol 10 mg, as preservative, Water for Injection q.s.
pH adjusted with Sodium Hydroxide. pH 6.8-7.8.
Usual Dosage:
For dosage recommendations and
other important, prescribing information, see package insert.
Store at controlled room temperature 15°-30°C (59°-86°F).

Y29-064-002   400-588-01

PRESCRIPTION: bumetanide (Bumex) 0.75 mg intramuscular daily.

Administer _____

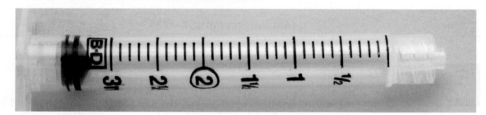

4.

Rx only

NDC 59676-320-01
6 - 1 mL
Multidose Vials

PROCRIT® **20**
EPOETIN ALFA   **M**

Sterile Solution — Preserved
20,000 Units/mL
For Intravenous or Subcutaneous
Use Only

THERMALERT® Insulated Container System

Manufactured by:
Amgen Inc. U.S. LIC. #1080
Thousand Oaks, California 91320-1789

Distributed by:
Ortho Biotech Products, L.P.
Raritan, New Jersey 08869-0670

PRESCRIPTION: epoetin alfa (Procrit) 7000 units subcutaneous three times per week.

Administer _____

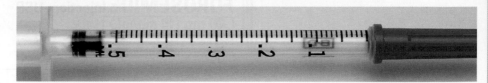

5.

> 542282
> **2 mL**
> **LANOXIN®**
> **(DIGOXIN)**
> **INJECTION**
> **500 μg (0.5 mg)**
> **in 2 mL**
> (250 μg [0.25 mg] per mL)
> **DILUTION NOT REQUIRED**
> PROPYLENE GLYCOL 40%
> ALCOHOL 10%
> Store at 15° to 25°C (59° to
> 77°F). Protect from light.
> FOR I.V. OR I.M. USE
> BURROUGHS WELLCOME CO.
> Research Triangle Park, NC 27709
> LOT   EXP.

PRESCRIPTION: digoxin (Lanoxin) 250 mcg intravenous push STAT (guideline: over 5 minutes).
Administer _____
How many mL/min will be administered? _____

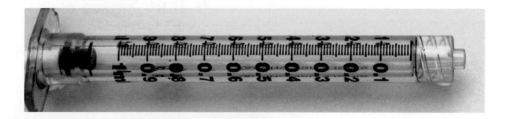

6.

> ⊡ **40 mEq** | **Potassium Chloride** for Inj. **Concentrate, USP (2 mEq/mL)**
> 25 Units/NDC 0074-6653-05
> **20 mL Single-dose**
> **For I.V. use.**
> **CONCENTRATE**
> *MUST BE DILUTED BEFORE USE.*
> ℞ only
> EXP
> LOT
> *ABBOTT LABORATORIES, NORTH CHICAGO, IL 60064, USA*
> 90

PRESCRIPTION: Add potassium chloride 20 mEq to each liter of intravenous fluids.
Add _____

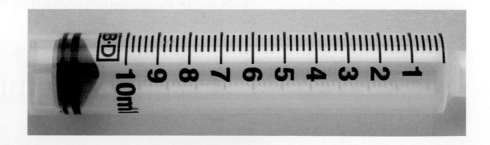

7.

4 mL Single-dose 25 Units/**NDC 0074-6102-04**

FUROSEMIDE Injection, USP

40 mg (10 mg/mL)

For I.V. or I.M. use. Protect from light.

ABBOTT LABORATORIES, NORTH CHICAGO, IL 60064, USA

EXP
LOT

82

Rx only

PRESCRIPTION: furosemide (Lasix) 30 mg slow intravenous push now (guideline: 40 mg/minute).

Administer _____

How many mL/min will be administered? _____

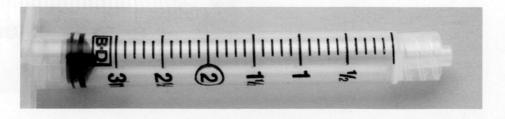

8.

NDC 0002-1675-01

20 mL VIAL No. 419

℞ *Lilly*

POISON

ATROPINE SULFATE

INJECTION, USP

0.4 mg per mL

CAUTION—Federal (U.S.A.) law prohibits dispensing without prescription.

Store at 59° to 86°F (15° to 30°C)

Usual Adult Dose—0.75 to 1.5 mL injected subcutaneously, intramuscularly, or slowly intravenously. See literature.

Each mL contains Atropine Sulfate, 0.4 mg with Chlorobutanol (Chloroform Derivative), 0.5 percent.

YA 9206 AMX

Eli Lilly & Co., Indianapolis, IN 46285, U.S.A.

APPROXIMATE EQUIVALENTS

0.4 mL	0.16 mg
0.5 mL	0.2 mg
0.6 mL	0.24 mg
0.8 mL	0.32 mg
1 mL	0.4 mg
1.25 mL	0.5 mg
1.6 mL	0.65 mg
2.5 mL	1.0 mg
3.1 mL	1.25 mg

Exp. Date/Control No.

PRESCRIPTION: atropine sulfate 0.4 mg subcutaneous 30 minutes prior to surgery.

Administer _____

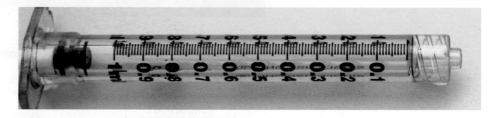

9.

NDC 0703-7041-03 *Rx only*

Haloperidol Injection, USP

5 mg/mL

(For Immediate Release)

For IM Use Only

1 mL Single Dose Vial

Sterile

GensiaSicor® PHARMACEUTICALS

Irvine, CA 92618

Each mL contains: 5 mg haloperidol (as the lactate) with 1.8 mg methylparaben, 0.2 mg propylparaben and lactic acid for pH adjustment to 3.0-3.6.

For Intramuscular Use

USUAL DOSAGE: See Package Insert.

Dispense in a light resistant container as defined in the official compendium.

Store at controlled room temperature 15°-30°C (59°-86°F). PROTECT FROM LIGHT. Do not freeze.

000045A

PRESCRIPTION: haloperidol (Haldol) 2.5 mg intramuscular now.

Administer _____

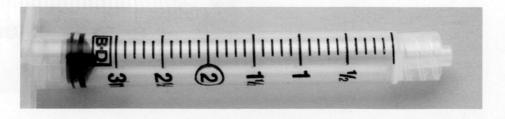

10.

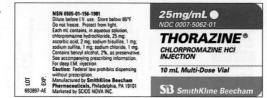

PRESCRIPTION: chlorpromazine hydrochloride (Thorazine) 12.5 mg intramuscular.
Administer _____

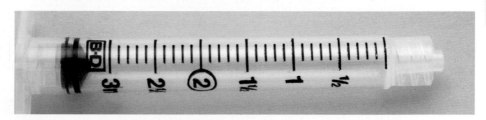

11.

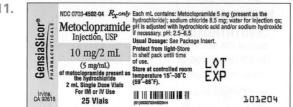

PRESCRIPTION: metoclopramide (Reglan) 15 mg intravenous push over 2 minutes now.
Administer _____
How many milliliters per minute will be administered? _____

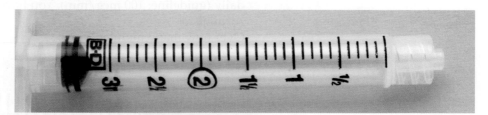

12.

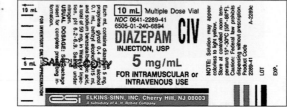

PRESCRIPTION: diazepam (Valium) 2 mg intramuscular every 6 hours.
Administer _____

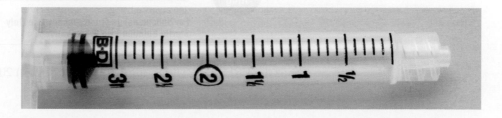

13.

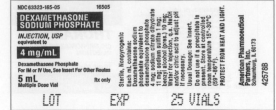

PRESCRIPTION: dexamethasone (Decadron) 6 mg intramuscular daily.
Administer _____

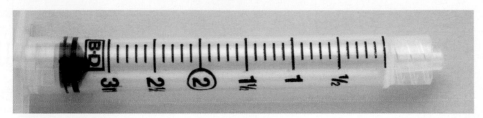

14.

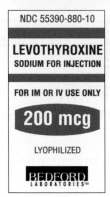

PRESCRIPTION: levothyroxine (Synthroid) 150 mcg intravenous push
daily (guideline: 100 mcg/min). You have 200 mcg/5 mL.
Administer _____
Over how many minutes? _____

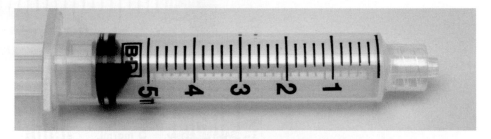

15.

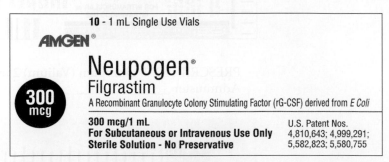

PRESCRIPTION: filgrastim (Neupogen) 200 mcg subcutaneous weekly.

Administer _____

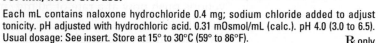

16.
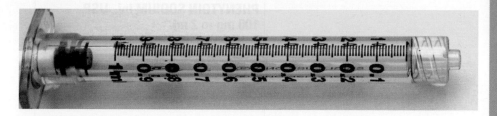

PRESCRIPTION: naloxone hydrochloride (Narcan) 0.6 mg intravenous push now (guideline: 0.4 mg/15 sec).
Administer _____
Over how many seconds? _____

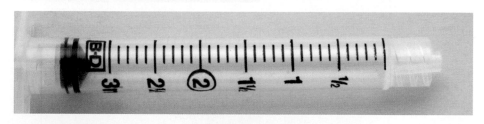

17.

NDC 0015-7403-20
NSN 6505-00-946-4700
EQUIVALENT TO

500 mg AMPICILLIN
STERILE AMPICILLIN SODIUM, USP
For IM or IV Use
CAUTION: Federal law prohibits dispensing without prescription.

For IM use, add 1.8 mL diluent (read accompanying circular). Resulting solution contains 250 mg ampicillin per mL. Use solution within 1 hour. This vial contains ampicillin sodium equivalent to 500 mg ampicillin. Usual Dosage: Adults—250 to 500 mg IM q. 6h. READ ACCOMPANYING CIRCULAR for detailed indications, IM or IV dosage and precautions. APOTHECON® A Bristol-Myers Squibb Company Princeton, NJ 08540 USA

7403200RL-2

Cont:
Exp. Date:

PRESCRIPTION: ampicillin (Omnipen) 400 mg intramuscular every 6 hours.
Administer _____

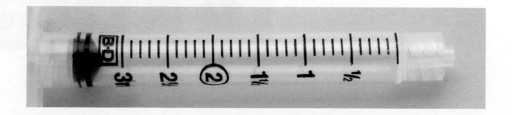

18.

2 mL Single-dose
5 Ampuls   NDC 0074-1317-01

PHENYTOIN SODIUM Inj., USP
100 mg in 2 mL
For I.M. or I.V. use (no infusion)   ℞ only

Each mL contains phenytoin sodium 50 mg; propylene glycol 40%
and alcohol 10%. Also contains sodium hydroxide for pH
adjustment. pH 11.5 (10.0 to 12.3). Administer slowly. **Do not exceed
50 mg per minute intravenously.** Usual dosage: See insert. **Note:** Do
not use Injection if it is hazy or contains a precipitate.

The addition of Phenytoin Sodium Injection to an intravenous
infusion is not recommended due to the lack of solubility and
resultant precipitation. Store at controlled room temperature 15° to
30°C (59° to 86°F). See USP.

©Abbott 2001   Printed in USA
ABBOTT LABORATORIES, NORTH CHICAGO, IL 60064, USA

58-2886-2/R4-2/02   EXP
                                     LOT

PRESCRIPTION: Administer 10 mg/kg phenytoin sodium (Dilantin) intra-
venous push now at a rate of 50 mg/min (patient weight = 60 kg).
Administer _____
Over how many minutes? _____

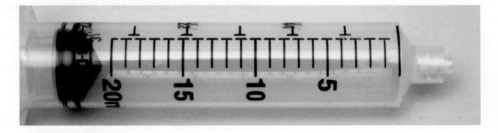

19.

⍲ NOVARTIS   NDC 0078-0181-01
                        Unit Dose Package

🔹**Sandostatin®**
octreotide acetate
INJECTION

Rx only

100 mcg/mL (0.1 mg/mL)
For Subcutaneous Injection   10 Ampuls/1 mL size

PRESCRIPTION: octreotide acetate (Sandostatin) 0.05 mg subcutaneous
every 12 hours.
Administer _____

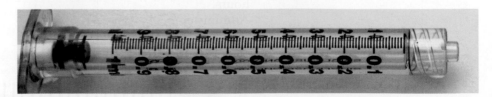

20.

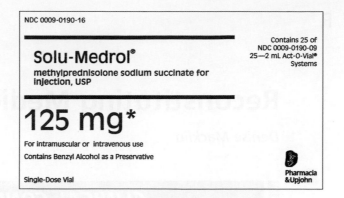

NDC 0009-0190-16

Solu-Medrol®
methylprednisolone sodium succinate for
injection, USP

125 mg*

For intramuscular or intravenous use

Contains Benzyl Alcohol as a Preservative

Single-Dose Vial

Contains 25 of
NDC 0009-0190-09
25—2 mL Act-O-Vial®
Systems

**Pharmacia
&Upjohn**

PRESCRIPTION: methylprednisolone sodium succinate (Solu-Medrol) 75 mg intramuscular.

Administer _____

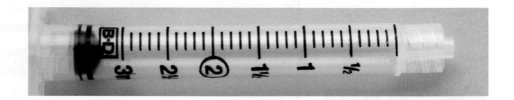

(Answers on pp. 459–460)

evolve **For additional practice problems, refer to the Basic Calculations section of the Drug Calculations Companion, version 4 on Evolve.**

Reconstituting Medications

Denise Macklin

CLINICAL CONNECTION

- Knowing the terms used with the reconstitution procedure enables understanding of the reconstitution process.
- Label interpretation is important to complete the reconstitution process, perform calculations, and promote optimal medication potency.
- Proper labeling of reconstituted medication is critical for safe administration.

INTRODUCTION

Some injectable and noninjectable medications come in a form that requires reconstitution. Reconstitution is necessary when the liquid form of an injectable medication has a short shelf life. Noninjectable solutions (e.g., oral medications, irrigating solutions) can come in either powders or liquid concentrates. Concentrates take up less shelf space. As a safety precaution, the pharmacy reconstitutes most medications under a laminar hood. However, it is important for nurses to know how to reconstitute, because a pharmacist is not always available and some medications must be reconstituted just prior to administration. In order to understand the use of powdered medications and liquid concentrates, a few terms must be defined.

- *Solute:* The powdered medication or liquid concentrate.
- *Solvent or diluent:* The liquid that is added to the powder or liquid concentrate for reconstitution. For parenteral medications, use normal saline or sterile water (bacteriostatic for multidose preparations). When a special diluent is required, it is supplied with the powdered medication. Oral medications can often but not always be reconstituted with tap water.
- *Solution:* The liquid that results from the diluent dissolving the solute.
- *Solution strength or concentration:* When reconstituting medications, remember that the solution strength or concentration is the relationship of solute to diluent. This is expressed as a ratio: solute/diluent (mg/mL). The more diluent added, the less concentrated the solution; the less diluent added, the more concentrated the solution. The amount of diluent may be altered, but the amount of the solute remains the same.
- *Reconstitution:* The process of adding a diluent to a solute to form a solution.

READING THE LABEL

Powdered medications can be administered by both the oral route and the parenteral route. The label and/or the package insert contain information about the reconstitution process. Reconstitution information can also be located on the Internet (using Google or another search engine) by drug name. (One information site is www.rxlist.com.) Reconstitution information includes the type of diluent, the total volume of diluent to be added, the total volume of the reconstituted solution (diluent plus powder), the dose/volume, storage guidelines, and length of time reconstituted medication can be used (not the same as expiration date, the date after which the medication cannot be reconstituted). Some medications have both room temperature and refrigeration guidelines. Storage guidelines determine the length of time the reconstituted medication can be used (Figure 12-1). Some medication can be recon-

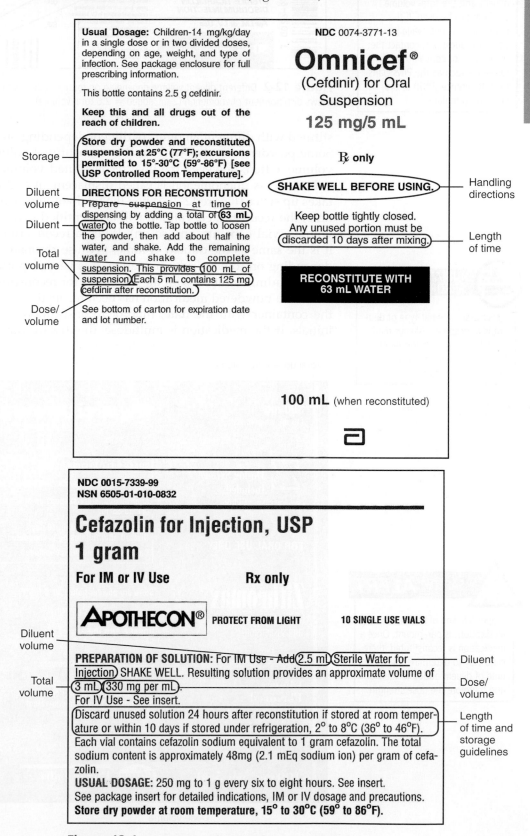

Figure 12-1 Reconstitution information found on drug label.

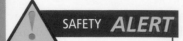
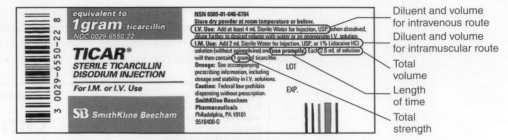

Diluent and volume for intravenous route
Diluent and volume for intramuscular route
Total volume
Length of time
Total strength

Figure 12-2 Different diluent volume depending on route of administration. Total intramuscular volume shows displacement phenomenon (2 mL added = 2.6 total volume).

stituted with different amounts of diluent depending on the route of administration. Some powders dissolve, making the reconstituted volume the same as the diluent volume. Often, however, the final reconstituted volume is greater than the diluent volume. This phenomenon is called displacement and occurs because the powder takes up space (Figure 12-2). When the total volume is different than the diluent volume, the reconstituted volume will be identified (available volume, withdrawable volume, vial contents, and so on). When a reconstituted volume is not identified, it is the same as the diluent volume. Because reconstitution information may vary depending on route of administration, it is very important to match the prescribed route of administration with the directions for reconstitution (see Figure 12-2).

Once a powdered medication has been reconstituted, it is very important to label the container with the date, time of reconstitution, storage guidelines, and your initials. If the medication is multidose, the discard date should be added. In some

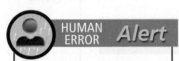
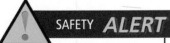
Total dose/total volume

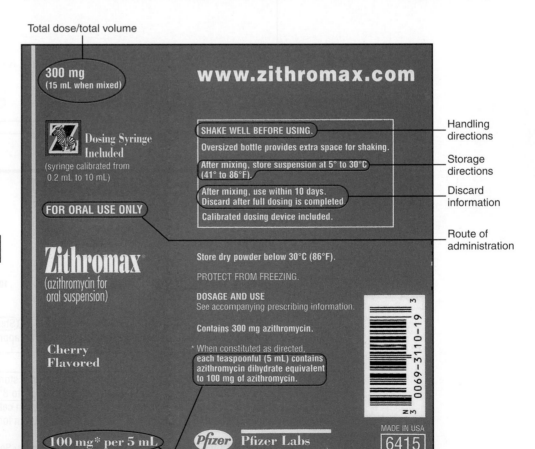

Handling directions
Storage directions
Discard information
Route of administration

Dose volume

Figure 12-3 Label information.

institutions there are set policies for how long a medication can be stored after reconstitution. Some institutions have storage guideline adhesive labels such as "Refrigerate" that can be affixed to the container. If there is not sufficient room on the label to clearly write the required information, you may add tape to the container. Apply it in such a manner as not to cover the medication name and dose. **When a container is not dated and timed, the medication should be discarded and a new one used.**

Review storage information and when to discard the medication in order to provide optimal medication potency for the patient (Figure 12-3).

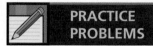
PRACTICE PROBLEMS

Directions: *Read the following labels and fill in the blanks.*

1.

Usual Dosage: Children-14 mg/kg/day in a single dose or in two divided doses, depending on age, weight, and type of infection. See package enclosure for full prescribing information.

This bottle contains 2.5 g cefdinir.

Keep this and all drugs out of the reach of children.

Store dry powder and reconstituted suspension at 25°C (77°F); excursions permitted to 15°-30°C (59°-86°F) [see USP Controlled Room Temperature].

DIRECTIONS FOR RECONSTITUTION
Prepare suspension at time of dispensing by adding a total of **63 mL** water to the bottle. Tap bottle to loosen the powder, then add about half the water, and shake. Add the remaining water and shake to complete suspension. This provides 100 mL of suspension. Each 5 mL contains 125 mg cefdinir after reconstitution.

See bottom of carton for expiration date and lot number.

NDC 0074-3771-13

Omnicef®
(Cefdinir) for Oral Suspension

125 mg/5 mL

℞ only

SHAKE WELL BEFORE USING.

Keep bottle tightly closed.
Any unused portion must be discarded 10 days after mixing.

RECONSTITUTE WITH 63 mL WATER

100 mL (when reconstituted)

Type of diluent to be added _____
Diluent volume to be added _____
Solution concentration _____
Storage requirements _____
Discard guidelines _____

2.

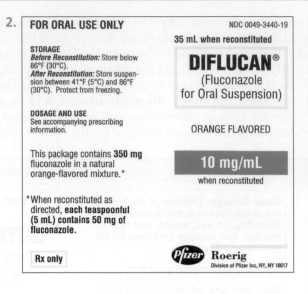

FOR ORAL USE ONLY

NDC 0049-3440-19

35 mL when reconstituted

DIFLUCAN®
(Fluconazole
for Oral Suspension)

ORANGE FLAVORED

10 mg/mL
when reconstituted

STORAGE
Before Reconstitution: Store below 86°F (30°C).
After Reconstitution: Store suspension between 41°F (5°C) and 86°F (30°C). Protect from freezing.

DOSAGE AND USE
See accompanying prescribing information.

This package contains **350 mg** fluconazole in a natural orange-flavored mixture.*

*When reconstituted as directed, **each teaspoonful (5 mL) contains 50 mg of fluconazole.**

Rx only

Pfizer Roerig
Division of Pfizer Inc, NY, NY 10017

0400K03A
EXP 1JUN 14

To the Pharmacist:

1. Mixing Directions:
   Tap bottle lightly to loosen powder. Add 24 mL of distilled water or Purified Water (USP) to the bottle. Shake well.

2. Store reconstituted suspension between 41°F (5°C) and 86°F (30°C). Protect from freezing.

   Shake well before each use. Discard unused portion after 2 weeks.

Type of diluent to be added _____
Diluent volume to be added _____
Solution concentration _____
Storage requirements _____
Expiration date _____

3.

DIRECTIONS FOR CONSTITUTION: Slowly add 46 mL of Purified Water. Shake vigorously for 5-10 seconds immediately after adding the water.

Inactive ingredients: citric acid, flavors, microcrystalline cellulose and carboxymethylcellulose sodium, sucrose, and xanthan gum, with sodium benzoate 0.1%, sodium methylparaben 0.1%, and sodium propylparaben 0.02% added as preservatives.

NDC 0006-3538-92

PEPCID®
(FAMOTIDINE) FOR
ORAL SUSPENSION

400 mg of famotidine

Constituted to 50 mL, each 5 mL contains 40 mg famotidine

SHAKE WELL BEFORE USING
NOT FOR INJECTION

Rx only

MERCK & CO., INC.
Whitehouse Station, NJ 08889, USA

For constitution and
USUAL ADULT DOSAGE:
See accompanying circular.

Notice to Patient: Bottle is oversized to allow for shaking.

KEEP CONTAINER TIGHTLY CLOSED.
Store dry powder and suspension at 25°C (77°F); excursions permitted to 15-30°C (59-86°F) [see USP Controlled Room Temperature]. Suspension: Protect from freezing. Discard unused suspension after 30 days.

9136308   400 mg | No. 3538

100% Recycled Paperboard
65% Post-Consumer Content

Type of diluent to be added _____
Diluent volume to be added _____
Solution concentration _____
Storage requirements _____
Discard guidelines _____

CHAPTER 12

4.

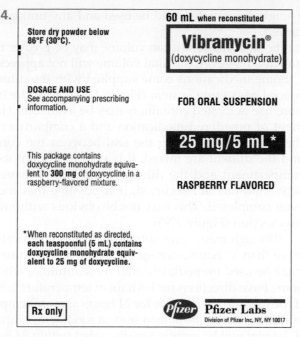

60 mL when reconstituted

Vibramycin®
(doxycycline monohydrate)

Store dry powder below
86°F (30°C).

FOR ORAL SUSPENSION

DOSAGE AND USE
See accompanying prescribing
information.

25 mg/5 mL*

This package contains
doxycycline monohydrate equivalent to **300 mg** of doxycycline in a
raspberry-flavored mixture.

RASPBERRY FLAVORED

*When reconstituted as directed,
each teaspoonful (5 mL) contains
doxycycline monohydrate equivalent to **25 mg** of doxycycline.

Rx only

Pfizer Labs
Division of Pfizer Inc, NY, NY 10017

0630K03A
EXP 1JUL 14

To the Pharmacist:

1. Mixing Directions:
Tap bottle lightly to loosen powder.
Add 47.6 mL of water to the bottle
to make a total volume of 60 mL.
Shake well.

2. This prescription, when in suspension, will maintain its potency
for two weeks when kept at room
temperature.

**DISCARD UNUSED PORTION
AFTER TWO WEEKS.**

Type of diluent to be added _____

Diluent volume to be added _____

Solution concentration _____

Storage requirements _____

Expiration date _____

5.

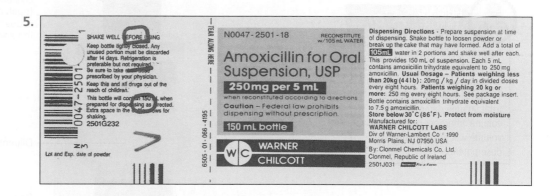

SHAKE WELL BEFORE USING
Keep bottle tightly closed. Any
unused portion must be discarded
after 14 days. Refrigeration is
preferable but not required.
Be sure to take entire dose
prescribed by your physician.
Keep this and all drugs out of the
reach of children.
This bottle will contain 150 mL when
prepared for dispensing as directed.
Extra space in the bottle allows for
shaking.
2501G232

Lot and Exp. date of powder

TEAR ALONG HERE

6505 - 01 - 066 - 4195

N0047 - 2501 - 18   RECONSTITUTE w/105mL WATER

**Amoxicillin for Oral
Suspension, USP**

250mg per 5 mL
when reconstituted according to directions

Caution – Federal law prohibits
dispensing without prescription.

150 mL bottle

W|C **WARNER
CHILCOTT**

Dispensing Directions - Prepare suspension at time
of dispensing. Shake bottle to loosen powder or
break up the cake that may have formed. Add a total of
105mL water in 2 portions and shake well after each.
This provides 150 mL of suspension. Each 5 mL
contains amoxicillin trihydrate equivalent to 250 mg
amoxicillin. **Usual Dosage – Patients weighing less
than 20kg (44lb):** 20mg / kg / day in divided doses
every eight hours. **Patients weighing 20 kg or
more:** 250 mg every eight hours. See package insert.
Bottle contains amoxicillin trihydrate equivalent
to 7.5 g amoxicillin.
Store below 30°C (86°F). Protect from moisture
Manufactured for:
WARNER CHILCOTT LABS
Div of Warner-Lambert Co © 1990
Morris Plains, NJ 07950 USA
By: Clonmel Chemicals Co. Ltd.
Clonmel, Republic of Ireland
2501J031

Type of diluent to be added _____

Diluent volume to be added _____

Solution concentration _____

Storage requirements _____

Discard guidelines _____

(Answers on p. 460)

PARENTERAL POWDERS

Reconstitution of parenteral medications requires close observation of reconstitution
directions. Diluents with parenteral medications must be sterile. Common diluents
include sterile 5% dextrose and water, sterile water, and sterile normal saline. When
reconstitution is required and the medication does not come with its own diluent,

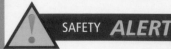

Use preservative-free diluent for single-use reconstitutions and bacteriostatic diluent for multi-dose vials.

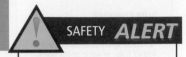

Never use tap water to reconstitute a medication that will be used parenterally. Always use a sterile solution.

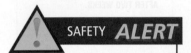

Never inject the reconstituted solution until all medication is completely dissolved.

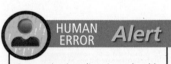

Reconstitution directions should be followed exactly for the total solution volume to be accurate. The total medication strength/total volume determines dose/volume. Improper reconstitution volume will result in improper dose potency.

a single-dose vial should be used and any unused portion after reconstitution discarded.

The final reconstitution volume may be greater than the diluent volume plus the powder; however, the total volume will not appreciably increase.

Some medications come supplied with the diluent either in the package or in a special packaging system (Figure 12-4). With the intravenous route of administration, use-activated containers may be available. These systems include a compartment of powdered medication and a compartment of diluent. You must activate the system by breaking the seal between the compartments so that the powder and the diluent are mixed. It is very important to make sure that the medication compartment and the diluent compartment have been successfully activated. If activation has not occurred, it is possible that the reconstitution process has not been completed. This may not be obvious without close inspection of the medication section (Figure 12-5).

Although many reconstituted parenteral medications are commonly not stored for more than 24 hours, storage information is included on the label. Some medications must be used immediately after reconstitution, whereas others can be stored longer. Some have directions for both room temperature (shorter) and refrigeration (longer). If the medication is stable for 24 hours at room temperature and 72 hours with refrigeration, you may be able to store at room temperature instead of under refrigeration if the vial will be emptied or discarded within 24 hours (Figure 12-6).

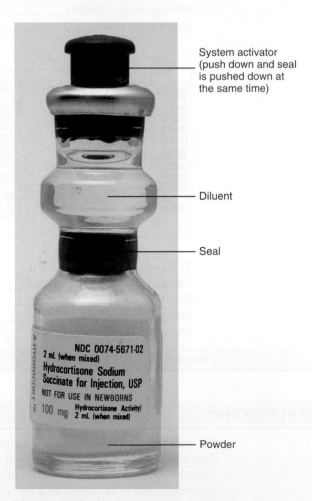

Figure 12-4 Medication supplied with diluent.

Step 1

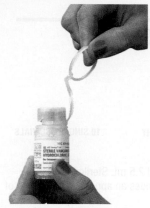 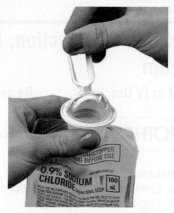 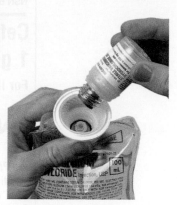

Swing the pull ring over the top of the vial and pull down far enough to start the opening. Then pull straight up to remove the cap. Avoid touching the rubber stopper and vial threads.

Hold diluent container and gently grasp the tab on the pull ring. Pull up to break the tie membrane. Pull back to remove the cover. Avoid touching the inside of the vial port.

Screw the vial into the vial port until it will go no further. Recheck the vial to assure that it is tight. Label appropriately.

Step 2

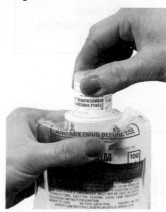 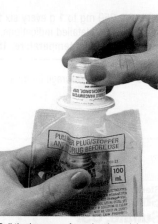 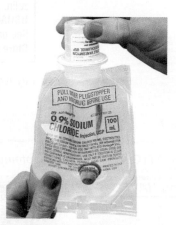

Hold the vial as shown. Push the drug vial down into container and grasp the inner cap of the vial through the walls of the container.

Pull the inner cap from the drug vial: allow drug to fall into diluent container for fast mixing. Do not force stopper by pushing on one side of inner cap at a time.

Verify that the plug and rubber stopper have been removed from the vial. The floating stopper is an indication that the system has been activated.

Step 3

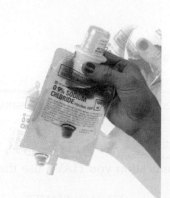 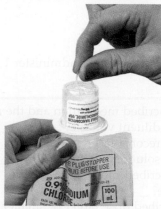 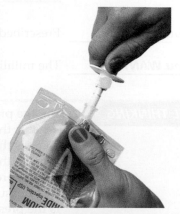

Mix container contents thoroughly to assure complete dissolution. Look through bottom of vial to verify complete mixing. Check for leaks by squeezing container firmly. If leaks are found, discard unit.

Pull up hanger on the vial.

Remove the white administration port cover and spike (pierce) the container with the piercing pin. Administer within the specified time.

Figure 12-5 Assembling and administering medication with the ADD-Vantage system. (Used with permission from Hospira, Inc., Lake Forest, IL.)

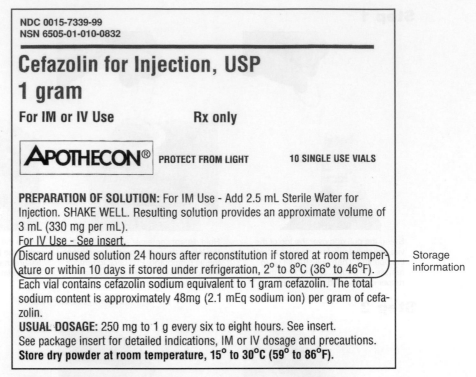

NDC 0015-7339-99
NSN 6505-01-010-0832

Cefazolin for Injection, USP
1 gram

For IM or IV Use   **Rx only**

APOTHECON® PROTECT FROM LIGHT   **10 SINGLE USE VIALS**

PREPARATION OF SOLUTION: For IM Use - Add 2.5 mL Sterile Water for Injection. SHAKE WELL. Resulting solution provides an approximate volume of 3 mL (330 mg per mL).
For IV Use - See insert.
Discard unused solution 24 hours after reconstitution if stored at room temperature or within 10 days if stored under refrigeration, 2° to 8°C (36° to 46°F).   — Storage information
Each vial contains cefazolin sodium equivalent to 1 gram cefazolin. The total sodium content is approximately 48mg (2.1 mEq sodium ion) per gram of cefazolin.
USUAL DOSAGE: 250 mg to 1 g every six to eight hours. See insert.
See package insert for detailed indications, IM or IV dosage and precautions.
Store dry powder at room temperature, 15° to 30°C (59° to 86°F).

Figure 12-6 Medication storage information.

Example 1

PRESCRIPTION	*Streptomycin 1 gram intramuscular daily.*

• **What You HAVE**

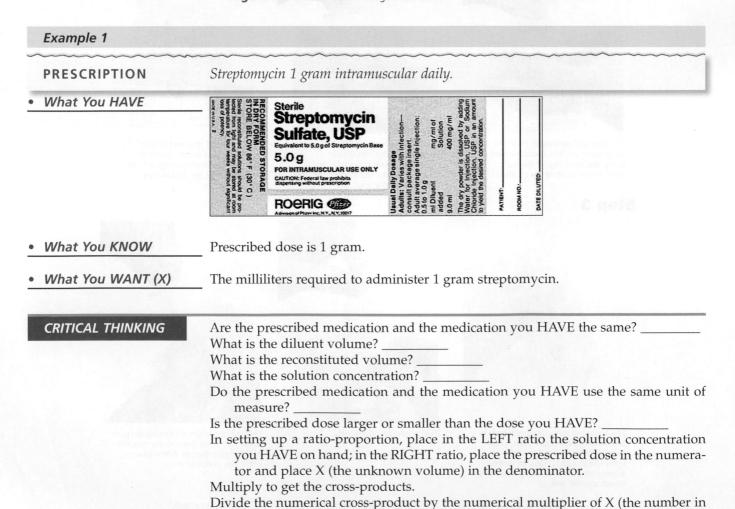

• **What You KNOW**   Prescribed dose is 1 gram.

• **What You WANT (X)**   The milliliters required to administer 1 gram streptomycin.

CRITICAL THINKING

Are the prescribed medication and the medication you HAVE the same? _____
What is the diluent volume? _____
What is the reconstituted volume? _____
What is the solution concentration? _____
Do the prescribed medication and the medication you HAVE use the same unit of measure? _____
Is the prescribed dose larger or smaller than the dose you HAVE? _____
In setting up a ratio-proportion, place in the LEFT ratio the solution concentration you HAVE on hand; in the RIGHT ratio, place the prescribed dose in the numerator and place X (the unknown volume) in the denominator.
Multiply to get the cross-products.
Divide the numerical cross-product by the numerical multiplier of X (the number in front of X).

The result is the answer for X.

Label answer properly in units (i.e., number of tablets, number of milliliters).

Check answer by placing the number obtained for X in the original equation. Cross-multiply. The cross-products should be approximately equal.

Label vial with reconstitution date, discard date, dose/volume, storage guidelines, and initials.

ANSWER FOR BEST CARE

Medication comparison? Yes.

Reconstitute with 9 mL.

Total volume? 9 mL (not identified on the label, so it is the same as diluent volume).

Solution concentration? 400 mg/mL.

Unit of measure comparison? No; prescribed in grams and HAVE milligrams.

Dose larger.

Perform calculation.

Convert grams to milligrams by moving the decimal three places to the right (1 gram = 1000 mg).

$$\frac{400\ mg}{1\ mL} = \frac{1000\ mg}{X\ mL}$$

400X = 1000

Reduce fraction.

4X = 10:

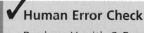

Label with the unit of measure.

2.5 mL

✔ **Human Error Check**

Replace X with 2.5.

$$\frac{400}{1} = \frac{1000}{2.5}$$

1000 = 1000

Guideline: 2.5 mL is less than the 3 mL maximum volume for an intramuscular dose.

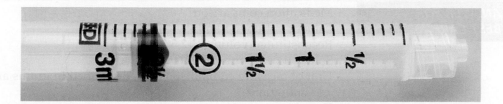

Drug Label

Date/time (reconstitution)

Discard date (4 weeks hence)

400 mg/mL

Room temperature

Initials

Example 2

PRESCRIPTION   *Cefepime (Maxipime) 1.4 gram intravenous every 12 hours.*

- **What You HAVE**

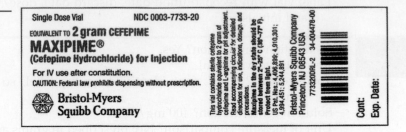

Cefepime Reconstitution Directions (Package Insert)			
Single-Dose Vials for Intravenous Administration	Amount of Diluent to be Added (mL)	Approximate Available Volume	Approximate Concentration (mg/mL)
2 g (IV)	10	12.5	160

- **What You KNOW**   Prescribed dose is 1.4 g.

- **What You WANT (X)**   The milliliters required to add cefepime 1.4 gram to the intravenous minibag.

CRITICAL THINKING

Are the prescribed medication and the medication you HAVE the same? _____

What is the diluent volume? _____

What is the reconstituted volume? _____

What is the solution concentration? _____

Do the prescribed medication and the medication you HAVE use the same unit of measure? _____

Is the prescribed dose larger or smaller than the dose you HAVE? _____

In setting up a ratio-proportion, place in the LEFT ratio the solution concentration you HAVE on hand; in the RIGHT ratio, place the prescribed dose in the numerator and place X (the unknown volume) in the denominator.

Multiply to get the cross-products.

Divide the numerical cross-product by the numerical multiplier of X (the number in front of X).

The result is the answer for X.

Label answer properly in units (i.e., number of tablets, number of milliliters).

Check answer by placing the number obtained for X in the original equation. Cross-multiply. The cross-products should be approximately equal.

ANSWER FOR BEST CARE

Medication comparison? Yes.

Diluent volume? 10 mL.

Reconstituted volume? 12.5 mL.

Solution concentration? 160 mg/mL.

Unit of measure comparison? No; prescribed in grams and HAVE milligrams.

Dose larger.

Perform calculation.

Convert grams to milligrams (1.4 gram = 1400 mg).

$$\frac{160 \text{ mg}}{1 \text{ mL}} = \frac{1400 \text{ mg}}{X \text{ mL}}$$

$$160X = 1400$$

$$\frac{8.75}{160)\overline{1400}} \text{ (round to the nearest tenth)}$$

$$-\underline{1280}$$
$$1200$$
$$\underline{1120}$$
$$800$$
$$800$$

Label with the units of measure.
8.8 mL.

✔ Human Error Check

Replace X with 8.8.

$$\frac{160}{1} = \frac{1400}{8.8}$$

$$1400 \approx 1408$$
The calculation is correct.

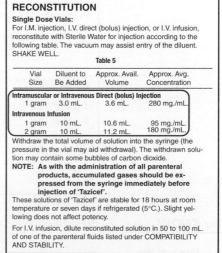

Drug Label
Date (reconstituted)
Discard date (24 hours)
160 mg/mL
Room temperature
Initials

Most parenteral medications have multiple reconstitution directions depending on the route of administration. Although the intravenous route is the most common in the acute care setting, intramuscular directions are also included (Figure 12-7).

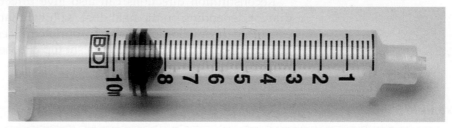

RECONSTITUTION

Single Dose Vials:
For I.M. injection, I.V. direct (bolus) injection, or I.V. infusion, reconstitute with Sterile Water for injection according to the following table. The vacuum may assist entry of the diluent. SHAKE WELL.

Table 5

Vial Size	Diluent to Be Added	Approx. Avail. Volume	Approx. Avg. Concentration
Intramuscular or Intravenous Direct (bolus) Injection			
1 gram	3.0 mL.	3.6 mL.	280 mg./mL.
Intravenous Infusion			
1 gram	10 mL.	10.6 mL.	95 mg./mL.
2 gram	10 mL.	11.2 mL.	180 mg./mL.

Withdraw the total volume of solution into the syringe (the pressure in the vial may aid withdrawal). The withdrawn solution may contain some bubbles of carbon dioxide.

NOTE: As with the administration of all parenteral products, accumulated gases should be expressed from the syringe immediately before injection of 'Tazicef'.

These solutions of 'Tazicef' are stable for 18 hours at room temperature or seven days if refrigerated (5°C.). Slight yellowing does not affect potency.

For I.V. infusion, dilute reconstituted solution in 50 to 100 mL. of one of the parenteral fluids listed under COMPATIBILITY AND STABILITY.

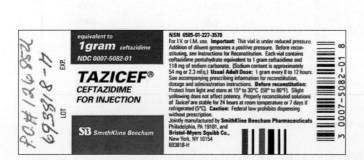

Figure 12-7 Different reconstitution directions depending on route of administration.

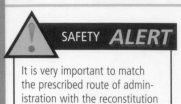

SAFETY **ALERT**

It is very important to match the prescribed route of administration with the reconstitution directions.

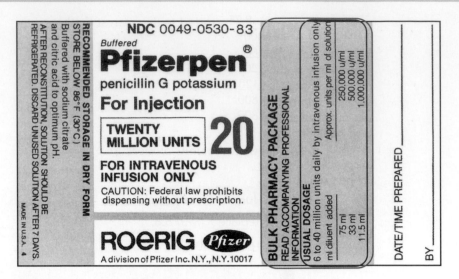

Figure 12-8 Different diluent volume alters final dose volume.

Reconstitution directions can also give directions to add different amounts of diluent depending on the final dose/volume that is needed. This enables you to reconstitute the medication to an appropriate concentration for the patient and closely approximates the prescription. You should choose the dose strength that is closest to what is prescribed (Figure 12-8).

Example 3

PRESCRIPTION   *Claforan 500 mg intramuscular every 6 hours.*

- **What You HAVE**

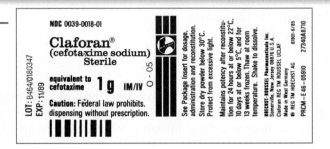

Preparation of Claforan Sterile (Package Insert)

CLAFORAN for IM or IV administration should be reconstituted as follows:

Strength	Diluent (mL)	Withdrawable Volume (mL)	Approximate Concentration (mg/mL)
1-g vial* (IM)	3	3.4	300
2-g vial* (IM)	5	6.0	330
1-g vial* (IV)	10	10.4	95
2-g vial* (IV)	10	11.0	180
1-g infusion	50-100	50-100	20-10
2-g infusion	50-100	50-100	40-20

- **What You KNOW**   Prescribed dose is Claforan 500 mg.

- **What You WANT (X)**   The milliliters required to administer 500 mg Claforan.

CRITICAL THINKING

Are the prescribed medication and the medication you HAVE the same? _____
What is the diluent volume? _____
What is the reconstituted volume? _____
What is the solution concentration? _____
Do the prescribed medication and the medication you HAVE use the same unit of measure? _____
Is the prescribed dose larger or smaller than the dose you HAVE? _____
In setting up a ratio-proportion, place in the LEFT ratio the solution concentration you HAVE on hand; in the RIGHT ratio, place the prescribed dose in the numerator and place X (the unknown volume) in the denominator.
Multiply to get the cross-products.
Divide the numerical cross-product by the numerical multiplier of X (the number in front of X).
The result is the answer for X.
Label answer properly in units (i.e., number of tablets, number of milliliters).
Check answer by placing the number obtained for X in the original equation. Cross-multiply. The cross-products should be approximately equal.
Label vial with reconstitution date, discard date, dose/volume, storage guidelines, and initials.

ANSWER FOR BEST CARE

Medication comparison? Yes.
Reconstitute with 3 mL.
Total volume? 3.4 mL (not identified on the label, so it is the same as diluent volume).
Solution concentration? 300 mg/mL.
Unit of measure comparison? Yes.
Dose larger.
Perform calculation.

$$\frac{300\ mg}{1\ mL} = \frac{500\ mg}{X\ mL}$$

$$300X = 500\ mg$$

$$300\overline{)500.00} \quad \underline{1.66}\ (round\ to\ the\ nearest\ tenth)$$
$$-300$$
$$2000$$
$$-1800$$
$$200$$

Label with unit of measure.
1.7 mL

✔ **Human Error Check**
Replace X with 1.7.

$$\frac{300}{1} = \frac{500}{1.7}$$

$$500 \approx 510$$

Guideline: 1.7 mL is less than the 3 mL maximum volume for an intramuscular dose.

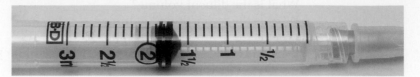

Drug Label
Date (reconstituted)
Discard date (24 hours)
300 mg/mL
Refrigerate
Initials

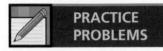

PRACTICE PROBLEMS

Directions: *Using the pictures of medication labels as what you HAVE, answer the questions, calculate the volume to be administered, and mark the syringe with the calculated volume.*

1.

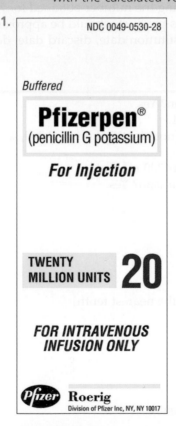

NDC 0049-0530-28

Buffered

Pfizerpen®
(penicillin G potassium)

For Injection

TWENTY MILLION UNITS **20**

FOR INTRAVENOUS INFUSION ONLY

Pfizer **Roerig**
Division of Pfizer Inc, NY, NY 10017

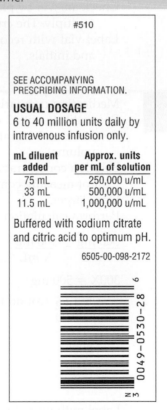

#510

SEE ACCOMPANYING PRESCRIBING INFORMATION.

USUAL DOSAGE
6 to 40 million units daily by intravenous infusion only.

mL diluent added	Approx. units per mL of solution
75 mL	250,000 u/mL
33 mL	500,000 u/mL
11.5 mL	1,000,000 u/mL

Buffered with sodium citrate and citric acid to optimum pH.

6505-00-098-2172

PRESCRIPTION: penicillin G potassium 4,000,000 units intravenous four times a day.
Diluent volume _____
Solution concentration _____
Administer _____

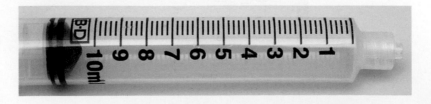

2.

NDC 0015-7403-20
NSN 6505-00-946-4700
EQUIVALENT TO
500 mg AMPICILLIN
STERILE AMPICILLIN
SODIUM, USP
For IM or IV Use
CAUTION: Federal law prohibits
dispensing without prescription.

For IM use, add 1.8 mL diluent
(read accompanying circular).
Resulting solution contains 250 mg
ampicillin per mL.
Use solution within 1 hour.
This vial contains ampicillin sodium
equivalent to 500 mg ampicillin.
Usual Dosage: Adults—250 to
500 mg IM q. 6h.
READ ACCOMPANYING CIRCULAR
for detailed indications, IM or IV
dosage and precautions.
APOTHECON®
A Bristol-Myers Squibb Company
Princeton, NJ 08540 USA

7403200RL-2

Cont:
Exp. Date:

PRESCRIPTION: ampicillin 500 mg intramuscular every 6 hours.
Diluent volume _____
Solution concentration _____
Administer _____

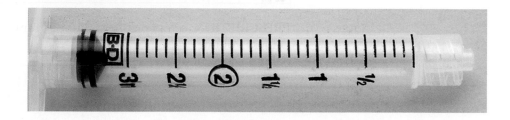

3.

NDC 0009-0233-01
6505-01-067-3977

Bacitracin for
Injection, USP

50,000
Units

For Intramuscular Use

PHARMACIA

℞ only
See package insert for
complete product
information.
Store unreconstituted
product in a refrigerator
2° to 8°C (36° to 46°F).
Reconstitution with 9.8 mL
of sodium chloride
injection containing 2 percent procaine hydro-
chloride will result in a
concentration of 5,000
units per mL. Diluents
containing parabens should
not be used.
Lyophilized in container.
Store solution in a
refrigerator 2° to 8°C
(36° to 46°F).
Discard after 1 week.
Each vial contains:
Bacitracin . . . 50,000 units

810 152 510

PHARMACIA

PRESCRIPTION: bacitracin 1000 units/kg/day. Give two equal doses every 12
hours intramuscular. Child weighs 21 kg.
Diluent volume _____
Solution concentration _____
Total daily dose _____
Each dose _____ units _____ mL

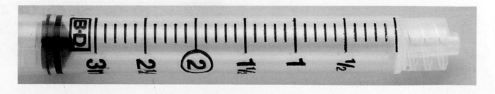

4.

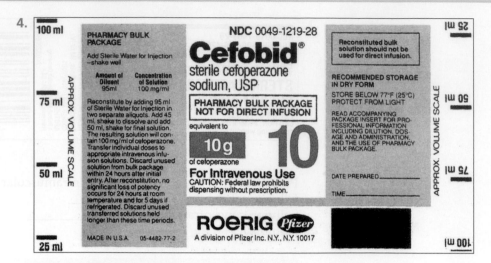

PRESCRIPTION: cefoperazone sodium 1 gram intravenous every 12 hours.

Diluent volume _____

Solution concentration _____

Administer _____

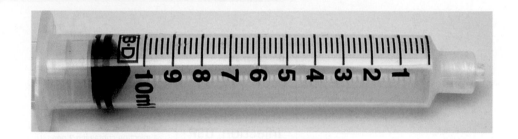

5.

PRESCRIPTION: streptomycin sulfate 1.5 gram intramuscular daily.

Diluent volume _____

Solution concentration _____

Administer _____

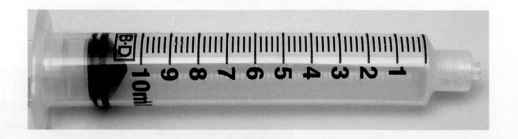

6.

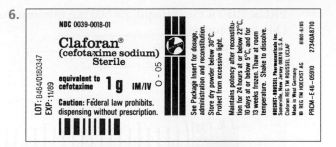

PREPARATION OF CLAFORAN STERILE

Claforan for IM or IV administration should be reconstituted as follows:

Strength	Diluent (mL)	Withdrawable Volume (mL)	Approximate Concentration (mg/mL)
1g vial (IM)*	3	3.4	300
2g vial (IM)*	5	6.0	330
1g vial (IV)*	10	10.4	95
2g vial (IV)*	10	11.0	180
1g infusion	50-100	50-100	20-10
2g infusion	50-100	50-100	40-20
10g bottle	47	52.0	200
10g bottle	97	102.0	100

*in conventional vials

Shake to dissolve; inspect for particulate matter and discoloration prior to use. Solutions of Claforan range from very pale yellow to light amber, depending on concentration, diluent used, and length and condition of storage.

PRESCRIPTION: Claforan 750 mg intramuscular every 8 hours.

Diluent volume _____

Solution concentration _____

Administer _____

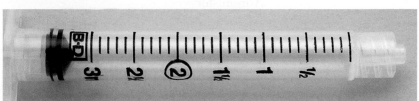

7.

TAZICEF®
CEFTAZIDIME
FOR INJECTION

equivalent to **1gram** ceftazidime
NDC 0007-5082-01

SB SmithKline Beecham

NSN 6505-01-227-3570
For I.V. or I.M. use. **Important:** This vial is under reduced pressure. Addition of diluent generates a positive pressure. Before reconstituting, see Instructions for Reconstitution. Each vial contains ceftazidime pentahydrate equivalent to 1 gram ceftazidime and 118 mg of sodium carbonate. (Sodium content is approximately 54 mg or 2.3 mEq.) **Usual Adult Dose:** 1 gram every 8 to 12 hours. See accompanying prescribing information for reconstitution, dosage and administration instructions. **Before reconstitution:** Protect from light and store at 15° to 30°C. (59° to 86°F). Slight yellowing does not affect potency. Properly reconstituted solutions of *Tazicef* are stable for 24 hours at room temperature or 7 days if refrigerated (5°C). **Caution:** Federal law prohibits dispensing without prescription.
Jointly manufactured by SmithKline Beecham Pharmaceuticals Philadelphia, PA 19101, and **Bristol-Myers Squibb Co.,** New York, NY 10154
693818-H

RECONSTITUTION

Single Dose Vials:
For I.M. injection, I.V. direct (bolus) injection, or I.V. infusion, reconstitute with Sterile Water for injection according to the following table. The vacuum may assist entry of the diluent. SHAKE WELL.

Table 5

Vial Size	Diluent to Be Added	Approx. Avail. Volume	Approx. Avg. Concentration
Intramuscular or Intravenous Direct (bolus) Injection			
1 gram	3.0 mL.	3.6 mL.	280 mg./mL.
Intravenous Infusion			
1 gram	10 mL.	10.6 mL.	95 mg./mL.
2 gram	10 mL.	11.2 mL.	180 mg./mL.

Withdraw the total volume of solution into the syringe (the pressure in the vial may aid withdrawal). The withdrawn solution may contain some bubbles of carbon dioxide.
NOTE: As with the administration of all parenteral products, accumulated gases should be expressed from the syringe immediately before injection of 'Tazicef'.
These solutions of 'Tazicef' are stable for 18 hours at room temperature or seven days if refrigerated (5°C.). Slight yellowing does not affect potency.

For I.V. infusion, dilute reconstituted solution in 50 to 100 mL. of one of the parenteral fluids listed under COMPATIBILITY AND STABILITY.

PRESCRIPTION: ceftazidime 500 mg intramuscular every 8 hours.

Diluent volume _____

Solution concentration _____

Administer _____

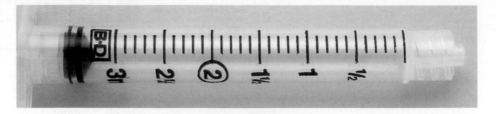

8.

NDC 0015-7226-20

Nafcil™

NAFCILLIN SODIUM
FOR INJECTION
Buffered—For I.M. or I.V. Use
EQUIVALENT TO

2 gram NAFCILLIN

CAUTION: Federal law prohibits
dispensing without prescription.

BRISTOL LABORATORIES
A Bristol-Myers Company
Evansville, IN 47721

When reconstituted with 6.6 ml diluent. (SEE INSERT—INTRAMUSCULAR
ROUTE), each vial contains 8 ml solution. Each ml of solution contains nafcillin sodium, as the monohydrate, equivalent to 250 mg nafcillin, buffered with 10
mg sodium citrate. Read accompanying
circular for complete stability data.

Usual Dosage: Adults—500 mg every 4
to 6 hours. Read accompanying circular
for directions for I.M. or I.V. use.

©Bristol Laboratories

72262DORL-06   LN 7226-99

Lot
Exp. Date

PRESCRIPTION: nafcillin 500 mg intramuscular every 6 hours.

Diluent volume _____

Solution concentration _____

Administer _____

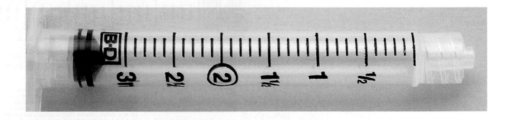

9.

NDC 0015-7970-20

EQUIVALENT TO

2 gram OXACILLIN

OXACILLIN SODIUM
FOR INJECTION, USP

Buffered For IM or IV Use
CAUTION: Federal law prohibits
dispensing without prescription.

APOTHECON®
A BRISTOL-MYERS SQUIBB COMPANY

This vial contains oxacillin
sodium monohydrate equivalent
to 2 grams oxacillin, and 40 mg
dibasic sodium phosphate,
For IM use add 11.5 mL Sterile
Water for Injection, USP. Each 1.5
mL of solution contains 250 mg
oxacillin.
Usual Dosage: Adults—250 mg
to 500 mg intramuscularly every
4 to 6 hours. See circular for
intravenous use.
READ ACCOMPANYING
CIRCULAR
Discard solution after 3 days at
room temperature or 7 days
under refrigeration.
APOTHECON®
A Bristol-Myers Squibb Company
Princeton, NJ 08540 USA   7970200DRL-2

Cont:
Exp. Date:

PRESCRIPTION: oxacillin 250 mg intramuscular every 4 hours.

Diluent volume _____

Solution concentration _____

Administer _____

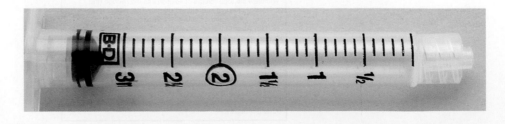

10.

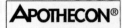

NDC 0015-7339-99
NSN 6505-01-010-0832

Cefazolin for Injection, USP
1 gram

For IM or IV Use   **Rx only**

APOTHECON® PROTECT FROM LIGHT   **10 SINGLE USE VIALS**

PREPARATION OF SOLUTION: For IM Use - Add 2.5 mL Sterile Water for Injection. SHAKE WELL. Resulting solution provides an approximate volume of 3 mL (330 mg per mL).
For IV Use - See insert.
Discard unused solution 24 hours after reconstitution if stored at room temperature or within 10 days if stored under refrigeration, 2° to 8°C (36° to 46°F).
Each vial contains cefazolin sodium equivalent to 1 gram cefazolin. The total sodium content is approximately 48mg (2.1 mEq sodium ion) per gram of cefazolin.
USUAL DOSAGE: 250 mg to 1 g every six to eight hours. See insert.
See package insert for detailed indications, IM or IV dosage and precautions.
Store dry powder at room temperature, 15° to 30°C (59° to 86°F).

PRESCRIPTION: cefazolin 500 mg intramuscular every 8 hours.
Diluent volume _____
Solution concentration _____
Administer _____

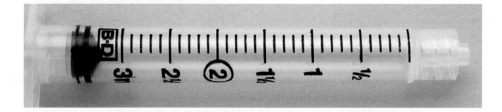

(Answers on pp. 460–461)

ORAL MEDICATIONS

Oral medications are commonly reconstituted with tap water, but the label or package insert must always be reviewed for directions prior to reconstitution. Read the package insert to determine the appropriate volume of diluent. The total volume of the diluent and the dissolved powder may be greater than the total volume of diluent added because the dissolved powder takes up space. It is important to understand that there is a diluent volume and a total volume (diluent + powder) of the container. The total volume is important if it is necessary to calculate how many total doses are available. The number of total doses will help you determine the length of time a bottle will last. The concentration is used for calculations. With liquids the common dose volume is 5 mL (similar to 1 mL with parenteral medications), but this is not always true (Figure 12-9).

Once the appropriate amount of diluent is added to the container, it is very important to shake the bottle to complete the suspension process. It may be necessary to add some diluent and shake, then add the remainder of the diluent and shake to complete the suspension process.

Because reconstituted oral medications are often multidose, always label the reconstituted oral medications with date, time of reconstitution, dose volume if a multidose container (if not visible on the container), storage information (if different

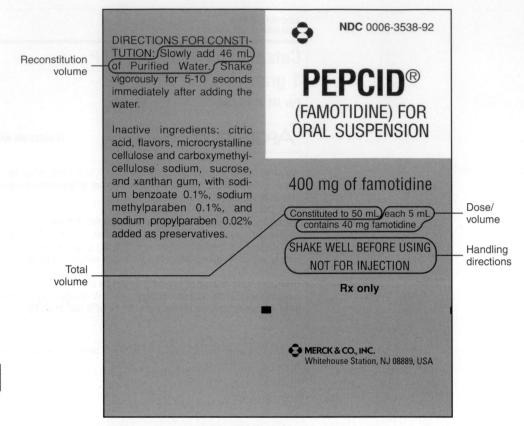

Reconstitution volume

DIRECTIONS FOR CONSTI-
TUTION: Slowly add 46 mL
of Purified Water. Shake
vigorously for 5-10 seconds
immediately after adding the
water.

Inactive ingredients: citric
acid, flavors, microcrystalline
cellulose and carboxymethylcellulose sodium, sucrose,
and xanthan gum, with sodium benzoate 0.1%, sodium
methylparaben 0.1%, and
sodium propylparaben 0.02%
added as preservatives.

Total volume

NDC 0006-3538-92

PEPCID®
(FAMOTIDINE) FOR
ORAL SUSPENSION

400 mg of famotidine

Constituted to 50 mL, each 5 mL
contains 40 mg famotidine

Dose/ volume

SHAKE WELL BEFORE USING
NOT FOR INJECTION

Handling directions

Rx only

MERCK & CO., INC.
Whitehouse Station, NJ 08889, USA

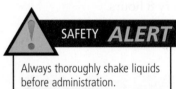

SAFETY **ALERT**

Always thoroughly shake liquids
before administration.

Figure 12-9 Label identifying reconstitution volume versus total volume
and dose/volume, as well as handling directions.

from refrigeration and not visible on label), discard date, and your first and last
initials.

Example 1

PRESCRIPTION	*Keflex 500 mg by mouth three times a day.*
• What You HAVE	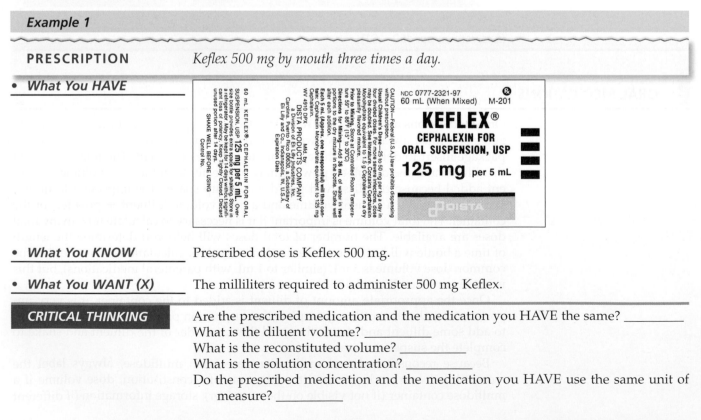
• What You KNOW	Prescribed dose is Keflex 500 mg.
• What You WANT (X)	The milliliters required to administer 500 mg Keflex.
CRITICAL THINKING	Are the prescribed medication and the medication you HAVE the same? _____ What is the diluent volume? _____ What is the reconstituted volume? _____ What is the solution concentration? _____ Do the prescribed medication and the medication you HAVE use the same unit of measure? _____

Is the prescribed dose larger or smaller than the dose you HAVE? _____

In setting up a ratio-proportion, place in the LEFT ratio the solution concentration you HAVE on hand; in the RIGHT ratio, place the prescribed dose in the numerator and place X (the unknown volume) in the denominator.

Multiply to get the cross-products.

Divide the numerical cross-product by the numerical multiplier of X (the number in front of X).

The result is the answer for X.

Label answer properly in units (i.e., number of tablets, number of milliliters).

Check answer by placing the number obtained for X in the original equation. Cross-multiply. The cross-products should be approximately equal.

Label vial with reconstitution date, discard date, dose/volume, storage guidelines, and initials.

ANSWER FOR BEST CARE

Medication comparison? Yes.

Reconstitute with 36 mL tap water. Add 18 mL tap water and shake. Repeat.

Solution concentration? 125 mg/5 mL.

Unit of measure comparison? Yes.

Dose larger.

Perform calculation.

$$\frac{125 \text{ mg}}{5 \text{ mL}} = \frac{500 \text{ mg}}{X \text{ mL}}$$

$$125X = 2500$$

$$125)\overline{2500} \quad \frac{20}{}$$

$$X = 20 \text{ mL}$$

✔ **Human Error Check**

Replace X with 20.

$$\frac{125}{5} = \frac{500}{20}$$

$$2500 = 2500$$

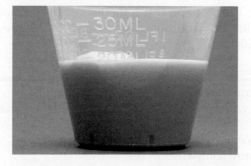

Drug Label
Date/time
Discard date
125 mg/5 mL
Refrigerate
Initials

Example 2

PRESCRIPTION   *Clarithromycin (Biaxin) 375 mg by mouth every 12 hours times 10 days.*

• *What You HAVE*

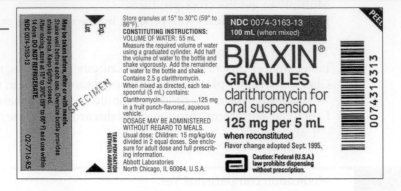

Store granules at 15° to 30°C (59° to 86°F).
CONSTITUTING INSTRUCTIONS:
VOLUME OF WATER: 55 mL
Measure the required volume of water using a graduated cylinder. Add half the volume of water to the bottle and shake vigorously. Add the remainder of water to the bottle and shake. Contains 2.5 g clarithromycin. When mixed as directed, each tea-spoonful (5 mL) contains:
Clarithromycin.................125 mg
in a fruit punch-flavored, aqueous vehicle.
DOSAGE MAY BE ADMINISTERED WITHOUT REGARD TO MEALS.
Usual dose: Children: 15 mg/kg/day divided in 2 equal doses. See enclo-sure for adult dose and full prescrib-ing information.
Abbott Laboratories
North Chicago, IL 60064, U.S.A.

NDC 0074-3163-13
100 mL (when mixed)
BIAXIN®
GRANULES
clarithromycin for oral suspension
125 mg per 5 mL
when reconstituted
Flavor change adopted Sept. 1995.
Caution: Federal (U.S.A.) law prohibits dispensing without prescription.

• *What You KNOW*   Prescribed dose is clarithromycin 375 mg.

• *What You WANT (X)*   The milliliters required to administer clarithromycin 375 mg.

CRITICAL THINKING

Are the prescribed medication and the medication you HAVE the same drug? _____
What is the diluent volume? _____
What is the reconstituted volume? _____
What is the solution concentration? _____
Do the prescribed medication and the medication you HAVE use the same unit of measure? _____
Is the prescribed dose larger or smaller than the dose you HAVE? _____
In setting up a ratio-proportion, place in the LEFT ratio the solution concentration you HAVE on hand; in the RIGHT ratio, place the prescribed dose in the numera-tor and place X (the unknown volume) in the denominator.
Multiply to get the cross-products.
Divide the numerical cross-product by the numerical multiplier of X (the number in front of X).
The result is the answer for X.
Label answer properly in units (i.e., number of tablets, number of milliliters).
Check answer by placing the number obtained for X in the original equation. Cross-multiply. The cross-products should be approximately equal.
Label vial with reconstitution date, discard date, dose/volume, storage guidelines, and initials.

ANSWER FOR BEST CARE

Medication comparison? Yes.
Reconstitute with 55 mL tap water. Add 25 mL and shake and repeat, adding 30 mL more.
Solution concentration? 125 mg/5 mL.
Unit of measure comparison? Yes.
Dose larger.
Perform calculation.

$$\frac{125 \text{ mg}}{5 \text{ mL}} = \frac{375 \text{ mg}}{X \text{ mL}}$$

$$125X = 1875$$

$$\frac{15}{125\overline{)1875}}$$
$$\frac{-\ 125}{625}$$
$$\frac{-\ 625}{0}$$

X = 15 mL

✓ **Human Error Check**

Replace X with 15.

$$\frac{125}{5} = \frac{375}{15}$$

1875 = 1875

Drug Label
Date/time (reconstituted)
Discard date (14 days)
125 mg/5 mL
Refrigerate
Initials

Example 3

~~~~~~

PRESCRIPTION	*Cefaclor (Ceclor) 300 mg by mouth every 8 hours.*

• **What You HAVE**

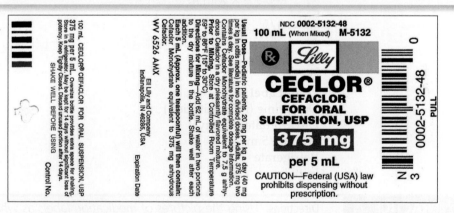

• **What You KNOW**   Prescribed dose is for cefaclor 300 mg.

• **What You WANT (X)**   The milliliters required to administer 300 mg cefaclor.

CRITICAL THINKING	Are the prescribed medication and the medication you HAVE the same drug? _____

What is the diluent volume? _____
What is the reconstituted volume? _____
What is the solution concentration? _____
Do the prescribed medication and the medication you HAVE use the same unit of measure? _____
Is the prescribed dose larger or smaller than the dose you HAVE? _____
In setting up a ratio-proportion, place in the LEFT ratio the solution concentration you HAVE on hand; in the RIGHT ratio, place the prescribed dose in the numerator and place X (the unknown volume) in the denominator.

Multiply to get the cross-products.

Divide the numerical cross-product by the numerical multiplier of X (the number in front of X).

The result is the answer for X.

Label answer properly in units (i.e., number of tablets, number of milliliters).

Check answer by placing the number obtained for X in the original equation. Cross-multiply. The cross-products should be approximately equal.

Label vial with reconstitution date, discard date, dose/volume, storage guidelines, and initials.

ANSWER FOR BEST CARE

Medication comparison? Yes.

Reconstitute with 62 mL tap water in two nearly equal portions. Shake after each of the two additions.

Solution concentration? 375 mg/5 mL.

Unit of measure comparison? Yes.

Dose smaller.

Perform calculation.

$$\frac{375 \text{ mg}}{5 \text{ mL}} = \frac{300 \text{ mg}}{X \text{ mL}} \qquad 375X = 1500$$

$$375\overline{)1500}^{4}$$

Label with the unit of measure.

4 mL

> ✔ **Human Error Check**
>
> Replace X with 4.
>
> $$\frac{375}{5} = \frac{300}{4}$$
>
> 1500 = 1500

Drug Label
Date/time (reconstitution)
Discard date (14 days)
375 mg/5 mL
Refrigerate
Initials

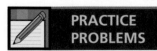

PRACTICE PROBLEMS

Directions: *Using the pictures of medication labels as what you HAVE, answer the questions, calculate the volume to be administered, and mark the medicine cup or the oral syringe (at the point you would pull the plunger back to) with this calculated volume.*

1.

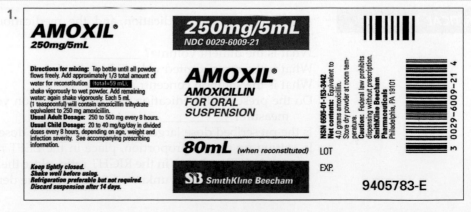

Prescription: amoxicillin oral suspension 500 mg by mouth every 8 hours.
Diluent volume _____
Solution concentration _____
Administer _____

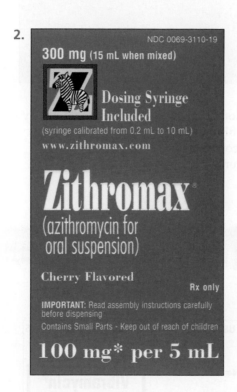

2.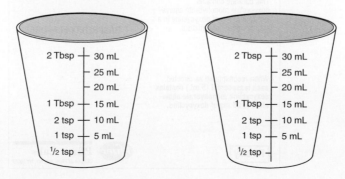

Prescription: Zithromax oral suspension 200 mg today and 100 mg once daily for the next 4 days.
Solution concentration _____
Total volume _____
Administer day 1 _____ Administer days 2-5 _____

3.

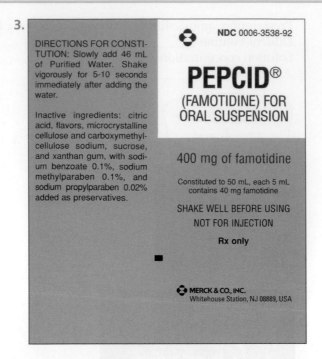

DIRECTIONS FOR CONSTI-
TUTION: Slowly add 46 mL
of Purified Water. Shake
vigorously for 5-10 seconds
immediately after adding the
water.

Inactive ingredients: citric
acid, flavors, microcrystalline
cellulose and carboxymethylcellulose sodium, sucrose,
and xanthan gum, with sodium benzoate 0.1%, sodium
methylparaben 0.1%, and
sodium propylparaben 0.02%
added as preservatives.

NDC 0006-3538-92

PEPCID®
(FAMOTIDINE) FOR
ORAL SUSPENSION

400 mg of famotidine

Constituted to 50 mL, each 5 mL
contains 40 mg famotidine

SHAKE WELL BEFORE USING
NOT FOR INJECTION

Rx only

MERCK & CO., INC.
Whitehouse Station, NJ 08889, USA

Prescription: famotidine suspension 20 mg by mouth twice daily.
Diluent volume _____
Solution concentration _____
Administer _____

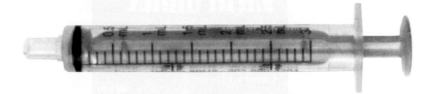

4. **FOR ORAL USE ONLY.**   NDC 0069-0970-65

Store dry powder below
86°F (30°C).

60 mL when reconstituted

Vibramycin®
(doxycycline monohydrate)

DOSAGE AND USE
See accompanying prescribing
information.

FOR ORAL SUSPENSION

25 mg/5 mL*

RASPBERRY FLAVORED

This package contains
doxycycline monohydrate equivalent to **300 mg** of doxycycline in a
raspberry-flavored mixture.

*When reconstituted as directed,
**each teaspoonful (5 mL) contains
doxycycline monohydrate equivalent to 25 mg of doxycycline.**

Rx only

Pfizer **Pfizer Labs**
Division of Pfizer Inc, NY, NY 10017

EXP

To the Pharmacist:

1. Mixing Directions:
Tap bottle lightly to loosen powder.
Add 47.6 mL of water to the bottle
to make a total volume of 60 mL.
Shake well.

2. This prescription, when in suspension, will maintain its potency
for two weeks when kept at room
temperature.

**DISCARD UNUSED PORTION
AFTER TWO WEEKS.**

Prescription: doxycycline monohydrate suspension 100 mg by mouth daily.
Diluent volume _____
Solution concentration _____
Administer _____

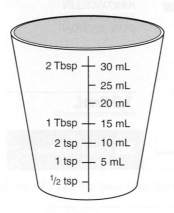

5.
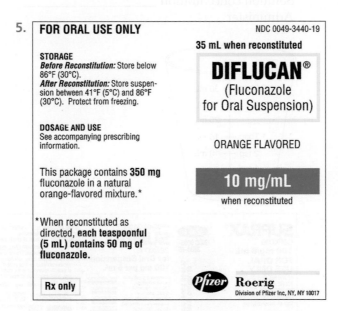

Prescription: fluconazole suspension 75 mg by mouth daily for 14 days.
Diluent volume _____
Solution concentration _____
Administer _____

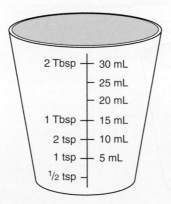

6.

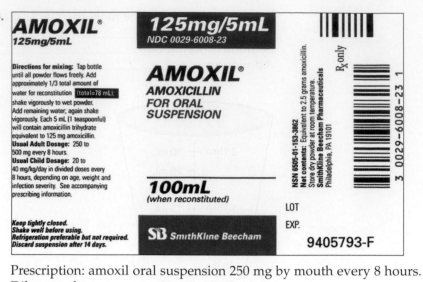

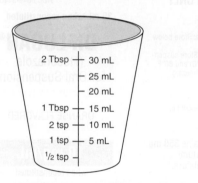

Prescription: amoxil oral suspension 250 mg by mouth every 8 hours.

Diluent volume _____

Solution concentration _____

Administer _____

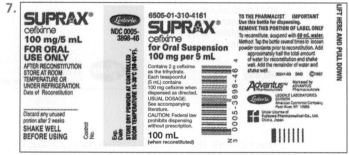

7.

Prescription: Suprax 400 mg by mouth daily.

Diluent volume _____

Solution concentration _____

Administer _____

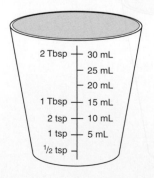

8.

NDC 0002-5136-18
75 mL (When Mixed)   M-5136

® *Lilly*

LORABID®
LORACARBEF
FOR ORAL
SUSPENSION, USP

200 mg
per 5 mL

CAUTION—Federal (USA)
law prohibits dispensing
without prescription.

0002-5136-18 PULL
N 3

75 mL LORABID® LORACARBEF FOR ORAL SUSPENSION, USP
200 mg per 5 mL. Oversize bottle provides extra space for shaking. Store at room temperature (59° to 86°F). May be kept for 14 days without significant loss of potency. Keep Tightly Closed. Discard unused portion after 14 days.
SHAKE WELL BEFORE USING

Usual Dose—Pediatric patients, 15 mg per kg per day (30 mg per kg per day for otitis media) in divided doses twice a day. Adults, 200 mg twice a day. See literature for complete dosage information.
Prior to Mixing, Store at Controlled Room Temperature 59° to 86°F (15° to 30°C).
Directions for Mixing—Add 45 mL of water in two portions to the dry mixture in the bottle. Shake well after each addition.
Contains Loracarbef equivalent to 3 g of activity in a dry pleasantly flavored mixture.
Each 5 mL (Approx. one teaspoonful) will then contain: Loracarbef equivalent to 200 mg of activity.

WW 4581 AMX
Eli Lilly and Company
Indianapolis, IN 46285, USA

Expiration Date

Control No.

Prescription: loracarbef 400 mg by mouth every 12 hours times 14 days.
Diluent volume _____
Solution concentration _____
Administer _____

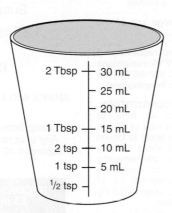

2 Tbsp — 30 mL
— 25 mL
— 20 mL
1 Tbsp — 15 mL
2 tsp — 10 mL
1 tsp — 5 mL
½ tsp —

9.

Cleocin Pediatric®
clindamycin palmitate
hydrochloride for oral
solution, USP

**75 mg
per 5 mL**

Equiv. to **75 mg per 5 mL**
clindamycin when reconstituted

**Pharmacia
&Upjohn**

100 mL
(when mixed)

NDC 0009-0760-04

Rx only

Usual child dosage - 5 mL
(1 teaspoonful) four times daily.
See package insert for complete
product information.

Warning - Not for injection

**DO NOT REFRIGERATE
SOLUTION**

Store solution at room
temperature

Store unreconstituted product at
controlled room temperature 20°
to 25°C (68° to 77°F)(see USP).

Reconstitute with a total of
75 mL of water as follows: Add a
large portion of the water and
shake vigorously; add remaining
water and shake until solution is
uniform.

Each 5mL (teaspoonful) of the
solution contains clindamycin
palmitate HCl equivalent to
75mg clindamycin. Each bottle
contains the equivalent of
1.5 grams clindamycin.

810 901 510

Prescription: clindamycin palmitate hydrochloride 100 mg by mouth every 8
hours.
Diluent volume _____

Solution concentration _____

Administer _____

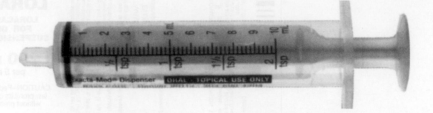

10.

Usual Dosage:	Children-14 mg/kg/day

Usual Dosage: Children-14 mg/kg/day in a single dose or in two divided doses, depending on age, weight, and type of infection. See package enclosure for full prescribing information.

This bottle contains 2.5 g cefdinir.

Keep this and all drugs out of the reach of children.

Store dry powder and reconstituted suspension at 25°C (77°F); excursions permitted to 15°-30°C (59°-86°F) [see USP Controlled Room Temperature].

DIRECTIONS FOR RECONSTITUTION
Prepare suspension at time of dispensing by adding a total of **63 mL** water to the bottle. Tap bottle to loosen the powder, then add about half the water, and shake. Add the remaining water and shake to complete suspension. This provides 100 mL of suspension. Each 5 mL contains 125 mg cefdinir after reconstitution.

See bottom of carton for expiration date and lot number.

NDC 0074-3771-13

Omnicef®
(Cefdinir) for Oral
Suspension
125 mg/5 mL

℞ only

SHAKE WELL BEFORE USING.

Keep bottle tightly closed.
Any unused portion must be
discarded 10 days after mixing.

**RECONSTITUTE WITH
63 mL WATER**

100 mL (when reconstituted)

Prescription: cefdinir 175 mg by mouth every 12 hours.

Diluent volume _____

Solution concentration _____

Administer _____

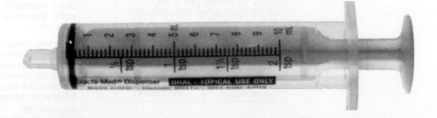

(Answers on pp. 461–462)

LIQUID CONCENTRATES

When reconstituting liquid concentrates, it is important to be able to understand what volume of concentrate is mixed with the solvent to result in a specific strength of solution. This may be expressed as a fraction, percentage, or a ratio ($\frac{1}{2}$ or 50% or 1:2). The numerator of the fraction is the parts of solute, and the denominator of the fraction is the parts of total solution volume. A $\frac{1}{4}$ solution is 1 part solute to 4 parts total solution volume. The amount of solvent/diluent is the difference between the solute and the total volume. When a liquid concentrate is added to a given amount of solvent, the finished solution is the sum of the two.

Example 1

PRESCRIPTION	*Begin tube feeding at $\frac{1}{4}$ strength for first 500 mL.*

- **What You HAVE**

  Full-strength formula 250 mL (solute).
  Water (solvent).

- **What You KNOW**

  The prescribed solution strength is $\frac{1}{4}$.
  Total solution volume prescribed is 500 mL.

- **What You WANT (X)**

  Volume of full-strength formula (solute) required to make 500 mL $\frac{1}{4}$-strength solution.
  Volume of water to be mixed with the formula (solute) to make 500 mL of $\frac{1}{4}$-strength solution.

CRITICAL THINKING

What is the prescribed solution strength? _____
What is the total prescribed solution volume? _____
In setting up a ratio-proportion, place in the LEFT ratio the prescribed solution strength; in the RIGHT ratio, X (the unknown solute volume) is the numerator and the total prescribed solution volume is the denominator.
The difference between the total solution volume (500 mL) and X is the amount of water (solvent) to be added.

ANSWER FOR BEST CARE

Prescribed solution strength? $\frac{1}{4}$.
Total prescribed solution volume? 500 mL.
Perform calculation.
(Prescribed strength)

$$\frac{1}{4} = \frac{X \text{ mL}}{500 \text{ mL}} \quad \frac{\text{(unknown solute volume)}}{\text{(total prescribed volume)}}$$

$$4\overline{)500} \text{(125)}$$

X = 125 mL of tube feeding

✔ **Human Error Check**

Replace X with 125.

$$\frac{1}{4} = \frac{125}{500}$$

$$500 = 500$$

Total water volume calculation:

$$
\begin{array}{ll}
500 \text{ mL} & \text{(total solution volume)} \\
- 125 \text{ mL} & \text{(X)} \\
\hline
375 \text{ mL} & \text{(total solvent volume)}
\end{array}
$$

You will mix 125 mL of full-strength tube feeding with 375 mL of water.

Example 2

PRESCRIPTION   *Give $\frac{2}{3}$-strength tube feeding 500 mL every 8 hours.*

• **What You HAVE**   Full-strength tube feeding 500 mL (solute).
Water (solvent).

• **What You KNOW**   The prescribed solution strength is $\frac{2}{3}$.
Total solution volume prescribed is 500 mL.

• **What You WANT (X)**   Volume of tube feeding (solute) required to make 500 mL $\frac{2}{3}$-strength solution.
Volume water to be mixed to the tube feeding to make 500 mL $\frac{2}{3}$-strength solution.

CRITICAL THINKING   What is the prescribed solution strength? _____
What is the total desired solution volume? _____
In setting up a ratio-proportion, place in the LEFT ratio the prescribed solution strength; in the RIGHT ratio, X (the unknown solute volume) is the numerator and the total desired solution volume is the denominator.
The difference between the total solution volume (500 mL) and X is the amount of solvent (water) to be added.

ANSWER FOR BEST CARE   Solution strength? $\frac{2}{3}$.
Total desired solution volume? 500 mL.
Perform calculation.

$$\frac{2}{3} = \frac{X \text{ mL}}{500 \text{ mL}}$$

$$3X = 1000$$

$$3\overline{)1000} \quad 333$$

X = 333 mL of full-strength tube feeding.

> ✓ **Human Error Check**
>
> Replace X with 333.
>
> $$\frac{2}{3} = \frac{333}{500}$$
>
> $1000 \approx 999$

Total water volume calculation:

$$
\begin{array}{ll}
500 \text{ mL} & \text{(total solution volume)} \\
- 333 \text{ mL} & \text{(X)} \\
\hline
167 \text{ mL} & \text{(total solvent volume)}
\end{array}
$$

You will add 333 mL of tube feeding to 167 mL of water.

Example 3

PRESCRIPTION	*Irrigate wound with 250 mL of $\frac{1}{2}$-strength irrigating solution three times a day.*

- **What You HAVE**

  Full-strength irrigant (solute).
  Normal saline (solvent).

- **What You KNOW**

  Prescribed total solution volume is 250 mL.
  Prescribed solution strength is $\frac{1}{2}$.

- **What You WANT (X)**

  Volume of irrigant needed to make 250 mL $\frac{1}{2}$-strength solution.
  Volume of normal saline to be mixed with the irrigant to make 250 mL $\frac{1}{2}$-strength solution.

CRITICAL THINKING

What is the solution strength? _____
What is the total desired solution volume? _____
In setting up a ratio-proportion, place in the LEFT ratio the prescribed solution strength; in the RIGHT ratio, X (the unknown solute volume) is the numerator and the total prescribed solution volume is the denominator.
The difference between the total solution volume (500 mL) and X is the amount of solvent (normal saline) to be added.

ANSWER FOR BEST CARE

Solution strength? $\frac{1}{2}$.
Total desired solution volume? 250 mL.
Perform calculation.

$$\frac{1}{2} = \frac{X \text{ mL}}{250 \text{ mL}} \quad 2X = 250$$

$$2\overline{)250} = 125$$

X = 125 mL (total volume of irrigant).

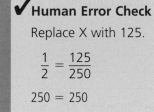

✔ **Human Error Check**

Replace X with 125.

$$\frac{1}{2} = \frac{125}{250}$$

$$250 = 250$$

Total water volume calculation:

$$\begin{array}{r} 250 \text{ mL (total desired solution volume)} \\ - 125 \text{ mL (X)} \\ \hline 125 \text{ mL (total solvent)} \end{array}$$

You will add 125 mL of wound irrigation and 125 mL of normal saline together.

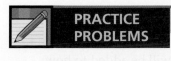

PRACTICE PROBLEMS

Directions: *Fill in the blanks with the appropriate information.*

1. You have been asked to prepare a 40% solution from 20 mL of mouthwash.
   Solution strength _____
   Total solution volume _____
   Total solute volume _____
   Total solvent volume _____

2. How much water would be required to prepare a 1:10 solution from 90 mL of skin cleanser?
   Solution strength _____
   Total solution volume _____
   Total solute volume _____
   Total solvent volume _____

3. How much water would be required to prepare a 2% solution from 1 level teaspoon (5 mL) of soda bicarbonate?
   Solution strength _____
   Total solution volume _____
   Total solute volume _____
   Total solvent volume _____

4. How much glucose would be required to make up 1 L of 5% glucose?
   Solution strength _____
   Total solution volume _____
   Total solute volume _____
   Total solvent volume _____

5. How much salt and how much water are in 500 mL of 3% NaCl?
   Solution strength _____
   Total solution volume _____
   Total solute volume _____
   Total solvent volume _____

6. You have a 300-mL can of Sustacal. You need to give 200 mL ¾-strength Sustacal via nasogastric tube. How much water will you add to the can of Sustacal?
   Solution strength _____
   Total solution volume _____
   Total solute volume _____
   Total solvent volume _____

7. You need to give 480 mL of ¼-strength tube feeding. What you have is a quart of full-strength tube feeding. How much water will you add to how much tube feeding to give 480 mL?
   Solution strength _____
   Total solution volume _____
   Total solute volume _____
   Total solvent volume _____

8. How much glucose is in 500 mL of 20% dextrose?
   Solution strength _____
   Total solution volume _____
   Total solute volume _____
   Total solvent volume _____

9. How much normal saline would you add to wound irrigant to make 100 mL of 75% solution?
   Solution strength _____
   Total solution volume _____
   Total solute volume _____
   Total solvent volume _____

10. You are to give 300 mL of ¼-strength Ensure over 4 hours via nasogastric tube. You have a 240-mL can of Ensure. How much water will be added to how much Ensure?
    Solution strength _____
    Total solution volume _____

Total solute volume _____
Total solvent volume _____

(Answers on p. 462)

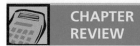 **CHAPTER REVIEW**

Using the pictures of medication labels as what you HAVE, calculate the volume to be administered, and mark the syringe or medicine cup with this volume.

1.

AMOXIL® 250mg/5mL

250mg/5mL
NDC 0029-6009-21

AMOXIL®
AMOXICILLIN
FOR ORAL
SUSPENSION

Directions for mixing: Tap bottle until all powder flows freely. Add approximately 1/3 total amount of water for reconstitution (total=59 mL); shake vigorously to wet powder. Add remaining water; again shake vigorously. Each 5 mL (1 teaspoonful) will contain amoxicillin trihydrate equivalent to 250 mg amoxicillin.
Usual Adult Dosage: 250 to 500 mg every 8 hours.
Usual Child Dosage: 20 to 40 mg/kg/day in divided doses every 8 hours, depending on age, weight and infection severity. See accompanying prescribing information.

80mL *(when reconstituted)*

Keep tightly closed.
Shake well before using.
Refrigeration preferable but not required.
Discard suspension after 14 days.

SB SmithKline Beecham

NSN 6505-01-153-3442
Net contents: Equivalent to 4.0 grams amoxicillin. Store dry powder at room temperature. Caution: Federal law prohibits dispensing without prescription. SmithKline Beecham Pharmaceuticals Philadelphia, PA 19101

LOT
EXP.

9405783-E

PRESCRIPTION: amoxicillin oral suspension 150 mg by mouth every 8 hours.
Administer _____

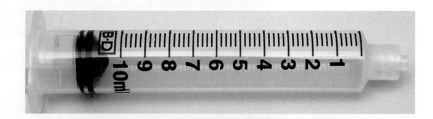

2.

300 mg
(15 mL when mixed)

www.zithromax.com

Dosing Syringe Included
(syringe calibrated from 0.2 mL to 10 mL)

FOR ORAL USE ONLY

Zithromax
(azithromycin for oral suspension)

Cherry Flavored

100 mg* per 5 mL

SHAKE WELL BEFORE USING.
Oversized bottle provides extra space for shaking.
After mixing, store suspension at 5° to 30°C (41° to 86°F).
After mixing, use within 10 days. Discard after full dosing is completed.
Calibrated dosing device included.

Store dry powder below 30°C (86°F).
PROTECT FROM FREEZING.
DOSAGE AND USE
See accompanying prescribing information.
Contains 300 mg azithromycin.
* When constituted as directed, each teaspoonful (5 mL) contains azithromycin dihydrate equivalent to 100 mg of azithromycin.

Pfizer Pfizer Labs
Division of Pfizer Inc, NY, NY 10017

MADE IN USA
6415

PRESCRIPTION: Zithromax oral suspension 260 mg by mouth once.
Administer _____

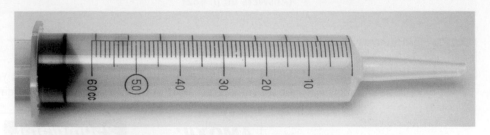

3.

DIRECTIONS FOR CONSTI-
TUTION: Slowly add 46 mL
of Purified Water. Shake
vigorously for 5-10 seconds
immediately after adding the
water.

Inactive ingredients: citric
acid, flavors, microcrystalline
cellulose and carboxymethylcellulose sodium, sucrose,
and xanthan gum, with sodium benzoate 0.1%, sodium
methylparaben 0.1%, and
sodium propylparaben 0.02%
added as preservatives.

NDC 0006-3538-92

PEPCID®
(FAMOTIDINE) FOR ORAL SUSPENSION

400 mg of famotidine

Constituted to 50 mL, each 5 mL
contains 40 mg famotidine

SHAKE WELL BEFORE USING

NOT FOR INJECTION

Rx only

MERCK & CO., INC.
Whitehouse Station, NJ 08889, USA

PRESCRIPTION: famotidine suspension 40 mg by mouth
twice daily.
Administer _____

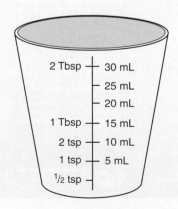

2 Tbsp — 30 mL
— 25 mL
— 20 mL
1 Tbsp — 15 mL
2 tsp — 10 mL
1 tsp — 5 mL
1/2 tsp —

4.

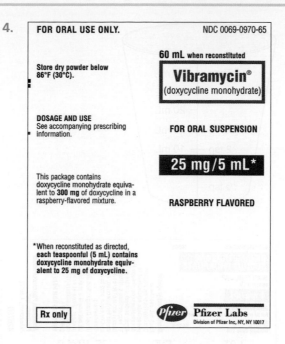

FOR ORAL USE ONLY.

NDC 0069-0970-65

Store dry powder below 86°F (30°C).

60 mL when reconstituted

Vibramycin®
(doxycycline monohydrate)

DOSAGE AND USE
See accompanying prescribing information.

FOR ORAL SUSPENSION

25 mg/5 mL*

This package contains doxycycline monohydrate equivalent to **300 mg** of doxycycline in a raspberry-flavored mixture.

RASPBERRY FLAVORED

*When reconstituted as directed, **each teaspoonful (5 mL) contains doxycycline monohydrate equivalent to 25 mg of doxycycline.**

Rx only

Pfizer **Pfizer Labs**
Division of Pfizer Inc, NY, NY 10017

PRESCRIPTION: doxycycline monohydrate suspension 35 mg by mouth daily.
Administer _____

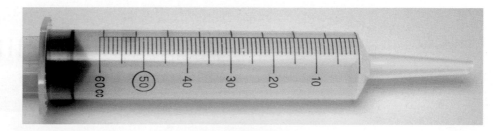

5.

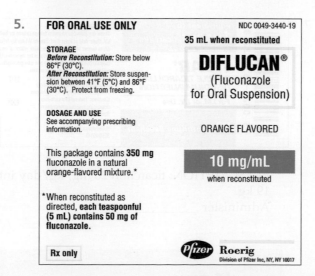

FOR ORAL USE ONLY

NDC 0049-3440-19

35 mL when reconstituted

STORAGE
Before Reconstitution: Store below 86°F (30°C).
After Reconstitution: Store suspension between 41°F (5°C) and 86°F (30°C). Protect from freezing.

DIFLUCAN®
(Fluconazole for Oral Suspension)

DOSAGE AND USE
See accompanying prescribing information.

ORANGE FLAVORED

This package contains **350 mg** fluconazole in a natural orange-flavored mixture.*

10 mg/mL
when reconstituted

*When reconstituted as directed, **each teaspoonful (5 mL) contains 50 mg of fluconazole.**

Rx only

Pfizer **Roerig**
Division of Pfizer Inc, NY, NY 10017

PRESCRIPTION: fluconazole suspension 200 mg by mouth daily for 14 days.
Administer _____

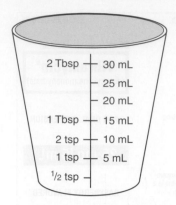

6.

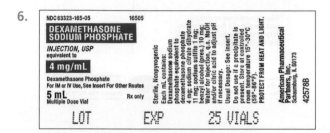

PRESCRIPTION: dexamethasone 9 mg intramuscular daily.
Administer _____

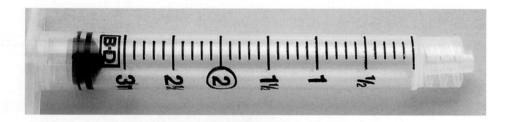

7.

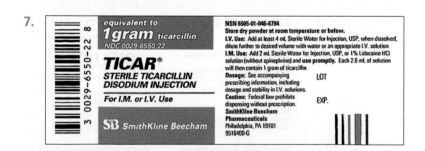

PRESCRIPTION: ticarcillin 20 mg/kg/day intramuscular. Baby weighs
19 kg.
Administer _____

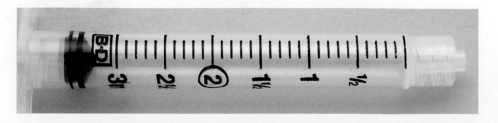

8.

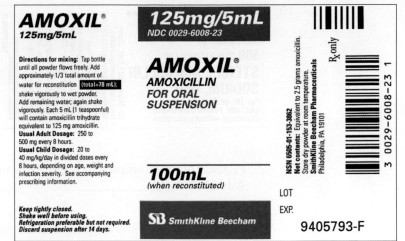

PRESCRIPTION: amoxil oral suspension 400 mg by mouth every 8 hours.
Administer _____

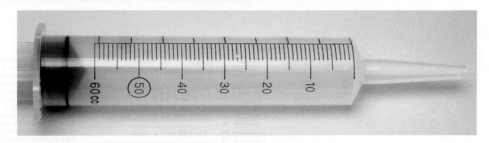

9.

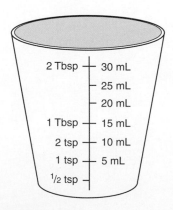

PRESCRIPTION: Suprax 200 mg by mouth daily.
Administer _____

10.

NDC 0015-7403-20
NSN 6505-00-946-4700
EQUIVALENT TO
500 mg AMPICILLIN
STERILE AMPICILLIN
SODIUM, USP
For IM or IV Use
CAUTION: Federal law prohibits
dispensing without prescription.

For IM use, add 1.8 mL diluent
(read accompanying circular).
Resulting solution contains 250 mg
ampicillin per mL.
Use solution within 1 hour.
This vial contains ampicillin sodium
equivalent to 500 mg ampicillin.
Usual Dosage: Adults—250 to
500 mg IM q. 6h.
READ ACCOMPANYING CIRCULAR
for detailed indications, IM or IV
dosage and precautions.
APOTHECON®
A Bristol-Myers Squibb Company
Princeton, NJ 08540 USA

7403200RL-2

Cont:
Exp. Date:

PRESCRIPTION: ampicillin 500 mg intramuscular every 6 hours.
Administer _____

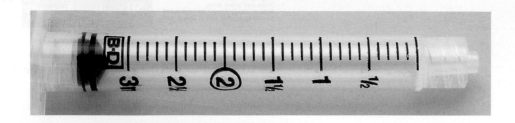

11.

equivalent to
1 gram *ticarcillin*
NDC 0029-6550-22

TICAR®
STERILE TICARCILLIN
DISODIUM INJECTION
For I.M. or I.V. Use

SB *SmithKline Beecham*

3 0029-6550-22 8

NSN 6505-01-046-6794
Store dry powder at room temperature or below.
I.V. Use: Add at least 4 mL Sterile Water for Injection, USP; when dissolved,
dilute further to desired volume with water or an appropriate I.V. solution.
I.M. Use: Add 2 mL Sterile Water for Injection, USP, or 1% Lidocaine HCl
solution (without epinephrine) and use promptly. Each 2.6 mL of solution
will then contain 1 gram of ticarcillin.
Dosage: See accompanying
prescribing information, including
dosage and stability in I.V. solutions.
Caution: Federal law prohibits
dispensing without prescription.
SmithKline Beecham
Pharmaceuticals
Philadelphia, PA 19101
9516400-G

LOT

EXP.

PRESCRIPTION: ticarcillin (Ticar) 0.5 gram intramuscular every 6 hours.
Administer _____

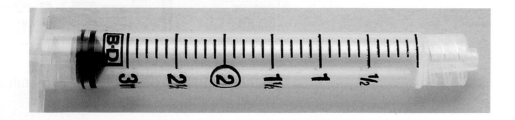

12.

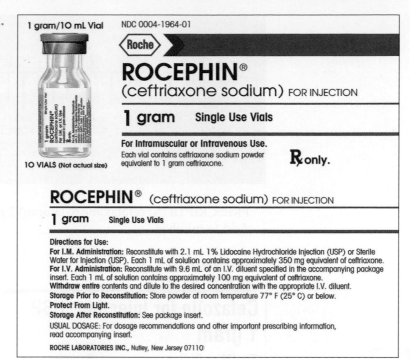

1 gram/10 mL Vial NDC 0004-1964-01

Roche

ROCEPHIN®
(ceftriaxone sodium) FOR INJECTION

1 gram Single Use Vials

For Intramuscular or Intravenous Use.
Each vial contains ceftriaxone sodium powder
equivalent to 1 gram ceftriaxone.

R only.

10 VIALS (Not actual size)

ROCEPHIN® (ceftriaxone sodium) FOR INJECTION

1 gram Single Use Vials

Directions for Use:
For I.M. Administration: Reconstitute with 2.1 mL 1% Lidocaine Hydrochloride Injection (USP) or Sterile
Water for Injection (USP). Each 1 mL of solution contains approximately 350 mg equivalent of ceftriaxone.
For I.V. Administration: Reconstitute with 9.6 mL of an I.V. diluent specified in the accompanying package
insert. Each 1 mL of solution contains approximately 100 mg equivalent of ceftriaxone.
Withdraw entire contents and dilute to the desired concentration with the appropriate I.V. diluent.
Storage Prior to Reconstitution: Store powder at room temperature 77° F (25° C) or below.
Protect From Light.
Storage After Reconstitution: See package insert.
USUAL DOSAGE: For dosage recommendations and other important prescribing information,
read accompanying insert.

ROCHE LABORATORIES INC., Nutley, New Jersey 07110

PRESCRIPTION: ceftriaxone sodium (Rocephin) 175 mg intramuscular
every 12 hours.
Administer _____

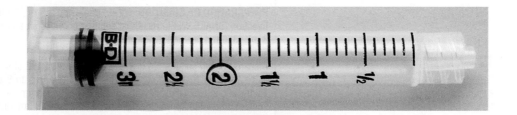

13.

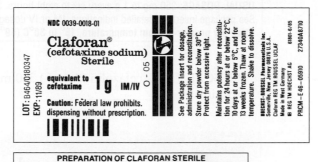

NDC 0039-0018-01

Claforan®
(cefotaxime sodium)
Sterile

equivalent to
cefotaxime **1 g** IM/IV

Caution: Federal law prohibits.
dispensing without prescription.

LOT: B464/0180347
EXP: 11/89

See Package Insert for dosage,
administration and reconstitution.
Store dry powder below 30°C.
Protect from excessive light.

Maintains potency after reconstitution for 24 hours at or below 22°C,
10 days at or below 5°C, and for
13 weeks frozen. Thaw at room
temperature. Shake to dissolve.

HOECHST-ROUSSEL Pharmaceuticals Inc.
Somerville, New Jersey 08876 U.S.A.
Claforan REG TM ROUSSEL UCLAF
Made in West Germany
REG TM HOECHST AG
PRCM—E46—05910

6180I-6/85
27340A8710

PREPARATION OF CLAFORAN STERILE
Claforan for IM or IV administration should be reconstituted as
follows:

Strength	Diluent (mL)	Withdrawable Volume (mL)	Approximate Concentration (mg/mL)
1g vial (IM)*	3	3.4	300
2g vial (IM)*	5	6.0	330
1g vial (IV)*	10	10.4	95
2g vial (IV)*	10	11.0	180
1g infusion	50-100	50-100	20-10
2g infusion	50-100	50-100	40-20
10g bottle	47	52.0	200
10g bottle	97	102.0	100

*in conventional vials

Shake to dissolve; inspect for particulate matter and discoloration
prior to use. Solutions of Claforan range from very pale yellow to
light amber, depending on concentration, diluent used, and length
and condition of storage.

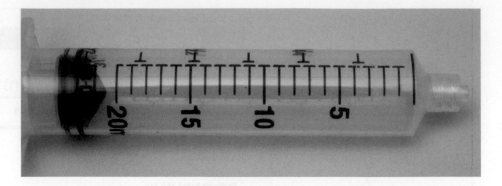

PRESCRIPTION: cefotaxime (Claforan) 2 gram intravenous every 8 hours. Add to minibag _____

14.

NDC 0015-7339-99
NSN 6505-01-010-0832

Cefazolin for Injection, USP
1 gram

For IM or IV Use   **Rx only**

APOTHECON®   PROTECT FROM LIGHT   10 SINGLE USE VIALS

PREPARATION OF SOLUTION: For IM Use - Add 2.5 mL Sterile Water for Injection. SHAKE WELL. Resulting solution provides an approximate volume of 3 mL (330 mg per mL).
For IV Use - See insert.
Discard unused solution 24 hours after reconstitution if stored at room temperature or within 10 days if stored under refrigeration, 2° to 8°C (36° to 46°F). Each vial contains cefazolin sodium equivalent to 1 gram cefazolin. The total sodium content is approximately 48mg (2.1 mEq sodium ion) per gram of cefazolin.
USUAL DOSAGE: 250 mg to 1 g every six to eight hours. See insert.
See package insert for detailed indications, IM or IV dosage and precautions.
Store dry powder at room temperature, 15° to 30°C (59° to 86°F).

PRESCRIPTION: cefazolin (Ancef) 500 mg intramuscular every 8 hours. Administer _____

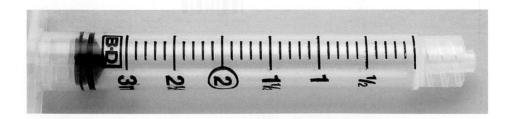

15.

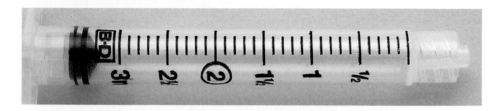

NDC 0015-7628-28
EQUIVALENT TO
1 gram CEPHAPIRIN
CEFADYL®
Sterile Cephapirin
Sodium, USP
For IM or IV Use
CAUTION: Federal law prohibits
dispensing without prescription.
APOTHECON®

PRESCRIPTION: cephapirin sodium (Cefadyl) 750 mg intramuscular every 6 hours.
Administer _____

16.

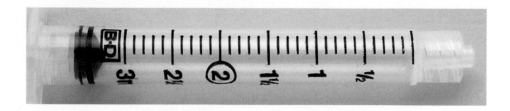

NDC 0015-7970-20
EQUIVALENT TO
2 gram OXACILLIN
OXACILLIN SODIUM
FOR INJECTION, USP
Buffered For IM or IV Use
CAUTION: Federal law prohibits
dispensing without prescription.
APOTHECON®

PRESCRIPTION: oxacillin sodium 400 mg intramuscular every 4 hours.
Administer _____

17.   PRESCRIPTION: Give 180 mL ⅔-strength tube feeding via gastrostomy tube every 3 hours.
 Tube feeding volume _____
 Water volume _____

18.   Prepare 360 mL ⅓ irrigation using normal saline as the solvent and wound irrigant concentrate.
 Normal saline volume _____
 Wound irrigation volume _____

19.   Prepare ¼ scalp cleanser using 50 mL water as the solvent and medicinal shampoo.
 Total volume _____
 Medicinal shampoo volume _____

20. How many 300-mL cans of Sustacal will you need to make 1000 mL of ¼-strength feeding? _____

(Answers on p. 463–464)

℮volve **For additional practice problems, refer to the Basic Calculations section of the Drug Calculations Companion, version 4 on Evolve.**

Methods of Administering and Recording Medications

Unit Dose, Card System, and Computerized Medication Administration System

Pat Revolinski

CLINICAL CONNECTION

- To administer medications effectively, the nurse must understand the unit dose, card, and computerized systems.
- Best clinical practice requires the nurse to compare the unit dose, card, and computerized systems for safety of administration.

HUMAN ERROR *Alert*

It is very important that the nurse is comfortable with the medication system used in the setting and follows the steps to ensure correct medication administration.

INTRODUCTION

The six rights of medication administration are right patient, right drug, right dose, right time, right route, and right documentation. The last four are directly affected by the nurse's comprehension of the facility's medication administration system. Depending on the setting and amount of medication dispensed by the staff, the facility may choose to use a unit dose system, the card system, or a computerized point-of-delivery system such as the Pyxis™ system.

UNIT DOSE SYSTEM

SAFETY *ALERT*

It is best not to borrow a medication from another patient's drawer, because it might result in that patient being charged twice for a drug if the borrower forgets to replace it, or it may delay that patient's medication if it is the last one in the drawer.

CLINICAL *ALERT*

There is an increased chance for clinical error if borrowing medications occurs. Although this realistically occurs in clinical practice, it should not be done.

Some settings utilize the unit dose system. This requires an area set aside, with designated bins or drawers for each patient's medications. Depending on the policy of the facility, these bins or drawers may be stored in a designated room or kept in a rolling medication cart.

When a medication prescription (order) is written and sent to the pharmacy, the pharmacy is responsible for bringing the medication to the floor and placing each individual dose in the patient's drawer. Generally, enough medication is provided for a 24-hour period. The medications can be prepackaged by the supplier or packaged within the pharmacy.

The nurse refers to the medication administration record (MAR) and then obtains the medication from the patient's drawer. The nurse then compares the medication label against the information on the MAR to verify that it is the right medication, the right dose, and the right route.

If the dose is not available, the nurse should contact the pharmacy to obtain the prescribed dose.

With the unit dose system, controlled substances are kept locked in a special drawer or cabinet. The medications are signed out to the patient, as they are given, on a special inventory sheet. The type of sheet may vary in different settings, but the nurse must document how many doses were used and how many doses remained.

Sometimes the prepackaged medication is a different dosage strength, resulting in the nurse having to calculate how to obtain the appropriate dosage.

Example 1

| PRESCRIPTION | *Loracarbef (Lorabid) 400 mg by mouth every 12 hours.* |

- **What You HAVE**

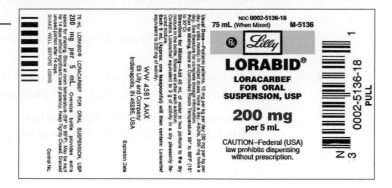

- **What You KNOW**   Prescribed dose is 400 mg.

- **What You WANT (X)**   How many milliliters needed to administer 400 mg loracarbef.

| CRITICAL THINKING | Are the prescribed medication and the medication you HAVE the same drug? _____ |

Does the prescribed dose use the same system of measurement as the medication you HAVE? _____

Does the prescribed dose use the same equivalent measurement within the same system? _____

Is the prescribed dose larger or smaller than the dose you HAVE? _____

In setting up a ratio-proportion, place in the LEFT ratio the medication dose strength per volume you HAVE on hand; in the RIGHT ratio, place what is prescribed in the numerator and place X in the denominator.

Multiply to get the cross-products.

Divide the numerical cross-product by the numerical multiplier of X (the number in front of X).

The result is the answer for X.

Label answer properly in units (i.e., number of tablets, number of milliliters).

Check answer by placing the number obtained for X in the original equation. Cross-multiply. The cross-products should be approximately equal.

| ANSWER FOR BEST CARE | Medication comparison? Yes.
System of measurement? Yes; metric.
Unit of measure comparison? Yes; milligrams.
Prescribed dose larger.
Perform calculation. |

$$\frac{200 \text{ mg}}{5 \text{ mL}} = \frac{400 \text{ mg}}{X \text{ mL}}$$

$$200X = 2000$$
$$X = 10 \text{ mL}$$

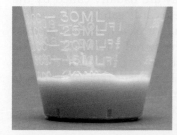

✓ Human Error Check

Replace X with 10.

$$\frac{200}{5} = \frac{400}{10}$$

$$2000 = 2000$$

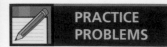

PRACTICE PROBLEMS

Directions: *Determine whether statements 1 through 6 are true or false.*

1. _____ With the unit dose system, all medications are always stored in the medication room.

2. _____ The pharmacy staff delivers medications to the floor at the beginning of each shift.

3. _____ The pharmacy staff restocks medications directly into the patient's drawer or bin.

4. _____ If the medication removed is not the exact dose ordered, the nurse should return the medication to the pharmacy.

5. _____ The nurse should not substitute another patient's medication if the needed dose is not available for his or her patient.

6. _____ Controlled substances are kept in each patient's drawer and removed as needed.

Directions: *Perform the necessary calculations to answer questions 7 through 10.*

7. PRESCRIPTION: phenytoin sodium (Dilantin) 100 mg by mouth three times a day. The patient's medication drawer contains vials of Dilantin 125 mg/5 mL. How many milliliters per dose will you administer to the patient? _____

8. PRESCRIPTION: digoxin (Digitek) 62.5 mcg every morning. Digoxin 0.125 mg per tablet is found in the drawer. How many tablets would you administer? _____

9. The patient has a PM order for codeine phosphate 30 mg intramuscular every 6 hours as needed for pain. The patient tells the physician that the medication does not relieve her pain. The physician instructs you to give the patient an additional 15 mg of codeine intramuscular now, and increase the evening dose to 45 mg intramuscular every 6 hours. The narcotics drawer contains prefilled cartridges that contain codeine 30 mg/mL. How many milliliters are needed to administer the additional 15-mg injection prescribed by the physician? _____

10. If the patient is to receive codeine 45 mg intramuscular every 6 hours as needed for pain, and you have codeine 30 mg/mL prefilled cartridges on hand, how many milliliters will you administer to the patient? _____

(Answers on p. 464)

CARD SYSTEM

When patients are residents in long-term care facilities, especially those not in close proximity to a hospital pharmacy, the card system may be used for medication administration. It involves the use of a card frame to store the patient/resident's supply of medications (Figure 13-1, A).

Each patient has a set of these frames, or cards as they are usually called by the nurses, for their routine and as-needed medications. These cards can be color-coded for the time of day that the medication is usually given. For example, the AM dosing card might be yellow, the midday dosing card might be red, and so forth. The as-needed card would also have a designated color. Each patient, or resident, has a set of these cards designated specifically to him or her. The larger rectangular slots will contain cards with the patient's name and the pharmacy used. The pharmacy is responsible for supplying the information on the cards each time that a card is changed out—that is, each time that a new supply of the patient/resident's medica-

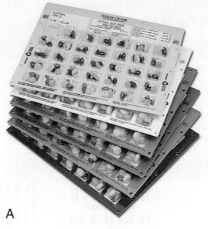
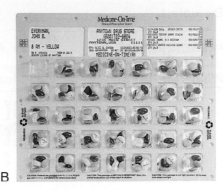

Figure 13-1 A, Card system. **B,** Reverse side of card frame. (Used with permission from Medicine-On-Time, Owings Mills, MD.)

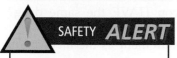
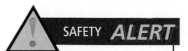
tions are brought in. A computerized MAR (see Chapter 14) usually accompanies the medications.

The reverse side will contain the exact medication prescription as written by the physician or advanced practice nurse and the name of the professional prescribing it (Figure 13-1, B).

There are 35 squares in each card, enough for at least a 31-day supply of the patient's medications. Each row contains seven squares, enough for the week. The card opens to allow the restocking of medications.

Within each square is a bubble pack of pills, usually all the medications due at a specific time. The pills are not individually packaged within the bubble pack (Figure 13-2, A).

Each blister pack contains the patient's name, medication name, and the date and time to be taken (Figure 13-2, B). Some systems have perforations between each dose, allowing the packet to be removed intact. If not, the medications must be removed and placed in another container to transport them to the resident. If the resident is going to be away from the facility and will need to take the medications while away, the medications will need to be placed in another container unless the package is intact.

If the medication prescription changes, the pharmacy will replace the entire card with new blister packs at their earliest convenience, so adjustments may have to be made at the point of delivery until this can be done.

Some units will keep bulk medication available to allow the nurse to administer a new medication prior to the arrival of the medication from the pharmacy. An inventory list for each bulk medication is kept, and each dose is signed out as being

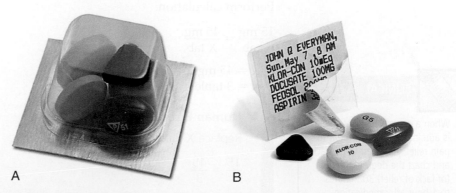

Figure 13-2 A, Bubble pack of pills. **B,** Reverse side of blister pack. (Used with permission from Medicine-On-Time, Owings Mills, MD.)

administered to the patient. Documentation that the patient has received the medication is done on the MAR used by the facility.

Example 1

| PRESCRIPTION | *Codeine 45 mg by mouth as needed for pain.* |

• **What You HAVE**   Individual blister pack.

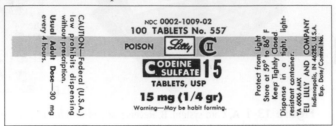

• **What You KNOW**   Prescribed dose is 45 mg.

• **What You WANT (X)**   How many tablets needed to administer codeine 45 mg.

CRITICAL THINKING

Are the prescribed medication and the medication you HAVE the same drug? _____

Does the prescribed dose use the same system of measurement as the medication you HAVE? _____

Does the prescribed dose use the same equivalent measurement within the same system? _____

Is the prescribed dose larger or smaller than the dose you HAVE? _____

In setting up a ratio-proportion, place in the LEFT ratio the medication dose strength per volume you HAVE on hand; in the RIGHT ratio, place what is prescribed in the numerator and place X in the denominator.

Multiply to get the cross-products.

Divide the numerical cross-product by the numerical multiplier of X (the number in front of X).

The result is the answer for X.

Label answer properly in units (i.e., number of tablets, number of milliliters).

Check answer by placing the number obtained for X in the original equation. Cross-multiply. The cross-products should be approximately equal.

ANSWER FOR BEST CARE

Medication comparison? Yes.
System of measurement? Yes; metric.
Unit of measure comparison? Yes, milligrams.
Prescribed dose larger.
Perform calculation.

$$\frac{15 \text{ mg}}{1 \text{ tab}} = \frac{45 \text{ mg}}{X \text{ tab}}$$

$$15X = 45 \text{ mg}$$
$$X = 3 \text{ tablets}$$

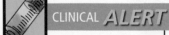
CLINICAL *ALERT*

When a controlled substance is administered to a patient for pain relief, you need to go back and chart the degree of relief (or lack of relief) 30 minutes to 1 hour after medication administration.

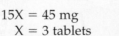**Human Error Check**

Replace X with 3.

$$\frac{15}{1} = \frac{45}{3}$$

$$45 = 45$$

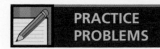

PRACTICE PROBLEMS

Directions: *Determine whether statements 1 through 7 are true or false.*

1. _____ Each patient has a set of cards for routine and as-needed medications.

2. _____ The cards are color-coded based on the time of day the medication is to be given.

3. _____ The nursing staff is responsible for filling in the information on the cards each day.

4. _____ The computerized MAR is usually printed at the nursing unit each day.

5. _____ Each card contains a 1-month supply of the medications.

6. _____ Pills are individually packed within each blister pack.

7. _____ Controlled substances are contained within each patient's PM card blister packs.

Directions: *Perform the necessary calculations to answer questions 8 through 10.*

8. Prescription: benztropine mesylate (Cogentin) 1.5 mg by mouth every morning. What you HAVE:

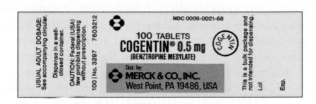

The nurse can expect to find how many tablets in the bubble pack on the patient's AM card? _____ Administer _____

9. The patient has been receiving phenobarbital 60 mg at bedtime. After the nurse reports to the physician that she believes that the patient is too drowsy during the day, the dose is reduced to 30 mg at bedtime. Upon receipt of the prescription, the pharmacy calls to notify the nurse that they do not have 30 mg in stock but will try to get some by the next day. Can the nurse use the medication in the bubble pack? _____ How? _____

10. The patient will begin receiving levothyroxine sodium (Synthroid [1 tab = 50 mcg]); the physician prescribes a daily dose of 1.6 mcg/kg/day based on the patient's admission weight, which was 62.5 kg. The patient will receive how much of the Synthroid sent by the pharmacy? _____

(Answers on p. 464)

COMPUTERIZED MEDICATION ADMINISTRATION SYSTEM

The point-of-use delivery system automates the distribution, management, and control of medications (meds). The medications are stored on the unit within a computer-operated console and are removed by the nurse as needed. Rather than each patient having a drawer with his or her ordered meds, a supply of each medication is kept within a drawer. The pharmacy usually collaborates with the unit administration to determine which medications are needed most frequently on a certain unit and provides a stock of them.

When a medication prescription (order) is written in the record, it is sent to the pharmacy. This can be done by hand, by facsimile, or on the computer, depending on the setting. The pharmacy personnel then enter the information into the patient's profile in the main console housed in the pharmacy using a computer software

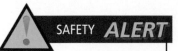

program. The information entered into the main console is also stored, via the computer network, in the station located in the clinical area where the patient is being managed. Any medication prescribed for routine administration or on an as-needed (PRN) basis can be stored in the station. When a medication needs to be administered, the nurse logs into the system using her personal identification code and password. The nurse then selects the patient from the patient profile on the screen by touching the screen or typing in the name of the patient. Once the patient is selected, the patient's list of profiled medications—that is, those medications entered into the system by the pharmacy when the patient's orders were sent to them—appears on the screen. Each profiled medication contains the name of the medication, the ordered dose, the route of administration to be used, the frequency of administration, and the last time that the medication was dispensed from the system.

There is also an area for special notes. This contains information that a nurse needs to know or needs to verify before giving a medication. This area will also tell you if a profiled medication is not available for some reason.

Although the software program usually alerts the pharmacy when a medication needs to be restocked, there can be a lag time between the notification and the time it takes the pharmacy personnel to replenish the stock within the machine. Also, a medication may not be on the formulary within the hospital, and so the pharmacy may need to make a substitution or obtain the medication from another source and package it individually for the patient. Patients who bring medications from home may also be allowed to use them, depending on the policy of the setting, and these are usually kept in a designated area and dispensed as needed. The pharmacy can also include this information in the special note area.

All medications prescribed for a patient can be entered into the profile regardless of whether the medication is kept within the machine. If a medication is on the MAR, it should be listed on the profile. If it is on the profile, it should be listed on the MAR. This provides a safety check for the nurse to prevent medication errors.

Once the nurse selects the medication, the drawer containing the medication will open, and the medication can be removed. Noncontrolled medications are kept in a matrix system within a large drawer. The large drawer opens to reveal several individual pockets containing various medications. When the medication is selected, the computer screen will display the drawer number and the pocket number for the selected medication.

The nurse verifies the right patient's profile, right drug, right dose, right route, and right time with the information contained on the MAR (see Chapter 14) and the machine screen, and then removes the medication. The nurse should verify that the medication and number of doses that she has removed, as instructed on the screen, is the correct medication and will deliver the correct dosage to the patient. Once the medication is removed, the drawer should be closed firmly, and the computer screen will return to the patient's list of profiled medications.

Example 1

PRESCRIPTION   *Dexamethasone (Decadron) 10 mg intramuscular every 6 hours.*

• **What You HAVE**

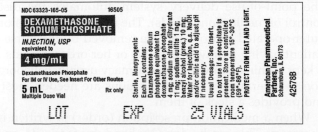

• **What You KNOW**   Prescribed dose is 10 mg.

- **What You WANT (X)**   How many milliliters needed to administer dexamethasone 10 mg.
How many vials should be removed to allow the nurse to administer the prescribed dose.

CRITICAL THINKING   Are the prescribed medication and the medication you HAVE the same drug? _____

Does the prescribed dose use the same system of measurement as the medication you HAVE? _____

Does the prescribed dose use the same equivalent measurement within the same system? _____

Is the prescribed dose larger or smaller than the dose you HAVE? _____

In setting up a ratio-proportion, place in the LEFT ratio the medication dose strength per volume you HAVE on hand; in the RIGHT ratio, place what is prescribed in the numerator and place X in the denominator.

Multiply to get the cross-products.

Divide the numerical cross-product by the numerical multiplier of X (the number in front of X).

The result is the answer for X.

Label answer properly in units (i.e., number of tablets, number of milliliters).

Check answer by placing the number obtained for X in the original equation. Cross-multiply. The cross-products should be approximately equal.

ANSWER FOR BEST CARE   Medication comparison? Yes.
System of measurement? Yes; metric.
Unit of measure comparison? Yes; milligrams.
Prescribed dose larger.
Perform calculation.

$$\frac{4 \text{ mg}}{1 \text{ mL}} = \frac{10 \text{ mg}}{X \text{ mL}}$$

$$4X = 10$$
$$X = 2.5 \text{ mL}$$

✔ **Human Error Check**

Replace X with 2.5.

$$\frac{4}{1} = \frac{10}{2.5}$$

$$10 = 10$$

Each vial contains 1 mL.
Determine the number of cartridges needed.

$$\frac{1 \text{ mL}}{1 \text{ cartridge}} = \frac{2.5 \text{ mL}}{X \text{ cartridge}}$$

$$X = 2.5 \text{ cartridges}$$

You will need to remove three cartridges. Two cartridges will be used, along with 0.5 mL of the third cartridge.

$$\begin{array}{r} 0\ 10 \\ \cancel{1}.0 \text{ mL} \text{ (total volume)} \\ - 0.5 \text{ mL} \text{ (desired dosage)} \\ \hline 0.5 \text{ mL} \text{ (discard prior to administration)} \end{array}$$

Controlled Substances

Controlled substances, such as narcotic analgesics, are kept in a carousel drawer. When the medication is selected, the screen will ask the nurse to enter the number of medications needing to be removed. After this is done, the carousel will turn to the selected medication, and the drawer will open, revealing only the supply of the selected medication. The screen will ask the nurse to verify the count—that is, to count the number of doses and verify that the number of doses in the drawer matches the number of doses expected to be there. The machine will request this information either by supplying the number expected and asking the nurse to select *Yes* or *No*, or by having the nurse type in the number of doses.

Any time that the amount within the drawer does not match the data in the machine's memory, the nurse will be prompted to count again and enter the information again. If the count does not match again, the machine will allow the medication to be removed; however, a discrepancy will be created. The policy of the institution dictates how these discrepancies are resolved, so the nurse should be aware of the institution's policy and notify the appropriate personnel.

Example 2

| PRESCRIPTION | *Hydromorphone hydrochloride (Dilaudid) 3 mg intravenous every 6 hours as needed for pain.* |

- **What You HAVE** Dilaudid 4 mg/mL in a prefilled cartridge.

- **What You KNOW** The prescribed dose is 3 mg.

- **What You WANT (X)** How many milliliters needed to administer hydromorphone 3 mg. How many cartridges needed.

CRITICAL THINKING

Are the prescribed medication and the medication you HAVE the same drug? _____

Does the prescribed dose use the same system of measurement as the medication you HAVE? _____

Does the prescribed dose use the same equivalent measurement within the same system? _____

Is the prescribed dose larger or smaller than the dose you HAVE? _____

Is the volume of hydromorphone contained in one cartridge more or less than the prescribed dose? _____

Will final volume be more or less than one cartridge? _____

In setting up a ratio-proportion, place in the LEFT ratio the medication dose strength per volume you HAVE on hand; in the RIGHT ratio, place what is prescribed in the numerator and place X in the denominator.

Multiply to get the cross-products.

Divide the numerical cross-product by the numerical multiplier of X (the number in front of X).

The result is the answer for X.

Label answer properly in units (i.e., number of tablets, number of milliliters).

Check answer by placing the number obtained for X in the original equation. Cross-multiply. The cross-products should be approximately equal.

ANSWER FOR BEST CARE

Medication comparison? Yes.
System of measurement? Yes; metric.
Unit of measure comparison? Yes; milligrams.
Prescribed dose smaller.
Cartridge volume? More.
Final volume? Less.

Perform calculation.

$$\frac{4\ mg}{1\ mL} = \frac{3\ mg}{X}$$

$$4X = 3$$

$$X = \frac{3}{4}$$

$$X = 0.75\ mL$$

> ✔ **Human Error Check**
>
> Replace X with 0.75.
>
> $$\frac{4}{1} = \frac{3}{0.75}$$
>
> $$3 = 3$$

One cartridge contains 1 mL. You will only need to remove one prefilled cartridge.

$$
\begin{array}{ll}
\overset{09\ 10}{1.\cancel{00}}\ mL & \text{(total volume)} \\
-\ 0.75\ mL & \text{(desired dosage)} \\
\hline
0.25\ mL & \text{(discard with witness prior to administration)}
\end{array}
$$

Whether removing medications from the matrix (noncontrolled) or carousel (controlled), the final screen in the process will display the patient's name and the medication and indicate the amount to be removed. The nurse will be given the option to accept or cancel the removal, as well as the option to review the original order that was entered into the system. If the nurse enters "Cancel," the screen will indicate that the drawer should be closed without removal of medicines, and the inventory will not reflect any change.

System Override

CLINICAL *ALERT*

If necessary, the nurse may have to remove an excessive amount and calculate the amount of what she has on hand to obtain the amount of medication she should administer.

Occasionally, the patient may have a medication prescribed that is not listed among the profiled medications, or a patient may need an immediate dose of a medication that is not included in the profile, such as a new order by the physician that has not yet been profiled by the pharmacy. The nurse logs into the system and selects the patient's name as previously described and then selects the "Override" function. This prompts the machine to display an alphabetized list of all medications available in the Pyxis, with their dosages. The nurse can then select the medication by scrolling down or by typing in the name of the medication. Before the machine will allow the medicine to be removed, it will display a screen requesting a reason for the override, with several options. If none of the options provided are appropriate, the nurse selects "Other," resulting in the screen asking the nurse to type in a reason. After this, the drawer will open and the medication can be removed.

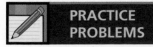
PRACTICE PROBLEMS

Directions: *Determine whether statements 1 through 7 are true or false.*

1. _____ The nursing personnel access the main console to enter medication orders for individual patients.

2. _____ Only routine medications can be stored in the station on the unit.

3. _____ The nurse can determine the last time a medication was administered by reviewing the profiled medication data.

4. _____ Only medications being kept within the console can be profiled by the system.

5. _____ The nurse must reenter the system to document administration once a medication has been administered to the patient.

6. _____ If the amount of drug in the drawer does not match the number expected according to the screen, the nurse must close the drawer immediately and notify the pharmacy.

7. _____ The nurse can obtain medications not yet profiled by the pharmacy by using the override function.

Directions: *Perform the necessary calculations to answer questions 8 through 10.*

8. You have received an order to give heparin 6000 units subcutaneous. The computer screen displays that you have three prefilled cartridges containing 10,000 units/mL.
   What would you remove to administer the dose? _____
   How many milliliters will you use to administer the correct dose of heparin? _____

9. The physician has ordered penicillin V potassium 2 grams for a patient who needs pretreatment with an antibiotic prior to a surgical procedure. The transporters have come for the patient, and pharmacy has not had time to profile the new medication. Using the override function, you determine that you have three capsules of 500 mg/capsule, and six capsules of 250 mg/capsule.
   What is the best way to administer the dose that will require the patient to swallow the least amount of capsules? _____

10. The physician prescribes phenobarbital elixir 50 mg by mouth at bedtime for the patient. The screen indicates that the medication is in a bulk supply that is not kept in the machine. The bottle of elixir labeled for the patient contains 20 mg/5 mL.
    How much of the elixir should you administer to this patient? _____

(Answers on pp. 464–465)

CHAPTER REVIEW

Determine whether the following statements are true or false.

1. _____ With the unit dose system, all prescribed medications are always stored in the medication room.

2. _____ The pharmacy staff delivers medications to the floor only when they are prescribed or daily at the beginning of each shift.

3. _____ The pharmacy staff restocks medications directly into the patient's drawer or bin.

4. _____ If the medication removed is not the exact dose as prescribed, the nurse should return the medication to the pharmacy.

5. _____ The cards are color-coded based on the time of day the medication is to be given.

6. _____ The nursing staff is responsible for filling in the information on the cards each day.

7. _____ The computerized MAR is usually printed at the nursing unit each day.

8. _____ Each card contains a 1-month supply of the medications.

9. _____ Only routine medications can be stored in the station on the unit.

10. _____ The nurse can determine the last time a medication was administered by reviewing the profiled medication data.

11. _____ Only medications being kept within the console can be profiled by the system.

12. _____ The nurse must reenter the system to document administration once a medication has been administered to the patient.

Answer the following questions.

13. PRESCRIPTION: carbamazepine (Tegretol) 300 mg by mouth.
    HAVE: carbamazepine 200-mg tablet(s) are available.
    How many tablet(s) will you administer? _____

14. PRESCRIPTION: thioridazine (Mellaril) 100 mg.
    HAVE: thioridazine 25-mg tablets.
    How many tablet(s) will you administer? _____

15. PRESCRIPTION: clonazepam (Klonopin) 1.25 mg.
    HAVE: clonazepam 0.5-mg tablets.
    How many tablet(s) will you administer? _____

16. PRESCRIPTION: haloperidol (Haldol) 2.5 mg.
    HAVE: haloperidol 0.5 mg.
    How many tablet(s) will you administer? _____

17. PRESCRIPTION: potassium chloride 40 mEq by mouth every morning.
    HAVE: potassium chloride 15 mEq/3 mL.
    How many milliliters will you need to administer? _____

18. PRESCRIPTION: cephalothin (Keflin) 250 mg.
    HAVE: The bottle says you must add 9.5 mL of sterile water to the vial to yield 0.5 g/mL.
    How many milliliters should you administer? _____

19. The physician has prescribed penicillin V potassium 1 gram for a patient who needs pretreatment with an antibiotic prior to a surgical procedure. The transporters have come for the patient, and the pharmacy has not had time to profile the new medication. Using the override function, you determine that you have one capsule of 500 mg/capsule, and six capsules of 250 mg/capsule.
    What is the best way to administer the dose that will require the patient to swallow the least amount of capsules? _____

20. The physician prescribes phenobarbital elixir 30 mg by mouth at bedtime for the patient. The screen indicates that the medication is in a bulk supply that is not kept in the machine.

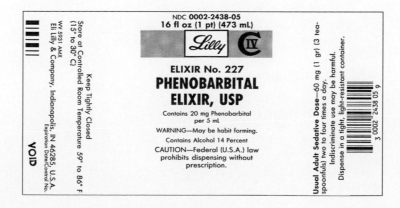

The bottle of elixir labeled for the patient contains 20 mg/5 mL. How much of the elixir should you administer to this patient? _____

(Answers on p. 465)

⊖volve **For additional practice problems, refer to the Safety in Medication Administration section of the Drug Calculations Companion, version 4 on Evolve.**

Medication Records

Pat Revolinski

CLINICAL CONNECTION

- Knowing the steps for safe documentation on the MAR is part of the medication administration process.
- Implementing a method for transcribing medication orders onto the MAR is necessary for safe and effective patient care.

INTRODUCTION

Documentation of medication administration is the final step of administering a medication. The medication administration record (MAR) is individualized to the setting and population being served, and it is considered a legal document to be contained with patient records once the patient is discharged from care.

PREPRINTED FORMS

CLINICAL *ALERT*

MARs usually have the times recorded, beginning with the first dose after midnight.

Some settings use a printed form that requires the staff to write in the patient's data, the medications prescribed, and the times that each dose is to be administered for routine medications. There will also be an area to document allergies.

MARs are usually color coded to distinguish routine and as-needed medication documentation. There may also be a different colored sheet used for one-time orders, as for preoperative medications.

Each sheet will have delineated areas corresponding to days of the week for each medication entered.

When a medication prescription is received, the information is transcribed onto the form exactly as written by the physician to avoid error.

Example 1

| PRESCRIPTION | *Hydrocortisone sodium succinate (Solu-Cortef) 250 mg intravenous every 6 hours times 8 doses beginning at 1600 hours.* |

- **What You HAVE**   Pharmacy has notified you that they will have to substitute Solu-Cortef 100 mg/mL vials overnight because they are out of Solu-Cortef 250-mg vials.

- **What You KNOW**   Prescribed dose is 250 mg.
  Dose frequency is every 6 hours, for a total of eight doses.
  Administration should begin at 1600 hours.

- **What You WANT (X)**   How many milliliters needed to administer Solu-Cortef 100 mg/mL.
  To mark the MAR with the administration times.

CRITICAL THINKING

Are the prescribed medication and the medication you HAVE the same drug? _____

Does the prescribed dose use the same system of measurement as the medication you HAVE? _____

Does the prescribed dose use the same equivalent measurement within the same system? _____

Is the prescribed dose larger or smaller than the dose you HAVE? _____

In setting up a ratio-proportion, place in the LEFT ratio the medication dose strength per volume you have on hand; in the RIGHT ratio, place what is prescribed in the numerator and place X in the denominator.

Multiply to get the cross-products.

Divide the numerical cross-product by the numerical multiplier of X (the number in front of X).

The result is the answer for X.

Label answer properly in units (i.e., number of tablets, number of milliliters).

Check answer by placing the number obtained for X in the original equation. Cross-multiply. The cross-products should be approximately equal.

Divide 24 hours by the dose frequency to determine number of entries on the MAR.

Add the frequency to 1600 to determine the second administration time. Repeat adding the frequency to the second administration time to determine the third dose. Continue to repeat the addition process for a 24-hour period.

ANSWER FOR BEST CARE

Medication comparison? Yes.
System of measurement? Yes.
Unit of measure comparison? Yes, milligrams.
Prescribed dose larger.
Perform calculation.

$$\frac{100 \text{ mg}}{1 \text{ mL}} = \frac{250 \text{ mg}}{X \text{ mL}}$$

$$100X = 250$$

$$X = \frac{250}{100}$$

Reduce by 25.

$$\frac{10}{4}$$

$$X = 2.5 \text{ mL}$$

✓ **Human Error Check**

Replace X with 2.5

$$\frac{100}{1} = \frac{250}{2.5}$$

$$250 = 250$$

How many entries per 24 hours on the MAR?

$$X = \frac{24 \text{ hours}}{6 \text{ hours}}$$

$$X = 4 \text{ entries}$$

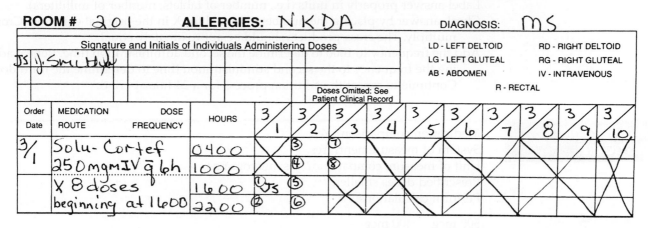

Everyman, John

** DOCUMENTING THE ADMINISTRA-
TION OF IVMB'S OR IV PUSH MEDS
INCLUDES DOCUMENTATION OF
SALINE FLUSHES BEFORE AND
AFTER EACH DOSE. ALL OTHER
FLUSHES MUST BE DOCUMENTED
ON THE MAR.

**ROUTINE MEDICATION
SHEET**

ROOM # 201   **ALLERGIES:** NKDA   **DIAGNOSIS:** MS

LD - LEFT DELTOID   RD - RIGHT DELTOID
LG - LEFT GLUTEAL   RG - RIGHT GLUTEAL
AB - ABDOMEN   IV - INTRAVENOUS
R - RECTAL

Figure 14-1 Written schedule for Solu-Cortef. (Used with permission from St Joseph Hospital, Augusta, GA.)

Times:
1600 (first dose time) + 6 = 2200
2200 (second dose time) + 6 = 0400
0400 (third dose time) + 6 = 1000
1000 (fourth dose time)

There will be four entries per 24-hour period: 1600, 2200, 0400, and 1000 (Figure 14-1).

Example 2

PRESCRIPTION	*Digoxin (Lanoxin) 400 mcg intravenous at 1000, 150 mcg intravenous in 6 hours, and then 75 mcg intravenous every 6 hours times 2 for a total of 4 doses.*

• **What You HAVE** — Digoxin 500 mcg/2 mL.

• **What You KNOW** — Prescription dose is 400 mcg for the first dose, 150 mcg for the second dose, and 75 mcg for the third and fourth doses.
Dose frequency is every 6 hours times 4.
Administration should begin at 1000 hours.

• **What You WANT (X)** — How many milliliters needed to administer digoxin 400 mg.
To mark the MAR with the administration times.

CRITICAL THINKING   Are the prescribed medication and the medication you HAVE the same drug?
_____
Does the prescribed dose use the same system of measurement as the medication you HAVE? _____
Does the prescribed dose use the same equivalent measurement within the same system? _____
Is the prescribed dose larger or smaller than the dose you HAVE? _____

In setting up a ratio-proportion, place in the LEFT ratio the medication dose strength per volume you have on hand; in the RIGHT ratio, place what is prescribed in the numerator and place X in the denominator.

Multiply to get the cross-products.

Divide the numerical cross-product by the numerical multiplier of X (the number in front of X).

The result is the answer for X.

Label answer properly in units (i.e., number of tablets, number of milliliters).

Check answer by placing the number obtained for X in the original equation. Cross-multiply. The cross-products should be approximately equal.

Add the frequency to 1000 to determine the second administration time. Repeat adding the frequency to the second administration time to determine the third dose. Continue to repeat the addition process for a 24-hour period.

ANSWER FOR BEST CARE

Medication comparison? Yes.

System of measurement? Yes.

Unit of measure comparison? Yes; micrograms.

Prescribed doses smaller.

Perform calculations.

$$\frac{500 \text{ mcg}}{2 \text{ mL}} = \frac{400 \text{ mcg}}{X \text{ mL}}$$

$500X = 800$

Reduce.

$5X = 8$

$X = 1.6 \text{ mL}$

✓ **Human Error Check**

Replace X with 1.6.

$$\frac{500}{2} = \frac{400}{1.6}$$

$500 \times 1.6 = 400 \times 2$
$800 = 800$

Second dose:

$$\frac{500 \text{ mcg}}{2 \text{ mL}} = \frac{150 \text{ mcg}}{X \text{ mL}}$$

$500X = 300$
$X = 0.6 \text{ mL}$

✓ **Human Error Check**

Replace X with 0.6.

$$\frac{500}{2} = \frac{150}{0.6}$$

$500 \times 0.6 = 150 \times 2$
$300 = 300$

Third and fourth doses:

$$\frac{500 \text{ mcg}}{2 \text{ mL}} = \frac{75 \text{ mcg}}{X \text{ mL}}$$

500X = 150

X = 0.3 mL

✓ **Human Error Check**

Replace X with 0.3.

$$\frac{500}{2} = \frac{75}{0.3}$$

$500 \times 0.3 = 75 \times 2$

150 = 150

Times:
1000 (first dose) + 6 = 1600
1600 (second dose) + 6 = 2200
2200 (third dose) + 6 = 0400
0400 (fourth dose)

There will be four entries per 24-hour period: 1000, 1600, 2200, and 0400.

PRACTICE PROBLEMS

Directions: *Determine whether statements 1 through 7 are true or false.*

1. _____ The forms are color-coded to distinguish between routine, as-needed, and one-time orders.

2. _____ Each form is used for documenting medications administered over a 1-month period.

3. _____ Medications are signed off with initials and/or the time as soon as the medication is taken by the patient.

4. _____ Medications that the patient self-administers cannot be documented by the nurse on the MAR.

5. _____ Only as-needed medications require documentation of the site of administration.

6. _____ Circled initials indicate that a medication was not given.

7. _____ Medication administration times cannot be individualized on the pre-printed MAR form.

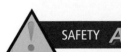

SAFETY ALERT

Never sign off a medication until you have actually seen the patient receive that medication.

CLINICAL ALERT

Never sign off a medication that you did not personally administer to the patient. If the patient administers the medication, as in the case of diabetic patients being taught to administer insulin, document this on the MAR and then initial it.

Directions: *Perform the calculations required for questions 8 through 10.*

8. PRESCRIPTION: Decadron 4 mg intramuscular today; on the second day, begin Decadron 3 mg by mouth twice a day for 2 days.
   How much total Decadron will the patient receive? _____

9. If you are using 0.75-mg Decadron tablets, how many will you administer to give each dose for days 2 and 3 in problem 8? _____

10. PRESCRIPTION: sertraline (Zoloft) 37.5 mg by mouth now.
    HAVE: 25-mg tablets.
    How many tablet(s) will you administer? _____

(Answers on p. 465)

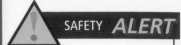
Some forms may have one large area for all doses for the 24 hours to be written within this area or a delineated block for each time to be written. If the times are entered individually, they will be crossed out after the dose is given, and the nurse's initials will be written next to them. If the times are not written individually for each time the dose is given, the nurse initials the MAR in the appropriate place.

In addition to the initials of the nurse administering the medication, all as-needed medications will require the time and the route used to be entered, as well as the site, if applicable (e.g., subcutaneous and intramuscular [IM] injections) (Figure 14-2). The site can and should be entered for routine medications, such as insulin and anticoagulant medications.

If additional information, such as a pulse rate or a glucose result, is required, there can be a designated area for that as well. This area can vary from setting to setting. If such an item is required, the nurse should enter the data each time the medication is given.

If a medication is withheld for any reason, this must be indicated on the MAR. Policies on this will vary with the setting. Some settings have the nurse initial in the appropriate place, but then circle the initials to identify that the medication was not given. If there is not enough space to indicate the reason the medication was withheld on the MAR, a notation should be made to check the nurses' notes and the reason should be documented there.

COMPUTERIZED MARs

As the health care industry moves more and more toward using computer technology, many settings are using records generated and maintained by computer software programs. In some settings, such as those using the card system for medication

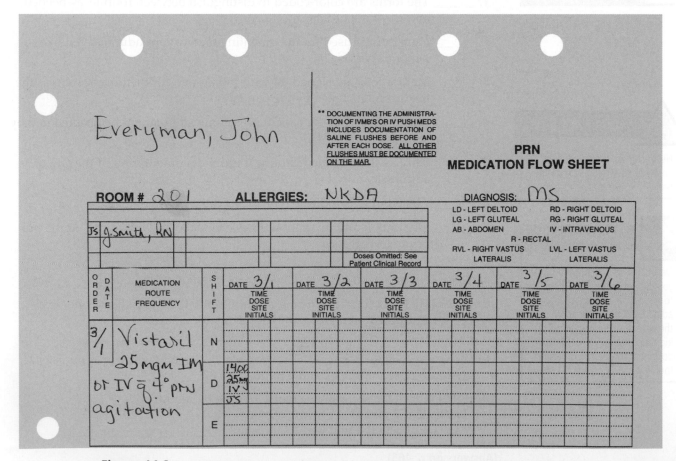

Figure 14-2 As-needed medication entry for Vistaril. (Used with permission from St Joseph Hospital, Augusta, GA.)

administration (see Chapter 13), the MAR will be printed out at the time that the medication is brought from the pharmacy to the point of administration. The patient data, including allergies, printed onto the sheet, as are the medications and the dose; the route, frequency, and time to be administered are printed on the MAR when it is received.

The nurse enters her initials in the appropriate area after administering the medication. These MARs also have an area for full signature and title. There may be areas designated for other patient data—such as pulse, blood pressure, and glucose readings—and an area to document any variations in the schedule, such as a missed dose.

Unlike the routine medication sheet, which has the times printed in the appropriate place by the computer, the MAR for as-needed medications has an additional area to enter the time of administration. This system still relies on the nurse to manually document that a medication was given.

Example 1

PRESCRIPTION	*Dilitiazem (Cardizem) 60 mg by mouth in the morning and 90 mg by mouth at hour of sleep.*
• **What You HAVE**	Dilitiazem 60-mg tablets.
• **What You KNOW**	Prescribed dose is 60 mg in the morning and 90 mg at the hour of sleep.
• **What You WANT (X)**	How many tablets needed to administer dilitiazem 60 mg, and how many tablets needed to administer 90 mg.

CRITICAL THINKING

Are the prescribed medication and the medication you HAVE the same drug? _____

Does the prescribed dose use the same system of measurement as the medication you HAVE? _____

Does the prescribed dose use the same equivalent measurement within the same system? _____

Is the prescribed dose larger or smaller than the dose you HAVE? _____

In setting up a ratio-proportion, place in the LEFT ratio the medication dose strength per volume you have on hand; in the RIGHT ratio, place what is prescribed in the numerator and place X in the denominator.

Multiply to get the cross-products.

Divide the numerical cross-product by the numerical multiplier of X (the number in front of X).

The result is the answer for X.

Label answer properly in units (i.e., number of tablets, number of milliliters).

Check answer by placing the number obtained for X in the original equation. Cross-multiply. The cross-products should be approximately equal.

ANSWER FOR BEST CARE

Medication comparison? Yes.
System of measurement? Yes.
Unit of measure comparison? Yes; milligrams.
Prescribed dose is the same for the morning and larger for the hour of sleep.
Perform calculation for the hour of sleep.

$$\frac{60 \text{ mg}}{1 \text{ tab}} = \frac{90 \text{ mg}}{X \text{ tab}}$$

$$60X = 90$$

$$X = 1.5 \text{ tablets.}$$

✓ **Human Error Check**

Replace X with 1.5.

$$\frac{60}{1} = \frac{90}{1.5}$$

$60 \times 1.5 = 1 \times 90$
$90 = 90$

The nurse would administer one tablet in the morning and 1.5 tablets at the hour of sleep.

Example 2

PRESCRIPTION

Ondansetron hydrochloride (Zofran) liquid solution 8 mg by mouth for nausea 30 minutes prior to radiation therapy. If patient is unable to swallow, give Zofran 2 mg intravenous.

• **What You HAVE**

NDC 0173-0489-00 *GlaxoWellcome*	Each 5 mL contains 5 mg of ondansetron HCl dihydrate equivalent to 4 mg of ondansetron.
Zofran® (ondansetron hydrochloride) Oral Solution **4 mg/5 mL** **Caution:** Federal law prohibits dispensing without prescription. **50 mL**	See package insert for Dosage and Administration. Store between 15° and 30°C (59° and 86°F). Protect from light. Store bottle upright in carton. Glaxo Wellcome Inc. Research Triangle Park, NC 27709 Made in England 4058968 Rev. 3/96

• **What You KNOW**

Prescribed dose is 8 mg.
The patient is able to swallow.

• **What You WANT (X)**

How many milliliters needed to administer Zofran 8 mg.

CRITICAL THINKING

Are the prescribed medication and the medication you HAVE the same drug? _____

Does the prescribed dose use the same system of measurement as the medication you HAVE? _____

Does the prescribed dose use the same equivalent measurement within the same system? _____

Is the prescribed dose larger or smaller than the dose you HAVE? _____

In setting up a ratio-proportion, place in the LEFT ratio the medication dose strength per volume you have on hand; in the RIGHT ratio, place what is prescribed in the numerator and place X in the denominator.

Multiply to get the cross-products.

Divide the numerical cross-product by the numerical multiplier of X (the number in front of X).

The result is the answer for X.

Label answer properly in units (i.e., number of tablets, number of milliliters).

Check answer by placing the number obtained for X in the original equation. Cross-multiply. The cross-products should be approximately equal.

ANSWER FOR BEST CARE

Medication comparison? Yes.
System of measurement? Yes.
Unit of measure comparison? Yes; milligrams.
Prescribed dose larger.

HUMAN ERROR *Alert*

Never assume that because there is no entry at a scheduled time that the medication was not given. If there is no information documented on the MAR or in the nurse's notes that verifies that the medication was with-held or missed, every effort should be made to reach the nurse who was supposed to give the medication. It is not a good idea to rely completely on the word of the patient, as he or she might be confused or might for-get having taken the medication.

Perform calculation.

$$\frac{40 \text{ mg}}{5 \text{ mL}} = \frac{8 \text{ mg}}{X \text{ mL}}$$

$$4X = 40$$

$$X = 10 \text{ mL}$$

✔ **Human Error Check**

Replace X with 10.

$$\frac{4}{5} = \frac{8}{10}$$

$$4 \times 10 = 8 \times 5$$
$$40 = 40$$

If the patient is unable to swallow, the nurse must use the virtual due list to enter this information and explain why the intravenous Zofran will be used. If a medication is not given for any reason, the nurse can select the missed medication box on a special menu and document the reason that the medication was missed or withheld.

BAR CODES

SAFETY *ALERT*

Never share your user codes with anyone, because these codes identify you as the person enter-ing data and administering a medication.

In 1996, the Veterans Health Administration (VHA) introduced the Veterans Health Information Systems and Technology Architecture (VISTA) computer application; this allows for the use of the Computerized Patient Record System, which maintains all patient records electronically. The VHA subsequently began using bar code scan-ning (BCMA) for medication administration. In March of 2003 the FDA proposed a rule that would recommend bar codes on all prescription medications and on some over-the-counter medications and vaccines, as well as recommend the use of the bar code scanning system, citing the reduction of medication errors in Veterans Ad-ministration Medical Centers using this system. In this medication administration system, the patient is given a bar-coded identification bracelet upon admission. All medications are then given bar codes, so before a patient receives a medication, the nurse uses a hand-held scanning device to scan the bracelet and medication (Figure 14-3). Each nurse has a user code and an electronic signature to verify the identity of the user of the scanner.

When the nurse scans the bar code on the patient's bracelet, the computer pulls up the patient's computerized medical record. The nurse then scans the medication

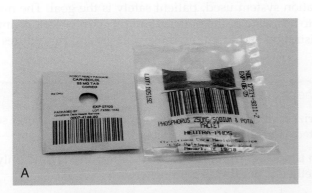

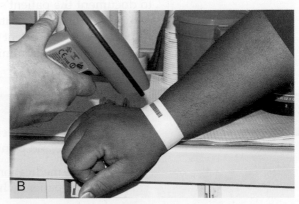

Figure 14-3 A, Bar code for unit drug dose. **B,** Bar code reader used to scan the patient's wristband. (From Kee J, Marshall S: *Clinical calculations: With applications to general and specialty areas*, ed 6, St Louis, 2009, Saunders.)

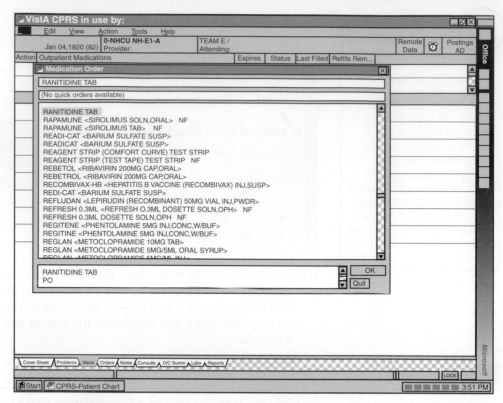

Figure 14-4 Medication screen for scrolling. (From Kee J, Marshall S: *Clinical calculations: With applications to general and specialty areas,* ed 6, St Louis, 2009, Saunders.)

that the pharmacy has provided for administration, which has been provided based on the orders entered into the computerized patient record upon admission. In this system, the MAR is referred to as the Medication Administration History (MAH).

If there is a problem—such as incorrect medication, incorrect dose, incorrect time, or a change in the medication order—the screen displays an error message. Using a virtual due list screen, the nurse can access tabs that display unit dose medications to be given routinely orally, intramuscularly, subcutaneously, topically, or intravenously (via piggyback or push method); as-needed medications; and one-time prescriptions (Figure 14-4).

When a medication requires special information, such as a heart rate, to be entered before administration or an injection site is recorded, special drop-down boxes appear that allow the nurse to select or type in the appropriate data. This system can also be configured with a command that displays a screen allowing the nurse to document the patient's response to the medication. Regardless of the medication administration documentation system used, patient safety is the goal. The nurse is responsible to the patient to be aware of the policies and procedures for documentation of medication administration and to follow those policies and procedures at all times.

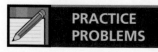

PRACTICE PROBLEMS

Directions: *Determine whether these statements are true or false.*

1. _____ With computerized MARs, the record is maintained by computer software and printed as needed.

2. _____ If a medication is not signed off on the MAR, the nurse should only ask the patient whether or not it was administered.

3. _____ With bar-scanning systems, the computerized medication record can be printed out, filled out manually, or maintained electronically.

4. _____ With bar-scanning systems, the patient receives a new identification bracelet each day.

Directions: *For the problems below, calculate the answers.*

5. PRESCRIPTION: chlorpromazine hydrochloride (Thorazine) 25 to 50 mg by mouth every 6 to 8 hours as needed for hiccups, not to exceed 100 mg in a 24-hour period. If unrelieved by this, switch patient to 35 mg intravenous every 6 hours as needed. If the patient is using 50 mg with each dose, what is the maximum number of doses the patient can receive not to exceed the limit for 24 hours? _____

6. PRESCRIPTION: chlorpromazine hydrochloride (Thorazine) 35 mg intravenous every 6 hours. You have a vial with 250 mg/10 milliliters. How many milliliters should you administer? _____

7. The order is gentamicin 6 mg/kg/24 hours intravenous in three divided doses. The patient weighs 18 kg. How many milligrams will the patient receive in 24 hours? _____

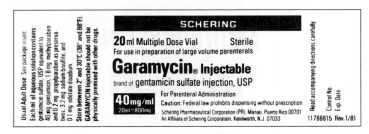

8. Based on problem 7, how many milligrams should the patient receive in each dose? _____

9. It is recommended that no more than 2.5 mg/kg of gentamicin be infused every 8 hours. Is the dosage for patient in problem 7 within the recommended guideline? _____

10. PRESCRIPTION: cefazolin 1 gram intravenous every 6 hours. The medication sent by the pharmacy is cefazolin 500 mg. When the patient's bar code is scanned against the medication, what can the nurse expect to see on the virtual due list screen? _____

(Answers on pp. 465–466)

CHAPTER REVIEW

Answer the questions as indicated.

1.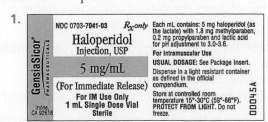

PRESCRIPTION: haloperidol 20 mg intramuscularly.
How many milliliters will you administer? _____

2.

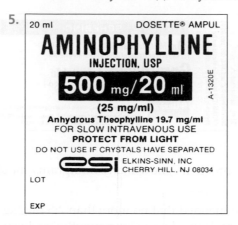

PRESCRIPTION: amoxicillin and potassium clavulanate (Augmentin) 200 mg by mouth.
How many milliliters will you administer? _____

3. **PRESCRIPTION:** sodium valproate 50 mg by mouth is ordered for a child.
HAVE: sodium valproate 200 mg/5 mL is available.
How many milliliters will you administer? _____

4. **PRESCRIPTION:** quinidine (Quinora) 0.6 g by mouth.
HAVE: quinidine 200-mg tablets.
How many tablet(s) will you need to administer? _____

5.

Aminophylline 50 mg intravenous is ordered.
How many milliliters will you add to the intravenous piggyback solution? _____

6. **PRESCRIPTION:** dicloxacillin 125 mg by mouth.
HAVE: dicloxacillin 62.5 mg per 5 milliliters on hand.
How many milliliters will you administer? _____

7. **PRESCRIPTION:** chlorpromazine hydrochloride (Thorazine) 25 to 50 mg by mouth every 6 to 8 hours as needed for hiccups, not to exceed 100 mg in a 24-hr period. If unrelieved by this, switch patient to 35 mg intravenous every 6 hours as needed.
If the patient is using 25 mg with each dose, what is the maximum number of doses the patient can receive not to exceed the limit for 24 hours? _____

8. **PRESCRIPTION:** chlorpromazine hydrochloride (Thorazine) 25 mg intravenous every 6 hours.
HAVE: 250 mg/10 mL.
How many milliliters should you administer? _____

9. The order is for gentamicin 4 mg/kg/24 hours intravenous in three divided doses. The patient weighs 20 kg. How many milligrams will the patient receive in 24 hours? _____

10. How many milligrams should the patient in problem 9 receive in each dose? _____

11. It is recommended that no more than 2.2 mg/kg of gentamicin be infused every 8 hours. Is the dose for the patient in problem 9 within the recommended guideline? _____

12. PRESCRIPTION: cefoxitin sodium (Mefoxin) 1 gram intravenous every 6 hours.
HAVE: cefoxitin 500 mg.
When the patient's bar code is scanned against the medication, what can the nurse expect to see on the virtual due list screen? _____

13. PRESCRIPTION: hydroxyzine hydrochloride (Vistaril) 50 mg intramuscularly.
HAVE: hydroxyzine hydrochloride 25 mg/mL intramuscular injection.
How many milliliters will you administer? _____

14. PRESCRIPTION: amoxicillin and potassium clavulanate (Augmentin) 200 mg by mouth.
HAVE: Augmentin 800 mg in 8 mL is available.
How many milliliters will you administer? _____

15. PRESCRIPTION: sodium valproate 40 mg by mouth is ordered for a child.
HAVE: sodium valproate 200 mg/5 mL is available.
How many milliliters will you administer? _____

16. PRESCRIPTION: quinidine (Quinora) 0.4 g by mouth is prescribed.
HAVE: quinidine 200-mg tablets.
How many tablet(s) will you need to administer? _____

17.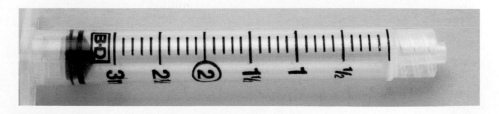

PRESCRIPTION: amoxicillin oral suspension 500 mg by mouth.
How many milliliters will you administer? _____

18. PRESCRIPTION: dicloxacillin 250 mg by mouth.
HAVE: dicloxacillin 62.5 mg per 5 mL oral suspension.
How many milliliters will you administer? _____

19. PRESCRIPTION: Solu-Cortef 250 mg intravenous now.
HAVE: 100 mg/mL vials.
How much medication do you draw up to administer your patient? _____

20.   PRESCRIPTION: dilitiazem (Cardizem) 180 mg by mouth now.
      HAVE: 60-mg tablets.
      How many tablet(s) will you administer? _____

(Answers on p. 466)

evolve   **For additional practice problems, refer to the Safety in Medication Administration section of the Drug Calculations Companion, version 4 on Evolve.**

BIBLIOGRAPHY

Food and Drug Administration. (2003, March). FDA proposes drug bar code regulation. *FDA News.* Accessed online February 12, 2004 at *http://www.fda.gov/oc/initiatives/barcode-sadr/fs-barcode.html.*

Hynes DM, Joseph G, & Pfeil C. (2002). Veterans Health Information Systems and Technology Architecture (VISTA): Computerized patient record system. VA information resource center, Hines, IL: Veterans Administration Information Resource Center. Available online at *www.virec.research.med.va.gov.*

Intravenous Fluid Calculations

Introduction to Intravenous Therapy

Denise Macklin

CLINICAL CONNECTION

- To accomplish the purposes of intravenous therapy, it is important to have a solid knowledge of infusion methods, fluid containers, types of solutions that can be infused, different administration sets, and different electronic infusion devices that can be used.
- To deliver a solution as prescribed, it is necessary to be able to calculate the flow rate to be administered to the patient.
- To calibrate an electronic pump effectively, you must be able to calculate milliliters per hour.
- To calculate intravenous infusions via gravity, you must be able to determine drops per milliliter (gtt/mL).
- To determine when to change or discontinue an intravenous bag, you will need to be able to anticipate when it will be completed by knowing the rate of flow.

INTRODUCTION

The purposes of intravenous therapy are to maintain daily fluid or electrolyte requirements, replace lost fluid and electrolytes, administer medications, and maintain a venous access for emergency purposes. Patients may be unable to meet their daily oral intake requirements, perhaps postoperatively or because they require nasogastric suction or have disorders that involve a large loss of fluid and electrolytes, such as hemorrhage, vomiting, chronic obstructive pulmonary disease, fluid overload, or burns. If any of these conditions exist, the bodily requirements must be replaced intravenously. The infusion of fluid into a patient's vein by means of a catheter is a primary responsibility of nurses.

INFUSION METHODS

Fluids are administered either continuously intermittently, or as direct intravenous push. If one solution is being administered continuously, a second solution can be added to the administration set. This is referred to as *piggybacking*. When an electronic pump is being used, this is referred to as *secondary solution*. Table 15-1 provides an overview of infusion methods.

FLUID CONTAINERS

Intravenous solutions are available in either glass bottles or plastic bags and come in sizes ranging from 25 mL to 1000 mL. Glass bottles are used less often than plastic bags. This is because plastic bags are lighter in weight, are easier to store and discard, do not break when dropped, are not sensitive to temperature fluctuations, and do not have a rubber stopper that can be cored during the spiking procedure. Because glass is inert (i.e., it does not react with contents), it is required that some drugs be

Table 15-1	Infusion Methods: Overview		
Method	**Description**	**Advantages**	**Disadvantages**
Continuous	Large-volume solutions: 250 mL to 1000 mL solution administered over 2-24 hours.	Constant serum levels can be maintained. Treat fluid volume deficit.	Drug incompatibility Accidental bolus (injected all at once) infusion Flow rate can be erratic if not infused with an electronic flow device
Intermittent	Small-volume solutions: 50 mL to 100 mL solution administered over 30 minutes to 2 hours. May be added to continuous fluid or hung alone through an as-needed (prn) adapter.	Risk of incompatibilities reduced. Large drug doses can be administered at a lower concentration/mL. Decreased risk of fluid overload.	Potential for speed shock Phlebitis when infused through a prn adapter
Intravenous push/bolus	Very small volume administered by syringe.	Administer medications rapidly. Ability to monitor response to medication.	Speed shock Phlebitis Infiltration Extravasation

supplied in glass bottles (e.g., nitroglycerin, single-use lipids). Fluid containers have a +/− overfill from 4% to 10%. It varies by size of the container, rising in volume from small to large containers, then leveling off with the largest containers. The overfill compensates for tubing that is filled with some volume during the intravenous line priming process. When using an electronic pump, overfill allows for the exact volume to be programmed and infused without having the container emptying completely. Some medications are manufactured in systems that have a vial of a given drug attached to a small bag (50 mL to 100 mL) of fluid. By activating these systems, the medication is added to the intravenous fluid and is reconstituted (Figure 15-1). This solution may need to be mixed by gently shaking the bag, and then it is ready for intravenous administration.

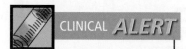

CLINICAL **ALERT**

Some self-activated bags need to be shaken vigorously to fully mix the medication in the solution (Figure 15-2).

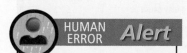

HUMAN ERROR **Alert**

Always remember to activate a self-activating system to mix the medication with the solution; otherwise, the patient will receive only the solution—not the medication.

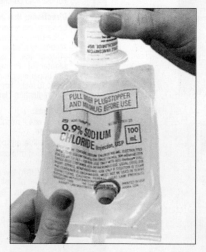

Figure 15-1 Medication manufactured in a system. (Used with permission from Hospira, Inc., Lake Forest, IL.)

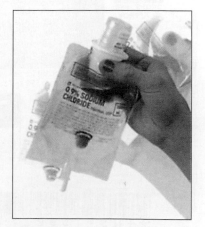

Figure 15-2 Activated piggyback bag. (Used with permission from Hospira, Inc., Lake Forest, IL.)

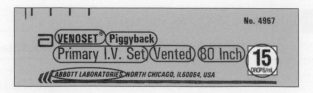

Figure 15-3 Administration set label. (From Gray Morris D: *Calculate with confidence*, ed 5, St Louis, 2010, Mosby.)

ADMINISTRATION SETS

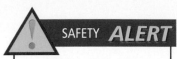

SAFETY *ALERT*

Use the higher bag configuration with all piggybacks, even when an electronic pump is being used.

Administration sets vary in length and in the size of the drip chamber. Each set is packaged individually. They are labeled with the name, description, length, drops/mL, lot number, usage description, and the manufacturer's name (Figure 15-3).

The administration sets are designed based on their usage and include the intravenous tubing and the associated parts required to allow fluid to flow from the container into the patient. The types of administration sets are *primary* (used for continuous infusion and intermittent infusions), *secondary* (used with piggybacks), *specialty* (blood administration), *pump-specific, low absorption,* and *meter-chambered* (Figure 15-4).

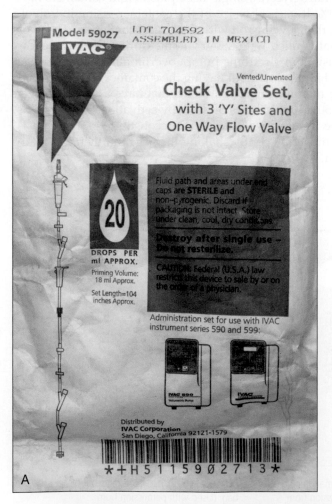

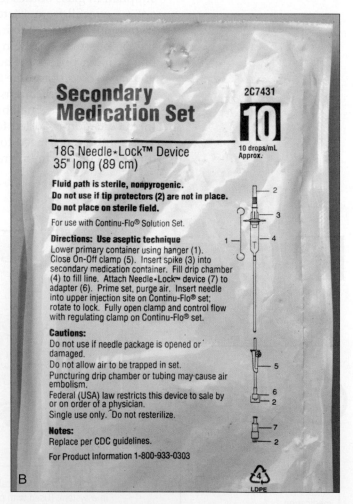

Figure 15-4 Types of administration sets. **A,** Pump specific. **B,** Piggyback.

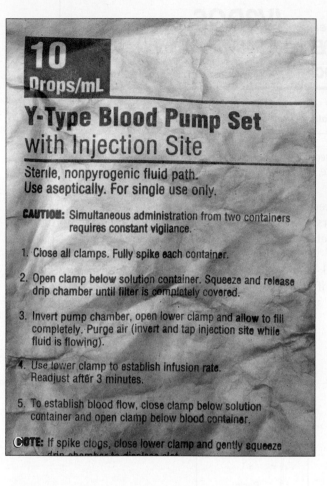

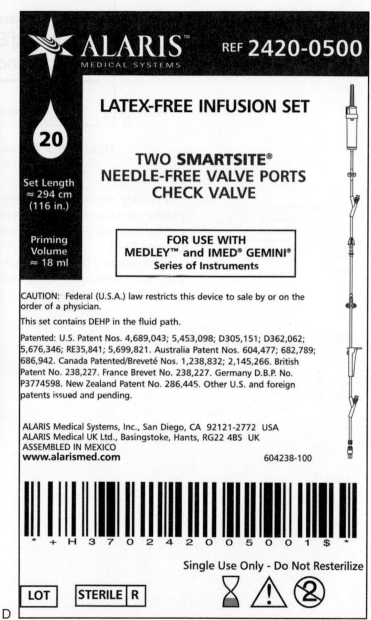

D

Figure 15-4, cont'd Types of administration sets. **C,** Specialty. **D,** Pump-specific.

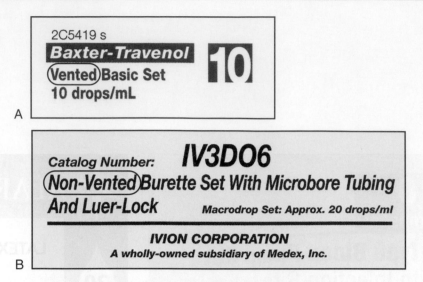

A,
```
2C5419 s
Baxter-Travenol      10
(Vented) Basic Set
10 drops/mL
```

B,
```
Catalog Number:    IV3DO6
(Non-Vented) Burette Set With Microbore Tubing
And Luer-Lock      Macrodrop Set: Approx. 20 drops/ml

IVION CORPORATION
A wholly-owned subsidiary of Medex, Inc.
```

Figure 15-5 A, Vented set label. **B,** Nonvented set label. (From Gray Morris D: *Calculate with confidence*, ed 5, St Louis, 2010, Mosby.)

Primary sets come in vented (use with glass containers), nonvented (use with plastic containers), and universal (open cap is vented and closed cap is nonvented) configurations. Whether the set is vented or nonvented is identified on the package (Figure 15-5).

Basic primary tubing (no back check valve), also referred to as *intermittent tubing*, is used for continuous infusions if no piggybacking is required or when a medication is given at specific intervals and a continuous infusion is not required (Figure 15-6).

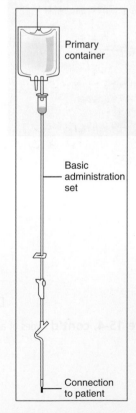

Primary container

Basic administration set

Connection to patient

Figure 15-6 Basic primary set to be used when no piggyback is prescribed. (Provided by Professional Learning Systems, Inc., Atlanta, GA.)

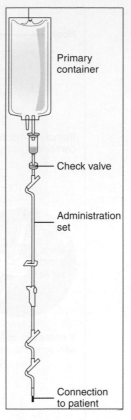

Primary
container

Check valve

Administration
set

Connection
to patient

Figure 15-7 Primary tubing configured to be used with piggybacks. (Provided by Professional Learning Systems, Inc., Atlanta, GA.)

Primary tubing also comes configured to be used with piggyback infusions. This type of tubing has a back check valve. It is used when a continuous infusion is required as well as additional medications that are infused at specific intervals, allowing one intravenous catheter to be used (Figure 15-7).

Secondary tubing is used when the patient requires both continuous intravenous infusion and additional medications at specified intervals (Figure 15-8). This tubing is designed to attach a piggyback medication onto a primary set. When a secondary set is added to the primary set, the secondary solution is hung on one side of the intravenous pole; then the metal or plastic extender that comes in the secondary tubing package is attached to the other side of the intravenous pole and the primary solution is hung on it.

The raised height of the secondary fluid increases the atmospheric pressure exerted on it. The fluid flowing from the secondary bag, therefore, has sufficient pressure to prevent fluid flow from the primary fluid (the lower one). You should notice that no drops are falling from the primary container's drop orifice. If, however, the primary container continues to drip, you need to lower the height of the primary container until the primary container's flow stops. This action will determine the correct distance between the two containers at which the secondary (higher) fluid flow is able to exert sufficient pressure to prevent flow from the primary (lower) container. Once the secondary solution is completely infused, the secondary fluid pressure decreases and the primary solution will again begin to flow. The flow rate must be reassessed at this point because the primary solution bag has been lowered and hence the primary flow rate has been decreased. Repositioning the primary bag to its original height will aid in reestablishing the flow rate.

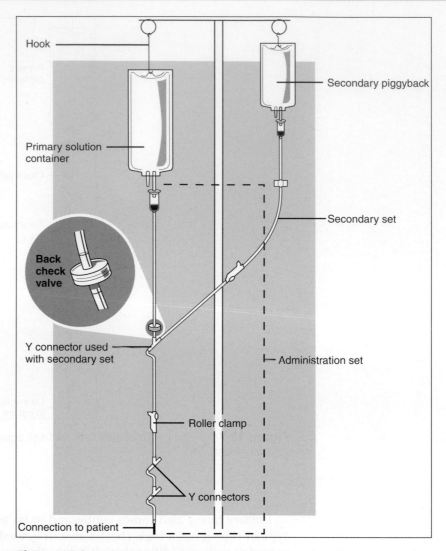

Hook

Primary solution
container

Back
check
valve

Y connector used
with secondary set

Roller clamp

Y connectors

Connection to patient

Secondary piggyback

Secondary set

Administration set

Figure 15-8   Secondary set. (From Macklin D, Chernecky C: *Real-world nursing survival guide: IV therapy*, St Louis, 2004, Saunders.)

TUBING COMPONENTS

Tubing differs in length, flexibility, clarity, and internal lumen diameter. Tubing is categorized by the internal lumen (bore) and comes in three types: standard, macro (larger internal lumen than standard), or micro (smaller lumen than standard). Macrobore tubing is stiffer than standard tubing and is used when high flow rates are required. Blood administration tubing is an example of macrobore tubing. Microbore tubing has a very small internal diameter; is kink-resistant; and is commonly used with very low flow rates, such as continuous administration of pain medication administered by an ambulatory pump (PCA) or because a lower priming volume is desired. Today most tubing is non-PVC (polyvinylchloride) tubing. However, with some drugs that can interact with plasticizers (such as paclitaxel [Taxol], an antineoplastic agent), non-PVC tubing is required.

Drip Chamber

At the top of the tubing is the flanged spike (Figure 15-9). It is designed to pierce the solution reservoir. Spikes are vented, nonvented, or universal. A universal spike allows the vent to be opened or closed. Vented spikes will work with most solution

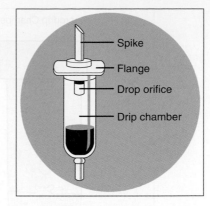

Figure 15-9 Flanged spike. (From Macklin D, Chernecky C: *Real-world nursing survival guide: IV therapy*, St Louis, 2004, Saunders.)

containers, but a nonvented set will only function with plastic, semirigid containers, or bottles with tubes (Figure 15-10).

The drop orifice, located at the top of the drip chamber, is designed to deliver large drops (macro) or small drops (micro). This is referred to as the *drop/drip factor*. The macrodrop configuration provides 10 gtt/mL (drops/milliliter), 15 gtt/mL, or 20 gtt/mL. The microdrop configuration provides 60 gtt/mL (Figure 15-11).

Back Check Valve

The back check valve prevents fluid from the secondary solution from entering the primary solution container. It is present on primary tubing configured to be used with a secondary set (see Figure 15-8).

Y-Site

These resealable entry points are placed at various distances along the tubing. The highest entry point is used to add secondary fluids. The lowest entry point is used to administer intravenous push medications (see Figure 15-8).

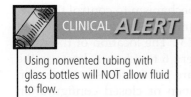

CLINICAL ALERT

Using nonvented tubing with glass bottles will NOT allow fluid to flow.

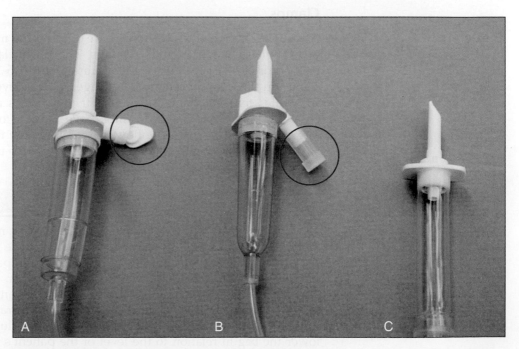

Figure 15-10 Types of spikes. **A,** Universal, **B,** Vented. **C,** Nonvented.

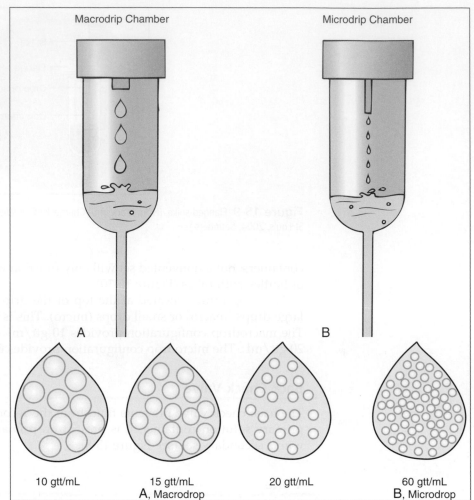

Figure 15-11 **A,** Macrodrip. **B,** Microdrip. (Modified from Gray Morris D: *Calculate with confidence,* ed 5, St Louis, 2010, Mosby.)

CLINICAL *ALERT*

You must know the drop factor for the intravenous administration set in order to do calculations for gravity infusions. The drop count is clearly identified on the tubing package (Figure 15-12).

Clamps

All administration sets have some type of clamping mechanism to control the flow rate. Primary sets have roller clamps. The roller clamp can be gradually rolled opened or closed to modify the flow rate (Figure 15-13). The location of the roller clamp on the tubing needs to be changed at least every 6 to 8 hours, because the flow rates tend to change over time if the clamps are left in the same location on the tubing. Slide or clip clamps have only an open or closed configuration (Figure 15-14). These do not allow incremental flow rate modification. Typically, a slide clamp is used with small solution bags that are used in ambulatory pumps or Buretrol tubing (Figure 15-15).

FLOW REGULATION

Three systems are used to regulate flow rate: gravity, mechanical, and electronic.

Gravity is the simplest method used to regulate flow (Figure 15-16). Placing the fluid container 36 inches above the level of the patient's heart exerts about 1.3 pounds per square inch (psi) on the fluid container. This pressure is greater than that of the patient's peripheral veins (0.2 to 0.6 psi) and central veins (0.1 to 0.4 psi) and is sufficient to provide the necessary pressure gradient (difference between the highest point of fluid flow and the lowest point of fluid flow) for the infusion. The lower the bag in relation to the level of the patient's heart, the lower the pressure exerted on the bag (the smaller the pressure gradient) and the slower the flow rate.

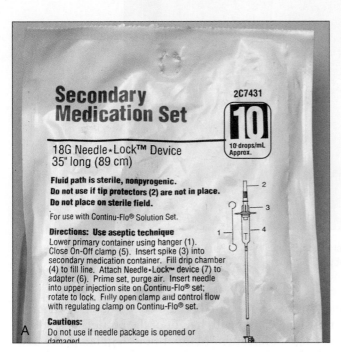

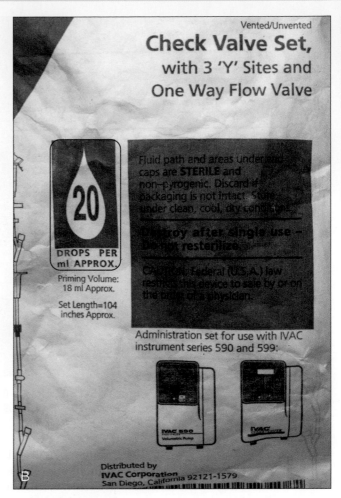

Figure 15-12 Drop count. **A,** 10 drops/mL. **B,** 20 drops/mL.

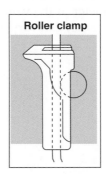

Figure 15-13 Roller clamp. (From Macklin D, Chernecky C: *Real-world nursing survival guide: IV therapy,* St Louis, 2003, WB Saunders.)

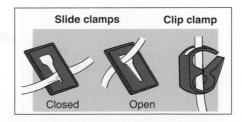

Figure 15-14 Slide and clip clamps. (From Macklin D, Chernecky C: *Real-world nursing survival guide: IV therapy,* St Louis, 2004, Saunders.)

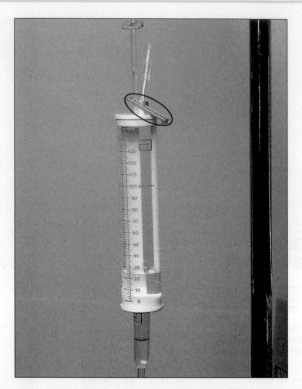

Figure 15-15 Slide clip on Buretrol tubing. (From Elkin MK, Perry AG, Potter PA: *Nursing interventions and clinical skills*, ed 4, St Louis, 2008, Mosby.)

The advantage of gravity is the low pressure exerted on the vein. The disadvantages are questionable accuracy (varies significantly with height of the bottle), lack of free-flow prevention, and no rate change notification. Manual flow regulators are add-ons that are labeled with specific flow rates (e.g., Dial-A-Flow®, Control-A-Flow®). The flow rate is adjusted by turning a dial to the prescribed flow rate. However, the labeled rate may not be the true flow rate owing to patient position, location of the catheter in the vein, and the height (also called head height) of the fluid container. Accuracy can vary $+/-$ 10% to 25%. In conditions such as fluid overload, right-side

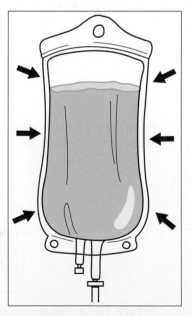

Figure 15-16 Gravity used to regulate flow.

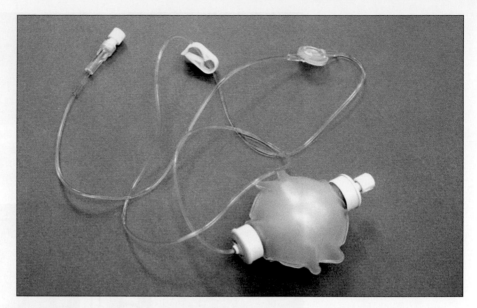

Figure 15-17 A mechanical system that requires no electricity. (From Professional Learning Systems, Inc., Atlanta, GA.)

heart failure, and pulmonary hypertension, the use of gravity flow as a regulatory system is not recommended.

Mechanical systems require no electricity to manage flow rate. For example, elastomeric pumps use a combination of atmospheric pressure and the addition of a flow-restricting orifice to the distal tip of the tubing to deliver a specific flow rate (Figure 15-17). A balloon is filled with the solution to be infused. The balloon collapses over a specified time period from 30 minutes to several days. Rate is determined by the caliber of opening in the orifice located either on the distal end of the tubing or at the outlet of the container. These pumps are used in home care settings with the ambulatory patient. Rate accuracy can be altered when there are changes to ambient temperature or pressure, such as when the solution is infused cold instead of at room temperature.

Another example of a mechanical system is the spring-loaded syringe pump, in which a spring is stretched when the syringe is loaded. As the spring returns to its original nonstretched configuration, it applies pressure to the syringe plunger, causing fluid to flow. The spring-coil type container has a stretched spring coil surrounded by two discs. As the coil returns to a nonstretched configuration, it pulls the two discs together. These discs collapse the fluid container. The fluid is then forced through restrictors.

Electronic systems require electricity, battery packs, or both. Electronic pumps are accurate, have free-flow prevention systems and initiate an alarm to sound when problems with the infusion occur. There are two types of electronic systems: nonvolumetric and volumetric.

- **Nonvolumetric:** These devices are commonly called *controllers*. They count drops while using gravity as the pressure source. These devices are not pumps. Because gravity is the pressure source, resistors such as head height of the fluid container and the viscosity of the fluid can alter accuracy. Optimal head height for the fluid container is 36 inches above the patient's heart. These devices sound an alarm when the drop rate changes, altering the preset flow rate.
- **Volumetric:** Volumetric pumps deliver a preset fluid rate over a specific time period using constant force to overcome resistance in the intravenous line (Figure 15-18). They are very accurate. Pumps require pump-specific tubing or cassette. They are programmable and many have additional program enhancements. They come in single-channel, dual-channel, and multichannel configurations, and in syringe, ambulatory, and patient-controlled analgesia (PCA) types. Common

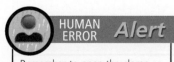

HUMAN ERROR *Alert*

Remember to open the clamp on the intravenous tubing before turning the electronic machine on or the pump will sound the occlusion alarm. Pump accuracy is dependent on a pump-specific administration set working in conjunction with the pump (see Figure 15-4, *D*).

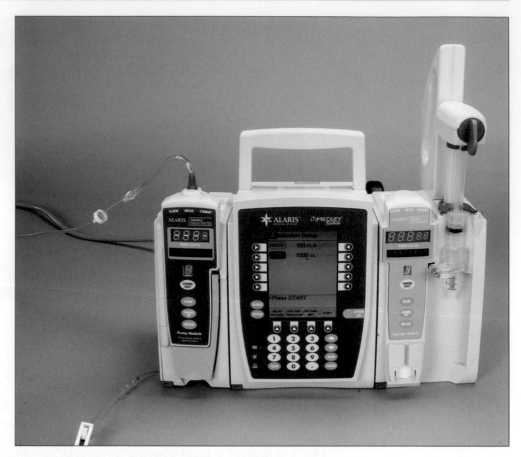

Figure 15-18 Volumetric pump.

alarms are "occlusion" (identifies that the preset psi limit has been surpassed), "air-in-line" (air bubbles pass through the pumping action), and "upstream" (pump is unable to meet the stroke volume requirement) alarms. Some additional pump alarms include "infusion complete," "low battery" or "low power," "not infusing," "nonfunctional," and "door open." These alarms notify personnel either that the pump is not programmed correctly or that there is a system problem.

Electronic pumps are used with all continuous fluids infusing through a central venous catheter, pediatric patients, geriatric patients, patients with a risk of fluid overload due to cardiac or renal conditions, parenteral nutrition solutions, and infusion of medications requiring accurate control (e.g., pitocin infusions during labor, magnesium sulfate, heparin, aminophylline, antihypertensive agents, vasoconstrictors, antiarrhythmic drugs, alteplase [tPA], insulin, potassium bolus infusions, narcotics and sedatives, cytotoxic agents). In the clinical setting, pumps are used with most infusions.

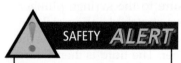

SAFETY ALERT

Most devices have free-flow protection, but the safest practice is to always close the clamp before removal. This action prevents any possibility that the solution will continue to flow (free-flow).

INTRAVENOUS SOLUTIONS

Intravenous solutions are a combination of water (solvent) and various additives (solutes). It is very important to be able to read and understand intravenous solution labels. Labels include the following:

1. **Solutes:** Dextrose, sodium chloride, and a few electrolytes are the most common. Lactated Ringer's (LR), or Ringer's lactate (RL), is an electrolyte solution that approximates plasma.
2. **Numbers:** Numbers are seen in percentage or decimal form and refer to the percentage or strength of solute (amount/100 mL of solution).

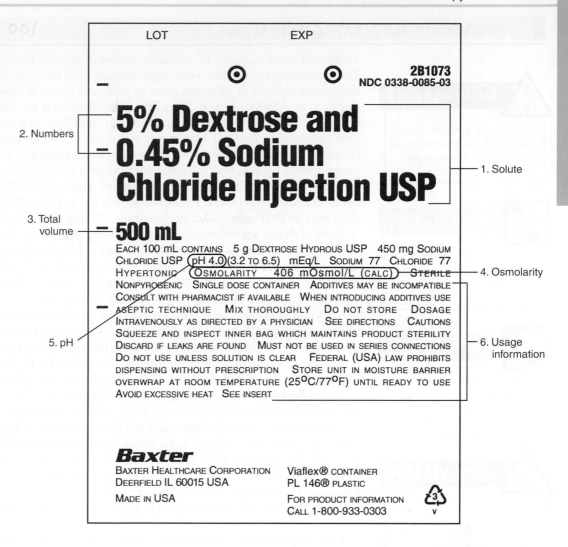

LOT   EXP

2B1073
NDC 0338-0085-03

2. Numbers

5% Dextrose and 0.45% Sodium Chloride Injection USP

1. Solute

3. Total volume

500 mL

EACH 100 mL CONTAINS   5 g DEXTROSE HYDROUS USP   450 mg SODIUM CHLORIDE USP pH 4.0 (3.2 TO 6.5) mEq/L SODIUM 77 CHLORIDE 77 HYPERTONIC OSMOLARITY   406 mOsmol/L (CALC) STERILE NONPYROGENIC SINGLE DOSE CONTAINER ADDITIVES MAY BE INCOMPATIBLE CONSULT WITH PHARMACIST IF AVAILABLE WHEN INTRODUCING ADDITIVES USE ASEPTIC TECHNIQUE MIX THOROUGHLY DO NOT STORE DOSAGE INTRAVENOUSLY AS DIRECTED BY A PHYSICIAN SEE DIRECTIONS CAUTIONS SQUEEZE AND INSPECT INNER BAG WHICH MAINTAINS PRODUCT STERILITY DISCARD IF LEAKS ARE FOUND MUST NOT BE USED IN SERIES CONNECTIONS DO NOT USE UNLESS SOLUTION IS CLEAR FEDERAL (USA) LAW PROHIBITS DISPENSING WITHOUT PRESCRIPTION STORE UNIT IN MOISTURE BARRIER OVERWRAP AT ROOM TEMPERATURE (25°C/77°F) UNTIL READY TO USE AVOID EXCESSIVE HEAT SEE INSERT

4. Osmolarity

5. pH

6. Usage information

Baxter

BAXTER HEALTHCARE CORPORATION
DEERFIELD IL 60015 USA

MADE IN USA

Viaflex® CONTAINER
PL 146® PLASTIC

FOR PRODUCT INFORMATION
CALL 1-800-933-0303

3. **Total volume:** Total volume (not including overfill) in milliliters is the volume that is programmed into the electronic pump or recorded as intake.

4. **Osmolarity:** Relationship of the fluid concentration to blood concentration (290 mOsm/L), with *isotonic* being the same as blood (250 to 375 mOsm/L); *hypotonic*, less than blood (<-50 mOsm/L); and *hypertonic*, more than blood (>375 mOsm/L). High osmolarity increases the risk of vein damage (phlebitis).

5. **pH:** Medications with a pH less than 5 or greater than 8 irritate veins.

6. **Usage information**

While solution component names are printed on the solution labels, prescriptions often use common abbreviations. Solution labels include the word "and" between components. With intravenous solutions, the percent signifies the number of grams of solute in 100 mL of solvent. $D_{20}W$ contains 20 grams of dextrose in each 100 mL of water. Prescriptions commonly eliminate this. Some common abbreviations are as follows:

- D_5W: 5% dextrose and water.
- NS: 0.9% sodium chloride.
- D_5NS: 5% dextrose and sodium chloride.
- ½ NS: 0.45% sodium chloride.
- D ¼ NS: 2.5% dextrose and 0.9% sodium chloride.
- D_5 ½ NS: 5% dextrose and 0.45% sodium chloride.
- D_5 ¼ NS: 5% dextrose and 0.2% sodium chloride.
- RL or LR: Ringer's lactate or lactated Ringer's.
- R: Ringer's.
- D_5LR: 5% dextrose and lactated Ringer's.

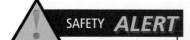

SAFETY ALERT

When infusing drugs that have a high risk of causing injury when administered incorrectly, pump settings should be independently checked by another nurse.

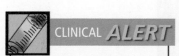

CLINICAL *ALERT*

When using more than one pump or dual-channel pumps with the capacity for multiple rate settings, close observation of tubing from pump to the patient must be used to determine that the solution, the pump, and the infusion site are all correct.

INTRAVENOUS FLOW RATE CALCULATIONS

Today the great majority of infusions are administered through an electronic pump. These pumps have become very sophisticated, with multiple channels that can deliver different solutions at different rates to different infusion sites, or through the same catheter, at different times. Adult infusions delivered by electronic pumps usually require the flow rate to be programmed in milliliters per hour (mL/hr), with most pumps allowing decimal increments per milliliter. Some pumps offer the option of choosing a drug set-up program within the device software. The medications can then programmed by selecting the drug name from a predetermined list of drugs selected by a hospital. Once the drug name is selected, a drug concentration and the prescribed drug amount are selected. Examples would be: heparin, 25,000 units/250 mL to be delivered at 1000 units/hour, or dopamine, 400 mg/500 mL at 5 mcg/minute.

Critical drugs administered in specialty care units may also be delivered in tenths of 1 mL. Other drugs, such as heparin and chemotherapeutic agents, may require fractions of a milliliter to be infused. Pediatric and infant fluid deliveries are often delivered in tenths of a milliliter. Pumps with a drug calculation feature will automatically calculate the rate if a prescribed dose is selected. Infant delivery is often given via a syringe pump. The syringe pump allows for a more accurate delivery and continuity of flow for very low rates. A common rate for infant delivery is 0.5 mL/hour. For infants, this is most often written as a prescription by the physician or advanced practice nurse and requires no calculation by the clinical nurse. The exception might be for blood delivery—for example, requiring 10 mL over 4 to 6 hours.

When large-volume intravenous fluids alone are prescribed, the prescription usually includes the total volume to be delivered over a total period of time, such as 1 L of normal saline every 12 hours and not the hourly infusion rate. Intravenous medication prescriptions that are to be infused intermittently, or as a secondary medication, specify the dose to be delivered and the frequency of administration, NOT the infusion rate or the infusion time (for example, ampicillin 500 mg intravenous every 8 hours). The pharmacy determines the solvent, the solvent volume, and the time to be infused. This information is included on the patient label affixed to the intravenous bag (Figure 15-19).

Certain pumps that are now available contain drug libraries that list drug names and standard concentrations that have been developed by the hospital purchasing

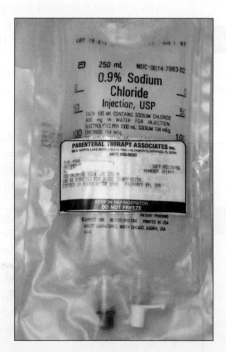

Figure 15-19 Patient label affixed to intravenous bag.

the device. This allows for the hospital's "best practice guidelines" to be included in the parameters. A device may also have minimum and maximum dosing limits that will give a warning should the programmed rate be below the minimum or above the maximum dosing parameter. An example of this might be the hospital parameter for heparin infusion is 5000 units (minimum limit) to 10,000 units (maximum limit) per hour. The programmed rate is heparin 500 unit/hour. In this example, a warning would appear on the device display to alert the nurse that the programmed rate is outside standard parameters.

CALCULATING LARGE VOLUME SOLUTION HOURLY INFUSION RATES

Even though some pumps today can complete the entire calculation when the prescription information is entered accurately, it is still important to know how to perform the calculations and to check your calculation against the pump calculation. This process may identify calculation errors and/or input errors when using a pump.

To calculate a flow rate for an electronic pump, it is necessary to identify the total volume of solution that is to be infused and the total time over which the infusion is to run. When using the ratio-proportion method to calculate infusion rates, the ratios are set up with volume (milliliters or drops) in the numerator and time (hours or minutes) in the denominator. Unlike medication dosage calculations, the complete ratio on the LEFT is written using information from what you KNOW. What you WANT is the correct hourly volume to be infused. Therefore X is placed in the numerator of the incomplete ratio on the RIGHT and 1 hour is written in the denominator.

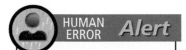

(Prescribed)

$$\frac{\text{(Total volume)}}{\text{(Total time)}} \qquad \frac{1000 \text{ mL}}{8 \text{ hr}} = \frac{X \text{ mL}}{1 \text{ hr}} \quad \text{(Unknown volume)}$$

Once the proportion is written, the calculation process is the same as with drug calculation. Because the interval is always 1 hour, you can simplify this process by just dividing the total volume by the total time.

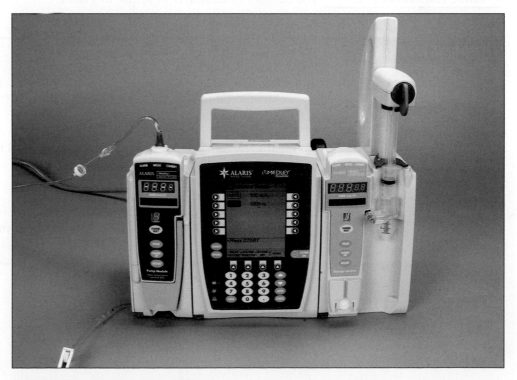

Figure 15-20 Electronic infusion pump.

Example 1

PRESCRIPTION   *1000 mL D₅ ½ NS every 12 hours.*

• **What You HAVE**

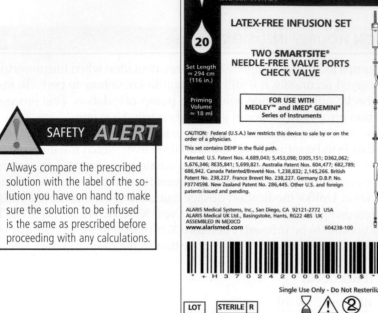

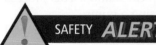

SAFETY ALERT

Always compare the prescribed solution with the label of the solution you have on hand to make sure the solution to be infused is the same as prescribed before proceeding with any calculations.

• **What You KNOW**   Prescribed volume is 1000 mL D₅ ½NS.
Prescribed infusion time is 12 hours.

• **What You WANT (X)**   The number of milliliters to infuse in 1 hour.

CRITICAL THINKING   What is the total fluid volume? _1000 mL_
What is the total infusion time? _12 hrs_
In setting up a ratio-proportion, place in the LEFT ratio what you KNOW (total volume/total time); in the RIGHT ratio, place X in the numerator and 1 hour in the denominator.
Multiply to get the cross-products.
Divide the numerical cross-product by the numerical multiplier of X (the number in front of X).
The result is the answer for X.
Label the answer with milliliters per hour.
Check the answer by placing the number obtained for X in the original equation. Cross-multiply. The cross-products should be approximately equal.

ANSWER FOR BEST CARE   Total volume? 1000 mL.
Total time? 12 hours.
Perform calculation.

$$\frac{1000 \text{ mg}}{12 \text{ hr}} = \frac{X \text{ mL}}{1 \text{ hr}}$$

$$12X = 1000 \quad X = \frac{1000 \text{ mg}}{12}$$

$$X = 83.3$$

Note that after setting up the proportion and cross-multiplying, X is equal to:

$$\frac{\text{Total volume}}{\text{Total time}}$$

Total volume/Total time

X = 83.3 mL/hr (Clinically appropriate 84 mL/hr)

> ✓ **Human Error Check**
>
> 83.3 × 12 × 999.6
> 996 ≈ 1000

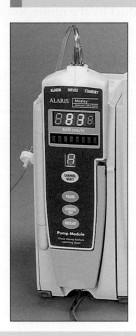

Example 2

PRESCRIPTION	*500 mL D₅ ¼ NS every 8 hours.*

- **What You HAVE** 500 mL D_5 ¼NS.

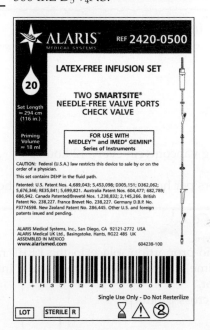

• **What You KNOW**	Prescribed volume is 500 mL D$_5$ ¼ NS.
	Prescribed infusion time is 8 hours.
• **What You WANT (X)**	The number of milliliters to infuse in 1 hour.

CRITICAL THINKING

What is the total fluid volume? *500 mL*

What is the total infusion time? *8 hrs*

In setting up a ratio-proportion, place in the LEFT ratio what you KNOW (total volume/total time); in the RIGHT ratio, place X in the numerator and 1 hour in the denominator.

Multiply to get the cross-products.

Divide the numerical cross-product by the numerical multiplier of X (the number in front of X).

The result is the answer for X.

Label the answer with milliliters per hour.

Check the answer by placing the number obtained for X in the original equation. Cross-multiply. The cross-products should be approximately equal.

ANSWER FOR BEST CARE

Total volume? 500 mL.

Total time? 8 hours.

Perform calculation.

$$\frac{500 \text{ mL}}{8 \text{ hr}} = \frac{X \text{ mL}}{1 \text{ hr}}$$

$$8X = 500 \qquad X = \frac{500 \text{ mL}}{8}$$

$$X = 62.5 \text{ (Clinically appropriate 63 mL/hr)}$$

✔ **Human Error Check**

62.5 × 8 = 500

Some intravenous medications are diluted in a large volume solution and infused over several hours. With these medications, the total volume will be found on the pharmacy label. The total time will also be on the label, as well as in the prescription.

Example 3

PRESCRIPTION *500 mg vancomycin intravenous every 12 hours.*

• **What You HAVE**	Pharmacy label:
	0.9% normal saline.
	Volume 750 mL.
	Vancomycin 500 mg.
	Rate 3 hours.
• **What You KNOW**	Prescribed is 500 mg vancomycin every 12 hours.
• **What You WANT (X)**	Number of milliliters per hour to infuse 750 mL in 3 hours.

CRITICAL THINKING

Total volume? 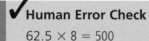 *750 mL*

Total time? *3 hrs*

In setting up a ratio-proportion, place in the LEFT ratio what you KNOW (total volume/total time); in the RIGHT ratio, place X in the numerator and 1 hour in the denominator.

Multiply to get the cross-products.

Divide the numerical cross-product by the numerical multiplier of X (the number in front of X).

The result is the answer for X.

Label the answer with milliliters per hour.

Check the answer by placing the number obtained for X in the original equation. Cross-multiply. The cross-products should be approximately equal.

ANSWER FOR BEST CARE	Total volume? 750 mL.

Total time? 3 hours.

Perform calculation.

$$X = \frac{750 \text{ mL}}{3 \text{ hr}} = \frac{X \text{ mL}}{1 \text{ hr}}$$

$$3X = 750 \qquad X = \frac{750 \text{ mL}}{3}$$

$$X = 250 \text{ mL/hr}$$

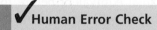

✔ **Human Error Check**

250 × 3 = 750

750 = 750

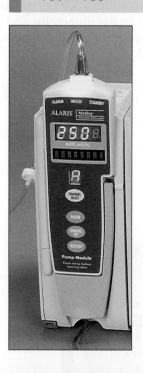

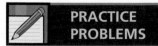 **PRACTICE PROBLEMS**	**Directions:** *Using the following intravenous prescriptions, determine the flow rate that you will program into the electronic infusion pump.*

1. PRESCRIPTION: 2000 mL D$_5$ ½ NS intravenous every 24 hours. ___84___ mL/hr

2. PRESCRIPTION: Ringer's lactate 500 mL over 8 hours. ___63___ mL/hr

3. PRESCRIPTION: D$_5$W 1000 mL intravenous over 12 hours. ___84___ mL/hr

4. PRESCRIPTION: Infuse 1500 mL of NS over 15 hours. ___100___ mL/hr

5. PRESCRIPTION: D$_5$W 500 mL with 25,000 units heparin sodium intravenous over 10 hours. ___50___ mL/hr.

6. PRESCRIPTION: 20% mannitol (Osmitrol 250 mL) over 2 hours. ___125___ mL/hr

7. PRESCRIPTION: D₅LR 1000 mL over 10 hours. ___100___ mL/hr

8. PRESCRIPTION: 250 mL Liposyn ll 20% over 6 hours. ___42___ mL/hr

9. PRESCRIPTION: A unit of packed cells (240 mL) over 4 hours. ___60___ mL/hr

10. PRESCRIPTION: Infuse 3000 mL TPN between 6 PM and 8 AM. ___215___ mL/hr

(Answers on p. 466)

CALCULATING SMALL VOLUME INFUSION RATES

With intermittent or secondary intravenous medication prescriptions, total solution volume and total time information are found on the pharmacy label, not the prescription. The infusion time is commonly written in minutes, not hours. Because pump programming requires time in hours, the total number of minutes must be converted to its hour decimal equivalent before the ratio-proportion method can be used. Some equivalents you will know by memory, such as 30 minutes equals 0.5 hours. However, you can always determine the appropriate equivalent by using the ratio-proportion method. The complete ratio (on the LEFT) is 60 minutes/hour, whereas the incomplete ratio (on the RIGHT) contains the minute rate found on the pharmacy label you HAVE in the numerator and X (hours) in the denominator. Once the hourly equivalent is determined, it can be substituted for minutes and the computation can be completed.

Example 1

PRESCRIPTION   *Ampicillin 500 mg intravenous every 6 hours.*

• **What You HAVE**   Pharmacy label:

NS.
Volume 50 mL.
Ampicillin 500 mg.
Rate 30 minutes.

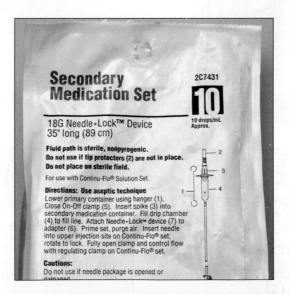

• **What You KNOW**   Prescribed is ampicillin 500 mg every 6 hours.

• **What You WANT (X)**   Milliliters required to infuse 50 mL in 30 minutes.

The medication is to be infused as a piggyback.

CRITICAL THINKING

Total volume? _____ 50 mL

Total time? _____ 30 min

Determine the hour equivalent by setting up a ratio-proportion: place in the LEFT ratio 60 minutes/hour; in the RIGHT ratio, place the rate you HAVE in the numerator and X in the denominator.

Multiply to get the cross-products.

Divide the numerical cross-product by the numerical multiplier of X (the number in front of X). The result is the answer for X.

Substitute the hour equivalent for the total time.

Divide the total volume by the total time in hours.

Label the answer with milliliters per hour.

To check the calculation, multiply the total time by the hourly volume (X). The product will be equal or approximately equal to the total fluid volume you HAVE.

ANSWER FOR BEST CARE

Total volume? 50 mL.

Total time? 30 minutes.

Perform calculation.

Convert minutes to hourly increment:

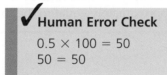

$$\frac{60 \text{ min}}{1 \text{ hr}} = \frac{30 \text{ min}}{X \text{ hr}} \qquad 60X = 30 \qquad 60)\overline{30} \quad ^{0.5 \text{ hr}}$$

$$X = \frac{50 \text{ mL}}{0.5 \text{ hr}} \qquad 5)\overline{500} \quad ^{100}$$

$$X = 100 \text{ mL/hr}$$

✔ **Human Error Check**

$0.5 \times 100 = 50$

$50 = 50$

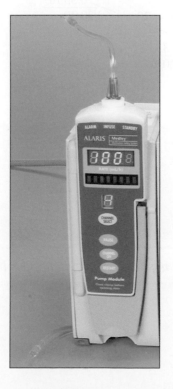

Example 2

PRESCRIPTION	*Rocephin (ceftriaxone sodium) 1 g intravenous piggyback before surgery.*
• **What You HAVE**	Pharmacy label: D_5W. Volume 100 mL. Rocephin 1 g. Rate 20 minutes.
• **What You KNOW**	Prescribed is Rocephin 1 g.
• **What You WANT (X)**	Milliliters required to infuse 100 mL in 20 minutes.

CRITICAL THINKING	Total volume? ___100 mL___ Total time? ___20 m___ Is the total time in hours or minutes? ___m___ Convert minutes to the hour decimal equivalent by setting up a ratio-proportion. Place in the LEFT ratio 60 minutes/hour; in the RIGHT ratio, place the rate you HAVE in the numerator and X in the denominator. Multiply to get the cross-products. Divide the numerical cross-product by the numerical multiplier of X (the number in front of X). The result is the answer for X. Substitute the hour equivalent for the total time. Divide the total volume by the total time in hours. Label the answer with milliliters per hour. To check the calculation, multiply the total time by the hourly volume (X). The product will be equal or approximately equal to the total HAVE fluid volume.

ANSWER FOR BEST CARE	Total volume? 100 mL. Total time? 20 minutes. Perform calculation. Convert minutes to the hourly increment:

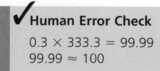

$$\frac{60 \text{ min}}{1 \text{ hr}} = \frac{20 \text{ min}}{X \text{ hr}} \qquad 60X = 20 \qquad 60\overline{)20.00} \quad 0.33 \text{ hr}$$

$$X = \frac{100 \text{ mL}}{0.3 \text{ hr}} \qquad 3\overline{)1000} \quad 333.3$$

$$X = 333.3 \text{ mL/hr}$$

> ✓ **Human Error Check**
>
> $0.3 \times 333.3 = 99.99$
> $99.99 \approx 100$

Example 3

PRESCRIPTION	*Cimetidine (Tagamet) 300 mg intravenous 90 minutes before surgery.*
• **What You HAVE**	Pharmacy label: NS. Volume 50 mL. Tagamet 300 mg. Rate 15 minutes.

- *What You KNOW*   Prescribed is Tagamet 300 mg.

- *What You WANT (X)*   Milliliters required to infuse 50 mL in 15 minutes.

CRITICAL THINKING
Total volume? _____ 50 mL
Total time? _____ 15 m
Convert minutes to the hour decimal equivalent by setting up a ratio-proportion. Place in the LEFT ratio 60 minutes/hour; in the RIGHT ratio, place the rate you HAVE in the numerator and X in the denominator.
Multiply to get the cross-products.
Divide the numerical cross-product by the number multiplier of X (the number in front of X). The result is the answer for X.
Substitute the hour equivalent for the total time.
Divide the total volume by the total time in hours.
Label the answer with milliliters per hour.
To check the calculation, multiply the total time by the hourly volume (X). The product will be equal or approximately equal to the total HAVE fluid volume.

ANSWER FOR BEST CARE
Total volume? 50 mL.
Total time? 15 minutes.
Perform calculation.
Convert minutes to the hourly increment:
60 min/1 hr = 15 min/X hr   60X = 15   0.25 hr/60/15.00

X = 50 mL/0.25 hr   200/25/500

X = 200 mL/hr

$$\frac{60 \text{ min}}{1 \text{ hr}} = \frac{15 \text{ min}}{X \text{ hr}} \qquad 60X = 15 \qquad 60\overline{)15.00}^{\,0.25 \text{ hr}}$$

$$X = \frac{50 \text{ mL}}{0.25 \text{ hr}} \qquad 25\overline{)5000}^{\,200}$$

X = 200 mL/hr

✔ **Human Error Check**
0.25 × 200 = 50
50 = 50

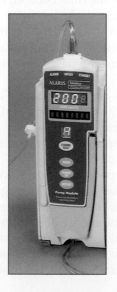

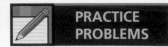

PRACTICE PROBLEMS

Directions: *Using the following intravenous prescriptions, determine the flow rate that you will program into the electronic infusion pump. The pharmacy label total volume and ratio confirmation is included. The medication information is excluded because it would be the same as the prescription.*

1. PRESCRIPTION: oxacillin sodium (Bactocill) 2 g intravenous piggyback every 6 hours (pharmacy label: D5W 250 mL; rate 60 minutes). ___250___ mL/hr

2. PRESCRIPTION: piperacillin (Pipracil) 1 g intravenous every 6 hours (pharmacy label: NS 250 mL; rate 30 minutes). ___500___ mL/hr

3. PRESCRIPTION: kanamycin sulfate (Kantrex) 900 mg intravenous every 12 hours (pharmacy label: D5W 180 mL; rate 45 minutes). ___240___ mL/hr

4. PRESCRIPTION: famotindine (Pepcid IV) 20 mg every 12 hours (pharmacy label: D5W 100 mL; rate 15 minutes). ___400___ mL/hr

5. PRESCRIPTION: Cefoxitin 3 g every 6 hours (pharmacy label: NS 50 mL; rate 15 minutes). ___200___ mL/hr

6. PRESCRIPTION: Infuse cimetidine (Tagamet) 300 mg intravenous 90 minutes before surgery (pharmacy label: solution volume NS 100 mL; rate 20 minutes). ___303___ mL/hr

7. PRESCRIPTION: (ceftriaxone sodium) Rocephin 1 g intravenous 30 minutes before surgery (pharmacy label: solution volume 250 mL; rate 30 minutes). ___500___ mL/hr

8. PRESCRIPTION: oxacillin sodium (Bactocill) 500 mg intravenous piggyback (pharmacy label: volume 50 mL; rate 10 minutes). ___301___ mL/hr

9. PRESCRIPTION: piperacillin (Pipracil) 3 g intravenous every 6 hours (pharmacy label: solution volume NS 50 mL; rate 30 minutes). ___100___ mL/hr

10. PRESCRIPTION: Amphotericin 70 mg daily (pharmacy label: solution volume D5W 100 mL; rate 90 minutes). ___67___ mL/hr

(Answers on pp. 466–467)

GRAVITY INFUSIONS: CALCULATING DROPS/MINUTE (gtt/min)

Gravity infusions are not as commonplace as in the past. However, because they still occur in certain settings—such as home care, combat, and rural health care—it is important to understand how to calculate infusion rates. In order to calibrate a gravity infusion, the nurse must be able to count the drops as they fall into the drop orifice in the drip chamber. This is accomplished by placing a watch that has a second hand up close to the drip chamber to monitor the passage of time while counting each drop for 1 full minute (Figure 15-21).

Intravenous administration sets come in different drop (gtt) factors (macrodrop factor provides 10 gtt/mL, 15 gtt/mL, or 20 gtt/mL; microdrop factor provides 60 gtt/mL). The drop factor information is located on the package of the intravenous administration set and identifies how many drops there are in 1 mL (Figure 15-22).

To determine how many drops per minute need to be counted, you must know how many milliliters per minute must infuse. With large-volume infusions, you must first identify the milliliters per hour. Then you can calculate the milliliters per minute by dividing the hourly milliliter volume by 60 minutes. Using the ratio-proportion method, the drop factor on the administration set package you HAVE is the complete ratio (on the left) (Figure 15-23). The right ratio contains X (the unknown drop factor) in the numerator and the rate/per minute in the denominator.

CHAPTER 15

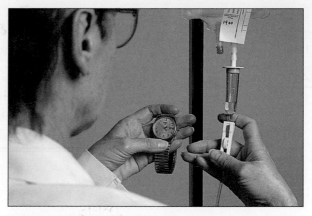

Figure 15-21 Nurse counting drops. (From Potter PA, Perry AG: *Fundamentals of nursing*, ed 7, St Louis, 2009, Mosby.)

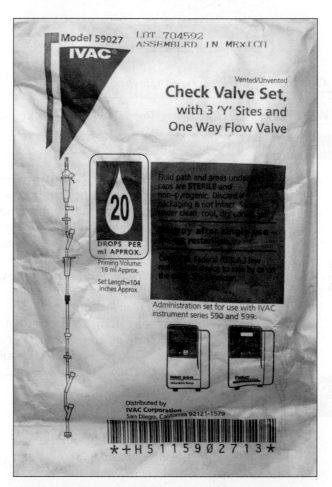

Figure 15-22 Drop factor information on administration set label.

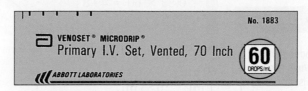

Figure 15-23 Drop factor information on administration set label. (From Gray Morris, D: *Calculate with confidence*, ed 5, St Louis, 2010, Mosby.)

Example 1

PRESCRIPTION	*Infuse D_5 ½ NS at 50 mL/hour to keep vein open.*

- **What You HAVE**

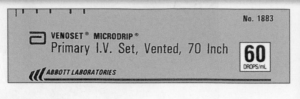

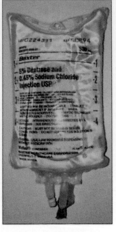

No. 1883

VENOSET® MICRODRIP®
Primary I.V. Set, Vented, 70 Inch **60** DROPS/mL

ABBOTT LABORATORIES

- **What You KNOW**   Prescribed rate is 50 mL/hr.

- **What You WANT (X)**   How many drops need to be counted to deliver the identified milliliters per minute.

CRITICAL THINKING

Total volume? ___50___
Total time? ___1 hr___
Is the prescribed rate in hours or minutes? ___50ml/hr___ ___60 gtt/1 mL___
What is the drop factor on administration set you HAVE? _____
Determine the minute rate by dividing the hourly rate by 60 minutes.
In setting up a ratio-proportion, place in the LEFT ratio the drop factor per minute; in the RIGHT ratio, place X in the numerator and the minute rate in the denominator.
Multiply to get the cross-products.
Divide the numerical cross-product by the numerical multiplier of X (the number in front of X).
The result is the answer for X.
Label the answer in drops per minute.
Check answer by placing the number obtained for X in the original equation. Cross-multiply. The cross-products should be approximately equal.

ANSWER FOR BEST CARE

Total volume? 50 mL.
Total time? 1 hour.
Perform calculation.
Convert 1 hour to 60 minutes.

$$\frac{50 \text{ mL (hourly volume)}}{60 \text{ min (1 hr)}} \quad \text{or} \quad 50 \div 60 = 0.83 \text{ mL/min}$$

✓ **Human Error Check**

$0.83 \times 60 = 49.8$
$49.8 \approx 50$

Drop factor:

$$\frac{60 \text{ gtt}}{1 \text{ mL}} = \frac{X \text{ gtt}}{0.83 \text{ mL}}$$

$X = 60 \times 0.83$
$X = 49.8 \text{ gtt/min}$

CLINICAL *ALERT*

When using a microdrip administration set, the gtt/min is equal to mL/hr. The mL/hr is divided by 60 to determine the mL/min and then the mL/min is multiplied by 60 to determine the gtt/min.

> ✔ **Human Error Check**
>
> Substitute 49.8 for X.
> 60 × 0.83 = 49.8

Example 2

PRESCRIPTION *Infuse 1000 mL D₅ ½ NS every 10 hours.*

• What You HAVE

> **Catalog Number: IV3DO6**
> **Non-Vented Burette Set With Microbore Tubing**
> **And Luer-Lock**   Macrodrop Set: Approx. 20 drops/ml
>
> ─────────────────────────────
>
> **IVION CORPORATION**
> **A wholly-owned subsidiary of Medex, Inc.**

• What You KNOW

Prescribed volume is 1000 mL.
Prescribed infusion time is 10 hours.

• What You WANT (X)

Rate in milliliters per minute.
How many drops need to be counted to deliver the identified milliliters per minute?

CRITICAL THINKING

Total volume? _1000 mL_
Total time? _10 hr_
Do you know the milliliters per hour? _100 mL_   _20 gtt/mL_
What is the drop factor on the administration set you HAVE? _____
Determine the minute rate by dividing the hourly rate by 60 minutes.
In setting up a ratio-proportion, place in the LEFT ratio the drop factor per minute; in the RIGHT ratio, place X in the numerator and the minute rate in the denominator.
Multiply to get the cross-products.
Divide the numerical cross-product by the numerical multiplier of X (the number in front of X).
The result is the answer for X.
Label the answer in drops per minute.
Check answer by placing the number obtained for X in the original equation. Cross-multiply. The cross-products should be approximately equal.

ANSWER FOR BEST CARE

Total volume? 1000 mL.
Total time? 10 hours.
Milliliters per hour known? No.
Drop factor? 20 gtt/mL.
Perform calculation.

$$\frac{1000 \text{ mL (total volume)}}{10 \text{ hr (total time)}}$$

Reduce $\frac{100}{1}$

Hourly rate is 100 mL/hr.

Convert 1 hour to 60 minutes.

$$\frac{100 \text{ mL}}{60 \text{ min}} = 1.66$$

> ✓ **Human Error Check**
>
> $60 \times 1.66 = 99.6$
> $99.6 \approx 100$

Minute rate is 1.66 mL.
Drop factor:

$$\frac{20 \text{ gtt}}{1 \text{ mL}} = \frac{X \text{ gtt}}{1.66 \text{ mL}} \quad 1 \times X = 20 \times 1.66 \quad X = 33.3 \text{ gtt/min}$$

> ✓ **Human Error Check**
>
> Substitute 34 for X.
> $20 \times 1.7 = 1 \times 34$
> $34 = 34$

Example 3

PRESCRIPTION	*Infuse 250-mL bag of packed red cells over 4 hours.*

- **What You HAVE**

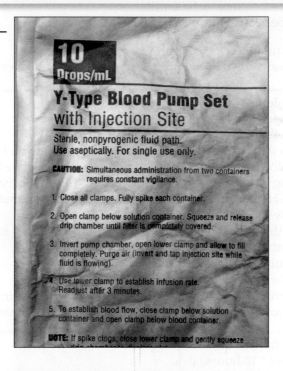

10 Drops/mL

Y-Type Blood Pump Set
with Injection Site

Sterile, nonpyrogenic fluid path.
Use aseptically. For single use only.

CAUTION: Simultaneous administration from two containers requires constant vigilance.

1. Close all clamps. Fully spike each container.
2. Open clamp below solution container. Squeeze and release drip chamber until filter is completely covered.
3. Invert pump chamber, open lower clamp and allow to fill completely. Purge air (invert and tap injection site while fluid is flowing).
4. Use lower clamp to establish infusion rate. Readjust after 3 minutes.
5. To establish blood flow, close clamp below solution container and open clamp below blood container.

NOTE: If spike clogs, close lower clamp and gently squeeze

- **What You KNOW**

Prescribed volume is 250 mL.
Prescribed infusion time is 4 hours.

- **What You WANT (X)**

Rate in milliliters per minute.
How many drops need to be counted to deliver the identified milliliters per minute?

CRITICAL THINKING	Total volume? _____ 250 mL

Total time? _____ 4 hr
Do you know the milliliters per hour? _____ 62.5
What is the drop factor on administration set you HAVE? _____ 10 g/1 mL
Determine the minute rate by dividing the hourly rate by 60 minutes.
In setting up a ratio-proportion, place in the LEFT ratio the drop factor per minute; in the RIGHT ratio, place X in the numerator and the minute rate in the denominator.

Multiply to get the cross-products.

Divide the numerical cross-product by the numerical multiplier of X (the number in front of X).

The result is the answer for X.

Label the answer in drops per minute.

Check answer by placing the number obtained for X in the original equation. Cross-multiply. The cross-products should be approximately equal.

ANSWER FOR BEST CARE	Total volume? 250 mL.

Total volume? 250 mL.

Total time? 4 hours.

Milliliters per hour known? No.

Drop factor? 10 gtt/mL.

Perform calculation.

$$\frac{250 \text{ mL (total volume)}}{4 \text{ hrs (total time)}} \quad 62.5 \text{ mL/min}$$

> ✔ **Human Error Check**
>
> $62.5 \times 4 = 250$

Convert 1 hour to 60 minutes.

$$\frac{62.5 \text{ mL}}{60 \text{ min}} \quad 1.04 \text{ (round to the nearest tenth)}$$

Minute rate is 1 mL/min.

> ✔ **Human Error Check**
>
> $60 \times 1.04 \neq 62.4$
> $62.4 \approx 62.5$

Drop factor:

$$\frac{10 \text{ gtt}}{1 \text{ mL}} = \frac{X \text{ gtt}}{1 \text{ mL}} \quad 1 \times X = 10 \times 1 \quad X = 10 \text{ gtt/min}$$

> ✔ **Human Error Check**
>
> Substitute 10 for X.
> $10 \times 1 = 10 \times 1$
> $10 = 10$

With small-volume infusions that are prescribed to infuse in minutes, you divide by the prescribed minutes into the total volume. Once the rate in milliliters per minute is known, it is multiplied by the drop factor associated with the administration set.

Example 4

PRESCRIPTION	*Infuse ampicillin (Omnipen) 1.5 g intravenous daily.*

• **What You HAVE**

2C5419 s
Baxter-Travenol
Vented Basic Set
10 drops/mL

Pharmacy label:
D_5W
Volume 100 mL.
Ampicillin (Omnipen) 1.5 g.
Rate 30 minutes.

- **What You KNOW**

Prescribed is ampicillin 1.5 g.

- **What You WANT (X)**

Rate in milliliters per minute.
How many drops need to be counted to deliver the identified milliliters per minute?

CRITICAL THINKING

Total volume? ___100 mL___
Total time? ___30___
What is the drop factor on the administration set you HAVE? ___10 gtt / 1 mL___
In setting up a ratio-proportion, place in the LEFT ratio the drop factor per minute; in the RIGHT ratio, place X in the numerator and the minute rate in the denominator.
Multiply to get the cross-products.
Divide the numerical cross-product by the numerical multiplier of X (the number in front of X).
The result is the answer for X.
Label the answer in drops per minute.
Check answer by placing the number obtained for X in the original equation. Cross-multiply. The cross-products should be approximately equal.

ANSWER FOR BEST CARE

Total volume? 100 mL.
Total time? 30 minutes.
Drop factor? 10 gtt/mL.
Perform calculation.

$$\frac{100 \text{ mL (total volume)}}{3}$$

Reduce.

$$3\overline{)10.0} \quad = 10$$

3.3 mL/min

$$\frac{10 \text{ gtt}}{1 \text{ mL}} = \frac{X \text{ gtt}}{3.3 \text{ mL}}$$

$$33 = X$$

> ✓ **Human Error Check**
> $3.3 \times 3 = 9.9$
> $9.9 \approx 10$

Drop factor:

$$\frac{10 \text{ gtt}}{1 \text{ mL}} = \frac{X \text{ gtt}}{3.3 \text{ mL}} \quad 1 \times X = 10 \times 3.3 \quad X = 3 \text{ gtt/min}$$

> ✓ **Human Error Check**
> Substitute 33 for X.
> $1 \times 33 = 10 \times 3.3$
> $33 = 33$

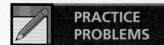

PRACTICE PROBLEMS

Directions: *Calculate drops per minute (gtt/min) and round rates to nearest whole number.*

1. PRESCRIPTION: Infuse D$_5$W at 125 mL/hr.

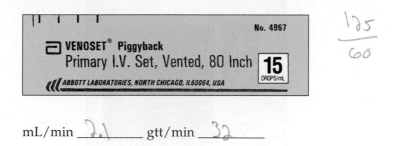

$$\frac{125}{60}$$

mL/min __2.1__ gtt/min __32__

2. PRESCRIPTION: Infuse NS 1000 mL at 100 mL/hr.

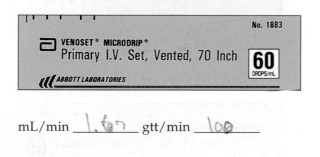

mL/min __1.67__ gtt/min __100__

3. PRESCRIPTION: Infuse gentamicin 70 mg every 8 hours (pharmacy label: NS 200 mL rate 1 hour).

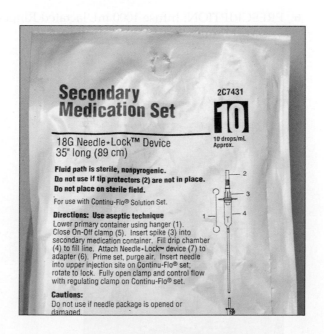

mL/min __3.33__ gtt/min __33__

4. PRESCRIPTION: Infuse D$_5$NS 2000 mL intravenous over 20 hours.

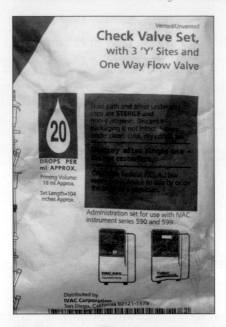

mL/min __1.7?__ gtt/min __34__

5. PRESCRIPTION: Infuse D$_5$ ½ NS intravenous at 50 mL/hr.

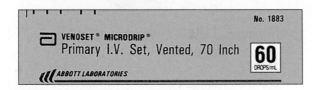

mL/min __.83__ gtt/min __50__

6. PRESCRIPTION: Infuse 1000 mL lactated Ringer's at 150 mL/hr.

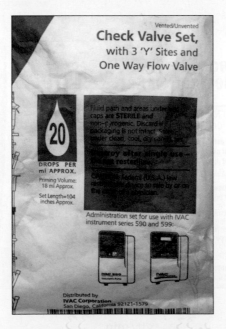

mL/min __2.5__ gtt/min __50?__

CHAPTER 15

7. PRESCRIPTION: Infuse 100 mL D$_5$W at 90 mL/hr.

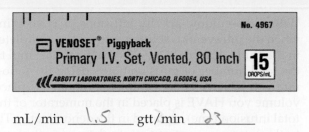

mL/min __1.5__ gtt/min __23__

8. PRESCRIPTION: Infuse 0.45% sodium chloride at 120 mL/hr.

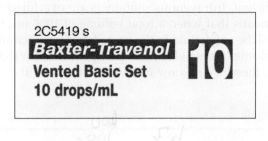

mL/min __2__ gtt/min __20__

9. PRESCRIPTION: cimetidine (Tagamet) 300 mg every 6 hours (pharmacy label: D$_5$W 50 mL; rate 20 minutes).

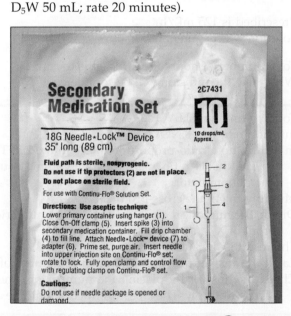

mL/min __2.5__ gtt/min __25__

10. PRESCRIPTION: cefazolin 1 g every 6 hours (pharmacy label: NS 100 mL; rate 30 minutes).

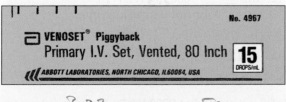

mL/min __3.33__ gtt/min __50__

(Answers on p. 467)

CALCULATING TOTAL INFUSION TIMES

CLINICAL ALERT

Allowing an intravenous solution to run dry may result in loss of intravenous access due to catheter occlusion.

SAFETY ALERT

Intravenous solutions cannot hang longer than 24 hours.

With large-volume gravity infusions, it is very important to know ahead of time when the intravenous solution bag will be complete. The prescription may be written in mL/hr (e.g., infuse D_5 ½ NS at 125 mL/hr until taking fluids orally). To determine the total number of infusion hours using the ratio-proportion method, the infusion rate you KNOW is the complete ratio and is placed on the left. The total solution volume you HAVE is placed in the numerator of the right ratio and X (the unknown total infusion time) is placed in the denominator. The total number of hours is added to the intravenous start time to determine the completion time. Although you can calculate the exact time of completion, an approximate time in 30-minute intervals is sufficient. Intravenous containers are overfilled +/− 10% from the manufacturer. This means that when a total volume of 1000 mL from a 1-L bag has infused, there will still be some fluid in the container. This phenomenon is seen when you program the volume into an electronic pump and, when the infusion sounds the "complete" alarm, there is still some fluid (<100 mL/L) left in the bag.

Example 1

PRESCRIPTION   *Infuse D_5 ½ NS 1000 mL intravenous at 125 mL until taking by-mouth fluids.*

- **What You HAVE**   1000 mL D_5 ½ NS.

- **What You KNOW**   Prescribed is 125 mL/hr.
  Solution was begun at 0800 hours (8 AM).

- **What You WANT (X)**   Total number of hours the infusion is to run.
  What time the infusion will be completed.

CRITICAL THINKING   Total volume you HAVE? _____ 125 ml
Infusion rate you KNOW? _____ 1 h
In setting up a ratio-proportion, place in the LEFT ratio what you KNOW (mL/hr); in the RIGHT ratio, place the total volume you HAVE in the numerator and X in the denominator.
Multiply to get the cross-products.
Divide the numerical cross-product by the numerical multiplier of X (the number in front of X).
The result is the answer for X.
Label the answer properly in units (i.e., number of tablets, number of milliliters).
Check the answer by placing the number obtained for X in the original equation. Cross-multiply. The cross-products should be approximately equal.

ANSWER FOR BEST CARE   Total volume? 1000 mL.
Infusion rate? 125 mL/hr.

(KNOW)

$$\frac{125 \text{ mL}}{1 \text{ hr}} = \frac{1000 \text{ mL (HAVE)}}{X \text{ hr (total infusion time)}}$$

125X = 1000

1000 ÷ 125

X = 8 hours

Infusion started at 0800 hours (8 AM).

0800 + 8 hours = 1600 hours (4 PM).

> **✓ Human Error Check**
>
> Replace X with 8.
>
> $$\frac{125}{1} = \frac{1000}{8}$$
>
> $125 \times 8 = 1 \times 1000$
> $1000 = 1000$

Example 2

PRESCRIPTION	*Infuse 2 L of D₅ ½ NS intravenous at 75 mL/hr.*

- **What You HAVE**   1000 mL D_5 ½ NS.

- **What You KNOW**   Prescribed rate is 75 mL/hr.
  Solution started at 1000 hours (10 AM).

- **What You WANT (X)**   Time at which infusion is complete.

CRITICAL THINKING   Total volume you HAVE? ___75 mL___
Infusion rate you KNOW? ___1 hr___
In setting up a ratio-proportion, place in the LEFT ratio what you KNOW (mL/hr); in the RIGHT ratio, place the total volume you HAVE in the numerator and X in the denominator.
Multiply to get the cross-products.
Divide the numerical cross-product by the numerical multiplier of X (the number in front of X).
The result is the answer for X.
Check the answer by placing the number obtained for X in the original equation. Cross-multiply. The cross-products should be approximately equal.
To determine completion time, take the start time and add the total number of hours to it.

ANSWER FOR BEST CARE

(KNOW)
$$\frac{75 \text{ mL}}{1 \text{ hr}} = \frac{1000 \text{ mL (HAVE)}}{X \text{ hr (total infusion time)}}$$

$75X = 1000$
$1000 \div 75 = 13.3$
$X = 13.3$ hours

> **✓ Human Error Check**
>
> Replace X with 13.
>
> $$\frac{75}{1} = \frac{1000}{13.3}$$
>
> $75 \times 13.3 = 1 \times 1000$
> $997.5 \approx 1000$

Solution started at 1000 hours (10 AM).

$1000 + 13$ hours = 2300 hours (11 PM).

The completion time can also be determined after the infusion has been started and the volume partially infused. The calculation uses the total volume at the present, which is divided by the known flow rate.

Example 3

PRESCRIPTION	*Infuse NS 1000 mL intravenous over 10 hr. At 0700 hours, 400 mL has infused.*

- **What You HAVE** — 600 mL remaining in the bag.

- **What You KNOW** — Rate is 100 mL/hr.
  Infusion begun at 0300 hours (3 AM).
  Current time is 0700 hours (7 AM).

- **What You WANT (X)** — Infusion completion time.

| **CRITICAL THINKING** | Partial volume you HAVE? ___600___
Infusion rate you KNOW? ___100 ml/hr___
In setting up a ratio-proportion, place in the LEFT ratio the infusion rate you KNOW; in the RIGHT ratio, place the partial volume you HAVE in the numerator and X in the denominator.
Multiply to get the cross-products.
Divide the numerical cross-product by the numerical multiplier of X (the number in front of X).
The result is the answer for X.
Label the answer properly.
Check the answer by placing the number obtained for X in the original equation. Cross-multiply. The cross-products should be approximately equal.
To determine completion time, take the current time and add the remaining infusion hours to it. |
|---|---|

| **ANSWER FOR BEST CARE** | Partial volume? 600 mL.
Infusion rate? 100 mL/hr.

(KNOW)
$$\frac{100 \text{ mL}}{1 \text{ hr}} = \frac{600 \text{ mL (HAVE)}}{X \text{ hr (total infusion time)}}$$

$100X = 600$

$600 \div 100$

$X = 6$ hours

Current infusion time is 0700 hours (7 AM).

$0700 + 6$ hours $= 1300$ hours (1 PM) |
|---|---|

> ✔ **Human Error Check**
>
> Replace X with 6.
>
> $$\frac{100}{1} = \frac{600}{6}$$
>
> $100 \times 6 = 600 \times 1$
> $600 = 600$

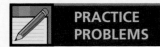

PRACTICE PROBLEMS

Directions: *Determine the infusion and completion times for each situation.*

1. 1000 mL D$_5$ 0.45 NS at 125 mL/hr; was hung at 1915 hours (7:15 PM).
   Infusion time ___8 hr___ Completion time ___~~0315~~ 3 AM___

2. 1000 mL NS at 50 mL/hr; was hung at 0845 hours (8:45 AM).
   Infusion time ___20 hr___ Completion time ___4:45 AM___

3. 1 unit packed cells (250 mL) to run at 80 mL/hr; was hung at 1300 hours (1 PM).
   Infusion time ___3.125___ Completion time ___4:20 p___

4. 380 mL remain in a bag of D$_5$W at 75 mL/hr; was hung at 0715 hours (7:15 AM).
   Infusion time ___5___ Completion time ___12:15 pm___

5. 500 mL NS at 75 mL/hr; was hung at 1400 hours (2 PM).
   Infusion time ___6.75___ Completion time ___845 p___

6. 500 mL 10% dextran at 42 mL/hr; was hung at 1000 hours (10 AM).
   Infusion time ___12___ Completion time ___10 p___

7. 200 mL packed cells at 50 mL/hr; was hung at 1415 hours (2:15 PM).
   Infusion time ___4___ Completion time ___1815___

8. 80 mL NS at 25 mL/hr is left to infuse at 1100 hours (11 AM).
   Infusion time ___40 m___ Completion time ___11:40___

9. 100 mL at 200 mL/hr; was hung at 1600 hours (4 PM).
   Infusion time ___30 m___ Completion time ___1630___

10. 100 mL at 400 mL/hr; was hung at 1400 hours (2 PM).
    Infusion time ___15 m___ Completion time ___14:15___

(Answers on p. 467)

CHAPTER REVIEW

For problems 1 through 5, determine the intravenous infusion rate in milliliters per hour.

1. PRESCRIPTION: D$_5$ ½ NS 3000 mL intravenous every 24 hours. ___125 mL/1 hr___

2. PRESCRIPTION: Ringer's lactate 500 mL intravenous over 6 hours. ___83 mL/hr___

3. PRESCRIPTION: D$_5$W 1000 mL intravenous over 10 hours. ___100 mL/hr___

4. PRESCRIPTION: Infuse D$_5$W 500 mL with 25,000 units heparin sodium over 10 hours. ___50 mL/hr___

5. PRESCRIPTION: Infuse NS 2000 mL intravenous over 15 hours. ___133 mL/h___

For questions 6 through 15, determine the milliliters per minute and the drops per minute for each intravenous infusion via gravity. Round rates to nearest whole number.

6. PRESCRIPTION: D$_5$W intravenous 125 mL/hr.

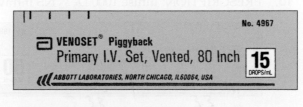

mL/min ___2.1___ gtt/min ___31.5___

7. PRESCRIPTION: Administer 2000 mL NS intravenous at 150 mL/hr.

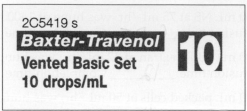

No. 1883
VENOSET® MICRODRIP®
Primary I.V. Set, Vented, 70 Inch   **60** DROPS/mL
ABBOTT LABORATORIES

mL/min _2.5_   gtt/min _150_

8. PRESCRIPTION: Infuse gentamicin 70 mg intravenous every 8 hours (pharmacy label: solution volume in NS 100 mL; rate 1 hour).

2C5419 s
Baxter-Travenol   **10**
Vented Basic Set
10 drops/mL

mL/min _1.7_   gtt/min _17_

9. PRESCRIPTION: Administer 3000 mL D₅NS intravenous over 20 hours.

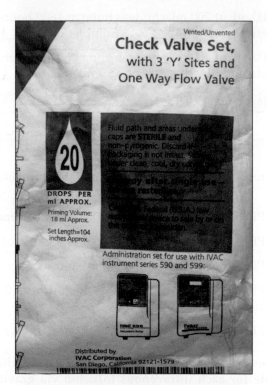

Vented/Unvented
Check Valve Set,
with 3 'Y' Sites and
One Way Flow Valve

20
DROPS PER
ml APPROX.
Priming Volume:
18 ml Approx.
Set Length=104
inches Approx.

Fluid path and areas under
caps are STERILE and
non-pyrogenic. Discard if
packaging is not intact. Store
under clean, cool, dry conditions.

...dy after single use—
...not resterilize.

Ca...n Federal (U.S.A.) law
res...s device to sale by or on
the ...f a physician.

Administration set for use with IVAC
instrument series 590 and 599.

Distributed by
IVAC Corporation
San Diego, California 92121-1579

mL/min _2.5_   gtt/min _50_

10. PRESCRIPTION: Infuse 1000 D₅ ½ NS intravenous at 75 mL/hr.

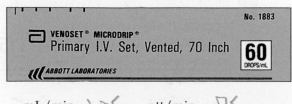

No. 1883
VENOSET® MICRODRIP®
Primary I.V. Set, Vented, 70 Inch   **60** DROPS/mL
ABBOTT LABORATORIES

mL/min _1.25_   gtt/min _75_

11.   PRESCRIPTION: Infuse 1 L of lactated Ringer's intravenous at 250 mL/hr.

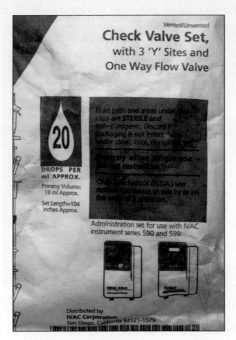

mL/min __42__ gtt/min __84__

12.   PRESCRIPTION: Infuse 500 mL D₅W at 60 mL/hr.

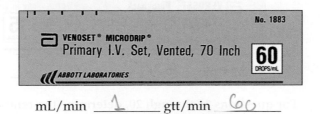

mL/min __1__ gtt/min __60__

13.   PRESCRIPTION: Infuse 0.45% sodium chloride intravenous at 300 mL/hr.

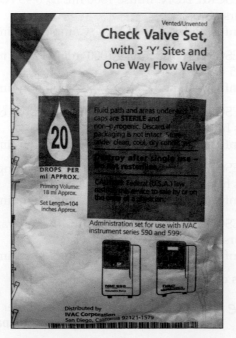

mL/min __5__ gtt/min __100__

14. PRESCRIPTION: Administer cimetidine (Tagamet) 300 mg every 6 hours (pharmacy label: solution volume D₅W 50 mL; rate 20 minutes).

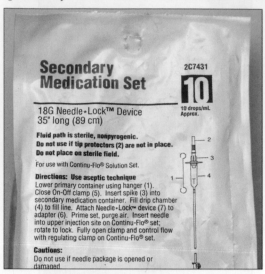

mL/min ___2.5___ gtt/min ___25___

15. PRESCRIPTION: Infuse cefazolin (Ancef) 1 g every 6 hours (pharmacy label: solution volume NS 250 mL; rate 30 minutes).

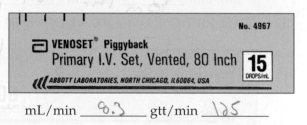

mL/min ___8.3___ gtt/min ___125___

For questions 16 through 20, determine the remaining infusion time in hours and the completion time in military time (and also convert to AM/PM).

16. PRESCRIPTION: Infuse 1000 mL D₅ 0.45 NS at 100 mL/hr; was hung at 0400 hours (4 AM).
    Infusion time ___10___ Completion time ___2pm___

17. PRESCRIPTION: Infuse 1000 mL NS at 75 mL/hr; was hung at 2045 hours (8:45 PM).
    Infusion time ___13___ Completion time ___9:45 A___

18. PRESCRIPTION: Infuse 1 unit packed red cells (300 mL) to run at 80 mL/hr; was hung at 0900 (9 AM).
    Infusion time ___3.75___ Completion time ___12:45 p___

19. PRESCRIPTION: There is 380 mL remaining in a bag of D₅W at 50 mL/hr; was hung at 1915 hours (7:15 PM).
    Infusion time ___7.6___ Completion time ___3:15 am___

20. PRESCRIPTION: Infuse 500 mL 10% dextran at 50 mL/hr; was hung at 2200 hours (10 PM).
    Infusion time ___10___ Completion time ___8 A___

(Answers on p. 467)

⊖volve **For additional practice problems, refer to the Intravenous Calculations section of the Drug Calculations Companion, version 4 on Evolve.**

Unique Calculations

CHAPTER

16

Calculating Intravenous Heparin Dosages

Cynthia Chernecky

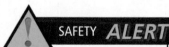

CLINICAL CONNECTION

- It is important to be able to identify the appropriate information in a prescription to mathematically determine medication dosages for persons receiving heparin by the intravenous route.
- Understanding the relationship of units of heparin to calculating heparin dosages is critical to successful computations.

SAFETY ALERT

NEVER administer heparin intramuscularly.

INTRODUCTION

Heparin is an anticoagulant medication that can be given by numerous routes, including subcutaneously, as an intravenous bolus, and as an intravenous drip. Heparin is commonly prescribed in a bolus dose followed by a heparin intravenous drip. The rate of the intravenous heparin drip is then adjusted based on the partial thromboplastin time (PTT) laboratory results or a weight-based heparin protocol. Some protocols also use PT/INR laboratory results to adjust heparin drips.

SAFETY ALERT

Always read the label carefully to determine the total amount of heparin in the intravenous solution and what the final concentration is in units/mL.

Heparin sodium injection is supplied in 1000 units/mL; 2000 units/mL; 5000 units/mL; 7500 units/mL; 10,000 units/mL; 20,000 units/mL; and 40,000 units/mL (Figure 16-1).

Dilute solutions of heparin (10 units/mL to 100 units/mL) are used to maintain patency of some central venous catheters (Figure 16-2).

Heparin, via a continuous intravenous route, is usually prescribed in units per hour (units/hr) and is available in specific premixed concentrations, such as 25,000 units of heparin/250 mL D₅W or 25,000 units/500 mL D₅W.

CALCULATING INFUSION RATES BASED ON HEPARIN UNITS/HOUR

HUMAN ERROR Alert

Some intravenous bags have the same volume of fluid, such as 250 mL D₅W, but differing units of heparin in the bag (i.e., different concentrations). Always read the units of heparin and the concentration on each bag of intravenous fluids.

The physician will prescribe the heparin units per hour (what you KNOW). You will HAVE from the pharmacy a bag of solution (total volume) with the total heparin unit dose strength (250 mL D₅W with 25,000 units heparin). What you WANT is the dose volume (mL) required to infuse the prescribed dose in 1 hour. With the ratio-proportion method, the LEFT (complete) ratio will contain what you HAVE (total dose/total volume) and the RIGHT (incomplete) ratio will contain what you KNOW (the prescribed dose) in the numerator and X mL (what you WANT) in the denominator. Although the total volume is larger than with small parenteral medication calculations, the method is the same: total strength/total volume = prescribed dose/dose volume.

316

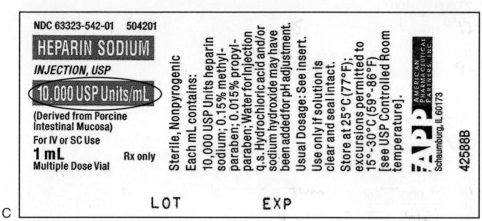

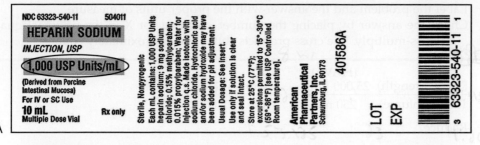

Figure 16-1 Heparin injection. **A,** 1000 units/mL. **B,** 5000 units/mL. **C,** 10,000 units/mL.

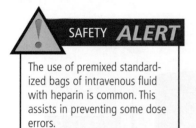

SAFETY **ALERT**

The use of premixed standard-ized bags of intravenous fluid with heparin is common. This assists in preventing some dose errors.

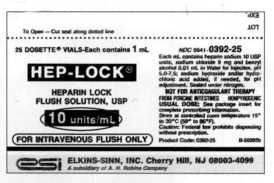

Figure 16-2 Heparin 10 units/mL.

Example 1

PRESCRIPTION	*Give heparin 600 units/hr intravenous.*
• **What You HAVE**	Total heparin strength is 25,000 units. Total volume is 250 mL D₅W.
• **What You KNOW**	Heparin dose strength is 600 units/hr.
• **What You WANT (X)**	Milliliters (dose volume) to administer prescribed heparin dose (mL/hr).
CRITICAL THINKING	In setting up a proportion, place what you HAVE (total strength/total volume) on the LEFT; on the RIGHT, place what you KNOW (the dose prescribed) in the numerator and X in the denominator. Cross-multiply to solve for X. Divide by the number in front of X to get the value for X.

Label the problem and the answer with the proper units of measure.

Check the answer by placing the number obtained for X in the original equation. Cross-multiply. The cross-products should be approximately equal.

$$\frac{\text{(Total strength)}}{\text{(Total volume)}} \quad \frac{\overset{\text{(HAVE)}}{25{,}000 \text{ units}}}{250 \text{ mL}} = \frac{600 \text{ units}}{X \text{ mL}} \quad \frac{\text{(KNOW)}}{\text{(WANT)}}$$

Reduce.

$$\frac{25{,}000}{250} = \frac{100}{1}$$

**HUMAN
ERROR** *Alert*

Do NOT confuse heparin to be administered intravenously with heparin lock solution used for intravenous catheter patency. The strengths are extremely different and can cause harm to patients.

$$\frac{100}{1} = \frac{600}{X} \qquad 100X = 600 \qquad 100\overline{)600}^{\,6}$$

$X = 6 \text{ mL/hr}$

Program pump.

SAFETY **ALERT**

An infusion pump is required for all intravenous heparin drips. Decimal pumps are particularly useful.

✔ **Human Error Check**

Substitute 6 for X.

$$\frac{25{,}000}{250} = \frac{600}{6}$$

$25{,}000 \times 6 = 600 \times 250$
$150{,}000 = 150{,}000$

SAFETY **ALERT**

Any discrepancy between the MAR, current dose, and your calculations warrants assistance from another professional.

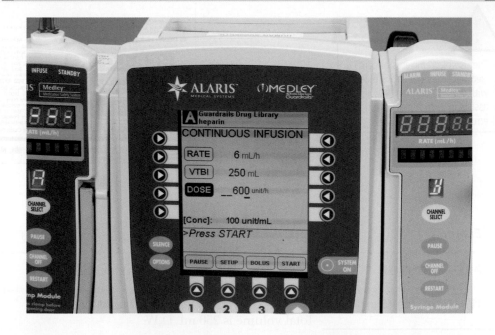

Example 2

PRESCRIPTION	*Infuse 2000 units heparin/hr intravenous.*
• **What You HAVE**	Total heparin strength is 25,000 units. Total volume is 250 mL NS.
• **What You KNOW**	Heparin dose is 2000 units/hr.
• **What You WANT (X)**	Milliliters to administer prescribed heparin dose (mL/hr).

| CRITICAL THINKING | In setting up a proportion, place what you HAVE (total strength/total volume) on the LEFT; on the RIGHT, place what you KNOW (the dose prescribed) in the numerator and X in the denominator. |

Cross-multiply to solve for X.

Divide by the number in front of X to get the value for X.

Label the problem and the answer with the proper units of measure.

Check the answer by placing the number obtained for X in the original equation. Cross-multiply. The cross-products should be approximately equal.

| ANSWER FOR BEST CARE | |

$$\underset{\text{(HAVE)}}{\frac{25{,}000 \text{ units}}{250 \text{ mL}}} \frac{\text{(total dose)}}{\text{(total volume)}} = \frac{2000 \text{ units}}{X \text{ mL}} \frac{\text{(KNOW)}}{\text{(WANT)}}$$

Reduce fraction

$$\frac{25{,}000}{250} = \frac{100}{1}$$

$$\frac{100}{1} = \frac{2000}{X} \qquad 100X = 2000 \qquad 100 \overline{)2000}^{\,20}$$

$X = 20$ mL/hr

Program pump.

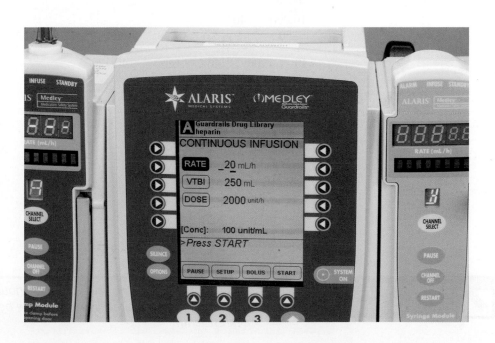

Example 3

| PRESCRIPTION | *Give heparin 1200 units/hr intravenous.* |

- **What You HAVE** Total heparin strength is 10,000 units.
  Total volume is 250 mL NS.

- **What You KNOW** Heparin dose is 1200 units/hr.

- **What You WANT (X)** Milliliters (volume) to administer prescribed heparin dose (mL/hr).

CRITICAL THINKING

In setting up a proportion, place what you HAVE (total strength/total volume) on the LEFT; on the RIGHT, place what you KNOW (the dose prescribed) in the numerator and X in the denominator.

Cross-multiply to solve for X.

Divide by the number in front of X to get the value for X.

Label the problem and the answer with the proper units of measure.

Check the answer by placing the number obtained for X in the original equation. Cross-multiply. The cross-products should be approximately equal.

ANSWER FOR BEST CARE

$$\underset{\text{(Total volume)}}{\overset{\text{(Total strength)}}{}}\ \frac{\overset{\text{(HAVE)}}{10{,}000 \text{ units}}}{250 \text{ mL}} = \frac{1200 \text{ units}}{X \text{ mL}}\ \frac{\text{(KNOW)}}{\text{(WANT)}}$$

Reduce.

$$\frac{10{,}000}{250} = \frac{40}{1}$$

$$\frac{40}{1} = \frac{1200}{X} \qquad 40X = 1200 \qquad 40\overline{)1200}^{\,30}$$

Answer is 30 mL.

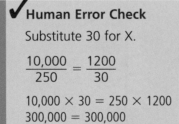

✔ **Human Error Check**

Substitute 30 for X.

$$\frac{10{,}000}{250} = \frac{1200}{30}$$

$10{,}000 \times 30 = 250 \times 1200$
$300{,}000 = 300{,}000$

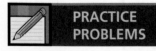

PRACTICE PROBLEMS

Directions: *Determine milliliters per hour for intravenous heparin drips. Assume that pumps that allow decimal increments are being used, and round to the nearest tenth.*

1. Heparin 600 units/hr from a solution of 25,000 units of heparin in 250 mL of D_5W.

2. Heparin 550 units/hr from a solution of 25,000 units of heparin in 250 mL of NS.

3. Heparin 400 units/hr from a solution of 50,000 units of heparin in 250 mL of D_5W.

4. Heparin 600 units/hr from a solution of 50,000 units of heparin in 250 mL of NS.

5. Heparin 800 units/hr from a solution of 25,000 units of heparin in 500 mL of NS.

6. Heparin 1800 units/hr from a solution of 50,000 units of heparin in 500 mL of D₅W.

7. Heparin 2400 units/hr from a solution of 25,000 units of heparin in 250 mL of D₅W.

8. Heparin 400 units/hr from a solution of 25,000 units of heparin in 250 mL of NS.

9. Heparin 1700 units/hr from a solution of 25,000 units of heparin in 250 mL of D₅W.

10. Heparin 1200 units/hr from a solution of 50,000 units of heparin in 500 mL of NS.

(Answers on pp. 468–469)

SAFETY *ALERT*

Always compare the solution you have from the pharmacy with the prescription before beginning any calculation. If there is a discrepancy, return the solution to the pharmacy.

Heparin is also prescribed in milliliters per hour (mL/hr), although not as often. When it is prescribed this way, it includes a specific diluted concentration, so you need to determine the dose (units/hr) the patient is to receive. You will KNOW the total heparin strength and volume and the prescribed dose volume (mL) to be infused in 1 hour. What you want is the heparin dose in units that will be infused with the prescribed dose volume in 1 hour. You will need to compare the prescription with the bag you HAVE on hand to verify that they are the same. With the ratio-proportion method, the LEFT (complete) ratio will be total dose of heparin/total solution volume; this information will be found in the prescription (what you KNOW) and on the solution bag you HAVE. In the RIGHT (incomplete) ratio will be an X (the unknown heparin dose) in the numerator (what you WANT) and the dose volume (what you KNOW) in the denominator.

In the following examples, the solution you HAVE and the solution prescribed are the same.

Example 1

PRESCRIPTION | *Infuse heparin at 22 mL/hr in 250 mL of D₅W with 25,000 units of heparin.*

• **What You HAVE** | Total heparin strength is 25,000 units.
Total volume is 250 mL D₅W.

• **What You KNOW** | Dose volume is 22 mL/hr.

• **What You WANT (X)** | Heparin dose to be infused in 1 hour, with a volume of 22 mL.

CRITICAL THINKING | In setting up a proportion, place what you HAVE (total strength/total volume) on the LEFT; on the RIGHT, place what you WANT (X) in the numerator and what you KNOW (prescribed dose volume) in the denominator.
Cross-multiply to solve for X.
Divide by the number in front of X to get the value for X.
Label the problem and the answer with the proper units of measure.
Check the answer by placing the number obtained for X in the original equation. Cross-multiply. The cross-products should be approximately equal.

ANSWER FOR BEST CARE |
(HAVE)
$$\frac{25{,}000 \text{ units}}{250 \text{ mL}} = \frac{\text{X units}}{22 \text{ mL}} \quad \frac{\text{(WANT)}}{\text{(KNOW)}}$$

Reduce.

$$\frac{25,000}{250} = \frac{100}{1}$$

$$\frac{100}{1} = \frac{X}{22}$$

1X = 2200

X = 2200 units/hour

Program pump.

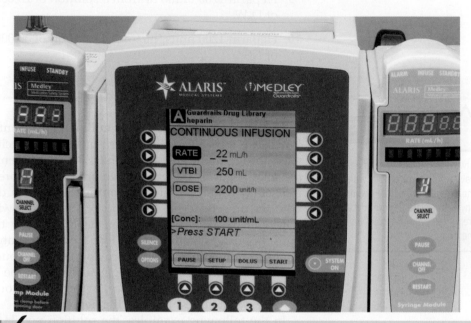

✔ **Human Error Check**

Substitute 2200 for X.

$$\frac{100}{1} = \frac{2200}{22}$$

100 × 22 = 2200 × 1
2200 = 2200

Example 2

PRESCRIPTION	*Infuse heparin at 35 mL/hr in 250 mL of D$_5$W with 25,000 units of heparin.*
• **What You HAVE**	Total heparin strength is 25,000 units. Total volume is 250 mL D$_5$W.
• **What You KNOW**	Dose volume is 35 mL/hr.
• **What You WANT (X)**	Heparin dose to be infused in 1 hour, with a volume of 35 mL.
CRITICAL THINKING	In setting up a proportion, place what you HAVE (total dose/total volume) on the LEFT; on the RIGHT, place what you WANT (X) in the numerator and what you KNOW (prescribed dose volume) in the denominator. Cross-multiply to solve for X. Divide by the number in front of X to get the value for X. Label the problem and the answer with the proper units of measure.

Check the answer by placing the number obtained for X in the original equation. Cross-multiply. The cross-products should be approximately equal.

ANSWER FOR BEST CARE	(HAVE) $\dfrac{25{,}000 \text{ units}}{250 \text{ mL}} = \dfrac{\text{X units}}{35 \text{ mL}}$ (WANT) (KNOW)

Reduce.

$$\frac{25{,}000}{250} = \frac{100}{1}$$

$$\frac{100}{1} = \frac{X}{35}$$

$$1X = 3500$$

$$X = 3500 \text{ units/hour}$$

Program pump.

> ✓ **Human Error Check**
>
> Substitute 3500 for X.
>
> $$\frac{100}{1} = \frac{3500}{35}$$
>
> $100 \times 35 = 3500 \times 1$
> $3500 = 3500$

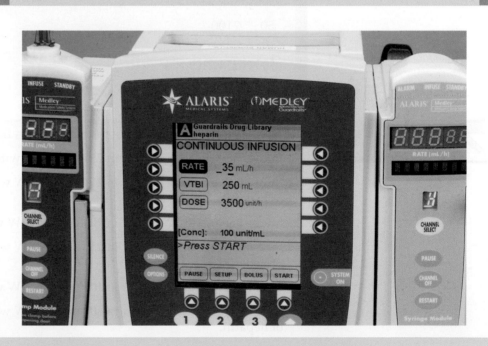

Example 3

PRESCRIPTION	*Infuse heparin at 42 mL/hr in 1000 mL of D₅W with 50,000 units of heparin.*
• **What You HAVE**	Total heparin strength is 50,000 units. Total volume is 1000 mL D₅W.
• **What You KNOW**	Dose volume is 42 mL/hr.
• **What You WANT (X)**	Heparin dose to be infused in 1 hour, with a volume of 42 mL.

CRITICAL THINKING	In setting up a proportion, place what you HAVE (total dose/total volume) on the LEFT; on the RIGHT, place what you WANT (X) in the numerator and what you KNOW (prescribed dose volume) in the denominator.

Cross-multiply to solve for X.

Divide by the number in front of X to get the value for X.

Label the problem and the answer with the proper units of measure.

Check the answer by placing the number obtained for X in the original equation. Cross-multiply. The cross-products should be approximately equal.

ANSWER FOR BEST CARE	

$$\frac{\text{(HAVE)}}{\underset{1000\text{ mL}}{50{,}000\text{ units}}} = \frac{X\text{ units}}{42\text{ mL}}\ \frac{\text{(WANT)}}{\text{(KNOW)}}$$

Reduce.

$$\frac{50{,}000}{1000} = \frac{50}{1}$$

$$\frac{50}{1} = \frac{X}{42}$$

$$1X = 2100$$

$$X = 2100\text{ units/hour}$$

There should be 2100 units infused each hour.

 Human Error Check

Substitute 2100 for X.

$$\frac{50}{1} = \frac{2100}{42}$$

$$50 \times 42 = 2100 \times 1$$
$$2100 = 2100$$

PRACTICE PROBLEMS	**Directions:** *Determine units per hour for intravenous heparin drip.*

1. Infuse heparin at 25 mL/hr in 250 mL of NS with 25,000 units of heparin.

2. Infuse heparin at 12 mL/hr in 250 mL of D_5W with 25,000 units of heparin.

3. Infuse heparin at 22 mL/hr in 1000 mL of D_5W with 50,000 units of heparin.

4. Infuse heparin at 20 mL/hr in 250 mL of D_5W with 25,000 units of heparin.

5. Infuse heparin at 40 mL/hr in 1000 mL of D_5W with 50,000 units of heparin.

6. Infuse heparin at 26 mL/hr in 500 mL of D_5W with 50,000 units of heparin.

7. Infuse heparin at 38 mL/hr in 250 mL of NS with 25,000 units of heparin.

8. Infuse heparin at 9 mL/hr in 250 mL of D_5W with 50,000 units of heparin.

9. Infuse heparin at 12 mL/hr in 250 mL of NS with 25,000 units of heparin.

10. Infuse heparin at 54 mL/hr in 500 mL of D_5W with 25,000 units of heparin.

(Answers on pp. 469–470)

HEPARIN BASED ON PROTOCOL AND PTT RESULTS

Heparin is also prescribed based on heparin protocols and partial thromboplastin time (PTT) laboratory results. Most protocols begin with an intravenous bolus of heparin, continue with an intravenous heparin drip, and then titrate (increase or decrease) the heparin drip based on the PTT results. These calculations look confusing at first glance. However, by breaking the calculation down into steps and using the ratio-proportion method, protocol prescriptions are very logical. The first step is to determine what information in the protocol is needed to perform each calculation. Protocols consist of bolus information, initial infusion rate information, and directions on what additional bolus and rate alterations must be made based on PTT results. The first step is to prepare the initial heparin bolus and the initial hourly infusion rate. A pump can be programmed to administer the initial bolus. Then, after a specified period of time, a PTT is drawn. An additional bolus and/or an intravenous rate change may be required based on the PTT result. You will compare the PTT result with the protocol parameters and complete a new set of calculations. Each time a PTT result is received, the protocol is referred to and alterations are made as required.

Weight-Based Heparin Protocol

1. Bolus heparin at 80 units/kg.
2. Begin intravenous infusion of heparin at 18 units/kg/hr using 25,000 units heparin in 500 mL D₅W or a concentration of 50 units/mL.
3. STAT PTT 6 hours after heparin bolus and then daily at 0700 hours (7 AM).
4. Adjust intravenous heparin daily based on PTT results and use the sliding scale that follows:
   PTT <35 seconds. Give 80 units/kg bolus and increase drip 4 units/kg/hr.
   PTT 35-45 seconds. Give 40 units/kg bolus and increase drip 2 units/kg/hr.
   PTT 46-70 seconds. No change.
   PTT 71-90 seconds. Reduce drip 2 units/kg/hr.
   PTT >90 seconds. Hold heparin drip for 1 hour, and then reduce drip 3 units/kg/hr.

Example 1

PRESCRIPTION *Use weight-based protocol for heparin. Patient weighs 90 kg.*

- **What You HAVE** Standing weight-based heparin protocol.
  Total heparin strength is 25,000 units.
  Total volume is 500 mL D₅W.
  Concentration is 50 units heparin/mL.

- **What You KNOW** Heparin bolus dose strength is 80 units/kg (protocol).
  Infusion rate dose strength is 18 units/kg/hr (protocol).
  Patient weight is 90 kg.

- **What You WANT (X)** Heparin dose strength and volume for initial bolus.
  Initial intravenous heparin infusion rate.

CRITICAL THINKING Determine heparin bolus dose strength by multiplying 80 units by patient weight in kilograms.
  Determine the bolus dose volume using the ratio-proportion method. The LEFT ratio contains the heparin concentration you HAVE, while the RIGHT ratio contains the heparin dose strength (which you calculated) in the numerator and X in the denominator.
  Cross-multiply to solve for X.

Divide by the number in front of X to get the value for X.

Label the problem and the answer with the proper units of measure.

Check the answer by placing the number obtained for X in the original equation. Cross-multiply. The cross-products should be approximately equal.

Determine heparin dose strength for infusion by multiplying 18 units by patient weight in kilograms.

Determine the infusion volume using the ratio-proportion method. The LEFT ratio contains the heparin concentration you HAVE, while the RIGHT ratio contains the heparin dose strength (which you calculated) in the numerator and X mL in the denominator.

Cross-multiply to solve for X.

Divide by the number in front of X to get the value for X.

Label the problem and the answer with the proper units of measure.

Check the answer by placing the number obtained for X in the original equation. Cross-multiply. The cross-products should be approximately equal.

ANSWER FOR BEST CARE	**Bolus calculation:**

Bolus calculation:

Dose strength (80 units/kg):

80 units $\times$ 90 kg = 7200 units intravenous heparin bolus

Dose volume:

$$\frac{\text{(Strength)}}{\text{(Volume)}} \quad \frac{50 \text{ units}}{1 \text{ mL}} = \frac{7200 \text{ units}}{X \text{ mL}} \text{ (Calculated dose strength)}$$

50X = 7200

X = 144

Bolus is 144 mL.

> ✔ **Human Error Check**
>
> Substitute 144 for X.
>
> $$\frac{50}{1} = \frac{7200}{144}$$
>
> 50 $\times$ 144 = 1 $\times$ 7200
> 7200 = 7200

Infusion rate:

Dose strength (18 units/kg/hr):

18 units $\times$ 90 kg = 1620 units

Dose volume:

$$\frac{50 \text{ units}}{1 \text{ mL}} = \frac{1620 \text{ units}}{X \text{ mL}}$$

50X = 1620

X = 32.4

> ✔ **Human Error Check**
>
> Substitute 32.4 for X.
>
> $$\frac{50}{1} = \frac{1620}{32.4}$$
>
> 50 $\times$ 32.4 = 1620 $\times$ 1
> 1620 = 1620

Patient STAT PTT result of 39 seconds.

• *What You HAVE*	Total heparin strength is 25,000 units. Total volume is 500 mL D₅W. Concentration is 50 units heparin/mL (protocol).
• *What You KNOW*	Give 40 units/kg bolus and increase drip 2 units/kg/hr (protocol). Patient weight is 90 kg. PTT result of 39.
• *What You WANT (X)*	Heparin dose strength and volume for the intravenous bolus based on PTT. Increase intravenous heparin infusion rate based on PTT.

CRITICAL THINKING

Determine dose strength for heparin intravenous bolus by multiplying 40 units by patient weight in kilograms.

Determine the bolus dose volume using the ratio-proportion method. The LEFT ratio contains the total heparin concentration you HAVE, while the RIGHT ratio contains the total heparin dose strength (you calculated) in the numerator and X mL in the denominator.

Cross-multiply to solve for X.

Divide by the number in front of X to get the value for X.

Label the problem and the answer with the proper units of measure.

Check answer by placing the number obtained for X in the original equation. Cross-multiply. The cross-products should be approximately equal.

Determine number of units for increasing infusion rate.

Determine increased infusion volume using the ratio-proportion method. The LEFT ratio contains the concentration you HAVE, while the RIGHT ratio contains the heparin dose strength (which you calculated) in the numerator and X mL in the denominator.

Cross-multiply to solve for X.

Divide by the number in front of X to get the value for X.

Label the problem and the answer with the proper units of measure.

Check the answer by placing the number obtained for X in the original equation. Cross-multiply. The cross-products should be approximately equal.

Determine the heparin dose for infusion by multiplying 18 units by the patient weight in kilograms.

Determine the infusion volume using the ratio-proportion method. The LEFT ratio contains the heparin concentration you HAVE, while the RIGHT ratio contains the heparin dose strength (which you calculated) in the numerator and X mL in the denominator.

Cross-multiply to solve for X.

Divide by the number in front of X to get the value for X.

Label the problem and the answer with the proper units of measure.

Check the answer by placing the number obtained for X in the original equation. Cross-multiply. The cross-products should be approximately equal.

**ANSWER FOR
BEST CARE**

Bolus calculation:
Dose strength (40 units/kg):

40 units × 90 kg = 3600 units

Dose volume:

$$\frac{50 \text{ units}}{1 \text{ mL}} = \frac{3600 \text{ units}}{X \text{ mL}}$$

50X = 3600

X = 72-mL bolus

✔**Human Error Check**

$$\frac{50}{1} = \frac{3600}{72}$$

$50 \times 72 = 1 \times 3600$
$3600 = 3600$

Infusion rate:

Strength increase:

$2 \text{ units} \times 90 \text{ kg} = 180 \text{ units/hr}$

Total volume increase:

$$\frac{50 \text{ units}}{1 \text{ mL}} = \frac{180 \text{ units}}{X \text{ mL}}$$

$50 X = 180$
$X = 3.6$

✔**Human Error Check**

$$\frac{50}{1} = \frac{180}{3.6}$$

$50 \times 3.6 = 180 \times 1$
$180 = 180$

Increase rate:

$$\begin{array}{r} 32 \text{ mL (current rate)} \\ + \ 3.6 \text{ mL (increase)} \\ \hline 35.6 \text{ mL (new rate)} \end{array}$$

New infusion rate is 35.6 mL/hr.

Example 2

PRESCRIPTION   *Use weight-based protocol for heparin. Patient weighs 108 kg.*

Weight-based heparin protocol:

1. Bolus heparin at 70 units/kg.
2. Begin intravenous heparin drip at 16 units/kg/hr using 25,000 units in 250 mL D$_5$W or concentration 100 units/mL.
3. STAT laboratory PTT 6 hours after initial heparin bolus (draw bloodwork from arm opposite to heparin infusion).
4. Adjust intravenous heparin based on PTT results, and use the following scale:
   PTT <41 seconds. Call physician STAT.
   PTT 41-50 seconds. Give 70 units/kg bolus of heparin and increase drip 4 units/kg/hr.
   PTT 51-59 seconds. Give heparin drip by 2 units/kg/hr.
   PTT 60-80 seconds. No change.
   PTT 81-100 seconds. Decrease heparin drip by 2 units/kg/hr.
   PTT > 100 seconds. Hold drip for 1 hour, then reduce heparin drip by 4 units/kg/hr.

- **What You HAVE**

Standing weight-based heparin protocol.
Total heparin dose is 25,000 units.
Total volume is 250 mL D₅W.
Concentration is 100 units/mL (protocol).

- **What You KNOW**

Heparin bolus dose strength is 70 units/kg (protocol).
Intravenous heparin drip dose strength is 16 units/kg/hr (protocol).
Patient weight is 108 kg.

- **What You WANT (X)**

Heparin dose strength and volume for initial bolus.
Initial intravenous heparin infusion rate.

CRITICAL THINKING

Determine bolus dose strength for heparin intravenous bolus by multiplying 70 units by patient weight in kilograms.

Determine the bolus dose volume using the ratio-proportion method. The LEFT ratio contains the heparin concentration you HAVE, while the RIGHT ratio contains the total heparin dose in the numerator and X mL in the denominator.

Cross-multiply to solve for X.

Divide by the number in front of X to get the value for X.

Label the problem and the answer with the proper units of measure.

Check answer by placing the number obtained for X in the original equation. Cross-multiply. The cross-products should be approximately equal.

Determine heparin dose strength for infusion by multiplying 16 units by patient weight in kilograms.

Determine the dose volume using the ratio-proportion method. The LEFT ratio contains the total heparin concentration you HAVE, while the RIGHT ratio contains the heparin dose (which you calculated) in the numerator and X mL in the denominator.

Cross-multiply to solve for X.

Divide by the number in front of X to get the value for X.

Label the problem and the answer with the proper units of measure.

Check the answer by placing the number obtained for X in the original equation. Cross-multiply. The cross-products should be approximately equal.

ANSWER FOR BEST CARE

Bolus calculation:
Total dose strength (70 units/kg):

70 units × 108 kg = 7560 units

Total dose volume:

$$\frac{100 \text{ units}}{1 \text{ mL}} = \frac{7560 \text{ units}}{X \text{ mL}}$$

100X = 7560

X = 75.6 mL (round to the nearest tenth mL)

The bolus is 75.6 mL.

✔ **Human Error Check**

Substitute 75.6 for X.

$$\frac{100 \text{ units}}{1 \text{ mL}} = \frac{7560 \text{ units}}{75.6}$$

100 × 75.6 = 7650 × 1
7560 = 7560

Heparin infusion:

Total dose strength (16 units/kg):

16 units × 108 kg = 1728 units

Total dose volume:

$$\frac{100 \text{ units}}{1 \text{ mL}} = \frac{1728 \text{ units}}{X \text{ mL}}$$

100X = 1728

X = 17.28 (round to the nearest tenth mL)

Infusion rate is 17.3 mL/hr.

> ✓ **Human Error Check**
>
> Substitute 17.3 for X.
>
> $$\frac{100}{1} = \frac{1730}{17.3}$$
>
> 100 × 17.3 = 1 × 1730
> 1730 = 1730

Patient STAT PTT result of 46 seconds.

- **What You HAVE**

  Standing weight-based heparin protocol.
  Total heparin strength is 25,000 units.
  Total volume is 250 mL D₅W.
  Concentration is 100 units heparin/mL (protocol).

- **What You KNOW**

  Give 70 units/kg bolus of heparin (protocol).
  Increase rate 4 units/kg/hour (protocol).
  Patient weight is 108 kg.
  PTT result of 46 seconds.

- **What You WANT (X)**

  Heparin dose strength and volume for the intravenous bolus based on PTT.
  Increase intravenous heparin infusion rate based on PTT.

CRITICAL THINKING	Determine bolus dose strength for heparin intravenous bolus by multiplying 70 units by patient weight in kilograms.

Determine bolus dose strength for heparin intravenous bolus by multiplying 70 units by patient weight in kilograms.

Determine the bolus dose volume using the ratio-proportion method. The LEFT ratio contains the heparin concentration you HAVE, while the RIGHT ratio contains the total heparin dose in the numerator and X mL in the denominator.

Cross-multiply to solve for X.

Divide by the number in front of X to get the value for X.

Label the problem and the answer with the proper units of measure.

Check answer by placing the number obtained for X in the original equation. Cross-multiply. The cross-products should be approximately equal.

Determine heparin dose strength for infusion by multiplying 4 units by patient weight in kilograms.

Determine the infusion dose volume using the ratio-proportion method. The LEFT ratio contains the total heparin concentration you HAVE, while the RIGHT ratio contains the heparin dose (which you calculated) in the numerator and X mL in the denominator.

Cross-multiply to solve for X.

Divide by the number in front of X to get the value for X.

Label the problem and the answer with the proper units of measure.

Check the answer by placing the number obtained for X in the original equation. Cross-multiply. The cross-products should be approximately equal.

Determine new infusion rate by adding the increased volume to the current infusion rate volume.

ANSWER FOR BEST CARE

Bolus calculation:

Dose strength:

$70 \times 108 = 7560$ units.

Dose volume:

$$\frac{100 \text{ units}}{1 \text{ mL}} = \frac{7560 \text{ units}}{X \text{ mL}}$$

$100X = 7560$

$X = 75.6$ (round to the nearest tenth number)

The bolus is 75.6 mL.

✔ **Human Error Check**

Substitute 75.6 for X.

$$\frac{100}{1} = \frac{7560}{75.6}$$

$100 \times 75.6 = 7560 \times 1$

$7560 = 7506$

Infusion rate:

Dose strength:

$4 \times 108 = 432$ units/hr.

Dose volume:

$$\frac{100 \text{ units}}{1 \text{ mL}} = \frac{432 \text{ units}}{X \text{ mL}}$$

$100X = 432$

$X = 4.32$ (round to the nearest tenth mL)

Increase rate 4.3 mL/hr.

✔ **Human Error Check**

Substitute 4.3 for X.

$$\frac{100}{1} = \frac{430}{4.3}$$

$100 \times 4.3 = 1 \times 430$

$430 = 430$

Increase rate:

17 mL/hr (current rate)
+ 4.3 (increase)
———————
21.3 (new rate)

New infusion rate is 21.3 mL/hr.

Example 3

PRESCRIPTION	*Use weight-based protocol for heparin. Patient weighs 72 kg.*

Weight-based heparin protocol:

1. Bolus heparin at 90 units/kg.
2. Begin intravenous heparin drip at 20 units/kg/hr using 25,000 units/250 mL of 0.45% NaCl (premixed) or concentration 100 units/mL.
3. STAT laboratory PTT 6 hours after initial heparin bolus (draw bloodwork from arm opposite to heparin infusion) and 6 hours after any adjustment.
4. Adjust intravenous heparin based on PTT results and use the sliding scale that follows:

   PTT <30 seconds. Call physician STAT.
   PTT 30-40 seconds. Give 90 units/kg bolus of heparin and increase drip 4 units/kg/hr.
   PTT 41-65 seconds. Give 45 units/kg bolus and increase heparin drip by 2 units/kg/hr.
   PTT 66-85 seconds. No change.
   PTT 86-95 seconds. Reduce heparin drip by 2 units/kg/hr.
   PTT >95 seconds. Hold drip for 1 hour, then reduce heparin drip by 3 units/kg/hr.

- **What You HAVE**

  Standing weight-based heparin protocol.
  Total heparin strength is 25,000 units.
  Total volume is 250 mL.
  Heparin concentration is 100 units/mL (protocol).

- **What You KNOW**

  Bolus dose strength is 90 units/kg (protocol).
  Infusion rate dose strength is 20 units/kg/hr (protocol).
  Patient weight is 72 kg.

- **What You WANT (X)**

  Heparin dose strength and volume for initial bolus.
  Initial intravenous heparin infusion rate.

CRITICAL THINKING

Determine bolus dose strength for heparin intravenous bolus by multiplying 90 units by patient weight in kilograms.

Determine the bolus dose volume using the ratio-proportion method. The LEFT ratio contains the heparin concentration you HAVE, while the RIGHT ratio contains the total heparin dose in the numerator and X mL in the denominator.

Cross-multiply to solve for X.

Divide by the number in front of X to get the value for X.

Label the problem and the answer with the proper units of measure.

Check answer by placing the number obtained for X in the original equation. Cross-multiply. The cross-products should be approximately equal.

Determine heparin dose strength for infusion by multiplying 20 units by patient weight in kilograms.

Determine the infusion dose volume using the ratio-proportion method. The LEFT ratio contains the total heparin concentration you HAVE, while the RIGHT ratio contains the heparin dose (which you calculated) in the numerator and X mL in the denominator.

Cross-multiply to solve for X.

Divide by the number in front of X to get the value for X.

Label the problem and the answer with the proper units of measure.

Check the answer by placing the number obtained for X in the original equation. Cross-multiply. The cross-products should be approximately equal.

ANSWER FOR BEST CARE

Bolus calculation:

Dose strength:

90 units × 72 kg = 6480 units

Dose volume:

$$\frac{100 \text{ units}}{1 \text{ mL}} = \frac{6480 \text{ units}}{X \text{ mL}}$$

100X = 6480

X = 64.8

The bolus is 65 mL.

✓ **Human Error Check**

Substitute 64.8 for X.

$$\frac{100}{1} = \frac{6480}{64.8}$$

100 × 64.8 = 6480 × 1
6480 = 6480

Infusion:

Dose strength:

20 units × 72 kg = 1440 units

Dose volume:

$$\frac{100 \text{ units}}{1 \text{ mL}} = \frac{1440 \text{ units}}{X \text{ mL}}$$

100X = 1440

X = 14.4

✓ **Human Error Check**

Substitute 14.4 for X.

$$\frac{100}{1} = \frac{1440}{14.4}$$

100 × 14.4 = 1440 × 1
1440 = 1440

Patient STAT PTT result of 88 seconds.

• **What You HAVE**	Standing weight-based heparin protocol. Total volume is 250 mL D$_5$W. Total heparin dose is 25,000 units. Concentration is 100 units/mL units heparin/mL (protocol).
• **What You KNOW**	Patient weight is 72 kg. PTT result of 88 seconds. Reduce heparin drip by 2 units/kg/hr.
• **What You WANT (X)**	Decrease intravenous heparin infusion rate based on PTT.

Determine total reduction number of units for heparin intravenous infusion rate by multiplying 2 units by patient weight in kilograms.

Determine reduction volume using the ratio-proportion method. In the LEFT ratio place the heparin concentration you HAVE; in the RIGHT ratio, place the total reduction units in the numerator and X mL in the denominator.

Cross-multiply to solve for X.

Divide by the number in front of X to get the value for X.

Label the problem and the answer with the proper units of measure.

Check the answer by placing the number obtained for X in the original equation. Cross-multiply. The cross-products should be approximately equal.

Determine new rate by subtracting calculated reduction volume from current rate volume.

Total unit reduction:

2 units $\times$ 72 kg = 144 units

Infusion volume reduction:

$$\frac{100 \text{ units}}{1 \text{ mL}} = \frac{144 \text{ units}}{\text{X mL}}$$

100 X = 144

X = 1.44 or 1.4 rounded to tenths

Decrease infusion rate by 1.4 mL/hr.

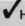 **Human Error Check**

Substitute 1.44 for X.

$$\frac{100}{1} = \frac{144}{1.44}$$

100 $\times$ 1.44 = 144 $\times$ 1
144 = 144

Decrease rate:

$$
\begin{array}{r}
14.0 \text{ mL/hr (current rate)} \\
- \quad 1.4 \text{ (decrease)} \\
\hline
12.6 \text{ (new rate)}
\end{array}
$$

Reprogram pump to 12.6 mL/hr.

 PRACTICE PROBLEMS

Directions: *Determine the bolus dose of heparin (in units) and the initial intravenous infusion of heparin, and then adjust the dose of heparin intravenous bolus (units) and intravenous drip (units/hr) up or down based on the PTT results using the weight-based heparin protocol that follows. For practice, instead of programming the pump for the bolus, use the heparin supplied by the pharmacy and mark the syringes (where provided).*

Bolus heparin at 80 units/kg.

Begin intravenous infusion of heparin at 18 units/kg/hr using 25,000 units heparin in 500 mL D₅W for 50 units/mL.

PTT <35 seconds. Give 80 units/kg bolus and increase drip 4 units/kg/hr.

PTT 35-45 seconds. Give 40 units/kg bolus and increase drip 2 units/kg/hr.

PTT 46-70 seconds. No change.

PTT 71-90 seconds. Reduce drip 2 units/kg/hr.

PTT >90 seconds. Hold heparin drip for 1 hour, and then reduce drip 3 units/kg/hr.

HAVE:

NDC 63323-540-11   504011

HEPARIN SODIUM
INJECTION, USP

1,000 USP Units/mL

(Derived from Porcine
Intestinal Mucosa)
For IV or SC Use
10 mL   Rx only
Multiple Dose Vial

Sterile, Nonpyrogenic
Each mL contains: 1,000 USP Units
heparin sodium; 9 mg sodium
chloride; 0.15% methylparaben;
0.015% propylparaben; Water for
Injection q.s. Made isotonic with
sodium chloride. Hydrochloric acid
and/or sodium hydroxide may have
been added for pH adjustment.
Usual Dosage: See Insert.
Use only if solution is clear
and seal intact.
Store at 25°C (77°F);
excursions permitted to 15°-30°C
(59°-86°F) [see USP Controlled
Room temperature].

American
Pharmaceutical
Partners, Inc.
Schaumburg, IL 60173

401586A

LOT
EXP

3 63323-540-11   1

1. Patient weight = 61 kg. PTT = 31.

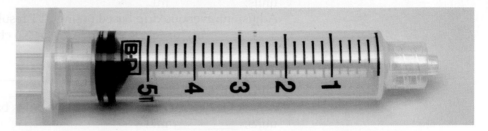

Bolus dose of heparin = _____ units; _____ mL.
Initial intravenous infusion of heparin = _____ units/hr; _____
mL/hr.
Adjust the dose of heparin intravenous bolus based on PTT results: _____
units; _____ mL.
Adjust intravenous drip based on the PTT results: _____ units/hr;
_____ mL/hr (circle either ↑ or ↓ or No change).

2. Patient weight = 77 kg. PTT = 26.
Bolus dose of heparin = _____ units; _____ mL.

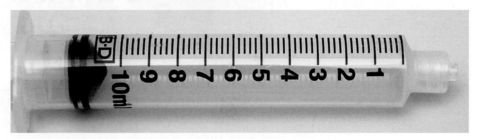

Initial intravenous infusion of heparin = _____ units/hr; _____ mL/hr.
Adjust the dose of heparin intravenous bolus based on PTT results: _____
units; _____ mL.
Adjust intravenous drip based on the PTT results: _____ units/hr;
_____ mL/hr (circle either ↑ or ↓ or No change).

3. Patient weight = 82 kg. PTT = 33.
Bolus dose of heparin = _____ units; _____ mL.
Initial intravenous infusion of heparin = _____ units/hr; _____
mL/hr.
Adjust the dose of heparin intravenous bolus based on PTT results: _____
units; _____ mL.
Adjust intravenous drip based on the PTT results: _____ units/hr;
_____ mL/hr (circle either ↑ or ↓ or No change).

4. Patient weight = 165 pounds. PTT = 34.
Bolus dose of heparin = _____ units; _____ mL.
Initial intravenous infusion of heparin = _____ units/hr; _____
mL/hr.

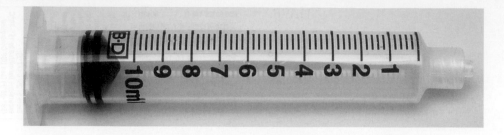

Adjust the dose of heparin intravenous bolus based on PTT results: _____ units; _____ mL.

Adjust intravenous drip based on the PTT results: _____ units/hr; _____ mL/hr (circle either ↑ or ↓ or No change).

5. Patient weight = 88 kg. PTT = 31.
   Bolus dose of heparin = _____ units; _____ mL.
   Initial intravenous infusion of heparin = _____ units/hr; _____ mL/hr.
   Adjust the dose of heparin intravenous bolus based on PTT results: _____ units; _____ mL.
   Adjust intravenous drip based on the PTT results: _____ units/hr; _____ mL/hr (circle either ↑ or ↓ or No change).

6. Patient weight = 96 kg. PTT = 42.
   Bolus dose of heparin = _____ units; _____ mL.

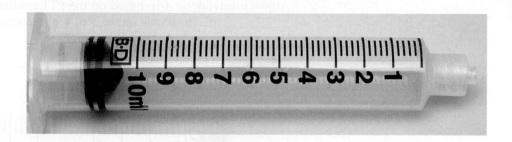

Initial intravenous infusion of heparin = _____ units/hr; _____ mL/hr.
Adjust the dose of heparin intravenous bolus based on PTT results: _____ units; _____ mL.

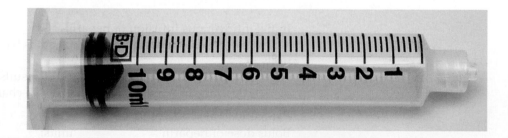

Adjust intravenous drip based on the PTT results: _____ units/hr; _____ mL/hr (circle either ↑ or ↓ or No change).

7. Patient weight = 72 kg. PTT = 79.
   Bolus dose of heparin = _____ units; _____ mL.
   Initial intravenous infusion of heparin = _____ units/hr; _____ mL/hr.
   Adjust the dose of heparin intravenous bolus based on PTT results: _____ units; _____ mL.
   Adjust intravenous drip based on the PTT results: _____ units/hr; _____ mL/hr (circle either ↑ or ↓ or No change).

8. Patient weight = 66 kg. PTT = 98.
   Bolus dose of heparin = _____ units; _____ mL.
   Initial intravenous infusion of heparin = _____ units/hr; _____ mL/hr.
   Adjust the dose of heparin intravenous bolus based on PTT results: _____
   units; _____ mL.
   Adjust intravenous drip based on the PTT results: _____ units/hr;
   _____ mL/hr (circle either ↑ or ↓ or No change).

9. Patient weight = 169.4 pounds. PTT = 88.
   Bolus dose of heparin = _____ units; _____ mL.
   Initial intravenous infusion of heparin = _____ units/hr; _____ mL/hr.
   Adjust the dose of heparin intravenous bolus based on PTT results: _____
   units; _____ mL.
   Adjust intravenous drip based on the PTT results: _____ units/hr;
   _____ mL/hr (circle either ↑ or ↓ or No change).

10. Patient weight = 82 kg. PTT = 93.
    Bolus dose of heparin = _____ units; _____ mL.
    Initial intravenous infusion of heparin = _____ units/hr; _____ mL/hr.
    Adjust the dose of heparin intravenous bolus based on PTT results: _____
    units; _____ mL.
    Adjust intravenous drip based on the PTT results: _____ units/hr;
    _____ mL/hr (circle either ↑ or ↓ or No change).

(Answers on pp. 470–472)

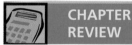

**CHAPTER
REVIEW**

Determine amount of heparin in units/hr or mL/hr as needed.

1. Heparin 400 units/hr from a solution of 25,000 units of heparin in 250 mL of
   D_5W.

2. Heparin 600 units/hr from a solution of 25,000 units of heparin in 250 mL of
   NS.

3. Heparin 550 units/hr from a solution of 50,000 units of heparin in 250 mL of
   D_5W.

4. Heparin 400 units/hr from a solution of 50,000 units of heparin in 250 mL of
   NS.

5. Heparin 600 units/hr from a solution of 25,000 units of heparin in 500 mL of
   NS.

6. Heparin 1200 units/hr from a solution of 50,000 units of heparin in 500 mL of
   D_5W.

7. Heparin 1100 units/hr from a solution of 25,000 units of heparin in 250 mL of
   D_5W.

8. Heparin 500 units/hr from a solution of 25,000 units of heparin in 250 mL of
   NS.

9. Heparin 1500 units/hr from a solution of 25,000 units of heparin in 250 mL of
   D_5W.

10. Heparin 1000 units/hr from a solution of 50,000 units of heparin in 500 mL of
    NS.

11. Infuse heparin at 20 mL/hr in 250 mL of NS with 25,000 units of heparin.

12. Infuse heparin at 10 mL/hr in 250 mL of D_5W with 25,000 units of heparin.

13. Infuse heparin at 17 mL/hr in 1000 mL of D$_5$W with 50,000 units of heparin.

14. Infuse heparin at 22 mL/hr in 500 mL of D$_5$W with 25,000 units of heparin.

15. Infuse heparin at 35 mL/hr in 1000 mL of D$_5$W with 50,000 units of heparin.

16. Infuse heparin at 24 mL/hr in 500 mL of D$_5$W with 50,000 units of heparin.

17. Infuse heparin at 34 mL/hr in 250 mL of NS with 25,000 units of heparin.

18. Infuse heparin at 12 mL/hr in 250 mL of D$_5$W with 50,000 units of heparin.

19. Infuse heparin at 7 mL/hr in 250 mL of NS with 25,000 units of heparin.

20. Infuse heparin at 24 mL/hr in 250 mL of D$_5$W with 25,000 units of heparin.

Determine the bolus dose of heparin (in units) and the initial intravenous infusion of heparin, and then adjust the dose of heparin intravenous bolus (units) and intravenous drip (units/hour) up or down based on the PTT results using the weight-based heparin protocol that follows. Mark the syringes (where provided). Use the heparin sodium supplied by the pharmacy.

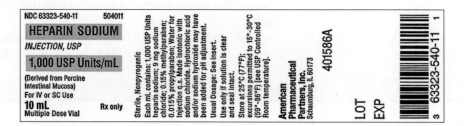

Bolus heparin at 80 units/kg.
Begin intravenous infusion of heparin at 18 units/kg/hr using 25,000 units heparin in 500 mL D$_5$W for 50 units/mL.
PTT <35 seconds. Give 80 units/kg bolus and increase drip 4 units/kg/hr.
PTT 35-45 seconds. Give 40 units/kg bolus and increase drip 2 units/kg/hr.
PTT 46-70 seconds. No change.
PTT 71-90 seconds. Reduce drip 2 units/kg/hr.
PTT >90 seconds. Hold heparin drip for 1 hour, and then reduce drip 3 units/kg/hr.

21. Patient weight = 64 kg. PTT = 31.
    Bolus dose of heparin = _____ units; _____ mL.

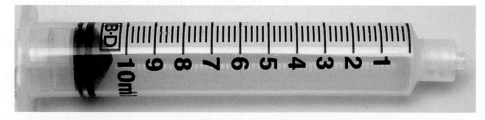

Initial intravenous infusion of heparin = _____ units/hr; _____ mL/hr.
Adjust the dose of heparin intravenous bolus based on PTT results: _____ units.
Adjust intravenous drip based on the PTT results: _____ units/hr (circle either ↑ or ↓ or No change).

22. Patient weight = 159.5 pounds. PTT = 58.
    Bolus dose of heparin = _____ units; _____ mL.

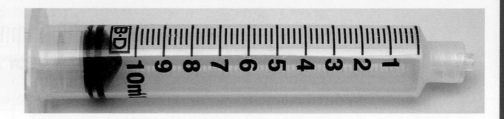

Initial intravenous infusion of heparin = _____ units/hr; _____ mL/hr.
Adjust the dose of heparin intravenous bolus based on PTT results:
_____ units.
Adjust intravenous drip based on the PTT results: _____ units/hr
(circle either ↑ or ↓ or No change).

23. Patient weight = 83 kg. PTT = 80.
     Bolus dose of heparin = _____ units; _____ mL.
     Initial intravenous infusion of heparin = _____ units/hr; _____ mL/hr.
     Adjust the dose of heparin intravenous bolus based on PTT results:
     _____ units.
     Adjust intravenous drip based on the PTT results: _____ units/hr
     (circle either ↑ or ↓ or No change).

24. Patient weight = 91 kg. PTT = 74.
     Bolus dose of heparin = _____ units; _____ mL.
     Initial intravenous infusion of heparin = _____ units/hr; _____ mL/hr.
     Adjust the dose of heparin intravenous bolus based on PTT results:
     _____ units.
     Adjust intravenous drip based on the PTT results: _____ units/hr
     (circle either ↑ or ↓ or No change).

25. Patient weight = 68 kg. PTT = 98.
     Bolus dose of heparin = _____ units; _____ mL.
     Initial intravenous infusion of heparin = _____ units/hr; _____ mL/hr.
     Adjust the dose of heparin intravenous bolus based on PTT results:
     _____ units.
     Adjust intravenous drip based on the PTT results: _____ units/hr
     (circle either ↑ or ↓ or No change).

26. Patient weight = 71 kg. PTT = 64.
     Bolus dose of heparin = _____ units; _____ mL.
     Initial intravenous infusion of heparin = _____ units/hr; _____ mL/hr.
     Adjust the dose of heparin intravenous bolus based on PTT results:
     _____ units.
     Adjust intravenous drip based on the PTT results: _____ units/hr
     (circle either ↑ or ↓ or No change).

27. Patient weight = 165 pounds. PTT = 76.
     Bolus dose of heparin = _____ units; _____ mL.

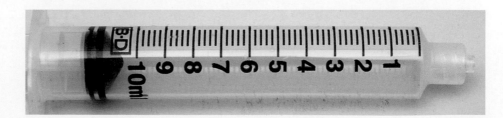

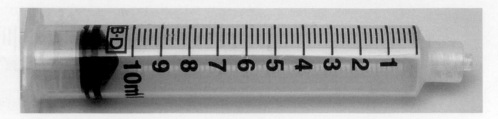

Initial intravenous infusion of heparin = _____ units/hr; _____ mL/hr.
Adjust the dose of heparin intravenous bolus based on PTT results:
_____ units.
Adjust intravenous drip based on the PTT results: _____ units/hr
(circle either ↑ or ↓ or No change).

28. Patient weight = 81 kg. PTT = 41.
    Bolus dose of heparin = _____ units; _____ mL.
    Initial intravenous infusion of heparin = _____ units/hr; _____ mL/hr.
    Adjust the dose of heparin intravenous bolus based on PTT results:
    _____ units.
    Adjust intravenous drip based on the PTT results: _____ units/hr
    (circle either ↑ or ↓ or No change).

29. Patient weight = 84 kg. PTT = 17.
    Bolus dose of heparin = _____ units; _____ mL.
    Initial intravenous infusion of heparin = _____ units/hr; _____ mL/hr.
    Adjust the dose of heparin intravenous bolus based on PTT results:
    _____ units.
    Adjust intravenous drip based on the PTT results: _____ units/hr
    (circle either ↑ or ↓ or No change).

30. Patient weight = 79 kg. PTT = 74.
    Bolus dose of heparin = _____ units; _____ mL.
    Initial intravenous infusion of heparin = _____ units/hr; _____ mL/hr.
    Adjust the dose of heparin intravenous bolus based on PTT results:
    _____ units.
    Adjust intravenous drip based on the PTT results: _____ units/hr
    (circle either ↑ or ↓ or No change).

(Answers on pp. 472–474)

evolve For additional practice problems, refer to the Advanced Calculations
section of the Drug Calculations Companion, version 4 on Evolve.

Insulin

Kathy Wren and Timothy Wren

CLINICAL CONNECTION

- Drawing up insulin correctly is critical to safely administering insulin.
- Understanding how to correctly calculate the doses ordered for bolus doses of insulin based upon the carbohydrate intake and the blood glucose level is necessary to correctly administer insulin to patients using an insulin pump.

HUMAN ERROR *Alert*

Every insulin dose needs to be assessed by another licensed professional before the medication is administered.

INTRODUCTION

Insulin comes in different forms and may be administered several ways. Depending on the form, it may be given via subcutaneous injections, via the intravenous route, or continuously through an insulin pump. Experimental administration routes include nasal sprays or inhalation. This chapter will address total subcutaneous insulin doses and insulin calculations based on blood glucose and food intake.

INSULIN TYPES

Insulin comes in many types of preparations that vary according to onset, peak, and duration of action. They are divided into four types of insulin: rapid or short-acting (lispro, aspart, glulisine, regular), intermediate-acting (NPH and lente), long-acting (ultralente, lantus, glargine, detemir), and mixtures (NPH 70/regular 30, 75% Lispro Protamine/25% Lispro, 70% Aspart protamine/30% Aspart). Table 17-1 lists most common types of insulin preparations and their associated time of onset, peak, and expected duration of action.

It is important to be able to read and understand the different parts of an insulin vial label. In addition to the items discussed in Chapter 12, insulin labels include a letter(s) after the trade name that represents the type of insulin and the origin of the insulin (Figure 17-1).

Insulin is packaged in two ways: vials containing 10 mL of solution with 100 units of insulin/mL and prepackaged syringes that contain smaller amounts of insulin. In the United States, insulin is usually standardized to 100 units/mL.

Insulin vials can combine NPH and regular insulin in one solution. The most common is 70/30, but 50/50 is also available (Figure 17-2).

PREPARING INSULIN INJECTIONS

Insulin syringes are available in 100-unit syringes, 50-unit syringes, and 30-unit syringes (low dose) (Figure 17-3).

The size of the dose to be given will determine the size of the syringe. For example, if you need to administer 17 units of regular insulin and 15 units of NPH, you would need a 50-unit syringe. Likewise, if you needed to administer only 8 units of lispro, it would be easier to use a 30-unit syringe. You may use a 100-unit syringe for smaller doses of insulin, but you must be very careful with the smaller increments

Table 17-1	Types of Insulin		
Type/Route of Administration	**Onset**	**Peak**	**Duration**
Lispro (Humalog) (subcut)	15-30 min	30-60 min	3-4 hr
Aspart (NovoLog) (subcut)	10-20 min	30-60 min	3-4 hr
Glulisine (Apidra) (subcut)	20-30 min	30-90 min	1-2.5 hr
Regular (subcut)	0.5-1 hr	2-4 hr	5-7 hr
Regular (IV)	10-30 min	15-30 min	30-60 min
Velosulin (external insulin pump)	0.5-1 hr	2-3 hr	2-3 hr
NPH (subcut)	1-4 hr	6-12 hr	18-24 hr
Lente (subcut)	1-2 hr	8-12 hr	18-28 hr
Ultralente (subcut)	4-6 hr	16-24 hr	36 hr
Lantus (subcut)	1.5 hr	Maintains constant	Up to 24 hr
Insulin glargine (subcut)	2-5 hr	Maintains constant	Up to 24 hr
Insulin determir (subcut)	1-3 hr	2-12 hrs, Maintains more of a constant	Up to 24 hr
NPH 70/regular 30 (subcut)	30 min	4-8 hr	Up to 24 hr
75% Lispro protamine/25% Lispro (subcut)	30 min	0.5-25 hr	16-20 hr
70% Aspart protamine/30% Aspart (subcut)	10-20 min	1-4 hr	Up to 24 hr

IV, Intravenous; *subcut*, subcutaneous; *h*, hour; *min*, minute.

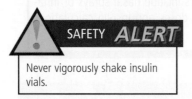

SAFETY ALERT

Never vigorously shake insulin vials.

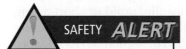

SAFETY ALERT

Always gently roll the insulin vials before drawing up the insulin dose to disperse the insulin throughout the solution. Insulin particles may adhere to the sides and bottom of the vial or may settle to the bottom of the vial, resulting in an inaccurate dose if not rotated. Check vial bottom before drawing up insulin to make sure the insulin has been mixed thoroughly.

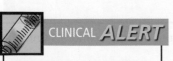

CLINICAL ALERT

One exception to long-acting insulins being cloudy is Lantus, which is clear. It should not be mixed with other insulin preparations.

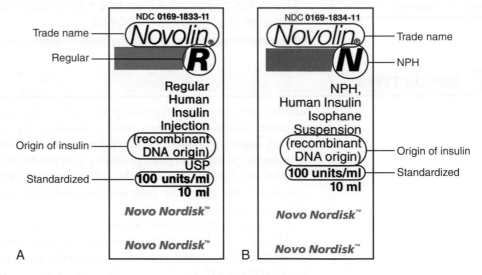

Figure 17-1 A, Novolin R insulin. **B,** Novolin N insulin.

on the syringe barrel as you draw up the insulin. It is always best to use the smallest syringe available when drawing up insulin. A smaller syringe will make it easier to see the unit markings on the syringe.

To successfully remove insulin from a vial, you must first inject the same quantity of air as the prescribed insulin volume (in each bottle if drawing up two types) before withdrawing the appropriate insulin quantity. This will prevent the creation of a vacuum in the vial after multiple doses have been removed. If two types of insulin are ordered to be given, some insulins may be combined in one syringe to allow for one injection. When mixing insulins, the nurse draws up the shorter-acting insulin first. For instance, if regular and NPH insulins have been ordered, the regular (or short-acting) insulin should be drawn up first. Another way to remember this sequence is to do "clear before cloudy." Short-acting insulin, such as regular or lispro, is clear whereas longer-acting types (NPH, lente) are cloudy suspensions.

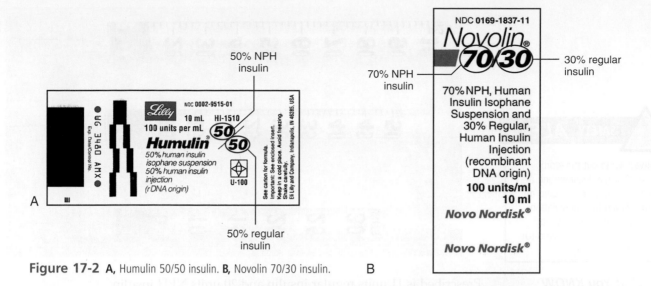

Figure 17-2 **A,** Humulin 50/50 insulin. **B,** Novolin 70/30 insulin.

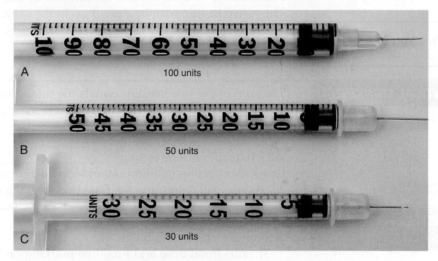

Figure 17-3 Insulin syringes. **A,** 100 units. **B,** 50 units. **C,** 30 units.

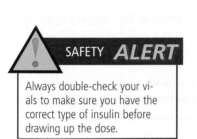

SAFETY ALERT

Always double-check your vials to make sure you have the correct type of insulin before drawing up the dose.

Example 1

PRESCRIPTION *11 units regular and 20 units NPH subcutaneous every* AM.

• *What You HAVE*

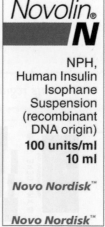

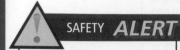

SAFETY ALERT

Always write out the word "units" when documenting a verbal order or transcribing an order. Using the abbreviation "U" to symbolize units may be misinterpreted as a zero (0) when handwritten.

- **What You KNOW**

  Prescribed is 11 units regular insulin and 20 units NPH insulin.
  These two insulins can be drawn up in the same syringe.

- **What You WANT**

  Total amount of insulin to be given.
  Size of syringe to be used.

CRITICAL THINKING

The sum of the two insulins equals the total dose.
Compare the total dose to the available syringes and choose the appropriate syringe.
Which insulin is short-acting? _____
Which insulin is long-acting? _____
Draw short-acting insulin first and long-acting insulin second.
Total dose will determine the final line marking on the syringe.

ANSWER FOR BEST CARE

    11 units short-acting regular
+ 20 units long-acting NPH
    31 units (total dose and final line marking on the syringe)

At least a 50-unit syringe will be required.

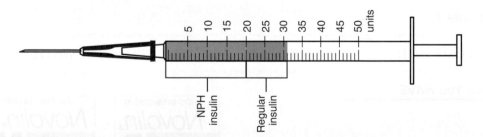

Example 2

PRESCRIPTION   *10 units regular and 36 units NPH subcutaneous every AM.*

- **What You HAVE**

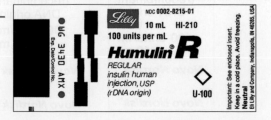

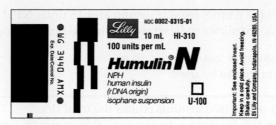

- *What You KNOW*

Prescribed is 10 units regular insulin and 36 units NPH insulin.
These two insulins can be drawn up in the same syringe.

- *What You WANT*

Total amount of insulin to be given.
Size of syringe to be used.

CRITICAL THINKING

The sum of the two insulins equals the total dose.
Compare the total dose to the available syringes and choose the appropriate syringe.
Which insulin is short-acting? _____
Which insulin is long-acting? _____
Draw short-acting insulin first and long-acting insulin second.
Total dose will determine the final line marking on the syringe.

ANSWER FOR BEST CARE

   10 units short-acting regular
+ 36 units long-acting NPH
   46 units (total dose and final line marking on the syringe)

At least a 50-unit syringe is required.

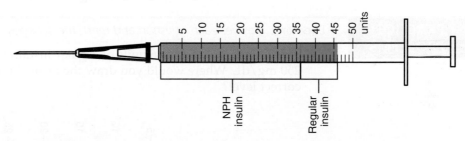

Example 3

PRESCRIPTION

8 units regular and 15 units NPH subcutaneous every AM.

- *What You HAVE*

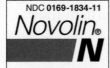

- *What You KNOW*

  Prescribed is 8 units regular insulin and 15 units NPH insulin.
  These two insulins can be drawn up in the same syringe.

- *What You WANT*

  Total amount of insulin to be given.
  Size of syringe to be used.

CRITICAL THINKING

The sum of the two insulins equals the total dose.
Compare the total dose to the available syringes and choose the appropriate syringe.
Which insulin is short-acting?_____
Which insulin is long-acting?_____
Draw short-acting insulin first and long-acting insulin second.
Total dose will determine the final line marking on the syringe.

ANSWER FOR BEST CARE

  8 units short-acting regular
+ 15 units long-acting NPH
  23 units (total dose and final line marking on the syringe)

At least a 30-unit syringe will be required.

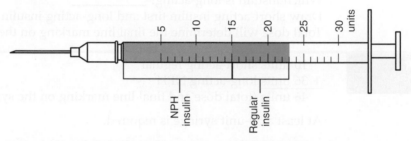

 PRACTICE PROBLEMS

Directions: *Answer each question and mark the syringes.*

1. The patient is to receive 6 units of regular insulin for a blood glucose level of 250 mg/dL. Where would you draw the arrow on the figure to represent the correct level?

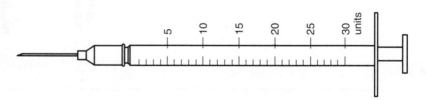

2. The patient is to receive 7 units of regular insulin and 13 units of NPH. Draw two arrows next to the syringe to indicate where the first insulin would be drawn up to and the total insulin dose arrow.

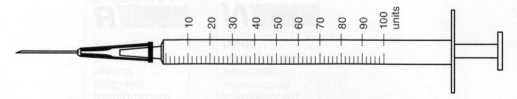

Indicate which insulin should be drawn up first.

3. What is the dose of regular insulin if you have a total dose of 65 units, with 42 units being NPH? Mark the syringe for both insulins.

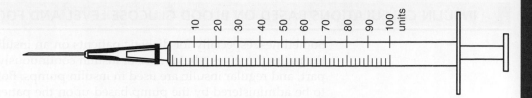

4. If you have a total dose of 47 units and you know 35 units are NPH, what is the dose of the regular insulin? _____

5. If you have a total dose of 65 units and you know 30 units are regular, what is the dose of the other insulin? _____

6. What size of insulin syringe would be the ideal to give the dose of 7 units of regular insulin? (a) 100-unit syringe, (b) 50-unit syringe, (c) 30-unit syringe. _____

7. The patient is to receive 20 units of regular insulin and 30 units of NPH. Draw two arrows next to the syringe to indicate where the first insulin would be drawn up to and the total insulin dose arrow. Also indicate which insulin should be drawn up first.

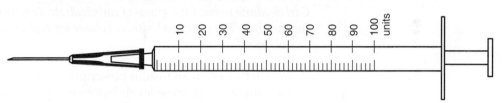

8. What size of syringe is needed to administer 18 units of regular insulin and 46 units of NPH? _____

9. The patient is to receive 28 units of regular insulin and 50 units of NPH. Draw two arrows next to the syringe to indicate where the first insulin would be drawn up to and the total insulin dose arrow. Also indicate which insulin should be drawn up first.

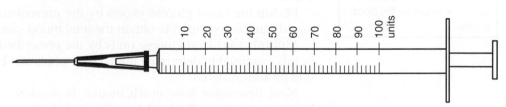

10. The patient is to receive 5 units of regular insulin and 11 units of NPH. Draw two arrows next to the syringe to indicate where the first insulin would be drawn up to and the total insulin dose arrow. Also indicate which insulin should be drawn up first.

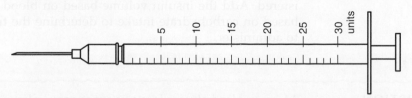

(Answers on pp. 474–475)

INSULIN CALCULATIONS BASED ON BLOOD GLUCOSE LEVEL AND FOOD INTAKE

Sometimes, especially for diabetic patients on an insulin pump and "tight" control, the patient receives a basal dose of insulin continuously through a pump. Lispro, aspart, and regular insulin are used in insulin pumps. Bolus doses of insulin will need to be administered by the pump based upon the patient's carbohydrate intake and the blood glucose level throughout the day. The physician will order a certain dose of insulin, based on the blood glucose level and the grams of carbohydrate that the patient eats, needed to bring the blood glucose level back to baseline (target blood glucose level). To use a prescription successfully and complete the required calculations, the following terms need to be understood.

Blood glucose target: Prescribed blood glucose level.
Blood glucose excess: The difference between the blood glucose target and the patient's blood glucose.
Blood glucose factor: The prescribed increment of blood glucose mg/dL used to determine insulin replacement volume.
Blood glucose units: Blood glucose excess divided by the blood glucose factor.
Carbohydrate factor: The prescribed increment of carbohydrate grams used to determine insulin replacement volume.
Carbohydrate units: Total grams of carbohydrate divided by the carbohydrate factor.
Insulin/unit: The prescribed insulin volume for replacement for the blood glucose units and carbohydrate units.

Now let's look at an insulin prescription for this type of administration:

Measure blood glucose levels before every meal and at bedtime. If the blood glucose is above 150 mg/dL (blood glucose target), administer 1 unit of insulin (insulin/unit) for every 30 mg/dL (blood glucose factor) increase in the blood glucose above 150. Administer 1 unit of insulin (insulin/unit) for every 15 grams of carbohydrate (carbohydrate factor) that is consumed.

To complete the calculations, first determine how much insulin will be required based on the blood glucose results. Subtract the target blood glucose (150 mg/dL in this example) from the patient's blood glucose to identify the blood glucose excess.

Divide the blood glucose excess by the prescribed blood glucose factor (each 30 mg/dL in this example) to obtain the total blood glucose units.

Multiply the blood glucose units by the prescribed insulin/unit (1 unit of insulin in this example) to determine the volume of insulin based on the blood glucose that will be administered.

Next determine how much insulin is needed to cover the amount of carbohydrates required. First, add up the carbohydrate content of all the foods. Then divide the total carbohydrate content of the food by the prescribed carbohydrate factor (15 grams in this example) to determine the carbohydrate units. Multiply the carbohydrate units by the prescribed insulin/unit (1 unit in this example) to determine the volume of insulin based on carbohydrate intake that will be administered. Add the insulin volume based on blood glucose and the insulin volume based on carbohydrate intake to determine the **total** amount of insulin you need to administer.

CLINICAL ALERT

If the patient's blood glucose is lower than the target blood glucose, you will not need to administer insulin for the blood glucose.

Example 1

PRESCRIPTION

Measure blood glucose levels before every meal and at bedtime. If the blood glucose is above 150 mg/dL, administer 1 unit of regular insulin for every 30 mg/dL increase in the blood glucose above 150. Administer 1 unit of regular insulin for every 15 grams of carbohydrate that is consumed.

• *What You HAVE*

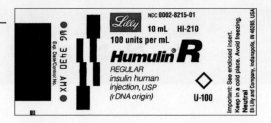

• *What You KNOW*

The patient's blood glucose is 270 mg/dL.
Breakfast was 1 bowl of cereal, 8 oz of milk, and a piece of toast.
Carbohydrate intake is as follows:

Item	Carbohydrate Content
Cereal	32 grams
8 oz milk	12 grams
1 piece toast	15 grams

Target blood glucose is 150 mg/dL.
Blood glucose unit is 30 mg/dL.
Carbohydrate unit is 15 grams.
Amount of insulin units required for each increased blood glucose unit is 1 unit of regular insulin.
Amount of insulin units required for each carbohydrate unit is 1 unit of regular insulin.

• *What You WANT*

The amount of insulin coverage based on blood glucose.
The amount of insulin coverage based on carbohydrate intake.
The total amount of insulin to be administered.

CRITICAL THINKING

What is the target blood glucose level? _____
What is the blood glucose factor? _____
What is the patient's blood glucose? _____
Subtract target blood glucose from patient's blood glucose.
Divide this answer by the blood glucose factor to determine blood glucose units.
Multiply blood glucose units by required insulin/unit.
What is the carbohydrate factor? _____
Add carbohydrate intake.
Divide total carbohydrate intake by carbohydrate factor to determine carbohydrate units.
Multiply carbohydrate units by required insulin/unit.
Add the insulin volume based on blood glucose and the insulin volume based on carbohydrate intake to determine the total amount of insulin.

ANSWER FOR BEST CARE

Target blood glucose level? 150 mg/dL.
Blood glucose factor? 30 mg/dL.
Patient's blood glucose? 270 mg/dL.
Carbohydrate factor? 15 grams.
Blood glucose calculation:

270 mg/dL − 150 mg/dL = 120
120 ÷ 30 = 4
4 × 1 unit = 4 units of regular insulin

Carbohydrate calculation:

32 g + 12 g + 15 g = 59 total grams of carbohydrate intake
59 ÷ 15 = 3.9; round to the nearest whole number
4 × 1 unit = 4 units

Total volume of insulin to be administered:

4 + 4 = 8 units of regular insulin

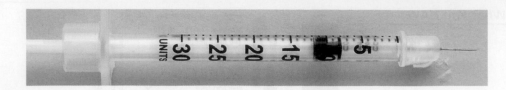

Example 2

PRESCRIPTION

Measure blood glucose levels before every meal and at bedtime. If the blood glucose is above 130 mg/dL, administer 1 unit of regular insulin for every 40 mg/dL increase in the blood glucose above 130. At mealtimes, administer 1 unit of regular insulin for every 8 grams of carbohydrate that is consumed.

- **What You HAVE**

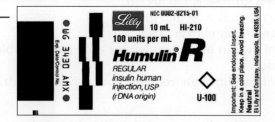

- **What You KNOW**

The patient's blood glucose is 128 mg/dL.
Breakfast was 1 muffin, 8 oz of milk, and half a banana.
Carbohydrate intake is as follows:

Item	Carbohydrate Content
Muffin	45 grams
8 oz milk	12 grams
½ banana	15 grams

Carbohydrate intake is the sum of the carbohydrate content for all foods eaten.
Target blood glucose is 130 mg/dL.
Blood glucose factor is 40 mg/dL.
Carbohydrate factor is 8 grams.
Amount of insulin required for each blood glucose unit is 1 unit.
Amount of insulin required for each carbohydrate unit is 1 unit.

- **What You WANT**

The amount of insulin based on blood glucose measurement.
The amount of insulin based on carbohydrate intake.
The total amount of insulin to be administered.

CRITICAL THINKING

What is the target blood glucose level? _____
What is the blood glucose factor? _____
What is the patient's blood glucose? _____
Subtract target blood glucose from patient's blood glucose.
Divide this answer by the blood glucose factor to determine blood glucose units.
Multiply blood glucose units by required insulin/unit.
What is the carbohydrate factor? _____
Add carbohydrate intake.
Divide total carbohydrate intake by carbohydrate factor to determine carbohydrate units.
Multiply carbohydrate units by required insulin/unit.
Add the insulin volume based on blood glucose and the insulin volume based on carbohydrate intake to determine the total amount of insulin.

ANSWER FOR BEST CARE	Target blood glucose level? 130 mg/dL.

Blood glucose factor? 40 mg/dL.

Patient's blood glucose? 128 mg/dL.

Carbohydrate factor? 8 grams.

Blood glucose calculation:

Because the patient's blood glucose (128 mg/dL) is below the target blood glucose (130 mg/dL), no insulin is required for blood glucose coverage.

Carbohydrate calculation:

45 g + 12 g + 15 g = 72 total grams of carbohydrate intake

72 ÷ 8 = 9 carbohydrate units

9 × 1 unit = 9 units regular insulin

Total amount of insulin to be administered:

0 + 9 = 9 units regular insulin

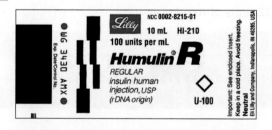

Example 3

PRESCRIPTION	*Measure blood glucose levels before every meal and at bedtime. If the blood glucose is above 130 mg/dL, administer 1 unit of regular insulin for every 30 mg/dL increase in the blood glucose above 130. At mealtimes, administer 1 unit of regular insulin for every 8 grams of carbohydrate that is consumed.*

• **What You HAVE**

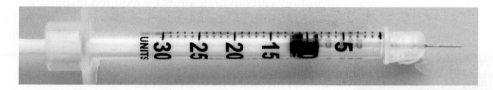

• **What You KNOW**

The patient's blood glucose is 155 mg/dL.

Lunch was 1 ground beef patty, 6 oz of french fries, 12 oz of diet soda, and ½ cup of baked beans.

Carbohydrate intake is as follows:

Item	Carbohydrate Content
Hamburger bun	20 grams
3 oz hamburger	0 grams
6 oz french fries	45 grams
½ cup baked beans	25 grams
12 oz diet soda	0 grams

Carbohydrate intake is the sum of the carbohydrate content for all foods eaten.

Target blood glucose level is 130 mg/dL.

Blood glucose factor is 30 mg/dL.

Carbohydrate factor is 8 grams.

Amount of insulin required for each blood glucose unit is 1 unit.

Amount of insulin required for each carbohydrate unit is 1 unit.

• **What You WANT**

The amount of insulin based on blood glucose measurement.
The amount of insulin based on carbohydrate intake.
The total amount of insulin to be administered.

CRITICAL THINKING

What is the target blood glucose level? _____
What is the blood glucose factor? _____
What is the patient's blood glucose? _____
Subtract target blood glucose from patient's blood glucose.
Divide this answer by the blood glucose factor to determine blood glucose units.
Multiply blood glucose units by required insulin/unit.
What is the carbohydrate factor? _____
Add carbohydrate intake.
Divide total carbohydrate intake by carbohydrate factor to determine carbohydrate
    units.
Multiply carbohydrate units by required insulin/unit.
Add the insulin volume based on blood glucose and the insulin volume based on
    carbohydrate intake to determine the total amount of insulin.

**ANSWER FOR
BEST CARE**

Target blood glucose level? 130 mg/dL.
Blood glucose factor? 30 mg/dL.
Patient's blood glucose level? 155 mg/dL.
Carbohydrate factor? 8 grams.
Blood glucose calculation:

155 mg/dL − 130 mg/dL = 25
25 ÷ 30 = 0.83; round to the nearest whole number.
1 × 1 unit of insulin = 1 unit of regular insulin

Carbohydrate calculation:

20 g + 0 g + 45 g + 25 g + 0 g = 90 total grams of carbohydrate intake
90 ÷ 8 = 11.25 (round to the nearest whole number)
11 × 1 unit = 11 units regular insulin

Total amount of insulin to be administered:

1 + 11 = 12 units of regular insulin

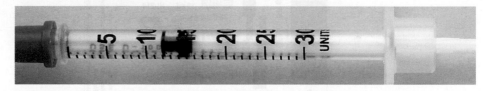

**PRACTICE
PROBLEMS**

Directions: *The following five practice problems use the following insulin orders and
are based on blood glucose readings taken throughout the day and carbohydrate intake. Mark the syringes.*

The patient is to receive insulin as follows:

Administer 0.8 units of insulin for every 15 grams of carbohydrate consumed. For
    a blood glucose reading > 150 mg/dL, administer 1 unit of insulin for every 30
    mg/dL increase in the blood glucose level above 150.

At lunch, your patient had a blood glucose level of 126 mg/dL and ate the following:

Item	Carbohydrate Content
1 apple	15 grams
8 oz milk	12 grams
3 oz ground beef patty	0 grams
1 hamburger bun	23 grams
4 oz french fries	25 grams

What is the target blood glucose level? _____

What is the blood glucose factor? _____

What is the patient's blood glucose? _____

How many units of insulin are to be administered based on glucose units? _____

What is the carbohydrate factor? _____

How many units of insulin are to be administered based on carbohydrate units? _____

1. How much insulin should you administer? _____

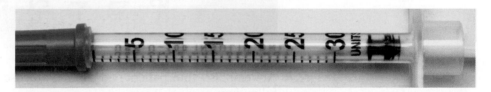

2. At supper, your patient had a blood glucose level of 175 mg/dL and ate 128 grams of carbohydrate. How much insulin should you administer? _____

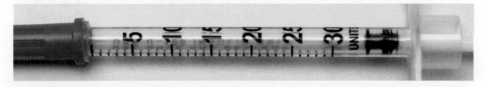

3. At bedtime, your patient's blood glucose level is 139 mg/dL. How much insulin should you administer? _____

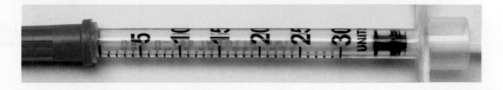

4. At breakfast, the patient's blood glucose level is 121 mg/dL. The patient is going to eat 98 grams of carbohydrate. How much insulin should you administer? _____

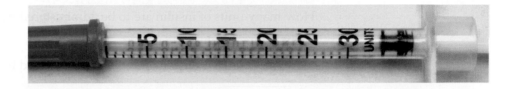

5. At lunch, the patient's blood glucose level is 248 mg/dL. The patient is going to eat 60 grams of carbohydrate. How much insulin should you administer?

_____

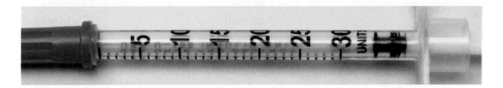

Directions: *Questions 6 through 8 use the following insulin prescriptions based on blood glucose readings taken throughout the day and carbohydrate intake. Mark the syringes.*

Your patient is to receive insulin as follows:

Administer 1 unit of insulin for every 8 grams of carbohydrate consumed. For a blood glucose reading >130 mg/dL, administer 1 unit of insulin for every 30 mg/dL increase in the blood glucose level above 130.

What is the target blood glucose level? _____

What is the blood glucose factor? _____

What is the patient's blood glucose? _____

How many units of insulin are to be administered based on glucose units? _____

What is the carbohydrate factor? _____

How many units of insulin are to be administered based on carbohydrate units? _____

6. At breakfast, your patient had a blood glucose level of 138 mg/dL and ate the following:

Item	Carbohydrate Content
1 apple	15 grams
8 oz milk	12 grams
1 bowl cereal	48 grams
1 piece toast	12 grams
3 strips bacon	0 grams

How much insulin should you administer? _____

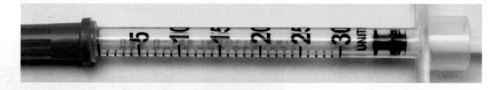

7. At breakfast, your patient had a blood glucose level of 126 mg/dl and ate the following:

Item	Carbohydrate Content
1 granola bar	26 grams
8 oz milk	12 grams
1 cheese sandwich	27 grams
2 oz potato chips	30 grams
Grapes	20 grams

How much insulin should you administer? _____

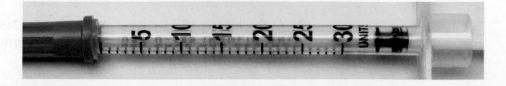

8. At lunch, the patient's blood glucose level is 149 mg/dL. The patient is going to eat 124 grams of carbohydrate. How much insulin should you administer?

_____

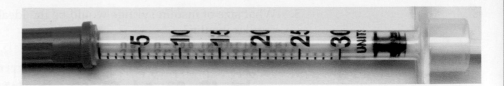

Directions: *Answer the following questions and mark the syringes.*

9. The patient is going to eat french fries (48 grams of carbohydrates) and is to take 1 unit of insulin for every 8 grams of carbohydrate consumed. How much insulin should the patient take to cover the french fries? _____

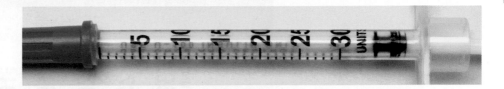

10. The patient's blood glucose is 198 mg/dL. The patient is to take 1 unit of insulin for every 25 mg/dL increase in blood glucose over 120 mg/dL. How much insulin should the patient take? _____

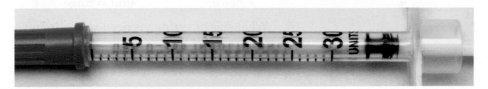

(Answers on pp. 475–476)

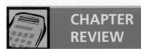 **CHAPTER REVIEW**

Write in the answer for each question and mark the syringes.

1. What would be the total dose for 8 units of regular insulin and 34 units of NPH?

_____ units of insulin

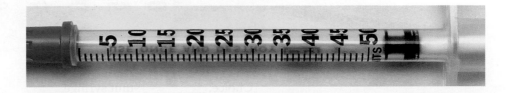

2. If you have a total dose of 62 units and you know that 28 units are regular, what is the dose of the other insulin?

_____ units of other insulin

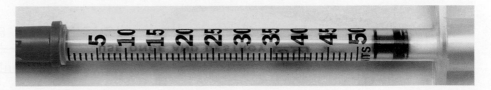

3.　What size of insulin syringe would be the ideal to give a dose of 14 units of regular insulin?

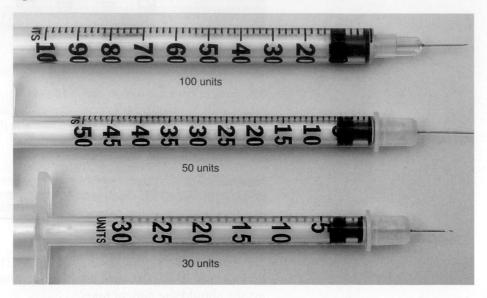

100 units

50 units

30 units

Choice: _____-unit syringe.

4.　What size of syringe is needed to administer 8 units of regular insulin and 46 units of NPH?

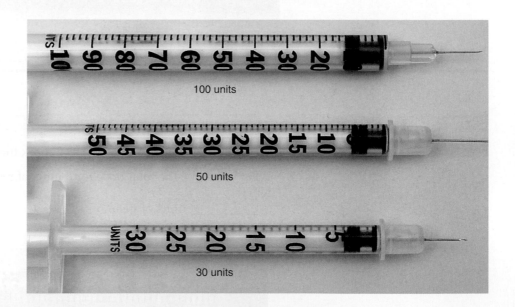

100 units

50 units

30 units

Choice: _____-unit syringe.

5.　The patient is to receive 24 units of regular insulin and 54 units of NPH. Draw two arrows next to the syringe to indicate where the first insulin would be drawn up to and the total insulin dose arrow. Also indicate which insulin should be drawn up first.

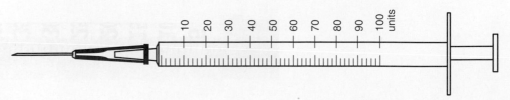

Questions 6 through 8 are based on the prescribed sliding insulin scale that follows. Mark the syringes.

> *<150 mg/dL.* Give 0 units of insulin.
> *150-200 mg/dL.* Give 4 units of regular insulin.
> *201-250 mg/dL.* Give 7 units of regular insulin.
> *251-300 mg/dL.* Give 10 units of regular insulin.
> *>300 mg/dL.* Give 13 units of regular insulin and contact physician on call.

6. The patient's blood glucose level before breakfast is 139 mg/dL. Draw an arrow on the following figure to indicate how much regular insulin you should give.

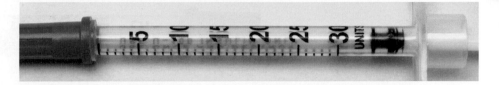

7. The patient's blood glucose level before lunch is 181 mg/dL. Draw an arrow on the following figure to indicate how much regular insulin you should give.

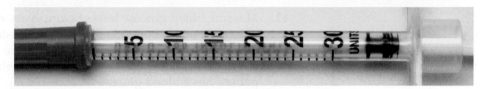

8. The patient's blood glucose level before supper is 314 mg/dL. Draw an arrow on the following figure to indicate how much regular insulin you should give. What should be another nursing intervention now?

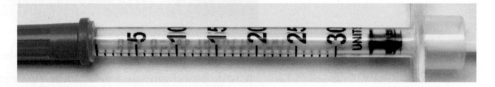

Problems 9 and 10 are based on the information that follows. Mark the syringes.

> Your patient is to receive insulin as follows:
> Administer 1 unit of insulin for every 8 grams of carbohydrate consumed.
> For a blood glucose reading >130 mg/dL, administer 1 unit of insulin for every 30 mg/dL increase in the blood glucose level above 130.

9. At breakfast, your patient had a blood glucose level of 135 mg/dL and ate the following:

Item	Carbohydrate Content
1 apple	15 grams
8 oz milk	12 grams
1 bowl cereal	48 grams
1 piece toast	12 grams
3 strips bacon	0 grams

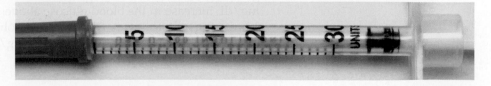

How much insulin should you administer? _____

10. At breakfast, your patient had a blood glucose level of 118 mg/dL and ate the following:

Item	Carbohydrate Content
1 granola bar	26 grams
8 oz milk	12 grams
1 cheese sandwich	27 grams
2 oz potato chips	30 grams
Grapes	20 grams

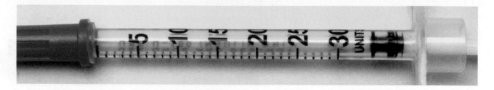

How much insulin should you administer? _____ units of insulin

For problems 11 through 20, answer the questions and mark the syringes.

11. Measure blood glucose levels before every meal and at bedtime. If the blood glucose level is above 130 mg/dL, administer 1 unit of insulin for every 30 mg/dL increase in the blood glucose above 130. At mealtimes, administer 1 unit of insulin for every 8 grams of carbohydrate that is consumed. Your patient has a blood glucose level of 124 mg/dL and ate 24 grams of carbohydrates.

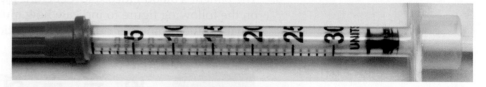

How much insulin should you administer? _____ units of insulin

12. Measure blood glucose levels before every meal and at bedtime. If the blood glucose level is above 130 mg/dL, administer 1 unit of insulin for every 30 mg/dL increase in the blood glucose above 130. At mealtimes, administer 1 unit of insulin for every 8 grams of carbohydrate that is consumed. Your patient has a blood glucose level of 166 mg/dL and ate 32 grams of carbohydrates.

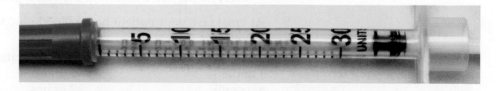

How much insulin should you administer? _____ units of insulin

13. Measure blood glucose levels before every meal and at bedtime. If the blood glucose level is above 130 mg/dL, administer 1 unit of insulin for every 30 mg/dL increase in the blood glucose above 130. At mealtimes, administer 1 unit of insulin for every 8 grams of carbohydrate that is consumed. Your patient has a blood glucose level of 140 mg/dL and ate 24 grams of carbohydrates.

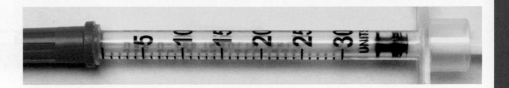

How much insulin should you administer? _____ units of insulin

14. Measure blood glucose levels before every meal and at bedtime. If the blood glucose level is above 130 mg/dL, administer 1 unit of insulin for every 30 mg/dL increase in the blood glucose above 130. At mealtimes, administer 1 unit of insulin for every 8 grams of carbohydrate that are consumed. Your patient has a blood glucose level of 242 mg/dL and ate 32 grams of carbohydrates.

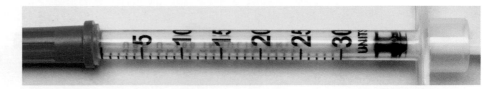

How much insulin should you administer? _____ units of insulin

15. Measure blood glucose levels before every meal and at bedtime. If the blood glucose reading is above 130 mg/dL, administer 1 unit of insulin for every 30 mg/dL increase in the blood glucose level above 130. Administer 1 unit of insulin for every 15 grams of carbohydrate that is consumed. Your patient has a blood glucose level of 194 mg/dL and ate 30 grams of carbohydrates.

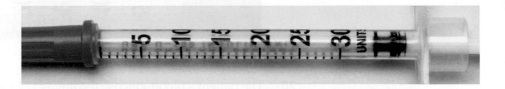

How much insulin should you administer? _____ units of insulin

16. Measure blood glucose levels before every meal and at bedtime. If the blood glucose reading is above 150 mg/dL, administer 1 unit of insulin for every 30 mg/dL increase in the blood glucose level above 150. Administer 1 unit of insulin for every 15 grams of carbohydrate that is consumed. Your patient has a blood glucose level of 128 mg/dL and ate 30 grams of carbohydrates.

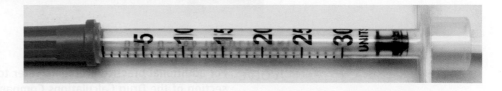

How much insulin should you administer? _____ units of insulin

17. Measure blood glucose levels before every meal and at bedtime. If the blood glucose reading is above 150 mg/dL, administer 1 unit of insulin for every 30 mg/dL increase in the blood glucose level above 150. Administer 1 unit of insulin for every 15 grams of carbohydrate that is consumed. Your patient has a blood glucose level of 198 mg/dL and ate 45 grams of carbohydrates.

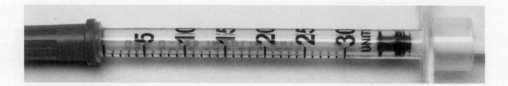

How much insulin should you administer? _____ units of insulin

18. Measure blood glucose levels before every meal and at bedtime. If the blood glucose reading is above 150 mg/dL, administer 1 unit of insulin for every 30 mg/dL increase in the blood glucose level above 150. Administer 1 unit of insulin for every 15 grams of carbohydrate that is consumed. Your patient has a blood glucose level of 210 mg/dL and ate 31 grams of carbohydrates.

How much insulin should you administer? _____ units of insulin

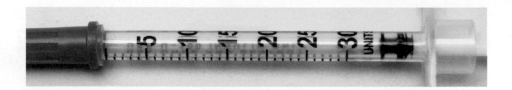

19. The patient is going to eat french fries (52 grams of carbohydrates) and is to take 1 unit of insulin for every 8 grams of carbohydrate consumed. How much insulin should the patient take to cover the french fries? _____ units of insulin

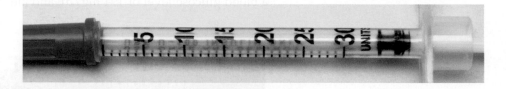

20. The patient's blood glucose reading is 174 mg/dL. The patient is to take 1 unit of insulin for every 25 mg/dL increase in blood glucose level over 120 mg/dL. How much insulin should the patient take? _____ units of insulin

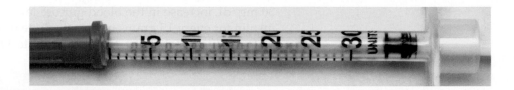

(Answers on p. 476)

⊖volve For additional practice problems, refer to the Intravenous Calculations section of the Drug Calculations Companion, version 4 on Evolve.

BIBLIOGRAPHY

Chernecky C, Berger B: Laboratory tests and diagnostic procedures, ed 5, Philadelphia, 2007, WB Saunders.
Deglin J, Vallerand A: Davis's drug guide for nurses, ed 11, Philadelphia, 2008, FA Davis, 520-523.
Hodgson B, Kizior R: Saunders nursing drug handbook 2010, Philadelphia, 2009, WB Saunders, 531-533.

Calculating Sliding-Scale Regular Insulin Dosages

Cynthia Chernecky, Kathy Wren, and Timothy Wren

CLINICAL CONNECTION

- Giving patients subcutaneous regular insulin based on a prescribed sliding scale offers excellent glucose control, which will aid in preventing or lessening damage from diabetes to the kidneys, circulation, and the heart.
- Mathematically determining sliding-scale regular insulin dosages based on the formula method is essential for quality diabetic patient care.

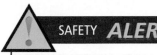

SAFETY ALERT

Not all insulin labels on the bottle of insulin say REGULAR or "R" on them, so be careful and ensure that you have the correct type of insulin.

INTRODUCTION

Patients often require subcutaneous regular insulin as coverage for blood glucose monitoring results, also called fingersticks, GLUMS, Accu-chek, BS, or blood sugars. At times, the physician or advanced practice nurse will prescribe insulin to be given on a "sliding-scale" schedule that is related to the current blood glucose level. Insulin prescriptions for this type of administration may take the following form:

Measure blood glucose levels before every meal and at bedtime. When rapid-acting insulin is given before bedtime, the blood glucose level must be checked in 2 hours.

SLIDING SCALE PRESCRIPTION

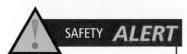

SAFETY ALERT

Insulin should ONLY be administered with an insulin syringe. The words "insulin" or "insulin syringe" are printed on each insulin syringe package.

The following three examples use the sliding scale and are based on blood glucose readings taken throughout the day. Administer insulin according to the following scale:

<150 mg/dL. Give 0 units of insulin.
150-200 mg/dL. Give 2 units of regular insulin.
201-250 mg/dL. Give 3 units of regular insulin.
251-300 mg/dL. Give 5 units of regular insulin.
>300 mg/dL. Give 6 units of regular insulin and contact physician immediately.

Example 1

The blood glucose level at 0730 (7:30 AM) is 268 mg/dL.

- **What You HAVE**

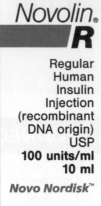

NDC 0169-1833-11
Novolin.
R
Regular
Human
Insulin
Injection
(recombinant
DNA origin)
USP
100 units/ml
10 ml
Novo Nordisk™

Novo Nordisk™

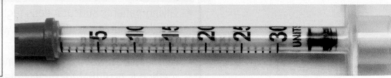

- **What You KNOW**

Give regular insulin based on the sliding scale.
Blood glucose level is 268 mg/dL.

- **What You WANT**

Amount of insulin to be administered.

CRITICAL THINKING

Compare the patient's blood glucose level with the prescribed sliding scale.

ANSWER FOR BEST CARE

251-300 mg/dL. Give 5 units of regular insulin.

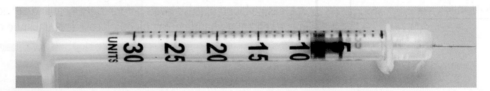

Example 2

Four hours later, at 1130 (11:30 AM), the blood glucose level is 126 mg/dL.

- **What You HAVE**

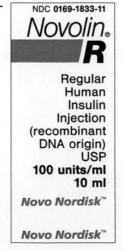

NDC 0169-1833-11
Novolin.
R
Regular
Human
Insulin
Injection
(recombinant
DNA origin)
USP
100 units/ml
10 ml
Novo Nordisk™

Novo Nordisk™

• **What You KNOW**   Give regular insulin based on the sliding scale.
Blood glucose level is 126 mg/dL.

• **What You WANT**   Amount of insulin to be administered.

CRITICAL THINKING   Compare the patient's blood glucose level with the prescribed sliding scale.

ANSWER FOR BEST CARE   <150 mg/dL. Give 0 units of insulin.
You do not administer any insulin.

Example 3

At 1730 (5:30 PM) the blood glucose level is 198 mg/dL.

• **What You HAVE**

NDC 0169-1833-11

Novolin.
R

Regular
Human
Insulin
Injection
(recombinant
DNA origin)
USP
100 units/ml
10 ml

Novo Nordisk™

Novo Nordisk™

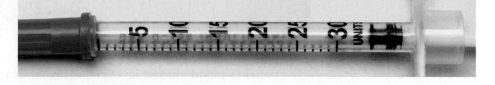

• **What You KNOW**   Give regular insulin based on the sliding scale.
Blood glucose level is 198 mg/dL.

• **What You WANT**   Amount of insulin to be administered.

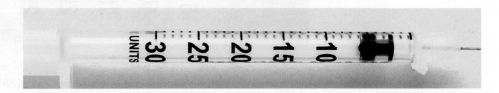

CRITICAL THINKING   Compare the patient's blood glucose level with the prescribed sliding scale.

ANSWER FOR BEST CARE   *150-200 mg/dL.* Give 2 units of regular insulin.

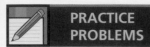

PRACTICE PROBLEMS

Your patient has the following sliding scale insulin prescription:

Measure blood glucose levels before every meal and at bedtime. When rapid-acting insulin is given before bedtime, the blood glucose level must be checked in 2 hours. Administer regular insulin based on the following blood glucose readings:

<150 mg/dL. Give 0 units of insulin.
150-200 mg/dL. Give 4 units of regular insulin.
201-250 mg/dL. Give 7 units of regular insulin.
251-300 mg/dL. Give 10 units of regular insulin.
>300 mg/dL. Give 13 units of regular insulin and contact physician immediately.

HAVE:

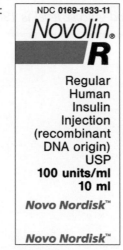

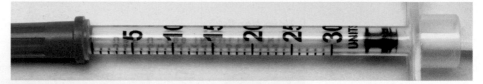

1. The patient's blood glucose level before breakfast is 128 mg/dL. Draw an arrow on the following figure to indicate how much regular insulin you should give.

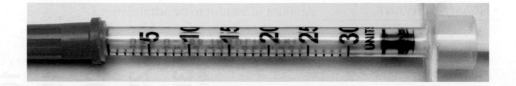

2. The patient's blood glucose level before lunch is 168 mg/dL. Draw an arrow on the following figure to indicate how much regular insulin you should give.

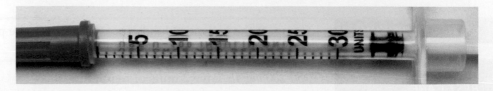

3. The patient's blood glucose level before supper is 306 mg/dL. Draw an arrow on the following figure to indicate how much regular insulin you should give.

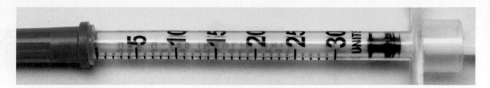

4. The patient's blood glucose level before bedtime is 238 mg/dL. Draw an arrow on the following figure to indicate how much regular insulin you should give.

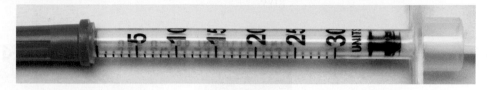

5. The patient's blood glucose level before breakfast is 162 mg/dL. Draw an arrow on the following figure to indicate how much regular insulin you should give.

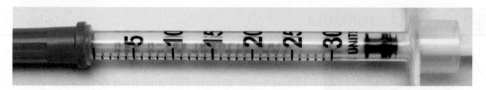

6. The patient's blood glucose level before breakfast is 152 mg/dL. Draw an arrow on the following figure to indicate how much regular insulin you should give.

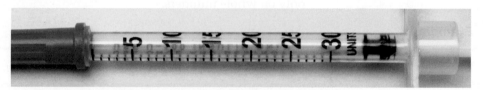

7. The patient's blood glucose level before lunch is 178 mg/dL. Draw an arrow on the following figure to indicate how much regular insulin you should give.

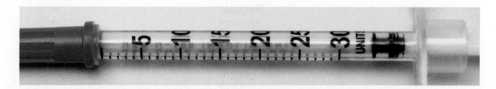

8. The patient's blood glucose level before supper is 122 mg/dL. Draw an arrow on the following figure to indicate how much regular insulin you should give.

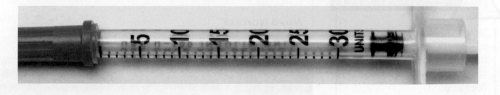

9. The patient's blood glucose level before bedtime is 150 mg/dL. Draw an arrow on the following figure to indicate how much regular insulin you should give.

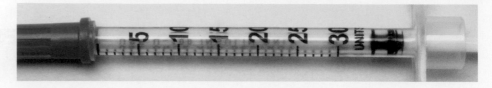

10. The patient's blood glucose level before breakfast is 121 mg/dL. Draw an arrow on the following figure to indicate how much regular insulin you should give.

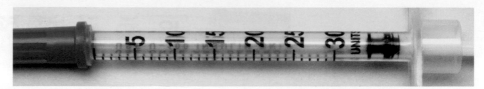

(Answers on p. 477)

UNIVERSAL FORMULA

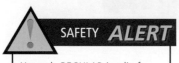

SAFETY **ALERT**

Use only REGULAR insulin for coverage or sliding-scale administration of insulin.

If a specific sliding scale is not provided, the following universal formula is used to determine total number of units of **regular** insulin to give the patient: Take patient's blood sugar minus 100, and then divide the difference by 30: (BS − 100)/30. Sliding scales are often used by patients who are known diabetics or by patients who have high blood glucose levels related to temporary conditions or as a result of medications. The answer when using the formula is always rounded to the nearest whole number because you can draw up the regular insulin in the insulin syringe based only on whole numbers.

Example 1

PRESCRIPTION *Cover blood sugar with sliding-scale regular insulin. BS is 340 mg/dL.*

• **What You HAVE**

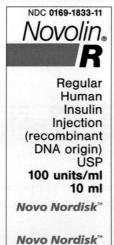

NDC **0169-1833-11**
Novolin.
R
Regular
Human
Insulin
Injection
(recombinant
DNA origin)
USP
100 units/ml
10 ml
Novo Nordisk™

Novo Nordisk™

SAFETY **ALERT**

More than 15 units of regular insulin for coverage is usually too much. If more coverage is needed, other interventions need to occur.

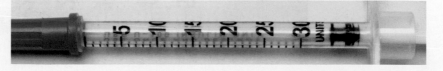

- *What You KNOW* — Patient's blood sugar is 340.

- *What You WANT* — Number of units of regular insulin to be administered.

CRITICAL THINKING — What is the patient's blood sugar? _____
Subtract 100 from the patient's blood sugar.
Divide the difference by 30.
Round your answer to the nearest whole number.

ANSWER FOR BEST CARE — Patient's blood sugar is 340.
340 − 100 = 240
240 ÷ 30 = 8 units of regular insulin

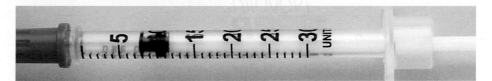

Example 2

PRESCRIPTION — *Cover blood sugar with sliding-scale regular insulin. BS is 260 mg/dL.*

- *What You HAVE* —

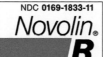

- *What You KNOW* — Patient's blood sugar is 260.

- *What You WANT* — Number of units of regular insulin to be administered.

CRITICAL THINKING — What is the patient's blood sugar? _____
Subtract 100 from the patient's blood sugar.
Divide the difference by 30.
Round your answer to the nearest whole number.

ANSWER FOR BEST CARE — Patient's blood sugar is 260.
260 − 100 = 160
160 ÷ 30 = 5.33 = 5 units of regular insulin

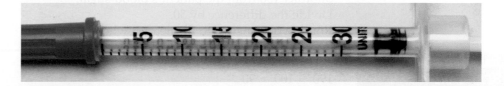

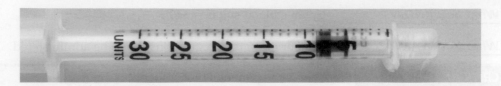

Example 3

PRESCRIPTION	*Cover blood sugar with sliding-scale regular insulin. BS is 190 mg/dL.*

• **What You HAVE**

NDC **0169-1833-11**

Novolin.
/R

Regular
Human
Insulin
Injection
(recombinant
DNA origin)
USP
100 units/ml
10 ml

Novo Nordisk™

Novo Nordisk™

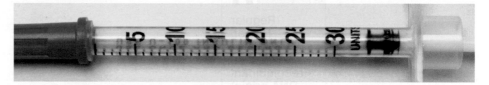

• **What You KNOW**   Patient's blood sugar is 190.

• **What You WANT**   Number of units of regular insulin to be administered.

CRITICAL THINKING	What is the patient's blood sugar? _____ Subtract 100 from the patient's blood sugar. Divide the difference by 30. Round your answer to the nearest whole number.

ANSWER FOR BEST CARE	Patient's blood sugar is 190. 190 − 100 = 90 90 ÷ 30 = 3 units of regular insulin

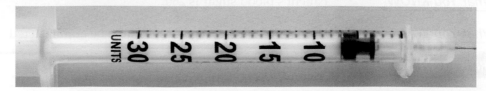

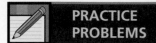

PRACTICE PROBLEMS

Directions: *Determine the number of units of regular insulin needed to cover the following blood sugar results using the universal coverage formula:*

$$\frac{Blood\ sugar\ -\ 100}{30}$$

Round your answer to the nearest whole number. Mark the syringes.

1. Blood sugar = 160 mg/dL.

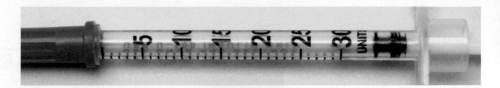

2. Blood sugar = 223 mg/dL.

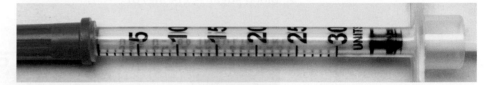

3. Blood sugar = 302 mg/dL.

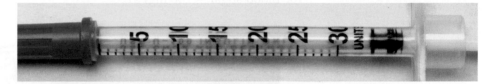

4. Blood sugar = 254 mg/dL.

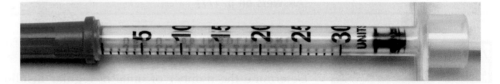

5. Blood sugar = 273 mg/dL.

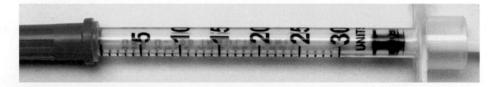

6. Blood sugar = 494 mg/dL.

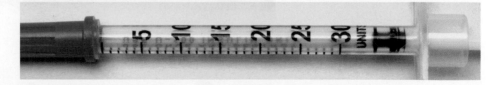

7. Blood sugar = 184 mg/dL.

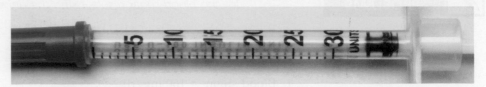

8. Blood sugar = 389 mg/dL.

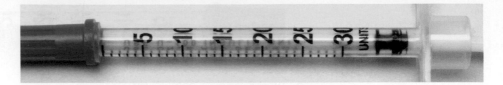

9. Blood sugar = 214 mg/dL.

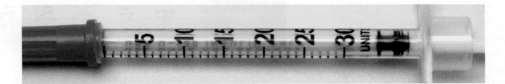

10. Blood sugar = 246 mg/dL.

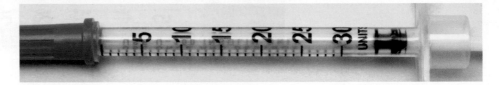

(Answers on p. 477)

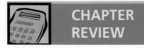

CHAPTER REVIEW

Determine the number of units of regular insulin needed to cover the following blood sugar results:

$$\frac{\text{Blood sugar} - 100}{30}$$

Round your answer to the nearest whole number. Mark the syringes.

1. Blood sugar = 138 mg/dL.

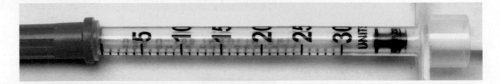

2. Blood sugar = 192 mg/dL.

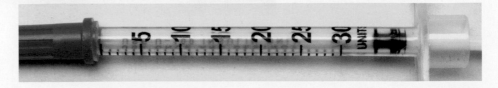

3. Blood sugar = 104 mg/dL.

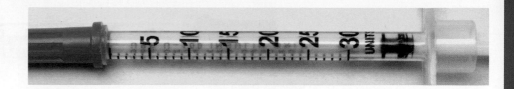

4. Blood sugar = 186 mg/dL.

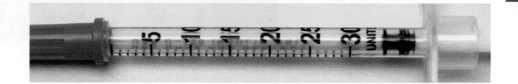

5. Blood sugar = 246 mg/dL.

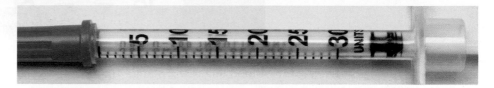

6. Blood sugar = 159 mg/dL.

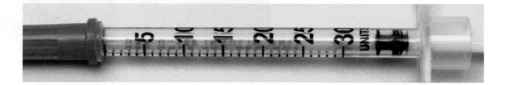

7. Blood sugar = 238 mg/dL.

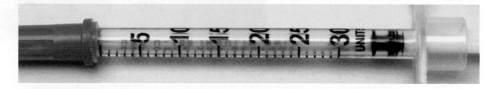

8. Blood sugar = 352 mg/dL.

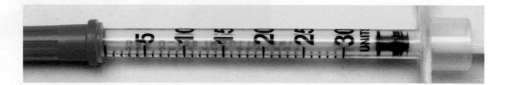

9. Blood sugar = 224 mg/dL.

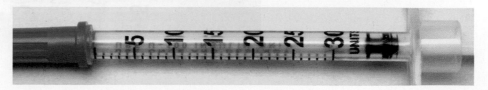

10.   Blood sugar = 288 mg/dL.

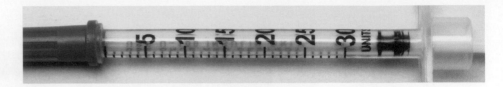

11.   Blood sugar = 136 mg/dL.

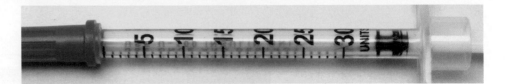

12.   Blood sugar = 315 mg/dL.

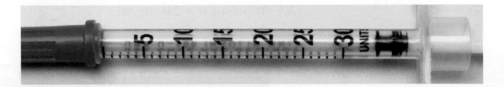

13.   Blood sugar = 247 mg/dL.

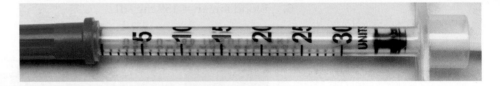

14.   Blood sugar = 274 mg/dL.

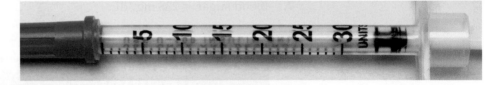

15.   Blood sugar = 183 mg/dL.

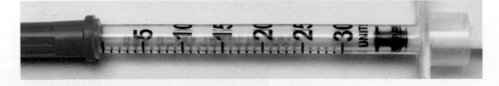

16.   Blood sugar = 199 mg/dL.

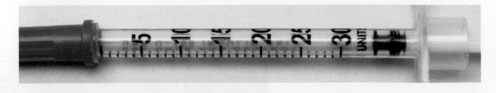

17.   Blood sugar = 268 mg/dL.

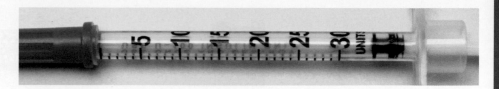

18.   Blood sugar = 245 mg/dL.

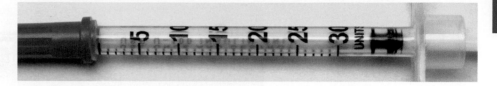

19.   Blood sugar = 320 mg/dL.

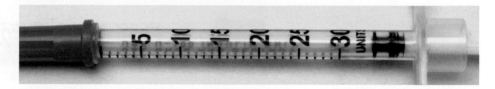

20.   Blood sugar = 366 mg/dL.

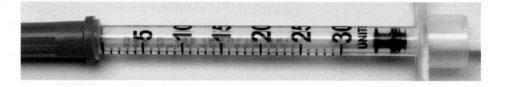

Based on the following sliding scale, determine the total regular insulin units to be administered and mark the syringe.

<150 mg/dL. Give 0 units of insulin.
150-200 mg/dL. Give 2 units of regular insulin.
201-250 mg/dL. Give 3 units of regular insulin.
251-300 mg/dL. Give 5 units of regular insulin.
>300 mg/dL. Give 6 units of regular insulin and contact physician immediately.

21.   Blood glucose level at 0800 hours is 244.

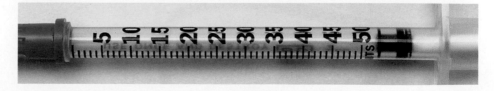

22.   Blood glucose level at 1200 hours is 86.

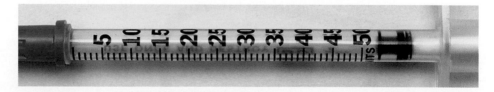

23. Blood glucose level at the hour of sleep is 269.

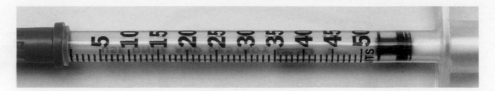

24. Blood glucose level at 0700 hours is 161.

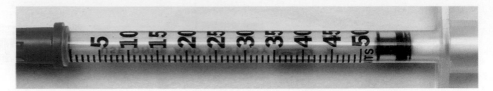

25. Blood glucose level at 1700 hours is 319.

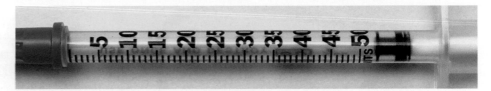

(Answers on pp. 478–479)

℮volve For additional practice problems, refer to the Advanced Calculations section of the Drug Calculations Companion, version 4 on Evolve.

Intake and Output

Cynthia Chernecky

CLINICAL CONNECTION

- Intake and output (I&O) is essential for intervention and monitoring in nursing care, particularly in pediatrics and with the elderly, and with trauma, burn, renal, and cardiac patients.

INTRODUCTION

Intake includes all methods of ingestion. Output includes all mechanisms of ridding the body of fluid and waste.

INTAKE

- Drinking fluids (baby bottle, coffee, soda, water, and so on)
- Primary intravenous fluids
- Secondary intravenous fluids via piggyback
- Intravenous push medications
- Intravenous blood products
- Tube feedings

OUTPUT

SAFETY *ALERT*

Improper maintenance of I&O will result in loss of homeostasis, resulting in problems with blood pressure, renal perfusions, proper brain activity, and cardiac function. Critical and lethal consequences are the result of alterations in homeostasis.

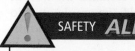

SAFETY *ALERT*

To maintain proper renal function in the adult patient, a urine output of 30 mL/hr to 50 mL/hr must be maintained.

- Urine (catheter, diaper, bedpan, and so on)
- Stool
- Sweat
- Vomit
- Ostomy (ileostomy, colostomy)
- Wound drainage
- Gastrointestinal drainage (nasogastric tube)
- Tracheostomy suctioning
- Drains
- Blood via hemorrhage or bleed
- Sputum expectoration
- Insensible loss (loss from breathing)

The purpose of monitoring I&O is to maintain homeostasis and improve patient condition. Identification of whether to expect an increase or decrease in either intake or output depending on patient condition will enable you to predict the cause of the potential deficit. For example, with a burn patient you can predict that the problem will be with maintaining adequate fluid intake and in patients with chronic renal failure you can predict the problem will be decreased output. This understanding is essential for planning appropriate nursing care.

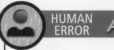

Conversion Review

5 mL = 1 teaspoon
15 mL = 1 tablespoon
30 mL = 1 ounce

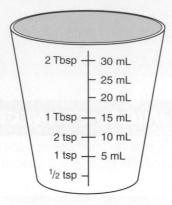

2 Tbsp	30 mL
	25 mL
	20 mL
1 Tbsp	15 mL
2 tsp	10 mL
1 tsp	5 mL
½ tsp	

500 mL = 1 pint (approximately)
1000 mL = 1 quart (approximately)

Using the ratio-proportion method for determining fluid replacement in non-burn patients is similar to using it for drug calculations. Before starting the calculation, all volumes must be converted to milliliters. With I&O, what you HAVE will be the urine output that has been collected during the prescribed period. What you KNOW is the prescribed output and replacement parameters. What you WANT is the replacement volume. The proportion is as follows:

$$\underbrace{\frac{\text{Prescribed output parameter}}{\text{Prescribed replacement parameter}}}_{\text{(KNOW)}} = \frac{\text{Total patient output}}{\text{X (replacement volume)}}\ \frac{\text{(HAVE)}}{\text{(WANT)}}$$

Example 1

PRESCRIPTION — *For every 100 mL of urine output, you replace with 30 mL of water through the percutaneous endoscopic gastrostomy (PEG) tube every 4 hours.*

- **What You HAVE** — Urine output for last 4 hours is 400 mL.

- **What You KNOW** — Prescribed output parameter is 100 mL.
  Prescribed replacement parameter is 30 mL.

- **What You WANT (X)** — Replacement fluid volume.

CRITICAL THINKING

Are all units in milliliters? _____
What is the prescribed output parameter? _____
What is the prescribed replacement parameter? _____
What is the total 4-hour patient output? _____
Using the ratio-proportion method, the LEFT (complete) ratio contains the output volume/replacement volume you KNOW, while the RIGHT (incomplete) ratio contains the urine output you HAVE in the numerator and X in the denominator.
Divide the numerical cross-product by the numerical multiplier of X (the number in front of X).
The result is the answer for X.
Label answer in milliliters.
Check answer by placing the number obtained for X in the original equation. Cross-multiply. The cross-products should be approximately equal.

ANSWER FOR BEST CARE	All units are in milliliters.

All units are in milliliters.
Output parameter? 100 mL.
Replacement volume? 30 mL.
Total patient output? 400 mL.
Perform calculation.

(KNOW)

$$\frac{100 \text{ mL}}{30 \text{ mL}} = \frac{400 \text{ mL}}{X \text{ mL}} \quad \frac{\text{(HAVE)}}{\text{(WANT)}}$$

Reduce.

$$\frac{10}{3} = \frac{400}{X}$$

$$10X = 1200$$

$$X = 120 \text{ mL}$$

Replacement volume is 120 mL.

✓ **Human Error Check**

$$\frac{100}{30} = \frac{400}{120}$$

$100 \times 120 = 30 \times 400$
$12{,}000 = 12{,}000$

Example 2

PRESCRIPTION — *For every 300 mL of urine output, you replace with 150 mL of water through the PEG tube every 8 hours.*

- **What You HAVE** — Urine output for last 8 hours is 900 mL.

- **What You KNOW** — Prescribed output parameter is 300 mL.
Prescribed replacement parameter is 150 mL.

- **What You WANT (X)** — Replacement fluid volume.

CRITICAL THINKING — Are all units in milliliters? _____
What is the prescribed output parameter? _____
What is the prescribed replacement parameter? _____
What is the total 8-hour patient output? _____
Using the ratio-proportion method, the LEFT (complete) ratio contains the output volume/replacement volume you KNOW, while the RIGHT (incomplete) ratio contains the urine output you HAVE in the numerator and X in the denominator.
Divide the numerical cross-product by the numerical multiplier of X (the number in front of X).
The result is the answer for X.
Label answer in milliliters.
Check answer by placing the number obtained for X in the original equation. Cross-multiply. The cross-products should be approximately equal.

ANSWER FOR BEST CARE — All units are in milliliters.
Output parameter? 300 mL.
Replacement volume? 150 mL.
Total patient output? 900 mL.

Perform calculation.

(KNOW)

$$\frac{300 \text{ mL}}{150 \text{ mL}} = \frac{900 \text{ mL}}{X \text{ mL}} \quad \begin{matrix} \text{(HAVE)} \\ \text{(WANT)} \end{matrix}$$

Reduce.

$$\frac{1}{2} = \frac{900}{X}$$

$2X = 900$

$X = 450 \text{ mL}$

Replacement volume is 450 mL.

> ✓ **Human Error Check**
>
> $$\frac{300}{150} = \frac{900}{450}$$
>
> $300 \times 450 = 150 \times 900$
> $135,000 = 135,000$

Example 3

PRESCRIPTION   *For every 200 mL of urine output, you replace with 75 mL of water through the PEG tube every 6 hours.*

- **What You HAVE**   Urine output for last 6 hours is 1200 mL.

- **What You KNOW**   Prescribed output parameter is 200 mL.
  Prescribed replacement parameter is 75 mL.

- **What You WANT (X)**   Replacement fluid volume.

CRITICAL THINKING   Are all units in milliliters? _____
What is the prescribed output volume? _____
What is the prescribed replacement volume? _____
What is the total 6-hour patient output? _____
Using the ratio-proportion method, the LEFT (complete) ratio contains the output volume/replacement volume you KNOW, while the RIGHT (incomplete) ratio contains the urine output you HAVE in the numerator and X in the denominator.
Divide the numerical cross-product by the numerical multiplier of X (the number in front of X).
The result is the answer for X.
Label answer in milliliters.
Check answer by placing the number obtained for X in the original equation. Cross-multiply. The cross-products should be approximately equal.

ANSWER FOR BEST CARE   All units are in milliliters.
Output parameter? 200 mL.
Replacement volume? 75 mL.
Total patient output? 1200 mL.
Perform calculation.

(KNOW)

$$\frac{200 \text{ mL}}{75 \text{ mL}} = \frac{1200 \text{ mL}}{X \text{ mL}} \quad \begin{matrix} \text{(HAVE)} \\ \text{(WANT)} \end{matrix}$$

$$200X = 90,000$$
$$X = 450 \text{ mL}$$

Replacement volume is 450 mL.

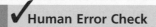

✔ Human Error Check

$$\frac{200}{75} = \frac{1200}{450}$$

$$200 \times 450 = 75 \times 1200$$
$$90,000 = 90,000$$

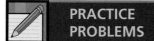

PRACTICE PROBLEMS

Directions: *Determine replacement fluids based on urinary output.*

1. PRESCRIPTION: For every 100 mL of urine output, you replace with 10 mL of water through the PEG tube every 8 hours. Patient output last 8 hours was 1000 mL.

2. PRESCRIPTION: For every 200 mL of urine output, you replace with 30 mL of water through the PEG tube every 8 hours. Patient output last 8 hours was 1400 mL.

3. PRESCRIPTION: For every 100 mL of urine output, you replace with 25 mL of water through the nasogastric tube every 4 hours. Patient output last 4 hours was 600 mL.

4. PRESCRIPTION: For every 200 mL of urine output, you replace with 40 mL of water through the jejunostomy (J-tube) tube every 8 hours. Patient output last 8 hours was 800 mL.

5. PRESCRIPTION: For every 200 mL of urine output, you replace with 50 mL of water through the PEG tube every 2 hours. Patient output last 2 hours was 500 mL.

6. PRESCRIPTION: For every 100 mL of urine output, you replace with 40 mL of water through the PEG tube every 4 hours. Patient output last 4 hours was 600 mL.

7. PRESCRIPTION: For every 300 mL of urine output, you replace with 25 mL of water through the J-tube every 8 hours. Patient output last 8 hours was 1200 mL.

8. PRESCRIPTION: For every 200 mL of urine output, you replace with 30 mL of water through the nasogastric tube every 4 hours. Patient output last 4 hours was 1000 mL.

9. PRESCRIPTION: For every 100 mL of urine output, you replace with 30 mL of water through the nasogastric tube every 8 hours. Patient output last 8 hours was 900 mL.

10. PRESCRIPTION: For every 300 mL of urine output, you replace with 50 mL of water through the PEG tube every 4 hours. Patient output last 4 hours was 1500 mL.

(Answers on p. 479)

FLUID RESUSCITATION FOR BURN PATIENTS

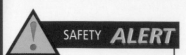

SAFETY **ALERT**

Resuscitation of burned patients with fluids requires massive amounts of fluids, thereby necessitating the largest intravenous line possible, or multiple lines.

There are several formulas for fluid resuscitation in burn patients. The Parkland formula—used with both adults and children (who are over age 10 years)—is a common choice and will be used in this section. The fluid replacement formula for infants who are burned is different, although it is very similar to the formula used for adults and children, and therefore will not be discussed.

The Parkland formula begins from the time of the burn injury and concludes at the end of the first 24 hours after the burn.

The Parkland formula is as follows:

$$2 \text{ to } 4 \text{ mL/kg} \times \% \text{ body surface area (BSA) burned} =$$
$$\text{Total fluid volume to be infused (lactated Ringer's)}$$

For the purposes of this book, 4 mL will be the constant for computing fluid resuscitation using the Parkland formula. In the first 24 hours after the burn injury, 50% of the total volume is given in the first 8 hours from the time of the burn (not the time of arrival at the hospital), and the remaining 50% of the total volume is given over the next 16 hours.

For the second 24 hours (hours 25 to 48) after the burn injury, the amount of intravenous fluid (usually D_5W) to be administered depends on maintaining urine output at a minimum; use the following formula:

$$1 \text{ mL/kg} \times \% \text{ BSA burned (15 to 20 mL/hr for a child and}$$
$$30 \text{ to } 50 \text{ mL/hr for an adult)}$$

This is the formula used in this book, although some institutions may use 0.5 mL/kg/hr for output for adults and 1 mL/kg/hr for children under 30 kg (66 pounds).

To complete these calculations, review the patient's chart to determine the patient's weight, the time the burn occurred, the time of admission, and the percentage of body surface burned. In the examples, this information is given to you as what you KNOW. Use the Parkland formula to determine the total amount of fluid volume to be replaced in a post-burn patient in the first 24 hours, including the first 8 hours and the next 16 hours; give the mL/hr for the intravenous solution. Also, using the post 24-hour formula for fluid replacement, based on urinary output, determine the hourly volume of fluid replacement for hours 25 to 48 post burn. Round all answers to the nearest whole number.

Example 1

PRESCRIPTION	*Lactated Ringer's intravenous to infuse per Parkland formula × 24 hours and, for post-burn hours 25 to 48, fluid replacement with D_5W based on the urinary output formula.*

- **What You HAVE**

  Lactated Ringers (LR) solution.
  D_5W solution.

- **What You KNOW**

  Weight is 220 lb.
  Percentage of body surface area burned is 45%.

- **What You WANT**

  Intravenous replacement total volume for the first 24 hours.
  Intravenous replacement total volume for the first 8 hours.
  Infusion rate (mL/hr) for the first 8 hours.
  Intravenous replacement total volume for the next 16 hours.
  Infusion rate (mL/hr) for the next 16 hours.
  Intravenous replacement total volume (mL/hr) for post-burn hours 25 through 48.
  Infusion rate (mL/hr) for post-burn hours 25 through 48.

CRITICAL THINKING	1. Is the weight in kilograms? _____ If not, convert to kg.
	2. What is the percentage of body surface area burned? _____
	3. Determine the 24-hour total LR volume to be infused using the formula 4 mL/kg × % BSA burned.
	4. Determine the first 8-hour replacement by converting 50% to a decimal equivalent and multiply by total volume.
	5. Determine the next 16 hours of volume.
	6. Determine infusion rate; divide the total 8-hour volume by the total time.
	7. Determine the infusion rate for the next 16 hours, divide total volume by total hours.
	8. Determine D_5W replacement based on output formula: 1 mL/kg × % BSA burned.
	9. Determine the infusion rate; divide total volume by total hours.

ANSWER FOR BEST CARE

1. No. Weight conversion:

$$\frac{220 \text{ lb}}{2.2} = 100 \text{ kg}$$

2. 45%
3. 24-Hour total LR volume:

(Constant)	(kg)	(% BSA)	(Total volume)
4 mL	× 100 kg ×	45	= 18,000 mL

4. 8-Hour and 16-hour volume calculation:
Decimal conversion:
50% = 0.5
5. 18,000 × 0.5 = 9000 mL (volume for first 8 hours)
18,000 − 9000 = 9000 mL (volume for next 16 hours)
6. Infusion rate calculation:

$$\frac{\text{(8-hour volume)}}{\text{(Total time)}} \frac{900 \text{ mL}}{8 \text{ hr}} = 1125 \text{ mL/hr}$$

7. (16-hour volume)/(Total time) 9000 mL/16 hr = 563 mL/hr
8. D_5W replacement based on urinary output:

(Constant)	(kg)	(% BSA)	
1 mL	× 100 kg ×	45	= 4500 mL/24 hr

9. Infusion rate:

$$\frac{\text{(24-hour volume)}}{\text{(Total time)}} \frac{4500 \text{ mL}}{24 \text{ hr}} = 188 \text{ mL/hr}$$

Example 2

PRESCRIPTION	*Lactated Ringer's intravenous to infuse per Parkland formula × 24 hours and, for post-burn hours 25 to 48, fluid replacement with D_5W based on the urinary output formula.*
• **What You HAVE**	LR solution. D_5W solution.
• **What You KNOW**	Patient weight is 204.6 lb Percentage of body surface area burned is 70%.
• **What You WANT**	Intravenous replacement total volume for the first 24 hours. Intravenous replacement total volume for the first 8 hours. Infusion rate (mL/hr) for the first 8 hours.

Intravenous replacement total volume for the next 16 hours.
Infusion rate (mL/hr) for the next 16 hours.
Intravenous replacement total volume (mL/hr) for post-burn hours 25 through 48.
Infusion rate (mL/hr) for post-burn hours 25 through 48.

CRITICAL THINKING

1. Is the weight in kilograms? _____ If not, convert to kg.
2. What is the percentage of body surface area burned? _____
3. Determine the 24-hour total LR volume to be infused using the formula 4 mL/kg × % BSA burned.
4. Determine the first 8-hour replacement by converting 50% to a decimal equivalent and multiply by total volume.
5. Determine the next 16 hours of volume.
6. Determine 8-hour infusion rate; divide total 8-hour volume by total time.
7. Determine the infusion rate for the next 16 hours; divide total volume by total hours.
8. Determine D_5W replacement based on output formula: 1 mL/kg × % BSA burned.
9. Determine infusion rate; divide total volume by total hours.

ANSWER FOR BEST CARE

1. No.   Weight conversion:
$$\frac{204.6}{2.2} = 93 \text{ kg}$$

2. 70%
3. Total 24-hour total LR volume

(Constant)	(kg)	(% BSA)	(Total volume)
4 mL ×	93 kg ×	70 =	26,040 mL

4. 8-Hour and 16-hour volume calculation:
Decimal conversion:
50% = 0.5
5. 26,040 × 0.5 = 13,020 mL (volume for first 8 hours)
26,040 − 13,020 = 13,020 mL (volume for next 16 hours)
6. Infusion rate calculation:
$$\frac{\text{(8-hour volume)}}{\text{(Total time)}} \frac{13,020 \text{ mL}}{8 \text{ hr}} = 1628 \text{ mL/hr}$$

7. (16-hour volume)/(Total time) 13,020 mL/16 hr = 814 mL/hr
8. D_5W replacement based on urinary output:

(Constant)	(kg)	(% BSA)	
1 mL ×	93 kg ×	70 =	6510 mL/24 hr

9. Infusion rate:
$$\frac{\text{(24-hour volume)}}{\text{(Total time)}} \frac{6510 \text{ mL}}{24 \text{ hr}} = 271 \text{ mL/hr}$$

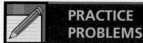

PRACTICE PROBLEMS

Directions: *Using the Parkland formula, determine the total amount of fluid volume to be replaced in a post-burn patient in the first 24 hours, including the first 8 hours and the next 16 hours, and the mL/hour for the intravenous solution. Also, using the post 24-hour formula for fluid replacement, based on urinary output, determine the hourly volume of fluid replacement for hours 25 to 48 post-burn. Round all weight conversions from pounds to kilograms to the nearest hundredth. Round all other final answers to the nearest tenth. Round to whole number.*

Parkland formula = 4 mL/kg × % BSA burn

Post 24-hour formula based on urinary output = 1 mL/kg × % BSA burned

1. PRESCRIPTION: Patient weight is 90 kg and % BSA burned is 30%.
   A. The 24-hour total of LR intravenous fluid to be replaced is _____.
   B. The 8-hour total of LR intravenous fluid to be replaced is _____.
   C. The mL/hr of the 8-hour LR intravenous fluid replacement is _____.
   D. The 16-hour total of LR intravenous fluid to be replaced is _____.
   E. The mL/hr of the 16-hour LR intravenous fluid replacement is _____.
   F. The post 24-hour total of D₅W intravenous fluid replacement is _____.

2. PRESCRIPTION: Patient is a 10-year-old child whose weight is 50 pounds and % BSA burned is 25%.
   A. The 24-hour total of LR intravenous fluid to be replaced is _____.
   B. The 8-hour total of LR intravenous fluid to be replaced is _____.
   C. The mL/hr of the 8-hour LR intravenous fluid replacement is _____.
   D. The 16-hour total of LR intravenous fluid to be replaced is _____.
   E. The mL/hr of the 16-hour LR intravenous fluid replacement is _____.
   F. The post 24-hour total of D₅W intravenous fluid replacement is _____.

3. PRESCRIPTION: Patient weight is 73 pounds and % BSA burned is 35%.
   A. The 24-hour total of LR intravenous fluid to be replaced is _____.
   B. The 8-hour total of LR intravenous fluid to be replaced is _____.
   C. The mL/hr of the 8-hour LR intravenous fluid replacement is _____.
   D. The 16-hour total of LR intravenous fluid to be replaced is _____.
   E. The mL/hr of the 16-hour LR intravenous fluid replacement is _____.
   F. The post 24-hour total of D₅W intravenous fluid replacement is _____.

4. PRESCRIPTION: Patient weight is 106 pounds and % BSA burned is 20%.
   A. The 24-hour total of LR intravenous fluid to be replaced is _____.
   B. The 8-hour total of LR intravenous fluid to be replaced is _____.
   C. The mL/hr of the 8-hour LR intravenous fluid replacement is _____.
   D. The 16-hour total of LR intravenous fluid to be replaced is _____.
   E. The mL/hr of the 16-hour LR intravenous fluid replacement is _____.
   F. The post 24-hour total of D₅W intravenous fluid replacement is _____.

5. PRESCRIPTION: Patient weight is 150 pounds and % BSA burned is 45%.
   A. The 24-hour total of LR intravenous fluid to be replaced is _____.
   B. The 8-hour total of LR intravenous fluid to be replaced is _____.
   C. The mL/hr of the 8-hour LR intravenous fluid replacement is _____.
   D. The 16-hour total of LR intravenous fluid to be replaced is _____.
   E. The mL/hr of the 16-hour LR intravenous fluid replacement is _____.
   F. The post 24-hour total of D₅W intravenous fluid replacement is _____.

6. PRESCRIPTION: Patient weight is 80 kg and % BSA burned is 35%.
   A. The 24-hour total of LR intravenous fluid to be replaced is _____.
   B. The 8-hour total of LR intravenous fluid to be replaced is _____.
   C. The mL/hr of the 8-hour LR intravenous fluid replacement is _____.
   D. The 16-hour total of LR intravenous fluid to be replaced is _____.

E. The mL/hr of the 16-hour LR intravenous fluid replacement is _____.

F. The post 24-hour total of D₅W intravenous fluid replacement is _____.

7. PRESCRIPTION: Patient weight is 96 kg and % BSA burned is 24%.

A. The 24-hour total of LR intravenous fluid to be replaced is _____.

B. The 8-hour total of LR intravenous fluid to be replaced is _____.

C. The mL/hr of the 8-hour LR intravenous fluid replacement is _____.

D. The 16-hour total of LR intravenous fluid to be replaced is _____.

E. The mL/hr of the 16-hour LR intravenous fluid replacement is _____.

F. The post 24-hour total of D₅W intravenous fluid replacement is _____.

8. PRESCRIPTION: Patient weight is 116 kg and % BSA burned is 70%.

A. The 24-hour total of LR intravenous fluid to be replaced is _____.

B. The 8-hour total of LR intravenous fluid to be replaced is _____.

C. The mL/hr of the 8-hour LR intravenous fluid replacement is _____.

D. The 16-hour total of LR intravenous fluid to be replaced is _____.

E. The mL/hr of the 16-hour LR intravenous fluid replacement is _____.

F. The post 24-hour total of D₅W intravenous fluid replacement is _____.

9. PRESCRIPTION: Patient weight is 109 kg and % BSA burned is 36%.

A. The 24-hour total of LR intravenous fluid to be replaced is _____.

B. The 8-hour total of LR intravenous fluid to be replaced is _____.

C. The mL/hr of the 8-hour LR intravenous fluid replacement is _____.

D. The 16-hour total of LR intravenous fluid to be replaced is _____.

E. The mL/hr of the 16-hour LR intravenous fluid replacement is _____.

F. The post 24-hour total of D₅W intravenous fluid replacement is _____.

10. PRESCRIPTION: Patient weight is 86 kg and % BSA burned is 60%.

A. The 24-hour total of LR intravenous fluid to be replaced is _____.

B. The 8-hour total of LR intravenous fluid to be replaced is _____.

C. The mL/hr of the 8-hour LR intravenous fluid replacement is _____.

D. The 16-hour total of LR intravenous fluid to be replaced is _____.

E. The mL/hr of the 16-hour LR intravenous fluid replacement is _____.

F. The post 24-hour total of D₅W intravenous fluid replacement is _____.

(Answers on p. 479)

CHAPTER REVIEW

Determine replacement fluids based on urinary output.

1. PRESCRIPTION: For every 100 mL urine output, replace with 20 mL water through PEG tube every 8 hours. Patient output last 8 hours was 1500 mL. Replacement is _____.

2. PRESCRIPTION: For every 200 mL urine output, replace with 20 mL water through PEG tube every 8 hours. Patient output last 8 hours was 800 mL. Replacement is _____.

3. PRESCRIPTION: For every 100 mL urine output, replace with 35 mL water through nasogastric tube every 4 hours. Patient output last 4 hours was 750 mL. Replacement is _____.

4. PRESCRIPTION: For every 250 mL urine output, replace with 50 mL water through J-tube tube every 8 hours. Patient output last 8 hours was 1000 mL. Replacement is _____.

5. PRESCRIPTION: For every 150 mL urine output, replace with 30 mL water through PEG tube every 2 hours. Patient output last 2 hours was 600 mL. Replacement is _____.

6. PRESCRIPTION: For every 100 mL urine output, replace with 25 mL water through PEG tube every 4 hours. Patient output last 4 hours was 600 mL. Replacement is _____.

7. PRESCRIPTION: For every 300 mL urine output, replace with 30 mL water through J-tube every 8 hours. Patient output last 8 hours was 1200 mL. Replacement is _____.

8. Your patient can be discharged once his intake exceeds 2200 mL in 24 hours. For the past 24 hours, your patient has drunk a half pint of milk, 8 oz of soda, 280 mL of iced tea, 3 cups of water, and 16 oz of juice. Has your patient had enough intake to be discharged? _____.

9. Your patient has to have an intravenous line started if her output in 4 hours is less than 4 oz or 1 oz/hr. Her output for the last 4 hours is 150 mL. Do you need to start the intravenous line? _____.

10. You must replace through your patient's PEG tube 10 mL of water for every 30 mL that the output is greater than the input. Your patient's intake is 4 oz of iced tea, 360 mL Ensure, 1 pt of skim milk, 8 oz of soda, 8 oz of gelatin, 380 mL of milkshake, and 1 pt of water. Your patient's output is 2200 mL. Is replacement necessary through the PEG tube? And if so, how much water will you replace? _____.

For problems 11 through 15, use the Parkland formula to determine the total amount of fluid volume to be replaced in a post-burn patient in the first 24 hours, including the first 8 hours and the next 16 hours, and the mL/hr for the intravenous solution. Also, use the post 24-hour formula for fluid replacement based on urinary output to determine the hourly volume of fluid replacement for hours 25 to 48 post-burn. Round all weight conversions from pounds to nearest kilograms to the hundredth. Round all other final answers to the nearest tenth. Round to whole numbers.

Parkland formula = 4 mL/kg × % BSA burn

Post 24-hr formula based on urinary output = 1 mL/kg × % BSA burn

11. PRESCRIPTION: Patient weight is 75 pounds and % BSA burned is 27%.
    A. The 24-hour total of LR intravenous fluid to be replaced is _____.
    B. The 8-hour total of LR intravenous fluid to be replaced is _____.
    C. The mL/hr of the 8-hour LR intravenous fluid replacement is _____.
    D. The 16-hour total of LR intravenous fluid to be replaced is _____.
    E. The mL/hr of the 16-hour LR intravenous fluid replacement is _____.
    F. The post 24-hour total of D_5W intravenous fluid replacement is _____.

12. PRESCRIPTION: Patient weight is 130 pounds and % BSA burned is 48%.
    A. The 24-hour total of LR intravenous fluid to be replaced is _____.
    B. The 8-hour total of LR intravenous fluid to be replaced is _____.
    C. The mL/hr of the 8-hour LR intravenous fluid replacement is _____.
    D. The 16-hour total of LR intravenous fluid to be replaced is _____.
    E. The mL/hr of the 16-hour LR intravenous fluid replacement is _____.
    F. The post 24-hour total of D5W intravenous fluid replacement is _____.

13. PRESCRIPTION: Patient weight is 262 pounds and % BSA burned is 55%.
    A. The 24-hour total of LR intravenous fluid to be replaced is _____.
    B. The 8-hour total of LR intravenous fluid to be replaced is _____.
    C. The mL/hr of the 8-hour LR intravenous fluid replacement is _____.
    D. The 16-hour total of LR intravenous fluid to be replaced is _____.
    E. The mL/hr of the 16-hour LR intravenous fluid replacement is _____.
    F. The post 24-hour total of D_5W intravenous fluid replacement is _____.

14.   PRESCRIPTION: Patient weight is 110 kg and % BSA burned is 40%.
   A.   The 24-hour total of LR intravenous fluid to be replaced is _____.
   B.   The 8-hour total of LR intravenous fluid to be replaced is _____.
   C.   The mL/hr of the 8-hour LR intravenous fluid replacement is _____.
   D.   The 16-hour total of LR intravenous fluid to be replaced is _____.
   E.   The mL/hr of the 16-hour LR intravenous fluid replacement is _____.
   F.   The post 24-hour total of D5W intravenous fluid replacement is _____.

15.   PRESCRIPTION: Patient weight is 65 kg and % BSA burned is 28%.
   A.   The 24-hour total of LR intravenous fluid to be replaced is _____.
   B.   The 8-hour total of LR intravenous fluid to be replaced is _____.
   C.   The mL/hr of the 8-hour LR intravenous fluid replacement is _____.
   D.   The 16-hour total of LR intravenous fluid to be replaced is _____.
   E.   The mL/hr of the 16-hour LR intravenous fluid replacement is _____.
   F.   The post 24-hour total of D$_5$W intravenous fluid replacement is _____.

(Answers on pp. 479–480)

evolve   For additional practice problems, refer to the Basic Calculations section of the Drug Calculations Companion, version 4 on Evolve.

Calculations in Special Care Units

Oncology

Cynthia Chernecky

CLINICAL CONNECTION

- Determining body surface area is necessary for calculating dosages of certain medications, particularly with chemotherapy for the treatment of cancer.
- Incorrect dosing based on body surface area can result in undertreatment or overtreatment in cancer, both of which can result in harm and even death.

INTRODUCTION

In oncology the majority of chemotherapy agents are prescribed based on the total area of the patient's body. This is referred to as *body surface area* (BSA). A medication prescribed based on BSA is a dosage based on current actual height and weight measurements. Once you know the actual height and weight, you can determine the meter-squared (m^2) area of the patient's body by using a special BSA slide ruler, BSA calculator, nomogram chart, or mathematical formula (Figure 20-1).

BSA RULER

The BSA slide ruler has two sides: a pediatric side and an adult side (Figure 20-2).

Once the correct side of the BSA slide ruler is determined, you locate the patient's weight in either pounds or kilograms by sliding the ruler up or down until the large arrows are aligned with the weight on either the kilogram side or the pound side of the scale.

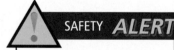

SAFETY ALERT

It is imperative that an actual height and weight be taken, not just estimated, because the final dosage of the chemotherapy agent to treat the cancer as well as the severity of side effects is linked to the BSA.

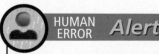

HUMAN ERROR Alert

Height and weight MUST use the same unit of measure—either metric (kilograms and centimeters) or household (pounds and inches). ALWAYS check to make sure that height and weight figures use the same unit of measure.

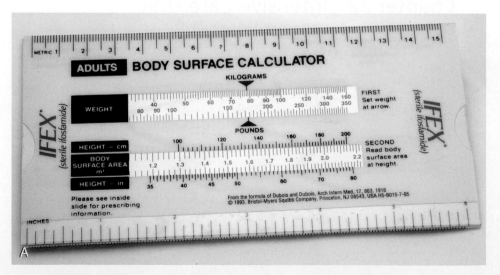

Figure 20-1 A, Adult body surface area slide ruler.

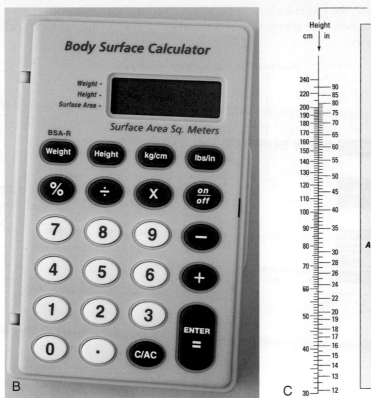

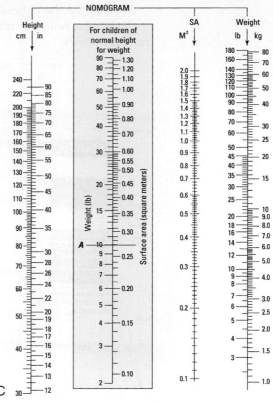

Figure 20-1, cont'd B, Body surface calculator. **C,** West nomogram for infants and children.
(**C** modified from data of E. Boyd by C.D. West, in Kleigman RM, Behrman RE, Jenson HB, Stanton BF: *Nelson textbook of pediatrics*, ed 18, Philadelphia, 2007, Saunders.)

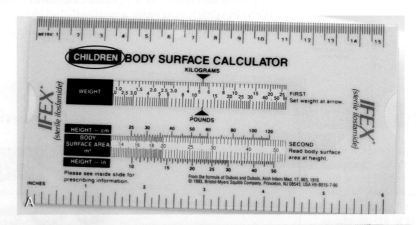

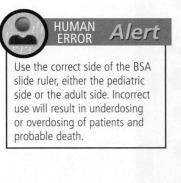

HUMAN ERROR *Alert*

Use the correct side of the BSA slide ruler, either the pediatric side or the adult side. Incorrect use will result in underdosing or overdosing of patients and probable death.

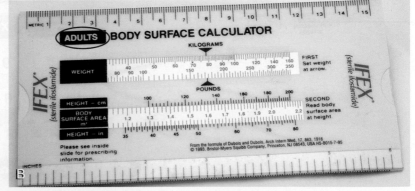

Figure 20-2 Body surface calculator. **A,** Children's side. **B,** Adult's side.

Next locate the patient's height on either the "cm" or "in" scale.

Then you note the meter-squared number in the center section and write this number down.

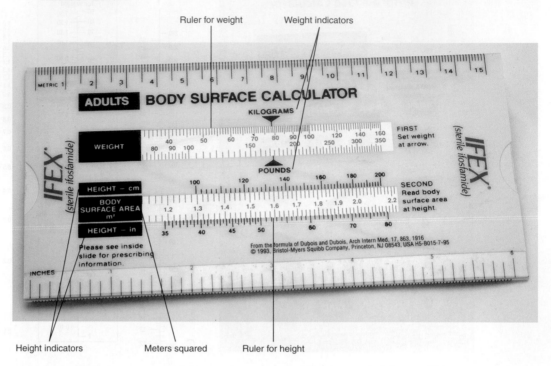

Ruler for weight · Weight indicators

Height indicators · Meters squared · Ruler for height

BSA CALCULATOR

The BSA calculator is a special calculator (which can be found on the World Wide Web) in which you enter a patient's height and weight in either kilograms and centimeters or pounds and inches, and it calculates the meter-squared number.

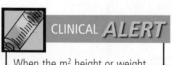

CLINICAL ALERT

When the m² height or weight is greater than the nomogram, using the method below will make you less likely to severely underdose if an error occurs and you forget to add the leftover value.

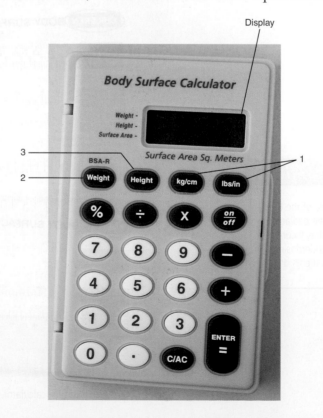

Display

Step 1: First you select either kg/cm or lb/in.
Step 2: Press the weight button, enter the weight, and press enter.
Step 3: Press the height button, enter the height, and press enter. The square meters will appear on the display. Write down the meter-squared number.

NOMOGRAMS

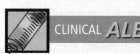

CLINICAL ALERT

Nomograms are the least accurate method but are used here as this is a book. In reality a BSA calculator, also found on the internet, should be used.

Nomograms come in pediatric versions and adult versions, so choose the correct side to avoid errors (Figure 20-3). To use the nomogram, you will need a straight-edge ruler. Place one end of the ruler on the patient's height (either centimeters or inches) and the other edge on the weight (either kilograms or pounds). Draw a line to connect these two points; where the line intersects on the line labeled meter-squared (m^2) is your meter-squared number. Write this number down. When the patient's height and/or weight is greater than is listed on the nomogram scale (75 in or 190 cm and 220 lb or 100 kg), take the patient's actual height and/or weight and subtract the maximum scale height/weight. Then using the difference, draw on the nomogram again to determine a second m^2. Add this second m^2 to the maximum nomogram scale m^2 value (2.3 m^2). This new total m^2 value is used in the dosage calculation.

Patient's weight 280 lb − 220 maximum scale weight = 60 pounds
Patient's height 79 inches − 75 inches = 4 inches
BSA = 0.8 + 2.3 (maximum scale m^2) = 3.1 m^2

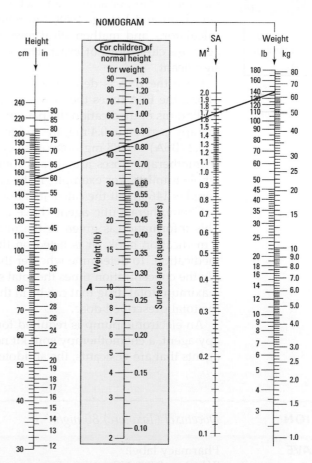

Figure 22-3 West nomogram for infants and children. Example: height, 60 inches; weight, 140 lb; m^2, 1.7. (Modified from data of E. Boyd by C.D. West, in Kleigman RM, Behrman RE, Jenson HB, Stanton BF: *Nelson textbook of pediatrics*, ed 18, Philadelphia, 2007, Saunders.)

FORMULA METHOD

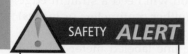

SAFETY ALERT

Determining amounts of medications based on BSA includes rounding the answer.

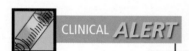

CLINICAL ALERT

Chemotherapy may be required to be administered by a certified or specially trained nurse.

You may also obtain the BSA by using a mathematical formula. Unlike nomograms and slide rulers, the formula can be used with both adults and children. The formula requires that the metric system (centimeters and kilograms) be used. If the height and weight measurements are written in inches and pounds, they will need to be converted to their metric equivalents. To convert inches to centimeters, multiply the number of inches by 2.54 (inches × 2.54) to obtain the number of centimeters. To convert pounds to kilograms, divide the number of pounds by 2.2 (pounds/2.2) to obtain the number of kilograms. For example, if a person weighs 143 pounds (lb), you divide 143 pounds by 2.2 kilograms/pound (143/2.2) and obtain the answer: 65 kilograms (kg). Weights calculated in kilograms when converted from pounds are rounded when determining chemotherapy dosages. You round up if the tenths column of the answer is equal to 5 or greater than 5, and you round down if the tenths column of the answer is equal to 4 or less than 4. For example, if the calculated weight is 59.6 kg, the weight used in calculating dosages is 60 kg. If the calculated weight is 52.4 kg, the weight used in calculating dosages is 52 kg.

Once you have obtained the patient's actual height in centimeters and weight in kilograms, you enter the numbers into the formula and complete the calculation. Using the metric system,

$$BSA\ (m^2) = \sqrt{\frac{Ht(cm) \times Wt(kg)}{3600}}$$

This mathematical formula is 99% accurate when compared to either the calculator, nomogram, or slide ruler methods and requires a calculator with a square-root key (Lam and Leung, 1988; Mosteller, 1987). Using nomograms, slide rulers, BSA calculators, and mathematical formulas, the final calculations for medication dosages are close but not exact. However, this difference is not considered clinically significant.

Once the BSA is determined, you figure the prescribed total dosage by multiplying the BSA times the dose written in mg/m² to determine the total number of milligrams of medication the patient is to receive. For example, if vincristine chemotherapy is given in 0.4 mg/m² and the patient's BSA is 2.2, the total dose is 0.4 (dose) × 2.2 (BSA) = 0.88 mg (total dose of the medication the patient is to receive). Final chemotherapy doses are always rounded when the mathematical answer is not a whole number. For example, if the calculated dosage is 146.47 mg, the dosage prepared is 146 mg. If the calculated dosage is 87.66 mg, the dosage prepared is 88 mg.

Chemotherapeutic agents have a maximum concentration (mg/mL) guideline. This information is given to the nurse by the pharmacist, found by the nurse in a medication book, or is listed on the intravenous bag that includes the prepared medication. To determine whether the total dose is within the guideline, you multiply the concentration times the total solution volume. This calculation gives you the maximum total drug that can be in the specific volume. This number is compared to the total prescribed dose.

An electronic pump is required for chemotherapy infusions. For any chemotherapy agent, a chemotherapy spill kit needs to be readily available. For chemotherapy agents that are vesicants, the antidote needs to be readily available.

Example 1

PRESCRIPTION   *Docetaxel (Taxotere) 80 mg/m².*

• **What You HAVE**   Pharmacy label:
Solution: 0.9% NS.
Total volume: 500 mL + docetaxel.
Rate: 1 hour.

CHAPTER 20

- **What You KNOW**   Docetaxel (Taxotere) 80 mg/m².
Patient: 48-year-old female.
Height: 5′ 5″.
Weight: 140 lb.
Maximum concentration is 0.9 mg/mL for this chemotherapeutic agent.

- **What You WANT**   Select adult side of nomogram or slide ruler, if using.
Height in total inches.
Weight in pounds.
Total Taxotere dosage.
Maximum Taxotere concentration for 500 mL.

CRITICAL THINKING

Are both height and weight in kg/cm or lb/in? _____
Convert 5′ 5″ to total inches.
Use an adult version of a nomogram, BSA calculator, or slide ruler to determine BSA.
Multiply BSA and the specific drug factor (noted in mg/m²) to obtain the total amount of medication to administer to the patient.
Multiply the maximum concentration by the total volume.
Is this total number of milligrams of Taxotere less than or equal to the maximum concentration?

ANSWER FOR BEST CARE

Height and weight same? No.
Convert feet to inches.

$$5 \text{ feet} \times \frac{12 \text{ inches}}{\text{foot}} = 60 \text{ inches} \quad 60 + 5 = 65 \text{ inches}$$

BSA based on adult height of 65 inches and 140 pounds = 1.7 m².

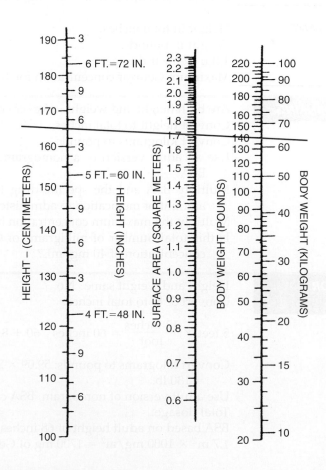

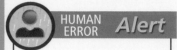

HUMAN
ERROR *Alert*

Be sure to use correct version for the BSA calculation.

Total dosage:

$$(\text{Drug dose}) \frac{80 \text{ mg}}{\text{m}^2} \times 1.7 \text{ m}^2 (\text{BSA}) = 136 \text{ mg of Taxotere}$$

Maximum concentration is 0.9 mg/mL × 500 mL = 450 mg.
Does your answer fit the general guideline? Yes; 136 mg is less than 450 mg.

> ✔ **Human Error Check**
>
> Always double- or triple-check your calculations with other professionals, such as nurses, pharmacists, and physicians.

Example 2

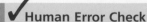

PRESCRIPTION	*Gemcitabine hydrochloride (Gemzar) 1000 mg/m² intravenous.*

- **What You HAVE**

Pharmacy label:
Solution type: 0.9% NS.
Volume total: 100 mL plus Gemzar.
Rate: 30 minutes.

- **What You KNOW**

Patient: 56-year-old male.
Height: 5' 8".
Weight: 59.09 kg.
Maximum concentration is 40 mg/mL for this chemotherapeutic agent (found in a medication textbook).
Adult side of nomogram or slide ruler.
Gemzar concentration of ≤0.9 mg/mL.

- **What You WANT**

Height in total inches.
Weight in pounds.
Total Gemzar dosage.
Maximum Gemzar concentration for 100 mL.

CRITICAL THINKING

Are both height and weight in kg/cm or lb/in? _____
Convert height to total inches.
Convert kilograms to pounds.
Use an adult version of a nomogram, BSA calculator, or slide ruler to determine BSA.
Multiply BSA and the specific drug factor (noted in mg/m²) to obtain the total amount of medication to administer to the patient.
Multiply the maximum concentration by the total volume.
Is this total number of milligrams of Gemzar less than or equal to the maximum concentration of 40 mg/mL?

ANSWER FOR BEST CARE

Height and weight same? No.
Convert 5' 8" to total inches:

$$5 \text{ feet} \times \frac{12 \text{ inches}}{\text{foot}} = 60 \text{ inches} \quad 60 + 8 = 68 \text{ inches}$$

Convert kilograms to pounds: 59.09 × 2.2 = 129.99 (round to nearest whole number) = 130 lb.
Use adult version of nomogram, BSA calculator, or slide ruler to determine BSA.
Total dosage:
BSA based on adult height of 68 inches and weight of 130 pounds = 1.7 m².
1.7 m² × 1000 mg/m² = 1700 mg of Gemzar.

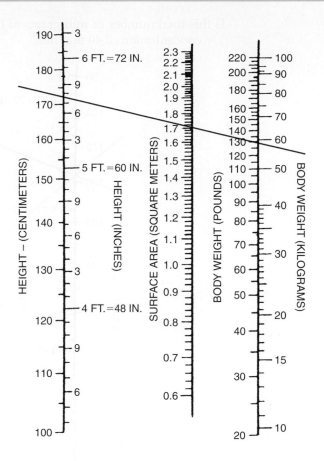

Maximum concentration is 40 mg/mL × 100 mL = 4000 mg.
Does your answer fit the general guideline? Yes; 1700 mg is less than 4000 mg.

Example 3	

PRESCRIPTION	*Carboplatin (Paraplatin) 360 mg/m^2 intravenous.*

• **What You HAVE**	Pharmacy label: D$_5$W. Volume total: 500 mL + Paraplatin. Rate: 4 hours.
• **What You KNOW**	Patient: 46-year-old female. Height: 5′ 4″. Weight: 270 lb. Maximum concentration is 10 mg/mL.
• **What You WANT**	Height in total inches. Weight in pounds. Total Paraplatin dosage. Maximum Paraplatin concentration for 500 mL.

CRITICAL THINKING	Are both height and weight in kg/cm or lb/in? _____
	Convert height to total inches.
	Use an adult version of a nomogram, BSA calculator, or slide ruler to determine BSA.
	     The BSA is based on 270 lb (220 lb + 50 lb).
	Multiply BSA and the specific drug factor (noted in mg/m^2) to obtain the total
	     amount of medication to administer to the patient.
	Multiply the maximum concentration by the total volume.

Is this total number of milligrams of Paraplatin less than or equal to the maximum concentration of 40 mg/mL?

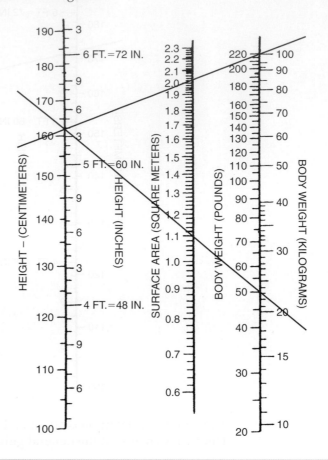

<table>
<tr><td>

ANSWER FOR BEST CARE

</td></tr>
</table>

ANSWER FOR BEST CARE

Height and weight same? No.
Convert 5′ 4″ to total inches:

$$5 \text{ feet} \times \frac{12 \text{ inches}}{\text{foot}} = 60 \text{ inches} \quad 60 + 4 = 64 \text{ inches}$$

BSA based on adult height of 64 inches and weighs 150 pounds = 1.72 m². Total dosage:

$$\frac{360 \text{ mg}}{\text{m}^2} \times 1.72 \text{ m}^2 \text{ BSA} = 619 \text{ mg of Paraplatin}$$

Maximum concentration is 12 mg/mL × 100 mL = 1200 mg.
Does your answer fit the general guideline? Yes; 619 mg is less than 1200 mg.

Example 4

PRESCRIPTION

Determine carboplatin (paraplatin) 360 mg/m² using the mathematical formula for BSA:

$$BSA\ (m^2) = \sqrt{\frac{Ht(cm) \times Wt(kg)}{3600}}$$

• **What You HAVE**

Pharmacy label is as follows:
Solution: D₅W.
Volume total: 500 mL + Paraplatin.
Rate: 4 hours.

- **What You KNOW**

  Patient: 46-year-old female.
  Height: 5′ 4″.
  Weight: 150 lb.
  Maximum concentration is 10 mg/mL.
  Formula method requires metric units of measure for height and weight.

- **What You WANT**

  Height in total centimeters.
  Weight in kilograms.
  Total Paraplatin dosage.
  Maximum Paraplatin concentration for 500 mL.

CRITICAL THINKING

Convert height to total centimeters.
Convert weight to kilograms.
Enter numbers into formula and complete computation.

ANSWER FOR BEST CARE

Convert 5′ 4″ or 64 inches to total centimeters: 64 × 2.54 = 162.6 cm.
Convert weight in pounds (150 lb) to kilograms: 150/2.2 = 68.2 kg.

$$\sqrt{\frac{Ht(cm) \times Wt(kg)}{3600}}$$

162.6 cm (Ht) × 68.2 kg (Wt) = 11,089.3
11,089.3 ÷ 3600 = 3.08

Square root of 3.08 (use calculator) is 1.75 m² for BSA.
Total number of milligrams of Paraplatin = 1.75 m² × 360 mg/m² = 631.8, or 632 total mg (rounded) of Paraplatin.
Note that when using a nomogram the total dose of Paraplatin is 619 mg, and when using the mathematical formula the total dose of Paraplatin is 632 mg. The difference of 13 mg (632 − 619) will not make any clinical difference to patient outcome. Also noteworthy, when the difference between the BSA calculations (i.e., nomograms verus mathematical formula) is less than 50 mg there is no clinical significance.

PRACTICE PROBLEMS

Directions: *Determine the total dose of medication for adults using a nomogram and the mathematical formula for BSA. Give your final answer by rounding and including units of measure. The mathematical formula for BSA follows.*
Note: *Use this one nomogram for questions 1 through 10.*

$$BSA\ (m^2) = \sqrt{\frac{Ht(cm) \times Wt(kg)}{3600}}$$

1. Vincristine sulfate (Oncovin) 1.2 mg/m². Height = 6′ 0″; weight = 75 kg.

2. Rituximab (Rituxan) 375 mg/m². Height = 5′ 8″; weight = 180 lb.

3. Irinotecan hydrochloride (Camptosar) 125 mg/m². Height = 6′ 2″; weight = 278 lb.

4. Paclitaxel (Taxol) 135 mg/m². Height = 5′ 7″; weight = 185 lb.

5. Doxorubicin hydrochloride (Adriamycin) 20 mg/m². Height = 5′ 6″; weight = 72.72 kg.

6. Cisplatin (CDDP) 100 mg/m². Height = 5′ 9″; weight = 166 lb.

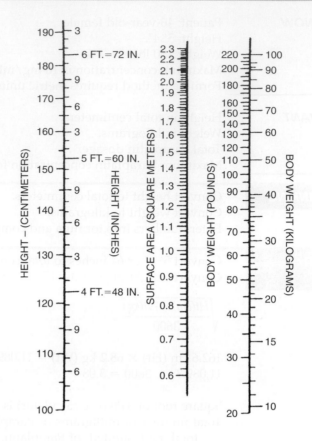

7. Fluorouracil (5-FU) 370 mg/m². Height = 5′ 9″; weight = 236 lb.

8. Methotrexate (MTX) 3.3 mg/m². Height = 6′ 1″; weight = 212 lb.

9. Epirubicin hydrochloride (Pharmorubicin) 100 mg/m². Height = 5′ 11″; weight = 144 lb.

10. Cyclophosphamide (Cytoxan) 500 mg/m². Height = 6′ 3″; weight = 275 lb.

(Answers on pp. 480–483)

CHAPTER REVIEW

Determine the total dose of medication for adults using a nomogram and the mathematical formula for BSA. Give your final answer by rounding and including units of measure. The mathematical formula for BSA follows. **Note:** Use this one nomogram for questions 1 through 20.

$$\sqrt{\frac{Ht(cm) \times Wt(kg)}{3600}}$$

1. Vincristine sulfate (Oncovin) 1.2 mg/m². Height = 6′ 0″; weight = 86 kg.

2. Rituximab (Rituxan) 375 mg/m². Height = 5′ 8″; weight = 136 lb.

3. Irinotecan hydrochloride (Camptosar) 125 mg/m². Height = 5′ 4″; weight = 164 lb.

4. Paclitaxel (Taxol) 135 mg/m². Height = 5′ 7″; weight = 127 lb.

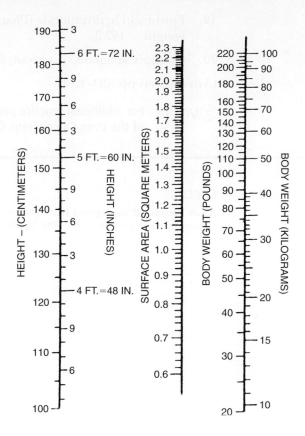

5. Doxorubicin hydrochloride (Adriamycin) 20 mg/m². Height = 5′ 6″; weight = 62 kg.

6. Cisplatin (CDDP) 100 mg/m². Height = 5′ 9″; weight = 142 lb.

7. Fluorouracil (5-FU) 370 mg/m². Height = 5′ 5″; weight = 168 lb.

8. Methotrexate (MTX) 3.3 mg/m². Height = 6′ 1″; weight = 152 lb.

9. Epirubicin hydrochloride (Pharmorubicin) 100 mg/m². Height = 5′ 11″; weight = 116 lb.

10. Cyclophosphamide (Cytoxan) 500 mg/m². Height = 5′ 7″; weight = 198 lb.

11. Vincristine sulfate (Oncovin) 1.2 mg/m². Height = 5′ 6″; weight = 66 kg.

12. Rituximab (Rituxan) 375 mg/m². Height = 5′ 8″; weight = 134 lb.

13. Irinotecan hydrochloride (Camptosar) 125 mg/m². Height = 6′ 2″; weight = 174 lb.

14. Paclitaxel (Taxol) 135 mg/m². Height = 5′ 5″; weight = 160 lb.

15. Doxorubicin hydrochloride (Adriamycin) 20 mg/m². Height = 5′ 2″; weight = 66 kg.

16. Cisplatin (CDDP) 100 mg/m². Height = 5′ 9″; weight = 144 lb.

17. Fluorouracil (5-FU) 370 mg/m². Height = 5′ 6″; weight = 112 lb.

18. Methotrexate (MTX) 3.3 mg/m². Height = 5′ 8″; weight = 150 lb.

19. Epirubicin hydrochloride (Pharmorubicin) 100 mg/m². Height = 5′ 11″; weight = 192 lb.

20. Cyclophosphamide (Cytoxan) 500 mg/m². Height = 5′ 4″; weight = 168 lb.

(Answers on pp. 483–488)

ⓔvolve **For additional practice problems, refer to the Pediatric Calculations section of the Drug Calculations Companion, version 4 on Evolve.**

CREDIT

Adult version of nomograms from Thelan LA, Urden LD, et al: *Critical care nursing: Diagnosis and management,* ed 3, St Louis, 1998, Mosby.

Pediatrics

Barbara Kiernan

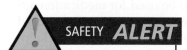

SAFETY ALERT

Any discrepancy between the MAR, current dose, and your calculations, warrants assistance from another professional.

SAFETY ALERT

It is important to obtain accurate measurements of both weight and height to use in calculating the doses of individual drugs.

INTRODUCTION

The administration of medications to children differs from that of adults in several ways. Children are not "little adults"; the physiology that makes them different must be considered when medications are part of the total nursing intervention and health care plan. The younger the infant or child is, the greater his or her metabolic rate, percentage of extracellular body fluid, and the body surface area. There are functional differences in the cardiovascular, renal, neurological, and gastrointestinal systems. These systems reach adult functioning at different chronological ages. All of these differences can alter the pharmacokinetics and pharmacodynamics of individual medications. *Pharmacokinetics*, or the movement of drugs through the body, is composed of absorption, distribution, biotransformation (or metabolism), and excretion. Pharmacodynamics is concerned with the effects of drugs on the body and the ways in which this process occurs. Nurses need to review and consult pharmacology texts and the specific drug literature to understand how individual infants and children, based on body weight and age, are affected by physiological and functional differences, then incorporate this knowledge into drug administration.

Medications for infants, children, and adolescents are prescribed on the basis of body weight or body surface area (see Chapters 8 and 20).

Infants and toddlers should be weighed nude, children and adolescents can be weighed with either underpants or lightweight undergarments. Children less than 2 years of age should be measured using the recumbent position (length), whereas older children can be measured using a stadiometer for accuracy. Height and weight are the important components of the body surface area.

In addition, nurses need to apply the principles of the "Six Rights" of drug administration (right drug, right dose, right time, right route, right client, right documentation) when working with pediatric patients and families. Nurses are responsible not only for administering medications to infants, children, and adolescents; they are also responsible for teaching the families and patients how to administer medications using these principles. Family education occurs during the period of hospitalization and after discharge to the home.

MEDICATION ADMINISTRATION

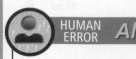

HUMAN ERROR *Alert*

Note that many medications should not be crushed because they can harm the patient due to altered drug effect or increased risk of clogging an enteral tube.

CLINICAL *ALERT*

Flavorings, such as bubble gum, grape, or orange, can often be added to liquid medications to increase the ease of taking medications. However, be careful that the flavoring is not psychologically correlated with other foods that the child may currently like to eat.

CLINICAL *ALERT*

The use of EMLA (eutectic mixture of local anesthetics) can be useful in decreasing the pain of intravenous starts.

Prescribed medications for infants and children are given by the oral, enteral, or parenteral routes. Oral medications can be liquids, powders, tablets, or capsules. The vehicle depends upon the child's age and ability to swallow. When taking a medicine by mouth becomes difficult or impossible because of oral problems; inability to chew, suck, or swallow; or upper gastrointestinal disorders, an enteral method of delivery may be used. Other enteral methods include oral gastric tubes (OG), nasogastric tubes (NG), nasojejunal tubes (NJ), gastrostomy tubes (GT), or suppository. The use of enteral methods will depend on the anticipated length of the regimen. If the medications are prescribed for chronic use, the health care team may decide that enteral methods are indicated. Liquids are recommended for enteral administration, although some tablets can be finely crushed, dissolved in a liquid vehicle such as a small amount of water or juice, and given through the appropriate tube. All tubes should be flushed with a few millimeters of water to clear the medication.

Parenteral medications may be given subcutaneously, intramuscularly, or intravenously. When giving parenteral medications, the correct route must be noted in the physician's prescription.

Oral Medications

Liquid preparations are used for infants and young children. They may be given by mouth or through an enteral tube. Some older children prefer liquids to pills because liquids are easier to swallow and may be more palatable. As children get older, the volume dose of a particular medication will increase to keep pace with either the kilograms or body surface area required by changes in growth (height and weight).

As children grow, it is important to continually assess their ability to swallow, because they may be ready to take medication as either tablets or capsules. For chronically ill children who are on daily medication regimens, making the administration of medicine as easy as possible promotes adherence to complex regimens. Children may be taught how to swallow tablets and capsules through a simple training process using graduated sizes of placebo or "sugar" pills. The process, called *shaping* (Czyzewski et al., 2000), is used when children demonstrate readiness to graduate to pills or tablets.

When preparing liquids for oral administration, it is critical that they be measured accurately. Oral medication syringes or droppers should be used for medication administration (Figure 21-1). These are calibrated in millimeters, as well as household measurements such as teaspoons. When the dose is less than 1 millimeter, it is helpful to use a 1-mL oral syringe to measure to the nearest hundredth. Liquid medication that has been measured can be placed in an empty nursing bottle nipple for the infant to suck as another possible way to ease administration.

Parenteral Medications

Some of the medications for parenteral use come prepared in liquid form and can be measured and drawn up in a syringe ready to administer according to the physician's order. Others come prepared as powders and will need to be diluted with sterile water, saline solution, or 1% lidocaine. Lidocaine 1% can be used according to the manufacturer's recommendations when specific drugs for intramuscular injection are particularly painful. It is important to read the drug insert that accompanies the drug to know exactly how much *diluent* to add (see Chapter 14). Knowing the concentration of drug in solution is necessary before proceeding with the calculation.

Pediatric medications are frequently administered intravenously for a number of reasons: medications are more effective using this route, children might be on a nothing-by-mouth regimen, the duration of a particular therapy is long term, immediate and continuous pain relief is needed, high serum concentrations of the medication are indicated, and gastrointestinal absorption is poor. Methods of intravenous

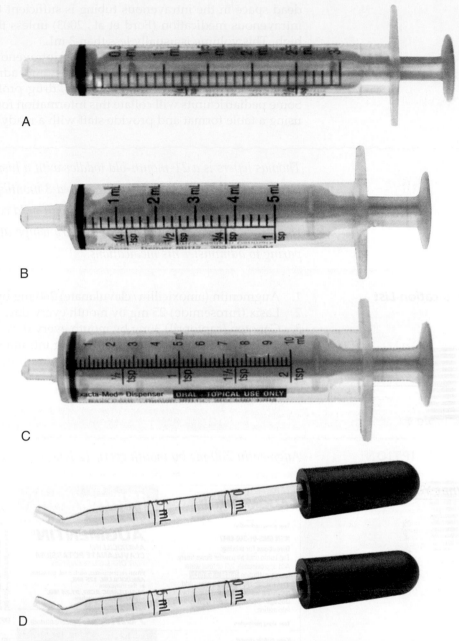

Figure 21-1 A, 3-mL oral syringe. B, 5-mL oral syringe. C, 10-mL oral syringe. D, Calibrated droppers.

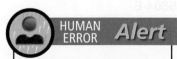

HUMAN ERROR *Alert*

When giving medications, it is important—regardless of the route—to verify that the drug prescribed is within the range for weight or body surface area. Checking the current *Physicians' Desk Reference* (2009), package insert, or reliable drug source for kilograms per recommended doses is helpful for assessing whether the drug and dose is within a safe range and for comparing the prescribed amount to the calculated maximum dose.

infusion include peripheral intravenous catheters, peripherally inserted central catheters (PICC lines), central lines, and long-term central venous access devices (VADs). The method used depends on the age and size of the child, duration of therapy, and desired accessibility for therapy.

The total fluid volume of children is based on individual age and size. Medications should use the least possible fluid volume to prevent fluid overload. Many of the intravenous medications are further diluted once the correct dose is calculated. Many individual medications list a maximum concentration per milliliter. The minimum fluid volume needed should be used.

A metered-volume chamber set (e.g., Buretrol) calibrated for a volume of 100 milliliters or less is often used as a safeguard as well as for providing a chamber for medication administration. After the medication has infused, the intravenous tubing can be flushed with intravenous fluid or normal saline. The tradition in practice has been to flush peripheral lines using 15 mL of solution or to flush central lines using 20 mL of solution, but research has recommended that using twice the volume of dead space in the intravenous tubing is sufficient to administer at least 95% of the intravenous medication (Ford et al., 2003) unless the viscosity of the medication is high. This volume is usually less than 3 mL.

Before administering any medication intravenously, it is important to carefully check the dosages, appropriate dilutions, and administration rates. These can be found in the manufacturer's guidelines, drug protocols, and hospital formularies. Some pediatric units will collate this information for the most commonly used drugs using a table format and provide staff with a ready reference tool.

Thomas Jeffers is a 21-month-old toddler with a history of congenital heart disease. He had a ventricular septal defect repaired 8 months before this admission. He was admitted to the pediatric unit yesterday with mild congestive heart failure and croup. He weighs 9.5 kg. Today he has an axillary temperature of 38° C. The nurse is preparing to administer his medications.

- **Medication List**
  1. Augmentin (amoxicillin/clavulanate) 200 mg by mouth every 12 hours.
  2. Lasix (furosemide) 25 mg by mouth every day.
  3. Capoten (captopril) 3 mg by mouth every day.
  4. Decadron (dexamethasone) 0.6 mg/kg intramuscular once at time of admission.
  5. Tylenol (acetaminophen) 120 mg by mouth every 6 hours when necessary for fever.

Example 1

PRESCRIPTION   *Augmentin 200 mg by mouth every 12 hours.*

- **What You HAVE**

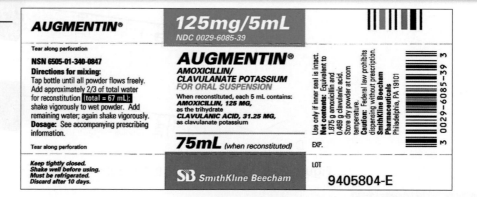

- **What You KNOW**

  Prescribed dose strength is Augmentin 200 mg.
  Patient is able to take a dose of medication by mouth.
  Weight is 9.5 kg.
  The range of medication dosing for this drug is 25 to 45 mg/kg/day.
  The medication is administered twice a day.

- **What You WANT**

  The total daily dose.
  Compare total daily dose with dose range.
  Dose volume required to administer Augmentin 200 mg.

CRITICAL THINKING   Are the prescribed medication and the medication you HAVE the same drug?

What is the diluent volume? _____

What is the solution strength? _____

Do the prescribed medication and the medication you HAVE use the same unit of measure? _____

Is the prescribed dose larger or smaller than the dose you HAVE? _____

Determine dose range by multiplying minimum and maximum range by patient weight in kilograms.

Compare total daily dose with dose range.

Determine dose volume by setting up a ratio-proportion. In the LEFT ratio, place the solution strength you HAVE; in the RIGHT ratio, place the dose strength you KNOW (what is prescribed) in the numerator and X in the denominator.

Multiply to get the cross-products.

Divide the numerical cross-product by the numerical multiplier of X (the number in front of X).

The result is the answer for X.

Label answer properly in milliliters.

Check answer by placing the number obtained for X in the original equation. Cross-multiply. The cross-products should be approximately equal.

Label bottle with reconstitution date, discard date, dose/volume, storage guidelines, and your initials.

ANSWER FOR BEST CARE

Medication comparison? Yes.

Reconstitute with 67 mL tap water.

Solution strength? 125 mg/5 mL.

Unit of measure comparison? Yes.

Dose larger.

Perform calculation.

To calculate the range of dosage, multiply by each range:

Low range: 9.5 kg × 20 mg = 190 mg.

High range: 9.5 kg × 50 mg = 475 mg.

The range of dosage is 190 to 475 mg/day.

Child receives 200 mg twice a day or every 12 hours, so the child receives 400 mg/day. Total dose is within dose range.

Dose volume calculation:

$$\frac{125 \text{ mL}}{5 \text{ mL}} = \frac{200 \text{ mg}}{X \text{ mL}}$$

Reduce.

$$\frac{25}{1} = \frac{200}{X}$$

125 X = 200   X = 8

Dose volume is 8 mL.

> ✔ **Human Error Check**
>
> Replace X with 8.
>
> $$\frac{125}{5} = \frac{200}{8}$$
>
> 1000 = 1000

SAFETY ALERT

Always check patient's identification band with identifying information found on the chart and compare with medication orders.

SAFETY ALERT

Always double- or triple-check your calculations with other professionals such as nurses, pharmacists, and physicians.

SAFETY ALERT

Check medication for interactions with other medications the patient may be taking.

SAFETY ALERT

Shake suspensions well just before measuring.

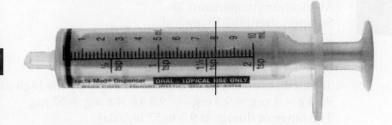

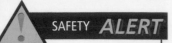

SAFETY ALERT

Use a medication syringe that will measure the dose correctly.

Bottle label:
Date/Time
Discard date 60 days hence
125 mg/5 mL
Room temperature
Initials
Does your answer fit the general guideline? The amount given each day (400 mg) does not exceed the acceptable range (190 to 450 mg/day).

Example 2

PRESCRIPTION *Lasix 25 mg by mouth daily.*

- **What You HAVE** Lasix oral solution 10 mg/mL.

- **What You KNOW** Prescribed dose strength is 25 mg.
  Patient is able to take a dose of medication by mouth.
  Weight is 9.5 kg.
  The range of medication dosing for this drug is 1 to 6 mg/kg/day.
  The medication is administered once a day.
  Store at controlled room temperature (59° F to 86° F).
  Discard opened bottle after 60 days.

- **What You WANT** The total daily dose.
  Compare total daily dose with dose range.
  Dose volume necessary to administer Lasix 25 mg.

CRITICAL THINKING Are the prescribed medication and the medication you HAVE the same drug? _____

What is the solution strength? _____
Do the prescribed medication and the medication you HAVE use the same unit of measure? _____
Is the prescribed dose larger or smaller than the dose you HAVE? _____
Determine dose range by multiplying minimum and maximum range by patient weight in kilograms.
Compare total daily dose with dose range.
Determine dose volume by setting up a ratio-proportion. In the LEFT ratio, place the solution strength you HAVE; in the RIGHT ratio, place the dose strength you KNOW (what is prescribed) in the numerator and X in the denominator.
Multiply to get the cross-products.
Divide the numerical cross-product by the numerical multiplier of X (the number in front of X).
The result is the answer for X.
Label answer properly in milliliters.
Check answer by placing the number obtained for X in the original equation. Cross-multiply. The cross-products should be approximately equal.
Label bottle with reconstitution date, discard date, dose/volume, storage guidelines, and your initials.

ANSWER FOR BEST CARE Medication comparison? Yes.
Solution strength? 10 mg/mL.
Unit of measure comparison? Yes.
Dose larger.
Perform calculation.
To calculate the range of dosage, multiply by the high and low range:
9.5 kg × 1 mg = 9.5 mg   9.5 kg × 6 mg = 57 mg
The range of dosage is 9.5 to 57 mg/day.

- **What You KNOW**

Prescribed dose strength is 0.6 mg/kg.
The range of medication dosing for this drug is 0.5 to 9 mg for the initial dose.
Weight is 9.5 kg.
The medication is administered as a one-time dose.

- **What You WANT**

Total dose strength based in milligrams.
Compare dose with dose range.
Dose volume necessary to administer calculated dose strength.

CRITICAL THINKING

Are the prescribed medication and the medication you HAVE the same drug? _____

Do the prescribed medication and the medication you HAVE use the same unit of measure? _____

Is the prescribed dose larger or smaller than the dose you HAVE? _____

Determine dose range by multiplying minimum and maximum range by patient weight in kilograms.

Compare total daily dose with dose range.

Determine total dose strength in milligrams by multiplying dose strength by patient weight in kilograms.

Determine dose volume by setting up a ratio-proportion. In the LEFT ratio, place the solution strength you HAVE; in the RIGHT ratio, place the dose strength you KNOW (what is prescribed) in the numerator and X in the denominator.

Multiply to get the cross-products.

Divide the numerical cross-product by the numerical multiplier of X (the number in front of X).

The result is the answer for X.

Label answer properly in milliliters.

Check answer by placing the number obtained for X in the original equation. Cross-multiply. The cross-products should be approximately equal.

Label bottle with reconstitution date, discard date, dose/volume, storage guidelines, and your initials.

ANSWER FOR BEST CARE

Medication comparison? Yes.
Solution strength? 4 mg/mL.
Unit of measure comparison? Yes.
Dose larger.
Perform calculation.
Total dose strength calculation:
9.5 kg × 0.6 mg = 5.7 mg
Child receives 5.7 mg once upon admission.
Initial dose is within range (0.5 to 9 mg).
Total volume calculation:

$$\frac{4 \text{ mg}}{1 \text{ mL}} = \frac{5.7 \text{ mg}}{X \text{ mL}}$$

4X = 5.7

X = 1.42 mL (round to the nearest tenth)

Dose is 1.4 mL.

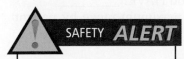

SAFETY ALERT

The FDA warned parents not to give children younger than 1 year over-the-counter cough or cold medicines unless given specific directions to do so by a health care provider.

✓ **Human Error Check**

Replace X with 1.4.

$$\frac{4}{1} = \frac{5.7}{1.42}$$

5.68 ≈ 5.7

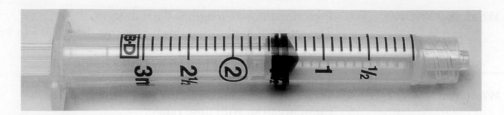

Example 5

PRESCRIPTION	*Tylenol 120 mg by mouth every 6 hours when necessary for fever.*

- **What You HAVE**

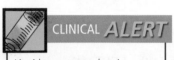

CLINICAL ALERT

Liquid acetomenophen is commonly sold in two strengths: infant drops (1.6 mL = 160 mg) and children's suspension (5 mL = 160 mg).

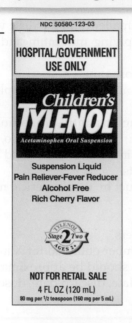

NDC 50580-123-03

FOR HOSPITAL/GOVERNMENT USE ONLY

Children's TYLENOL
Acetaminophen Oral Suspension

Suspension Liquid
Pain Reliever-Fever Reducer
Alcohol Free
Rich Cherry Flavor

Stage **2** Two
AGES 2+

NOT FOR RETAIL SALE
4 FL OZ (120 mL)
80 mg per ¹/₂ teaspoon (160 mg per 5 mL)

- **What You KNOW**

Prescribed dose strength is 120 mg.
Patient is able to take a dose of medication by mouth.
Weight is 9.5 kg.
The medication dosing for this drug is 10 to 15 mg/kg/dose every 4 to 6 hours.
The medication is administered every 6 hours as necessary to treat fever.

- **What You WANT**

Calculate dose range.
Compare dose with dose range.
Dose volume necessary to administer Tylenol 120 mg.

CRITICAL THINKING	Are the prescribed medication and the medication you HAVE the same drug? _____

Do the prescribed medication and the medication you HAVE use the same unit of measure? _____
Is the prescribed dose larger or smaller than the dose you HAVE? _____
Determine dose range by multiplying minimum and maximum range by patient weight in kilograms.
Compare dose with dose range.
Determine dose volume by setting up a ratio-proportion. In the LEFT ratio, place the solution strength you HAVE; in the RIGHT ratio, place the dose strength you KNOW (what is prescribed) in the numerator and X in the denominator.
Multiply to get the cross-products.
Divide the numerical cross-product by the numerical multiplier of X (the number in front of X).
The result is the answer for X.

Label answer properly in milliliters.

Check answer by placing the number obtained for X in the original equation. Cross-multiply. The cross-products should be approximately equal.

Label bottle with reconstitution date, discard date, dose/volume, storage guidelines, and your initials.

ANSWER FOR BEST CARE	Medication comparison? Yes.

Solution strength? 160 mg/5 mL.

Unit of measurement comparison? Yes.

Dose smaller.

Perform calculation.

Calculate the range of dosage by multiplying:

9.5 kg × 10 mg = 95 mg   9.5 kg × 15 mg = 142.5 mg

The range of dosage is 95 to 142.5 mg/dose.

Child receives 120 mg/dose. This is within the dose range.

Dose volume calculation:

$$\frac{160 \text{ mg}}{5 \text{ mL}} = \frac{120 \text{ mg}}{X \text{ mL}}$$

Reduce:

$$\frac{32}{1} = \frac{120}{X}$$

$$32X = 120$$

$$X = 3.75 \text{ (round to the nearest tenth)}$$

$$X = 3.8$$

✓ **Human Error Check**

Replace X with 3.75.

$$\frac{160}{5} = \frac{120}{3.75}$$

$$600 = 600$$

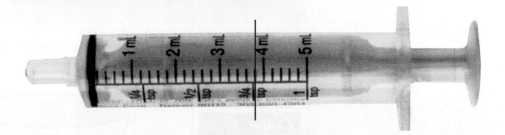

Does your answer fit the general guideline? The amount given in each dose (120 mg) does not exceed the acceptable range of 95 to 142.5 mg/dose.

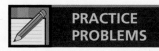 **PRACTICE PROBLEMS**	Directions: *Read the following patient scenarios and then answer each question. Mark the oral syringe where you would pull the plunger back to, mark the syringe, or mark the medicine cup.*

1. Merilee Bennington is a 12-year-old girl who was diagnosed with cystic fibrosis at age 4. She is admitted to the pediatric unit with a diagnosis of pulmonary exacerbation, weight loss, and thrush. She has an intravenous line of D_5 ½ NS to keep the vein open (KVO). Her weight is 31.4 kg. Last week during a clinic visit, she weighed 74 pounds. The nurse is preparing to administer her medications.

Medication list:
Vancomycin, 400 mg intravenous every 8 hours.
Ranitidine hydrochloride (Zantac), 75 mg by mouth twice a day.
Piperacillin sodium and tazobactam sodium (Zosyn), 2 grams intravenous every 8 hours; infuse over 30 minutes.
Pancrease MT 20, 3 capsules by mouth with meals; can give 1 to 3 capsules with snacks.
Vitamin ADEK, 1 capsule by mouth every day.
Fluticasone propionate (Flonase) nasal spray, 2 sprays each nostril twice a day.
Dornase alfa recombinant (Pulmozyme), 2.5 mg by mouth twice a day.
Advair 250/50, 1 spray twice a day.
Nystatin, 4 mL by mouth 4 times a day swish and swallow.

A. How much weight has Merilee lost since last week? _____
B. PRESCRIPTION: vancomycin 400 mg intravenous every 8 hours.
    HAVE: 20 mL sterile water added to reconstitute powder.

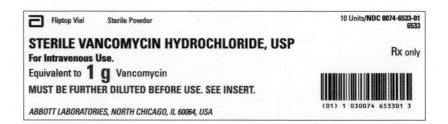

Fliptop Vial	Sterile Powder	10 Units/NDC 0074-6533-01

STERILE VANCOMYCIN HYDROCHLORIDE, USP
For Intravenous Use.   Rx only
Equivalent to **1 g** Vancomycin
MUST BE FURTHER DILUTED BEFORE USE. SEE INSERT.

ABBOTT LABORATORIES, NORTH CHICAGO, IL 60064, USA   (01) 1 030074 653301 3

How many milliliters of medication are added to minibag? _____

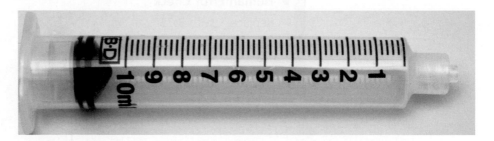

C. PRESCRIPTION: Zantac 75 mg by mouth twice a day.
    HAVE:

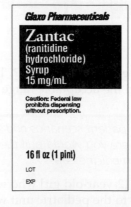

Glaxo Pharmaceuticals
Zantac
(ranitidine hydrochloride)
Syrup
15 mg/mL

Caution: Federal law prohibits dispensing without prescription.

16 fl oz (1 pint)
LOT
EXP

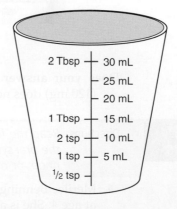

How many milliliters will you give? _____
D. PRESCRIPTION: Zosyn 2 g intravenous every 9 hours.
    HAVE: Zosyn 2.5 g/10 mL for intravenous infusion.

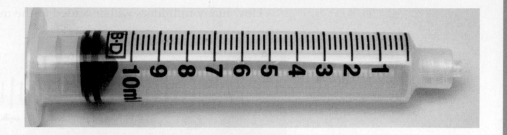

How many milliliters of intravenous medication do you administer? _____

E. Pancrease MT 20 is an enzyme preparation—consisting of 20,000 units of lipase; 56,000 units of amylase; and 44,000 units of protease—that aids in the digestion of food. The dose is based on the lipase fraction. The dose can range from 400 lipase units/kg/meal to 2500 lipase units/kg/meal. Merilee is receiving 3 capsules with each meal; is her dose within the normal range? _____

2. Zachary Simmons is an 8-month-old who is admitted with respiratory distress. He was born at 25 weeks' gestation and subsequently developed bronchopulmonary dysplasia. He has a tracheostomy tube that is connected to a ventilator for part of the day as well as a nasogastric (NG) tube for feedings. He weighs 6 kg. The nurse is preparing to administer medications to Zachary.

Medication list:
Clindamycin (Cleocin), 60 mg intravenous every 6 hours for 10 days.
Tobramycin (Nebcin), 15 mg intravenous every 8 hours for 10 days.
Rifampin, 75 mg via the nasogastric tube once a day.
Pulmicort, 0.5 mg by inhalation twice a day.
Albuterol, 2.5 mg by inhalation 4 times a day.
Ibuprofen (Motrin), 60 mg per nasogastric tube every 6 hours for fever or pain.
Palivizumab (Synagis), 90 mg intramuscular before discharge.

A. PRESCRIPTION: rifampin 75 mg per nasogastric tube.
HAVE: rifampin 20 mg/mL suspension.
How much will you give via the nasogastric tube? _____

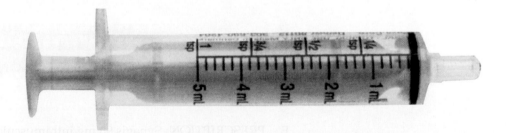

B. PRESCRIPTION: clindamycin 60 mg intravenous every 6 hours.
HAVE:

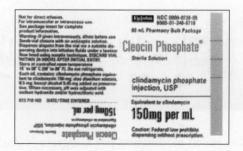

How many milliliters will be added to the minibag intravenous line? _____

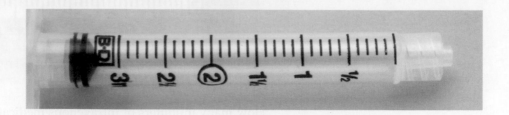

C. PRESCRIPTION: tobramycin 15 mg intravenous every 8 hours.
    HAVE:

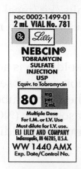

NDC 0002-1499-01
2 mL VIAL No. 781
℞ *Lilly*
NEBCIN®
TOBRAMYCIN
SULFATE
INJECTION
USP
Equiv. to Tobramycin
80 mg
per
2 mL
Multiple Dose
For I.M. or I.V. Use
Must dilute for I.V. use.
ELI LILLY AND COMPANY
Indianapolis, IN 46285, U.S.A.
WW 1440 AMX
Exp. Date/Control No.

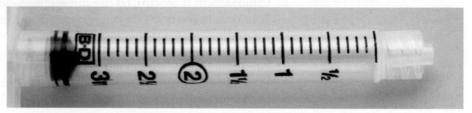

D. PRESCRIPTION: Motrin 60 mg via nasogastric tube.
    HAVE: Motrin 40 mg/mL suspension.
    How much will you give via the nasogastric tube? _____

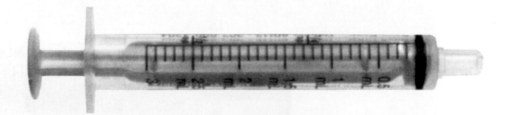

E. PRESCRIPTION: Synagis 90 mg intramuscular before discharge.
    HAVE: Synagis 100 mg/mL.
    How much will you give by injection? _____

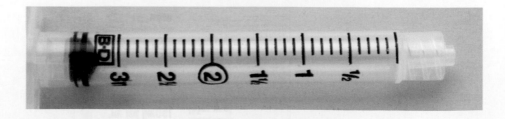

How much medication per kilogram is Zachary receiving? _____

3. Maxine Talbot is a 15-year-old with end-stage renal disease (ESRD) who is admitted with vomiting and fever. She has the following comorbidities: pancreatitis, anemia, depression, and hypertension. She has an intravenous line of D₅ ½ NS running at 40 mL/hour. She weighs 42.8 kg. The nurse is preparing to administer medications to Maxine.

Medication list:
Ondansetron hydrochloride (Zofran) 4 mg by mouth three times a day whenever necessary for nausea.
Vancomycin, 430 mg intravenous piggyback once after admission.
Gentamicin (Garamycin), 35 mg intravenous piggyback once after admission.
Amlodipine (Norvasc), 10 mg by mouth every day.
Metoclopramide (Reglan), 5 mg by mouth every 6 hours.
Sertraline hydrochloride (Zoloft), 75 mg by mouth every day.
Omeprazole (Prilosec), 20 mg by mouth twice a day.

A. PRESCRIPTION: vancomycin 440 mg intravenous piggyback for one dose after admission.
HAVE: Reconstituted with 20 mL sterile water.

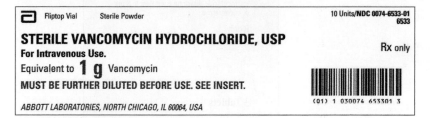

Vancomycin label:
Fliptop Vial   Sterile Powder   10 Units/NDC 0074-6533-01   6533
STERILE VANCOMYCIN HYDROCHLORIDE, USP
For Intravenous Use.   Rx only
Equivalent to **1 g** Vancomycin
MUST BE FURTHER DILUTED BEFORE USE. SEE INSERT.
ABBOTT LABORATORIES, NORTH CHICAGO, IL 60064, USA
(01) 1 030074 653301 3

How many milliliters are added to the 100-mL minibag? _____

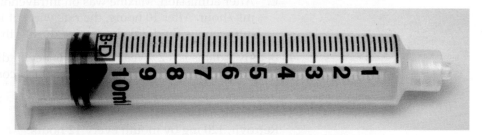

B. PRESCRIPTION: gentamicin 35 mg intravenous piggyback once after admission.
HAVE:

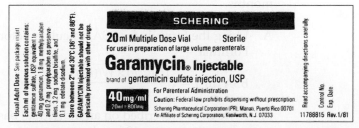

Garamycin label:
Usual Adult Dose See package insert
Each ml of aqueous solution contains: gentamicin sulfate, USP equivalent to 40 mg gentamicin, 1.8 mg methylparaben and 0.2 mg propylparaben as preservatives, 3.2 mg sodium bisulfite, and 0.1 mg edetate disodium.
Store between 2° and 30°C (36° and 86°F). GARAMYCIN Injectable should not be physically premixed with other drugs.
SCHERING
20 ml Multiple Dose Vial   Sterile
For use in preparation of large volume parenterals
Garamycin® Injectable
brand of gentamicin sulfate injection, USP
40mg/ml   For Parenteral Administration
20ml = 800mg   Caution: Federal law prohibits dispensing without prescription.
Schering Pharmaceutical Corporation (PR), Manati, Puerto Rico 00701
An Affiliate of Schering Corporation, Kenilworth, N.J. 07033
11788815 Rev.1/81
Read accompanying directions carefully.
Control No   Exp. Date

How many milliliters of medication are added to the 50-mL minibag? ____

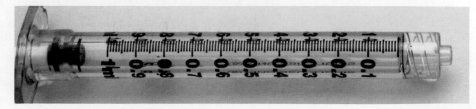

C. PRESCRIPTION: Zoloft 75 mg by mouth every day.
   HAVE: Zoloft 50-mg scored tablets.
   How many tablets will you give? _____

D. PRESCRIPTION: Zofran 4 mg by mouth three times a day whenever necessary for nausea.
   HAVE:

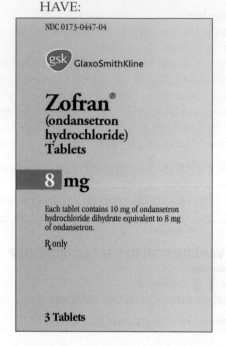

How many tablets will you give? _____

E. After admission, Maxine was on intravenous fluids running at 40 mL/hour. After 10 hours, the rate was cut to 35 mL/hour. How much intravenous fluid did she receive during the first 24-hour period? _____

4. Betony Adams is a 2½ year old who is newly diagnosed with HIV infection. She is to be started on antiretroviral therapy consisting of retrovir, Videx, and Kaletra. She weighs 13 kg and is 90 cm long.

Medication list:
Retrovir, 120 mg by mouth every 12 hours.
Didanosine (Videx), 70 mg by mouth every 12 hours on an empty stomach.
Kaletra, 2 mL by mouth every 12 hours.
Amantadine (Symmetrel), 65 mg by mouth every day during the winter months.

A. Using the formula for BSA, calculate Betony's body surface area. _____
   Formula =

   $$BSA\ (m^2) = \sqrt{\dfrac{Ht(cm) \times Wt(kg)}{3600}}$$

B. Retrovir is prescribed on an individual basis ranging from 180 to 240 mg/m² per dose every 12 hrs. It comes as a syrup with a concentration of 10

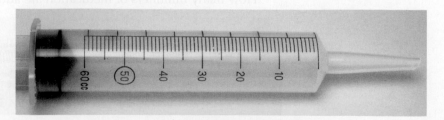

mg/mL. She is prescribed 120 mg every 12 hours. Is this dose within the acceptable range? _____
How much will the nurse administer? _____

C. Videx is prescribed on an individual basis ranging from 90 to 150 mg/m² per dose. It comes as a solution with a concentration of 10 mg/mL. She is prescribed 70 mg every 12 hours. Is this dose within the acceptable range? _____
How much will the nurse administer? _____

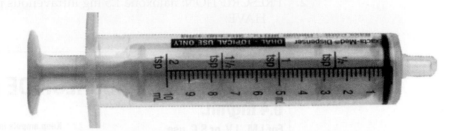

D. PRESCRIPTION: amantadine 65 mg.
HAVE: amantadine 50 mg/5 mL.
How much will you give? _____

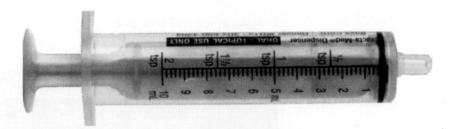

E. Betony is to receive Kaletra, which is a combination drug composed of two medications: lopinavir and ritonavir. Each milliliter of Kaletra has 80 milligrams of lopinavir and 20 milligrams of ritonavir. How many milligrams of each medication is she receiving with each dose? _____

(Answers on pp. 488–490)

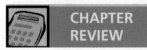 **CHAPTER REVIEW**

Answer the following questions. Mark the syringes.

1. PRESCRIPTION: meperidine 29 mg intramuscular.
HAVE:

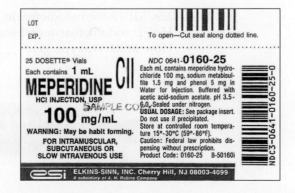

How much will you give? _____

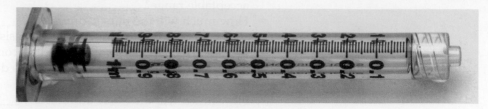

2. PRESCRIPTION: naloxone 1.5 mg intravenous push now.
    HAVE:

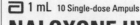

▱ 1 mL 10 Single-dose Ampuls	NDC 0074-1212-01

NALOXONE HYDROCHLORIDE Injection, USP
0.4 mg/mL
For I.M., I.V. or S.C. use.

Protect from light.
Keep ampuls in tray until time of use.

Each mL contains naloxone hydrochloride 0.4 mg; sodium chloride added to adjust
tonicity. pH adjusted with hydrochloric acid. 0.31 mOsmol/mL (calc.). pH 4.0 (3.0 to 6.5).
Usual dosage: See insert. Store at 15° to 30°C (59° to 86°F).   ℞ only

©Abbott 1996, 2002   Printed in USA

ABBOTT LABORATORIES, NORTH CHICAGO, IL 60064, USA   58-2852-2/R8-11/01   EXP
                                                                        LOT

How much will you give? _____

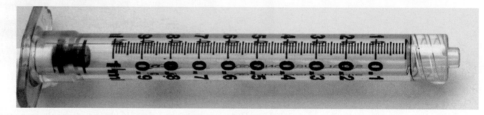

3. PRESCRIPTION: lamivudine 75 mg by mouth.
    HAVE: lamivudine oral solution = 10 mg/mL.
    How much will you give? _____

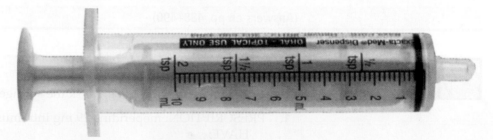

4. PRESCRIPTION: indomethacin 14 mg by mouth.
    HAVE: indomethacin oral suspension = 25 mg/5 mL.
    How much will you give? _____

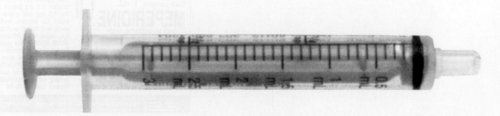

5.   PRESCRIPTION: pseudoephedrine 13 mg by mouth.
     HAVE: pseudoephedrine oral syrup = 15 mg/5 mL.
     How much will you give? _____

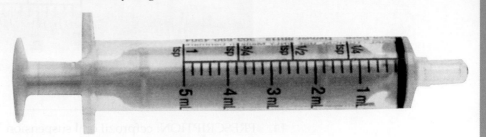

6.   PRESCRIPTION: promethazine 9.25 mg by mouth.
     HAVE: promethazine oral syrup = 6.25 mg/5 mL.
     How much will you give? _____

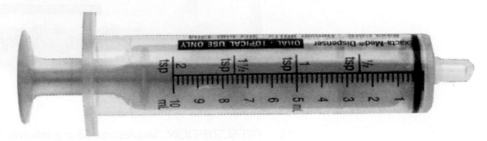

7.   PRESCRIPTION: valproic acid 367.5 mg by mouth.
     HAVE: valproic acid oral syrup = 250 mg/5 mL.
     How much will you give? _____

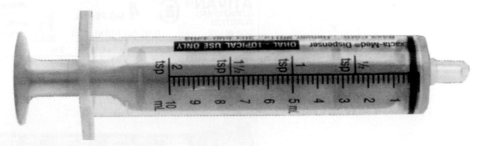

8.   PRESCRIPTION: griseofulvin 400 mg by mouth.
     HAVE: griseofulvin oral suspension = 125 mg/5 mL.
     How much will you give? _____

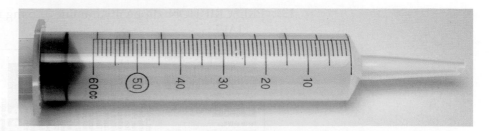

9.   PRESCRIPTION: fosamprenavir 1400 mg by mouth.
     HAVE: fosamprenavir 700 mg per capsules.
     How much will you give? _____

10.   PRESCRIPTION: albuterol 1.6 mg by mouth.
      HAVE: albuterol oral syrup = 2 mg/5 mL.

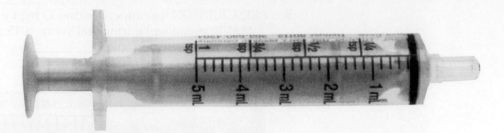

How much will you give? _____

11. PRESCRIPTION: cefprozil oral suspension 330 mg by mouth.
    HAVE: cefprozil oral suspension = 250 mg/5 mL.
    How much will you give? _____

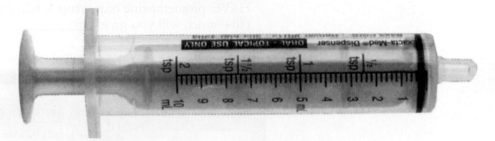

12. PRESCRIPTION: lorazepam 1.8 mg intramuscular.
    HAVE:

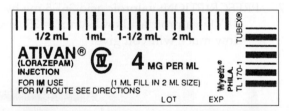

How much will you give? _____

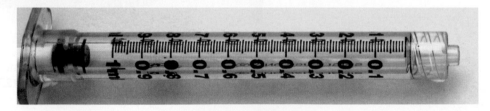

13. PRESCRIPTION: diphenhydramine 32.5 mg intramuscular.
    HAVE:

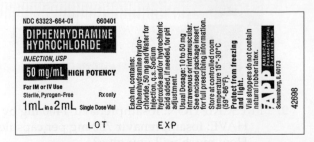

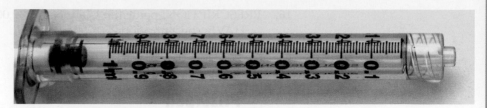

How much will you give? _____

14. PRESCRIPTION: fentanyl citrate 42 mcg intramuscular.
    HAVE:

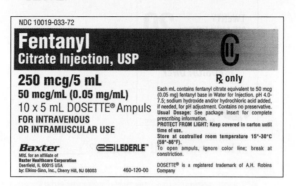

How much will you give? _____

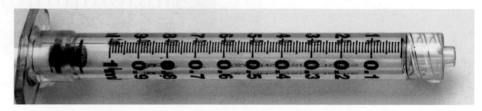

15. PRESCRIPTION: acyclovir 240 mg intravenous.
    HAVE: acyclovir solution for intravenous infusion = 500 mg/10 mL.
    How much will you give? _____

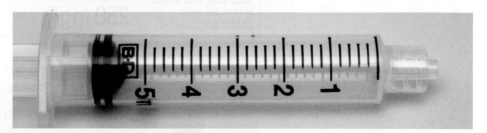

16. PRESCRIPTION: penicillin G aqueous 230,000 units intravenous.
     HAVE: concentration 250,000 units/mL.

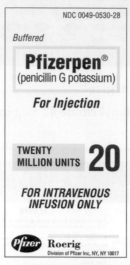

NDC 0049-0530-28

Buffered

Pfizerpen®
(penicillin G potassium)

For Injection

TWENTY
MILLION UNITS **20**

*FOR INTRAVENOUS
INFUSION ONLY*

Pfizer **Roerig**
Division of Pfizer Inc, NY, NY 10017

How much will you give? _____

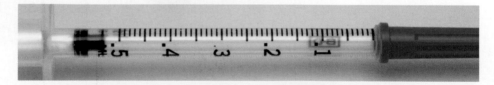

17. PRESCRIPTION: hydrocortisone sodium succinate 60 mg intravenous.
     HAVE:

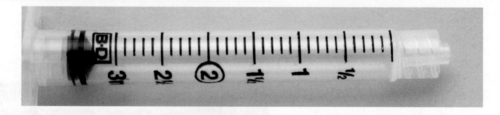

Single-Dose Vial   For IV or IM use
Contains Benzyl Alcohol as a Preservative
See package insert for complete
product information.
Per 2 mL (when mixed):
• hydrocortisone sodium succinate equiv.
to hydrocortisone, 250 mg. Protect
solution from light. Discard after 3 days.

814 070 205 Reconstituted ....

The Upjohn Company
Kalamazoo, MI 49001, USA

2 mL Act-O-Vial®   NDC 0009-0909-08

Solu-Cortef® Sterile Powder
hydrocortisone sodium succinate
for injection, USP

250 mg*

How much will you give? _____

18. PRESCRIPTION: metaclopramide 0.68 mg by mouth.
     HAVE: metaclopramide syrup = 5 mg/5 mL.
     How much will you give? _____

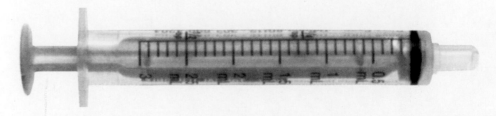

19. PRESCRIPTION: phenytoin 67.5 mg.
     HAVE:

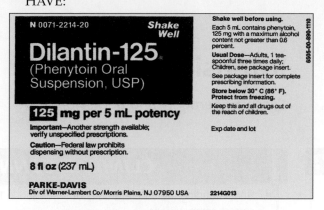

How much will you give? _____

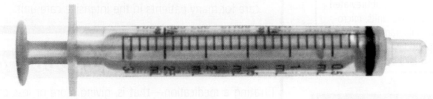

20. PRESCRIPTION: erythromycin 300 mg by mouth.
     HAVE:

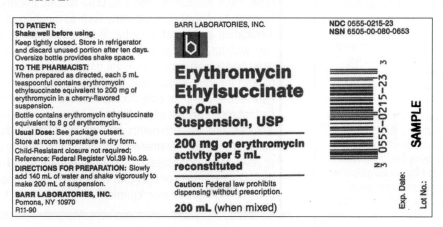

How much will you give? _____

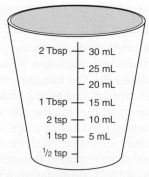

(Answers on pp. 490–491)

⊖volve   **For additional practice problems, refer to the Pediatric Calculations section
            of the Drug Calculations Companion, version 4 on Evolve.**

Intensive Care Unit

Cynthia Chernecky and Becki Hodges

SAFETY ALERT

Note that the unit called the *microgram*, also known by the abbreviation mcg, is different from the milligram, abbreviated as mg. These two units, microgram and milligram, are often misinterpreted when written and spoken, so take extra caution.

HUMAN ERROR Alert

In general, medications that are titrated hold a greater risk of lethality if errors occur than medications that do not require titration. Therefore, it is not unusual to have institutional policies requiring double- or triple-checking of all drug dosages and the associated mathematical computations. You may also double-check your calculation by using the World Wide Web site http://www.globalrph.com/drip.htm. Some electronic pumps have ready-access calculators attached within the pump to make calculations easier.

CLINICAL CONNECTION

- Understanding the different units of time used in titrating medications is critical to correct computations.
- Calculating titrations based on prescriptions is absolutely critical to following a plan of care for many patients in the intensive care unit.

INTRODUCTION

Titrating a medication—that is, giving more or less of a medication based on assessment parameters—requires knowing the prescription, the solution concentration (strength/volume) that you have on hand, and the infusion rate required to administer the prescribed dose. Each medication also has drug-specific information that is necessary for the nurse to know to deliver effective care, such as duration of onset of the medication, peak effect, medication antagonist, time frame for reassessment, and consequences of sudden medication withdrawal. Titration prescriptions should include the purpose for titrating (i.e., chest pain) and a maximum dose. From this information, a titration table that includes increments of both the intravenous infusion rate and the drug dosage is often designed and kept on the intravenous pump for easy access. Increments are determined by the relationship of dose to patient response. Usually, if the dose range is small, increments are small; if the dose range is wider, then the increments used for the titration chart are larger. Most titration prescriptions also include parameters (i.e., blood pressure, respiratory rate, pulse rate, temperature, or level of consciousness), or parameters are found in specific facility protocols. Typically the administration consists of a dose per unit of time—either in mcg/min, mg/min, mg/hr, units/hr, mg/kg/hr or mcg/kg/min.

TITRATION

SAFETY ALERT

Never exceed the prescribed upper dose limit. Notify the physician when the maximum limit is reached, and be prepared because a different medication may be prescribed.

The majority of titrated medications are prescribed in mcg/min or mg/hr. Each prescription should include a minimum infusion dose (the dose at which the infusion is started) and the dose rate. The infusion rate is then adjusted based on the parameters defined in the prescription. Just as important as the correct dosage is the knowledge regarding the frequency of making the adjustments based upon patient assessment and prescribed parameters. Electronic pumps are used with critical drugs that are titrated.

Titration problems can, like all drug calculations, be computed using the ratio-proportion method demonstrated throughout this book. Understanding this method permits anyone to solve a computation without recalling a memorized formula. This is particularly helpful if the formula is not being used on a regular basis and has been forgotten. The following problems will be solved using both the ratio-proportion method and the common formula. This will enable you to see that—although the problem looks complicated—you can determine the information required even when you have forgotten the formula. As discussed in Chapter 16, knowing mL/hr

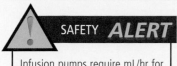

SAFETY ALERT

Infusion pumps require mL/hr for programming.

is required to program electronic pumps. Critical medications are always infused by electronic pump and can accept one decimal place. Final answers should be rounded to the nearest tenth.

Reading the prescription carefully is very important in intensive care. Units of measure, weight, and/or time will often need conversion in order to complete the calculation for determining mL/hr. In the following examples, computations will use the ratio-proportion method, followed by the common formula method. When using the common formula instead of ratio-proportion, the total volume (mL) is placed in the numerator instead of the denominator. As shown, either method results in the correct answer.

Example 1

PRESCRIPTION | *Start nitroglycerin at 10 micrograms/minute (mcg/min) for chest pain for acute myo-cardial infarction (AMI) and titrate for chest pain to maximum 80 mcg/min and also keep systolic blood pressure greater than 100 mm Hg (torr).*

• **What You HAVE** | Pharmacy label:
Solution NS.
Volume 250 mL.
Nitroglycerin 50 mg.

• **What You KNOW** | Prescribed is nitroglycerin; dose range is 10 mcg/min to 80 mcg/min.

• **What You WANT** | Nitroglycerin dose volume per hour.
Compute a minimum/maximum titration table of intravenous rate for each incremental dose.

CRITICAL THINKING | Are the units of measure of what you HAVE and what you KNOW the same? _____

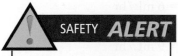

SAFETY ALERT

Any discrepancy between the MAR, current dose and your calculations, warrants assistance from another professional.

Will conversion calculations be necessary? _____
In setting up a ratio-proportion, place the nitroglycerin total strength per volume you HAVE on the LEFT; on the RIGHT, place the mg/hr you calculated in the numerator and X in the denominator.
Multiply to get the cross-products.
Divide the numerical cross-product by the numerical multiplier of X (the number in front of X).
The result is the answer for X.
Label the answer properly in mL/hr.
To develop a titration table at 10-mcg increases using the ratio-proportion method, place the dose strength per volume you HAVE on the LEFT; on the RIGHT, place the incremental dose strength in the numerator and X in the denominator. Complete the calculation. Repeat for each increment to the maximum limit (80 mcg).
Check all answers by placing the number obtained for X in the original equation. Cross-multiply. The cross-products should be approximately equal.
Alternately, use the formula: mL/mg × mcg/min × min/hr × mg/mcg.

ANSWER FOR BEST CARE | Units of measure are not the same.
Conversions are necessary for units of measure and time.
Convert micrograms to milligrams.
10 mcg = 0.01 mg (remember that you drop zeros to the right of the last digit to the right of the decimal point).
Convert mg/min to mg/hr by multiplying by 60.

0.01 mg × 60 minutes = 0.6 mg/hr

(HAVE)

$$\frac{50 \text{ mg}}{250 \text{ mL}} = \frac{0.6 \text{ mg}}{X \text{ mL}}$$

50X = 150

X = 3 mL/hr

✔ **Human Error Check**

Replace X with 3.

$$\frac{50}{250} = \frac{0.6}{3}$$

50 × 3 = 250 × 0.6
150 = 150

The dose volume for 10 mcg/min is 3 mL/hr.
Alternately, use the formula: mL/mg × mcg/min × min/hr × mg/mcg.

	(Prescribed start rate)	(Hourly conversion)	(mg/mcg conversion)		

(HAVE)

$$\frac{250 \text{ mL (Total volume)}}{50 \text{ mg (Total strength)}} \times \frac{10 \text{ mcg}}{1 \text{ min}} \times \frac{60 \text{ min}}{1 \text{ hr}} \times \frac{1 \text{ mg}}{1000 \text{ mcg}} = \frac{150,000}{50,000} = \frac{3 \text{ mL}}{1 \text{ hr}}$$

Titration table for NTG: 50 mg/250 mL concentration.
Develop a titration chart using 10-mcg increments.

HAVE

$$\frac{10 \text{ mcg}}{3 \text{ mL}} = \frac{20 \text{ mcg}}{X \text{ mL}}$$ (10-mcg increase) 10 X = 60 mcg X = 6 mL/hr

$$\frac{10 \text{ mcg}}{3 \text{ mL}} = \frac{30 \text{ mcg}}{X \text{ mL}}$$ (10-mcg increase) 10 X = 90 mcg X = 9 mL/hr

$$\frac{10 \text{ mcg}}{3 \text{ mL}} = \frac{40 \text{ mcg}}{X \text{ mL}}$$ (10-mcg increase) 10 X = 120 mcg X = 12 mL/hr

$$\frac{10 \text{ mcg}}{3 \text{ mL}} = \frac{50 \text{ mcg}}{X \text{ mL}}$$ (10-mcg increase) 10 X = 1500 mcg X = 15 mL/hr

$$\frac{10 \text{ mcg}}{3 \text{ mL}} = \frac{60 \text{ mcg}}{X \text{ mL}}$$ (10-mcg increase) 10 X = 180 mcg X = 18 mL/hr

$$\frac{10 \text{ mcg}}{3 \text{ mL}} = \frac{70 \text{ mcg}}{X \text{ mL}}$$ (10-mcg increase) 10 X = 210 mcg X = 21 mL/hr

$$\frac{10 \text{ mcg}}{3 \text{ mL}} = \frac{80 \text{ mcg}}{X \text{ mL}}$$ (10-mcg increase) 10 X = 240 mcg X = 24 mL/hr

✔ **Human Error Check**

With each calculation, the answer for X should be substituted for X and the equation repeated. This process ensures that each calculation is correct.

Titration Table

Intravenous Rate	Nitroglycerin Dose
3 mL/hr	10 mcg/min (minimum)
6 mL/hr	20 mcg/min
9 mL/hr	30 mcg/min
12 mL/hr	40 mcg/min
15 mL/hr	50 mcg/min
18 mL/hr	60 mcg/min
21 mL/hr	70 mcg/min
24 mL/hr	80 mcg/min (maximum)

Example 2

PRESCRIPTION

Start Levophed (norepinephrine bitartrate) at 3 mcg/min to maintain blood pressure and titrate to keep systolic blood pressure greater than 100 mm Hg to a maximum of 12 mcg/min.

• **What You HAVE**

Pharmacy label:
Solution D_5W.
Volume 250 mL.
Levophed 2 mg.

• **What You KNOW**

Prescribed is Levophed; dose range is 3 mcg/min to 12 mcg/min.

• **What You WANT**

Levophed dose volume per hour.
Compute a minimum/maximum titration table of intravenous rate for each
    incremental dose.

CRITICAL THINKING

Are the units of measure of what you HAVE and what you KNOW the same? _____

Will conversion calculations be necessary? _____
In setting up a ratio-proportion, place the Levophed total strength per volume you
    HAVE on the LEFT; on the RIGHT, place the mg/hr you calculated in the nu-
    merator and X in the denominator.
Multiply to get the cross-products.
Divide the numerical cross-product by the numerical multiplier of X (the number in
    front of X).
The result is the answer for X.
Label the answer mL/hr.
To develop a titration table at 1-mcg increases using the ratio-proportion method,
    place the dose strength per volume you HAVE on the LEFT; on the RIGHT,
    place the incremental dose strength in the numerator and X in the denomina-
    tor. Complete the calculation. Repeat for each increment to the maximum limit
    (12 mcg).
Check the answer by placing the number obtained for X in the original equation.
    Cross-multiply. The cross-products should be approximately equal.
Alternately, use the formula: mL/mg × mcg/min × min/hr × mg/mcg.

**ANSWER FOR
BEST CARE**

Units of measure are different.
Conversions are necessary for units of measure and time.
3 mcg = 0.003 mg
Convert mg/min to mg/hr by multiplying by 60.

0.003 mg × 60 minutes = 0.18 mg.
Determine dose volume per hour.

(HAVE)

$$\frac{2\ mg}{250\ mL} = \frac{0.18\ mg}{X\ mL}$$

2X = 45

X = 22.5 mL/hr

> ✔ **Human Error Check**
>
> Replace X with 22.5.
>
> $$\frac{2}{250} = \frac{0.18}{22.5}$$
>
> 2 × 22.5 = 250 × 0.18
> 45 = 45

There is also a formula that can be used: mL/mg × mcg/min × min/hr × mg/mcg.

$$\underset{\text{(HAVE)}}{\frac{250\ mL\ (Total\ volume)}{2\ mg\ (Total\ strength)}} \times \underset{\substack{\text{(Prescribed}\\\text{start rate)}}}{\frac{3\ mcg}{1\ min}} \times \underset{\substack{\text{(Hourly}\\\text{conversion)}}}{\frac{60\ min}{1\ hr}} \times \underset{\substack{\text{(mg/mcg}\\\text{conversion)}}}{\frac{1\ mg}{1000\ mcg}} = \frac{45,000}{2000} = \frac{22.5\ mL}{1\ hr}$$

Dose 3 mcg/min = 22.5 mL/hr
Develop a titration chart using 1-mcg increments.

HAVE

$$\frac{3\ mcg}{22.5\ mL} = \frac{4\ mcg}{X\ mL}$$ (1-mcg increase) 3 X = 90 mcg X = 30 mL/hr

$$\frac{3\ mcg}{22.5\ mL} = \frac{5\ mcg}{X\ mL}$$ (1-mcg increase) 3 X = 112.5 mcg X = 37.5 mL/hr

$$\frac{3\ mcg}{22.5\ mL} = \frac{6\ mcg}{X\ mL}$$ (1-mcg increase) 3 X = 135 mcg X = 45 mL/hr

$$\frac{3\ mcg}{22.5\ mL} = \frac{7\ mcg}{X\ mL}$$ (1-mcg increase) 3 X = 157.5 mcg X = 52.2 mL/hr

$$\frac{3\ mcg}{22.5\ mL} = \frac{8\ mcg}{X\ mL}$$ (1-mcg increase) 3 X = 180 mcg X = 60 mL/hr

$$\frac{3\ mcg}{22.5\ mL} = \frac{9\ mcg}{X\ mL}$$ (1-mcg increase) 3 X = 202.5 mcg X = 67.5 mL/hr

$$\frac{3\ mcg}{22.5\ mL} = \frac{10\ mcg}{X\ mL}$$ (1-mcg increase) 3 X = 225 mcg X = 75 mL/hr

$$\frac{3\ mcg}{22.5\ mL} = \frac{11\ mcg}{X\ mL}$$ (1-mcg increase) 3 X = 247.5 mcg X = 82.5 mL/hr

$$\frac{3\ mcg}{22.5\ mL} = \frac{12\ mcg}{X\ mL}$$ (1-mcg increase) 3 X = 270 mcg X = 90 mL/hr

> ✔ **Human Error Check**
>
> With each calculation, the answer for X should be substituted for X and the equation repeated. This process ensures that each calculations is correct.

Titration Table

Intravenous Rate	Levophed Dose
22.5 mL/hr	3 mcg/min (minimum)
30 mL/hr	4 mcg/min
37.5 mL/hr	5 mcg/min
45 mL/hr	6 mcg/min
52.5 mL/hr	7 mcg/min
60 mL/hr	8 mcg/min
67.5 mL/hr	9 mcg/min
75 mL/hr	10 mcg/min
82.5 mL/hr	11 mcg/min
90 mL/hr	12 mcg/min (maximum)

Example 3

PRESCRIPTION	*Lidocaine hydrochloride 4 mg/min intravenous infusion for treatment of ventricular tachycardia STAT.*
• **What You HAVE**	Pharmacy label: Solution D$_5$W. Volume 250 mL. Lidocaine 1 g.
• **What You KNOW**	Prescribed is lidocaine hydrochloride; dosage is 4 mg/min.
• **What You WANT**	Lidocaine dose volume per hour.

CRITICAL THINKING	Are the units of measure of what you HAVE and what you KNOW the same? _____ Will conversion calculations be necessary? _____ In setting up a ratio-proportion, place the lidocaine hydrochloride total strength per volume you HAVE on the LEFT; on the RIGHT, place the mg/hr you calculated in the numerator and X in the denominator. Multiply to get the cross-products. Divide the numerical cross-product by the numerical multiplier of X (the number in front of X). The result is the answer for X. Label the answer properly in mL/hr. Check the answer by placing the number obtained for X in the original equation. Cross-multiply. The cross-products should be approximately equal. Alternately, use the formula: mL/mg × mg/min × min/hr (note that mL is placed in the numerator, not the denominator).
ANSWER FOR BEST CARE	Units of measure and time are different. Conversions are necessary. 1g = 1000 mg The prescription is in mg/min. Convert to mg/hr. 4 mg × 60 minutes = 240 mg/hr (HAVE) $$\frac{1000 \text{ mg}}{250 \text{ mL}} = \frac{240 \text{ mg}}{\text{X mL}}$$ Reduce. $$\frac{4}{1} = \frac{240}{\text{X}}$$ X = 60 mL

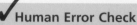

Human Error Check

Replace X with 60.

$$\frac{1000}{250} = \frac{240}{60}$$

$1000 \times 60 = 250 \times 240$
$60,000 = 60,000$

Alternate formula:

$$\frac{250 \text{ mL}}{1000 \text{ mg}} \times \frac{4 \text{ mg}}{1 \text{ min}} \times \frac{60 \text{ min}}{1 \text{ hr}} = \frac{60 \text{ mL}}{1 \text{ hr}}$$

Example 4

PRESCRIPTION	*Diltiazem hydrochloride (Cardizem) 2 to 15 mg/hr for atrial fibrillation.*

- **What You HAVE**

  Pharmacy label:
  Solution: D_5W.
  Volume: 100 mL.
  Cardizem 100 mg.

- **What You KNOW**

  Prescribed is diltiazem hydrochloride; dosage is 2 to 15 mg/hr.

- **What You WANT**

  Minimum and maximum milliliters per hour to deliver the prescribed dose.

CRITICAL THINKING

Are the units of measure of what you HAVE and what you KNOW the same?

In setting up a ratio-proportion, place the total strength/total volume you HAVE on the LEFT; on the RIGHT, place the minimum dose strength you KNOW in the numerator and X in the denominator.
Multiply to get the cross-products.
Divide the numerical cross-product by the numerical multiplier of X (the number in front of X).
The result is the answer for X.
Label the answer properly in mL/hr.
Check answer by placing the number obtained for X in the original equation. Cross-multiply. The cross-products should be approximately equal.

ANSWER FOR BEST CARE

Units are the same.

(HAVE)   (Prescribed)

$$\frac{100 \text{ mg}}{100 \text{ mL}} = \frac{2 \text{ mg}}{X \text{ mL}}$$

Reduce.

$$\frac{1}{1} = \frac{2}{X}$$

X = 2 mL/hr minimum rate

$$\frac{1 \text{ mg}}{1 \text{ mL}} = \frac{15 \text{ mg}}{X \text{ mL}}$$

X = 15 mL/hr maximum rate

✓ **Human Error Check**

Replace X with 15 mL.

$$\frac{1}{1} = \frac{15}{15}$$

$1 \times 15 = 1 \times 15$
$15 = 15$

Alternately, use the formula: mL/mg × mg/hr.

$$\frac{100 \text{ mL}}{100 \text{ mg}} \times \frac{2 \text{ mg}}{1 \text{ hr}} \times \frac{200 \text{ mL}}{100 \text{ hr}} = \frac{2 \text{ mL}}{1 \text{ hr}}$$

Example 5

PRESCRIPTION	*Aminophylline 0.5 mg/kg/hr.*

• **What You HAVE**
Pharmacy label:
Solution: D_5W.
Volume: 250 mL.
Aminophylline 50 mg.

• **What You KNOW**
Prescribed is aminophylline; dosage is 0.5 mg/kg/hr.
Patient weight is 154 pounds.

• **What You WANT**
Aminophylline dose strength based on weight.
Milliliters per hour required to administer aminophylline dose strength.

CRITICAL THINKING

Will conversion calculations be necessary? _____

In setting up a ratio-proportion, place the total strength/total volume you HAVE on the LEFT; on the RIGHT, place the minimum dose strength you KNOW in the numerator and X in the denominator.

Multiply to get the cross-products.

Divide the numerical cross-product by the numerical multiplier of X (the number in front of X).

The result is the answer for X.

Label the answer properly in units.

Check answer by placing the number obtained for X in the original equation. Cross-multiply. The cross-products should be approximately equal.

Alternately, use the formula: mL/mg × mg/hr = mL/hr.

ANSWER FOR BEST CARE

The prescription requires kilograms, so there is a conversion for weight.
Convert pounds to kilograms.
154 pounds ÷ 2.2 = 70 kg.
Determine milligrams/hour.
0.5 mg × 70 kg = 35 mg/hr
(HAVE)

$$\frac{50 \text{ mg}}{250 \text{ mL}} = \frac{35 \text{ mg}}{X \text{ mL}}$$

Reduce.

$$\frac{1}{5} = \frac{35}{X}$$

$X = 175$

> ✔ **Human Error Check**
>
> Replace X with 175.
>
> $$\frac{50}{250} = \frac{35}{175}$$
>
> 50 × 175 = 250 × 35
> 8750 = 8750

Alternately, use the formula: mL/mg × mg/hr = mL/hr.

$$\frac{5 \text{ mL}}{1 \text{ mg}} \times \frac{35 \text{ mg}}{1 \text{ hr}} = 175 \text{ mL/hr}$$

Example 6

PRESCRIPTION	*Dopamine at 4 mcg/kg/min.*

- **What You HAVE**

Pharmacy label:
Solution: D₅W.
Volume: 250 mL.
Dopamine 400 mg.

- **What You KNOW**

Prescribed is dopamine; dose is 4 mcg/kg/min.
Patient weight is 154 pounds.

- **What You WANT**

Dopamine dose strength based on weight.
Milliliters per hour required to administer dopamine dose.

CRITICAL THINKING

Will conversion calculations be necessary? _____
In setting up a ratio-proportion, place the total strength/total volume you HAVE on
the LEFT; on the RIGHT, place the minimum dose strength you KNOW in the
numerator and X in the denominator.
Multiply to get the cross-products.
Divide the numerical cross-product by the numerical multiplier of X (the number in
front of X).
The result is the answer for X.
Label the answer properly in mL/hr.
Check answer by placing the number obtained for X in the original equation. Cross-
multiply. The cross-products should be approximately equal.
Alternately, use the formula: mL/mg (concentration) × mcg/min × min/hr × mg/
mcg = mL/hr.

**ANSWER FOR
BEST CARE**

Conversion for weight and time is needed.
Weight conversion from pounds to kilograms: 154/2.2 = 70 kg.
Convert micrograms to milligrams.
4 mcg = 0.004 mg
Determine mg/min: 0.004 mg × 70 = 0.28 mg/min.
Determine mg/hr: 0.28 mg × 60 min = 16.8 mg/hr.
Calculate mL/hr

$$\frac{400 \text{ mg}}{250 \text{ mL}} \times \frac{16.8 \text{ mg}}{X \text{ mL}} \qquad \frac{16.8 \text{ mg}}{1 \text{ mL}} = \frac{16.8 \text{ mg}}{X \text{ mL}} \qquad 1.6 \text{ X} = 16.8 \qquad 16\overline{)168.0}^{\,10.5 \text{ mL/hr}}$$

✔ **Human Error Check**

Replace X with 175.

$$\frac{400}{250} = \frac{16.5}{10.5}$$

400 × 10.5 = 250 × 16.8
4200 = 4200

Alternately, use the formula: mL/mg × mcg/min × min/hr × mg/mcg = mL/hr.

$$\frac{1.6 \text{ mL}}{1 \text{ mg}} \times \frac{280 \text{ mg}}{1 \text{ min}} \times \frac{60 \text{ min}}{1 \text{ hr}} \times \frac{1}{1000 \text{ mcg}} = 10.5 \text{ mL/hr}$$

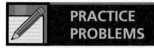

PRACTICE PROBLEMS

Directions: *Give each answer in mL/hr unless otherwise indicated.*

1. Bumetanide (Bumex) 0.5 mg/hr is infusing. You need to give a one-time STAT dose equal to 2 hours of dosages as an intravenous push over 2 minutes.

   How many milligrams do you need to give the patient? _____

2. Propranolol hydrochloride (Inderal) used in operating room setting for dysrhythmias during anesthesia. The initial infusion rate is 1 mg/hr and the maximum infusion rate is 3 mg/hr.
   HAVE: Inderal intravenous 15 mg in 500 mL D₅W.
   What are the initial infusion rate _____ and the maximum infusion rate _____?

3. PRESCRIPTION: nitroglycerin at 10 mcg/min for chest pain for acute myocardial infarction and titrate for chest pain to maximum 60 mcg/min, keeping systolic blood pressure >100 mm Hg (torr).
   HAVE: NTG 100 mg in 250 mL D₅W.
   Develop a titration table from minimum to maximum dose in 10 mcg/min increments.

4. PRESCRIPTION: nitroglycerin at 5 mcg/min for chest pain for acute myocardial infarction and titrate for chest pain to maximum 50 mcg/min, keeping systolic blood pressure greater than 100 mm Hg (torr).
   HAVE: NTG 100 mg in 500 mL D₅W.
   Develop a titration table from minimum to maximum dose in 10 mcg/min increments.

5. PRESCRIPTION: procainamide hydrochloride (Pronestyl) 2 mg/min for maintenance drip after conversion from ventricular tachycardia.
   HAVE: procainamide hydrochloride 2 g in 500 mL D₅W.
   What is the infusion rate? _____

6. PRESCRIPTION: procainamide hydrochloride (Pronestyl) 4 mg/min for sustained ventricular tachycardia.
   HAVE: procainamide hydrochloride 1 g in 250 mL D₅W.
   What is the infusion rate? _____

7. PRESCRIPTION: lidocaine 2 mg/min as intravenous infusion now for unstable ventricular tachycardia.
   HAVE: lidocaine 1 g in 250 D₅W.
   What is the infusion rate? _____

8. PRESCRIPTION: morphine sulfate 25 mg/hr continuous infusion for pain control.
   HAVE: 100 mg morphine sulfate in 250 mL NS.

What is the infusion rate? _____

9. PRESCRIPTION: morphine sulfate 40 mg/hr. Maximum dose for this patient is 120 mg/hr continuous infusion for pain control.
   HAVE: 100 mg morphine sulfate in 250 mL NS.
   Develop a titration table in 40 mg/hr increments up to the maximum dose.

10. PRESCRIPTION: atropine sulfate 3 mg/hr intravenous until respiratory effects decrease as adult treatment for organophosphate poisoning.
    HAVE: atropine 0.3 mg/mL.
    What is the infusion rate? _____ mL/hr.

(Answers on pp. 491–492)

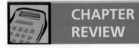

CHAPTER REVIEW

Give each answer in mL/hr unless otherwise indicated. Complete titration charts as directed.

1. PRESCRIPTION: atropine sulfate 2 mg/hr intravenous until respiratory effects decrease as adult treatment for organophosphate poisoning.
   HAVE: atropine 0.8 mg/mL.
   What is the infusion rate? _____

2. PRESCRIPTION: procainamide hydrochloride 2 mg/min. Maximum maintenance dose is 6 mg/min.
   HAVE: procainamide 2 g in 250 mL D_5W.
   Develop a titration table in 2 mg/min increments up to maximum maintenance dose.

3. PRESCRIPTION: fosphenytoin sodium (Cerebyx) 2 mg/kg/min.
   HAVE: fosphenytoin sodium 5 g in 100 mL 0.9% NS.
   Patient weight is 74 kg.
   What is the infusion rate? _____

4. PRESCRIPTION: morphine sulfate 0.2 mg/kg/hr. Maximum dose is 1 mg/kg/hr.
   HAVE: morphine 100 mg in 100 mL 0.9% NS.
   Patient weight is 116 kg.
   Develop a titration table in 0.2 mg/kg/hr increments up to the maximum dose.

5. PRESCRIPTION: 0.5 mg/kg/hr of theophylline-ethylenediamine (aminophylline).
   HAVE: aminophylline 500 mg in 500 mL D_5W.
   Patient weight is 110 pounds.
   What is the infusion rate? _____

6. PRESCRIPTION: dexmedetomidine hydrochloride 0.02 mg/kg/hr.
   HAVE: dexmedetomidine hydrochloride 4 mg in 100 mL 0.9% NS.
   Patient weight is 198 pounds.
   What is the infusion rate? _____

7. PRESCRIPTION: esmolol 150 mcg/kg/min.
   HAVE: esmolol 500 mg in 50 mL D_5 0.9% NaCl.
   Patient weight is 268.4 pounds (122 kg).
   What is the infusion rate? _____

8. PRESCRIPTION: remifentanil (Ultiva) 0.05 mcg/kg/min intravenous infusion for 2 minutes.
   HAVE: Ultiva 50 mg in 50 mL 0.9% NaCl.
   Patient weight is 68 kg.
   How many micrograms will be infused? _____

9. PRESCRIPTION: dobutamine hydrochloride (Dobutrex) 5 mcg/kg/min for a patient in heart failure.
   HAVE: dobutamine 500 mg in 500 mL D_5W.
   Patient weight is 154 pounds.
   What is the infusion rate? _____

10. Nitroglycerin (NTG) is infusing at 28 mL/hr when you assess the patient.
    HAVE: nitroglycerin 50 mg in 250 mL D_5W.
    What is the dose in mcg/min? _____

11. PRESCRIPTION: heparin at 500 units/hr intravenous.
    HAVE: heparin 20,000 units 1000 mL D_5W.
    What is the rate in mL/hr? _____

12. Dopamine is infusing at 16.8 mL/hr when you assess the patient.
    HAVE: dopamine 400 mg in 250 mL D_5W.
    Patient weight is 56 kg.
    What is the rate in mcg/kg/min? _____

13. Dobutrex is infusing at 9.8 mcg/kg/min when you assess the patient.
    HAVE: Dobutrex 500 mg in 250 mL D_5W.
    Patient weight is 68 kg.
    What is the rate in mL/hr? _____

14. Dopamine is infusing at 8 mcg/kg/min when you assess the patient.
    HAVE: dopamine 400 mg in 250 mL D_5W.
    Patient weight is 56 kg.
    What is the rate in mL/hr? _____

15. Esmolol is infusing at 500 mcg/kg/min when you assess the patient.
    HAVE: esmolol (Brevibloc) 5 g in 500 mL D_5 0.9% NS.
    Patient weight is 62 kg.
    What is the rate in mL/hr? _____

16. Dopamine is infusing at 14 mL/hr when you assess the patient.
    HAVE: dopamine 500 mg in 250 mL D_5W.
    Patient weight is 60 kg.
    What is the dose in mcg/kg/min? _____

17. Nitroglycerin (NTG) is infusing at 20 mL/hr when you assess the patient.
    HAVE: nitroglycerin 50 mg in 250 mL D_5W.
    What is the dose in mcg/min? _____

18. PRESCRIPTION: Start Levophed (norepinephrine bitartrate) at 4 mcg/min to maintain blood pressure and titrate to keep systolic blood pressure greater than 100 mm Hg to a maximum of 12 mcg/min.
    HAVE: Levophed 8 mg in 1000 mL D_5W.
    Develop a titration table from minimum to maximum dose in 2 mcg/min increments.

19. PRESCRIPTION: midazolam (Versed) 10 mcg/kg intravenous as sedation in critical care. Patient weight is 123.2 pounds.
    How many micrograms do you give this patient for sedation?
    _____

20. PRESCRIPTION: Start nitroglycerin at 40 mcg/min for chest pain for acute myocardial infarction and titrate for chest pain to maximum 120 mcg/min and also keep systolic blood pressure greater than 100 mm Hg (torr).

HAVE: 100 mL D$_5$W with 40 mg nitroglycerin.

What is the dose volume/per hour? _____

Develop a titration table from minimum to maximum dose in 20-mcg increments.

(Answers on p. 492)

𝒆volve   For additional practice problems, refer to the Advanced Calculations section of the Drug Calculations Companion, version 4 on Evolve.

Answer Key

CHAPTER 1
Decimals: Relative Value, Addition, and Subtraction
Relative Value of a Decimal Number, pp. 5-6

1. 3.75
   2.50
   3.55
   3.75

2. 1.5
   1.25
   1.50
   1.35

3. 0.175
   0.175
   0.125
   0.150

4. 1 tablet exactly
   0.4 mg
   0.4 mg

5. Less than 1 tablet; 2.5 (HAVE) has greater value.
   2.50 mg
   1.25 mg

6. More than 1 tablet; 0.05 mg (Prescription) has greater value.
   0.050 mg
   0.025 mg

7. Less than 1 tablet; 2.5 mg (HAVE) has greater value.
   2.50 mg
   1.25 mg

8. More than 1 tablet; 0.5 mg (Prescription) has greater value.
   0.50 mg
   0.25 mg

9. More than 1 tablet; 1 mg (Prescription) has greater value.
   1.0 mg
   0.5 mg

10. More than 1 tablet; 7.5 mg (Prescription) has greater value.
    7.5 mg
    2.5 mg

Addition of Decimal Numbers, p. 11

1.   1.50
   +1.25
     2.75

   Human Error Check

   1.5 = 2
   1.25 = 2
   2 + 2 = 4

   Answer is less than or equal to 4.

2.   ¹
     0.350
   +1.275
     1.625

   Human Error Check

   0.35 = 1
   1.275 = 2
   1 + 2 = 3

   Answer is less than or equal to 3.

3.   12.5
   +00.4
     12.9 mg

   Human Error Check

   12.5 = 13
   0.4 = 1
   13 + 1 = 14

   Answer is less than or equal to 14.

4.   0.50
   +0.25
     0.75 mg

   Human Error Check

   .5 = 1
   0.25 = 1
   1 + 1 = 2

   Answer is less than or equal to 2.

5.   ¹
     1.500
     0.125
   +0.125
     1.750 mg
   Answer is 1.75 mg (last zero does not change value of number and is dropped).

   Human Error Check

   1.5 = 2
   0.125 = 1
   0.125 = 1
   2 + 1 + 1 = 4

   Answer is less than or equal to 4.

6.   30.00
     00.05
   +00.40
     30.45 mg

Human Error Check

30 = 30
0.05 = 1
0.4 = 1
30 + 1 + 1 = 32

Answer is less than or equal to 32.

7. $\overset{1\ 1}{}$
    1.000
    0.375
    +0.750
    2.125 mg

Human Error Check

1 = 1
0.375 = 1
0.75 = 1
1 + 1 + 1 = 3

Answer is less than or equal to 3.

8. 2.5
    5.0
    + 5.0
    12.5 mg

Human Error Check

2.5 = 3
5 = 5
5 = 5
3 + 5 + 5 = 13

Answer is less than or equal to 13.

9. $\overset{1\ 1}{}$
    2.25
    0.75
    +0.75
    3.75 mg

Human Error Check

2.25 = 3
0.75 = 1
0.75 = 1
3 + 1 + 1 = 5

Answer is less than or equal to 5.

10. $\overset{1}{}$
    1.00
    1.00
    1.00
    0.25
    +0.25
    3.50 (drop the last zero)

Answer is 3.5 g.

Human Error Check

1 = 1
1 = 1
1 = 1
0.25 = 1
0.25 = 1
1 + 1 + 1 + 1 + 1 = 5

Answer is less than or equal to 5.

Subtraction of Decimal Numbers, pp. 15-16

1. 2.5
    −1.0
    1.5 mg

Human Error Check

2.5 = 3
1 = 1
3 − 1 = 2

Answer is less than or equal to 2.

2. 20
    −10
    10 mg

Human Error Check

20 = 20
10 = 10
20 − 10 = 10

Answer is less than or equal to 10.

3. $\overset{0910}{}$
    1̸0̸.0̸
    −07.5
    2.5 mg

Human Error Check

10 = 10
7.5 = 7
10 − 7 = 3

Answer is less than or equal to 3.

4. $\overset{2910}{}$
    3̸0̸.0̸
    −22.5
    7.5 mg

Human Error Check

30 = 30
22.5 = 22
30 − 22 = 8

Answer is less than or equal to 8.

5. $\overset{09910}{}$
    1̸0̸.0̸0̸
    − 7.25
    2.75 mg

Human Error Check

10 = 10
7.25 = 7
10 − 7 = 3

Answer is less than or equal to 3.

6. $\overset{410}{}$
    0.25̸0̸
    −0.125
    0.125 mg

Human Error Check

0.25 = 1
0.125 = 0
1 − 0 = 1

Answer is less than or equal to 1.

7. ⁴⁹10
    5̶.0̶0̶
    −2.25
    2.75 g

    Human Error Check

    5 = 5
    2.25 = 2
    5 − 2 = 3

    Answer is less than or equal to 3.

8. ¹¹2
    2̶.2̶5̶
    −1.75
    0.50 Answer 0.5 mg

    Human Error Check

    2.25 = 3
    1.75 = 1
    3 − 1 = 2

    Answer is less than or equal to 2.

9. ²⁹10
    3̶.0̶0̶
    −2.25
    0.75 mg

    Human Error Check

    3 = 3
    2.25 = 2
    3 − 2 = 1

    Answer is less than or equal to 1.

10. ⁰⁹10
    1̶.0̶0̶
    −0.75
    0.25 mg

    Human Error Check

    1 = 1
    0.75 = 0
    1 − 0 = 1

    Answer is less than or equal to 1.

Chapter Review, pp. 16-18

1. b
2. a
3. c
4. c
5. a
6. b
7. c
8. 0.75 mg
9. 1.75 mg
10. 30.45 mg
11. 2.5 mg
12. 0.225 mg
13. 0.25 mg
14. 2.9 mg

15. 1.5 mg
16. 17.5 mg
17. 2.5 mg
18. 7.5 mg
19. 25 mg
20. 0.125 mg
21. Yes. 3 grams is within the dose range.
22. The problem is written incorrectly. The decimal points are improperly aligned.
23. 76.9 mg
24. 2000 mg
25. 66 g
26. 2250 mg
27. 820 mg
28. 75.2 mg
29. 1375 mg
30. 150 mg

CHAPTER 2
Decimals: Multiplication and Division
Multiplication of Decimal Numbers, p. 22

1.   4
    ×   5
      2.0 (1 decimal place)

    Drop last zero. Answer is 2.

2.   15
    ×   1
      0.15 (2 decimal places)

3.   125
    × 35
      625
      375
    43.75 (2 decimal places)

4.   25
    × 5
    12.5 (1 decimal place)

5.   225
    ×   2
      0.450 (3 decimal places)

    Drop last zero. Answer is 0.45.

6.   15
    ×   3
      4.5 (1 decimal place)

7.   375
    × 15
     1875
      375
     5.625 (3 decimal places)

8.   125
    ×   5
     6.25 (2 decimal places)

9.
```
      65
×     15
     325
      65
```
9.75 (2 decimal places)

10.
```
    1225
×      3
```
36.75 (2 decimal places)

Division of Decimal Numbers, pp. 25-26

1. Dividend: 5.25 mg.
   Divisor: 1.5 mg.
```
       3.5 tablets
15)52.5
   45
   75
   75
```

   Human Error Check

   $3.5 \times 15 = 52.5$

2. Dividend: 0.75 mg.
   Divisor: 0.25 mg.
```
      3 tablets
25)75
   75
    0
```

   Human Error Check

   $25 \times 3 = 75$

3. Yes.
   Dividend: 4.5 mg.
   Divisor: 1.5 mg.
```
      3 tablets
15)45
   45
    0
```

   Human Error Check

   $15 \times 3 = 45$

4. Dividend: 125 mg.
   Divisor: 50 mg.
```
      2.5 tablets
50)125.0
   100
   250
   250
     0
```

   Human Error Check

   $50 \times 2.5 = 125.0$

5. Dividend: 1.25 mg.
   Divisor: 0.125 mg.
```
        10 tablets
125)1250
    125
      0
```

   Human Error Check

   $125 \times 10 = 1250$

6. Dividend: 1.25 mg.
   Divisor: 0.5 mg.
```
      2.5 tablets
5)12.5
  100
   25
   25
    0
```

   Human Error Check

   $5 \times 2.5 = 12.5$

7. Dividend: 1.2 mg.
   Divisor: 0.4 mg.
```
      3 tablets
4)12
  12
   0
```

   Human Error Check

   $4 \times 3 = 12$

8. Dividend: 8.75 mg.
   Divisor: 2.5 mg.
```
       3.5 tablets
25)87.5
   75
   125
   125
     0
```

   Human Error Check

   $25 \times 3.5 = 87.5$

9. Dividend: 0.625 mg.
   Divisor: 0.25 mg.
```
       2.5 tablets
25)62.5
   50
   125
   125
     0
```

   Human Error Check

   $25 \times 2.5 = 62.5$

10. No, this is not a correct dosage; there should be 1.5 tablets or 2 scored tablets.
    Dividend: 3.75 mg.
    Divisor: 2.5 mg.
```
        1.5 tablets
25)37.5
   25
   125
   125
     0
```

    Human Error Check

    $25 \times 1.5 = 37.5$

Chapter Review, pp. 26-28

1. 3

2. 0.18

3. 56.25

4. 17.5

5. 0.9

6. 7.5

7. 5.175

8. 9.25

9. 11.25

10. 36.45

11. 1.5 mg

12. 5.25 mg

13. 0.15 mg

14. 2.35 mg

15. 4 mg

16. 1.5 g

17. 45 mcg

18. 0.8 mg

19. 0.125 mg

20. 0.1875 mg

21. 7 tablets

22. 4 tablets

23. 3 tablets

24. 2 tablets

25. 2½ tablets

26. 3 tablets

27. No. There should be 2 tablets in the drawer.

28. 4 tablets

29. 5 tablets

30. 4 tablets

31. 29 ounces in 1 day

32. 7.6 liters

33. 1125 mL

34. 13.5 grams

35. When multiplying, the decimal in the answer is placed by counting the appropriate number of spaces, starting on the far *right* and moving toward the *left*.

CHAPTER 3
Fractions: Reduction and Equations

Relative Value of Fractions, p. 30

1. (b) Same numerator, so lowest denominator: $\frac{1}{2}$.

2. (c) Same denominator, so highest numerator: $\frac{5}{7}$.

3. (b) Change to decimals: 0.67, 0.83 (highest), 0.75.

4. (a) Same numerator, so lowest denominator: $\frac{3}{2}$.

5. (c) Same denominator, so highest numerator: $\frac{9}{6}$.

6. (c) Change to decimals: 0.25, 0.5, 0.87 (highest).

7. (b) Change to decimals: 0.2, 0.7 (highest), 0.6.

8. (a) Same numerator, lowest denominator, $\frac{1}{2}$.

9. (c) Change to decimals: 0.75, 0.87, 0.9 (highest).

10. (a) Change to decimals: 2.67 (highest), 2.5, 1.2.

11. 0.67, 0.75, 0.83 (highest) $= \frac{5}{6}$.

12. 0.38, 0.25 (lowest), 0.6 $= \frac{1}{4}$.

Multiplying and Reducing Fractions, p. 33

1. $\frac{1}{8}$, 0.1

$$\frac{1}{2} \times \frac{1}{4} = \frac{1}{8}$$

$$\begin{array}{r} 0.12 \text{ (round to nearest tenth)} \\ 8\overline{)1.00} \\ \underline{8} \\ 20 \\ \underline{16} \\ 4 \end{array}$$

2. $\frac{100}{10}$, 10

$$\frac{1}{10} \times \frac{100}{1} = \frac{100}{10}$$

$$\begin{array}{r} 10 \\ 10\overline{)100} \\ \underline{100} \end{array}$$

3. $\frac{1}{6}$, 0.2

$$\frac{\cancel{7}}{\cancel{8}} \times \frac{\cancel{4}}{\cancel{21}} = \frac{1}{2} \times \frac{1}{3} = \frac{1}{6}$$

$$\begin{array}{r} 0.16 \text{ (round to nearest tenth)} \\ 6\overline{)1.00} \\ \underline{6} \\ 40 \\ \underline{36} \\ 4 \end{array}$$

4. $\frac{8}{15}$, 0.5

$$\frac{8}{3} \times \frac{1}{5} = \frac{8}{15}$$

$$\begin{array}{r} 0.53 \text{ (round to nearest tenth)} \\ 15\overline{)8.0} \\ \underline{75} \\ 50 \\ \underline{45} \\ 5 \end{array}$$

5. $\frac{7}{10}$, 0.7

$$\frac{\cancel{3}}{\cancel{4}} \times \frac{\cancel{14}}{\cancel{15}} = \frac{1}{2} \times \frac{7}{5} = \frac{7}{10}$$

$$\begin{array}{r} 0.7 \\ 10\overline{)7.0} \\ \underline{70} \end{array}$$

6. $\frac{30}{2}$, 15

$$\frac{1\cancel{5}0}{\cancel{4}} \times \frac{\cancel{2}}{\cancel{5}} = \frac{30}{2} \times \frac{1}{1} = \frac{30}{2} = 15$$

7. $\frac{1}{1}$, 1

$$\frac{1000}{1} \times \frac{1}{1000} = \frac{1}{1} = 1$$

8. $\frac{14}{45}$, 0.3

$$\frac{2}{5} \times \frac{7}{9} = \frac{14}{45}$$

$$\begin{array}{r} 0.31 \text{ (round to nearest tenth)} \\ 45\overline{)14.00} \\ \underline{135} \\ 50 \\ \underline{45} \\ 5 \end{array}$$

9. $\frac{3}{10}$, 0.3

$$\frac{1}{5} \times \frac{3}{2} = \frac{3}{10}$$

$$\begin{array}{r} 0.3 \\ 10\overline{)3.0} \\ \underline{30} \end{array}$$

10. $\frac{25}{3}$, 8.3

$$\frac{2500}{3} \times \frac{1}{100} = \frac{25}{3} \times \frac{1}{1} = \frac{25}{3}$$

$$\begin{array}{r} 8.33 \text{ (round to nearest tenth)} \\ 3\overline{)25.00} \\ \underline{24} \\ 10 \\ \underline{9} \\ 10 \\ \underline{9} \\ 1 \end{array}$$

11. $\frac{1}{10}$, 0.1

$$\frac{1}{5} \times \frac{1}{2} = \frac{1}{10}$$

$$\begin{array}{r} 0.1 \\ 10\overline{)1.0} \end{array}$$

12. $\frac{1}{4}$, 0.3

$$\frac{1}{6} \times \frac{3}{2} = \frac{1}{2} \times \frac{1}{2} = \frac{1}{4}$$

$$\begin{array}{r} 0.25 \text{ (round to nearest tenth)} \\ 4\overline{)1.0} \end{array}$$

Dividing Fractions, p. 35

1. $\frac{3}{8}$, 0.4

Reduce by 25:

$$\frac{1}{200} \times \frac{75}{1} = \frac{1}{8} \times \frac{3}{1} = \frac{3}{8}$$

$$\begin{array}{r} 0.37 \text{ (round to nearest tenth)} \\ 8\overline{)3.00} \\ \underline{24} \\ 60 \\ \underline{56} \\ 4 \end{array}$$

2. $\frac{5}{3}$, 1.7

Reduce by 2:

$$\frac{1}{6} \times \frac{10}{1} = \frac{1}{3} \times \frac{5}{1} = \frac{5}{3}$$

$$\begin{array}{r} 1.66 \text{ (round to nearest tenth)} \\ 3\overline{)5.00} \\ \underline{3} \\ 20 \\ \underline{18} \\ 20 \\ \underline{18} \\ 2 \end{array}$$

3. $\frac{2}{1}$, 2

Reduce by 3:

$$\frac{1}{3} \times \frac{6}{1} = \frac{1}{1} \times \frac{2}{1} = \frac{2}{1}$$

4. $\frac{6}{7}$, 0.9

Reduce by 4:

$$\frac{3}{4} \times \frac{8}{7} = \frac{3}{1} \times \frac{2}{7} = \frac{6}{7}$$

$$\begin{array}{r} 0.85 \text{ (round to nearest tenth)} \\ 7\overline{)6.00} \\ \underline{56} \\ 40 \\ \underline{35} \end{array}$$

5. $\frac{12}{1}$, 12

Reduce by 250:

$$\frac{1000}{1} \times \frac{3}{250} = \frac{4}{1} \times \frac{3}{1} = \frac{12}{1}$$

6. $\frac{15}{4}$, 3.8

$$\frac{3}{2} \times \frac{5}{2} = \frac{15}{4}$$

$$\begin{array}{r} 3.75 \text{ (round to nearest tenth)} \\ 4\overline{)15.00} \\ \underline{12} \\ 30 \\ \underline{28} \\ 20 \\ \underline{20} \end{array}$$

7. $\frac{2}{9}$, 0.2

Reduce by 5:

$$\frac{2}{15} \times \frac{5}{3} = \frac{2}{3} \times \frac{1}{3} = \frac{2}{9}$$

$$\begin{array}{r} .22 \text{ (round to nearest tenth)} \\ 9\overline{)2.00} \\ \underline{18} \\ 20 \\ \underline{18} \\ 2 \end{array}$$

8. $\frac{5}{12}$, 0.4

Reduce by 25:

$$\frac{125}{3} \times \frac{1}{100} = \frac{5}{3} \times \frac{1}{4} = \frac{5}{12}$$

$$\begin{array}{r} 0.41 \text{ (round to nearest tenth)} \\ 12\overline{)5.00} \\ \underline{48} \\ 20 \\ \underline{12} \end{array}$$

9. $\frac{10}{1}$, 10

Reduce by 3:

$$\frac{15}{1} \times \frac{2}{3} = \frac{5}{1} \times \frac{2}{1} = \frac{10}{1}$$

10. $\frac{30}{1}$, 30

Reduce by 15, then by 2:

$$\frac{225}{2} \times \frac{4}{15} = \frac{15}{2} \times \frac{4}{1} = \frac{15}{1} \times \frac{2}{1} = \frac{30}{1}$$

11. $\frac{1}{3} \times \frac{6}{1} = \frac{6}{3} = 2$ pounds per week

12. $\frac{1}{3} \times \frac{4}{1} = \frac{4}{2} = 2$ mL reduction

Equations, pp. 37-38

1. $X = \dfrac{20}{50} \times 2$

   Reduce by 10: $\dfrac{2}{5} \times \dfrac{2}{1} = \dfrac{4}{5}$

   $$5)\overline{4.0}$$
   $$\underline{40}$$
   $$0$$
   quotient 0.8

   $X = 0.8$

2. $X = \dfrac{250}{1000} \times 1.3$

   Reduce by 250 and move decimals to convert to whole numbers:

   $\dfrac{1}{4} \times \dfrac{13}{10} = \dfrac{13}{40}$

   $$40)\overline{13.00}$$
   $$\underline{120}$$
   $$100$$
   $$\underline{80}$$
   $$20$$
   quotient 0.32

   $X = 0.3$

3. $X = \dfrac{0.25}{1.25} \times \dfrac{1.2}{1}$

   Move decimals to convert to whole numbers:

   $\dfrac{25}{125} \times \dfrac{12}{10}$

   Reduce: $\dfrac{1}{5} \times \dfrac{6}{5} = \dfrac{6}{25}$

   $$25)\overline{6.00}$$
   $$\underline{50}$$
   $$100$$
   $$\underline{100}$$
   $$0$$
   quotient 0.24

   $X = 0.2$

4. $X = \dfrac{1/60}{1/150} \times 2.1 = \dfrac{1}{60} \times \dfrac{150}{1} \times \dfrac{2.1}{1}$

   Move decimal:

   $\dfrac{1}{60} \times \dfrac{150}{1} \times \dfrac{21}{10}$

   Reduce:

   $\dfrac{1}{2} \times \dfrac{1}{1} \times \dfrac{21}{2} = \dfrac{21}{4}$

   $$4)\overline{21.00}$$
   $$\underline{20}$$
   $$10$$
   $$\underline{8}$$
   $$20$$
   $$\underline{20}$$
   $$0$$
   quotient 5.25

   $X = 5.3$

5. $X = \dfrac{2}{7} \times \dfrac{3.5}{1}$

   Move decimals to make whole numbers: $\dfrac{2}{7} \times \dfrac{35}{10}$

   Reduce: $\dfrac{2}{7} \times \dfrac{7}{2} = \dfrac{1}{1} \times \dfrac{1}{1} = 1$

   $X = 1$

6. $X = \dfrac{3}{5} \times \dfrac{25}{6} \times \dfrac{3}{1}$

   Reduce: $\dfrac{1}{1} \times \dfrac{5}{2} \times \dfrac{3}{1} = \dfrac{15}{2}$

   $$2)\overline{15.0}$$
   $$\underline{14}$$
   $$10$$
   $$\underline{10}$$
   $$0$$
   quotient 7.5

   $X = 7.5$

7. $X = \dfrac{125}{1} \times \dfrac{1}{75} \times \dfrac{6}{1}$

   Reduce: $\dfrac{5}{1} \times \dfrac{1}{1} \times \dfrac{2}{1} = 10$

   $X = 10$

8. $X = \dfrac{15}{20} \times \dfrac{35}{30}$

   Reduce: $\dfrac{1}{4} \times \dfrac{7}{2} = \dfrac{7}{8}$

   $$8)\overline{7.00}$$
   $$\underline{64}$$
   $$60$$
   $$\underline{56}$$
   $$4$$
   quotient 0.87

   $X = 0.9$

9. $X = \dfrac{1000}{1} \times \dfrac{1}{100} \times \dfrac{2.25}{1}$

   Reduce: $\dfrac{10}{1} \times \dfrac{1}{1} \times \dfrac{2.25}{1} = \dfrac{22.5}{1}$

   $X = 22.5$

10. $X = \dfrac{1}{100} \times \dfrac{1000}{1} \times \dfrac{3.75}{2}$

    Reduce: $\dfrac{1}{1} \times \dfrac{10}{1} \times \dfrac{3.75}{2} = \dfrac{37.5}{2} = 18.75$

    $X = 18.8$

Chapter Review, pp. 38–40

1. 2 tablets.
2. 2 tablets.
3. 1.5 mL.
4. 2 tablets.
5. 0.25 mg.
6. 2.5 mL.
7. 3.25 ounces.
8. 0.25 mL.
9. 7.5 mL.
10. 5 mL.
11. 1½ tablets.
12. 2 tablets.
13. 20 mL.
14. 5 mL.

15. 100 mL.

16. 1.5

17. 1

18. 20.3

19. 2

20. 105

21. 600 mL.

22. 1600-calorie diet.

23. 320 mL.

24. Day 2 is 600 mL; day 3 is 900 mL; day 4 is 1350 mL.

25. 3 units

CHAPTER 4
Units of Measure
Basic Units, pp. 43-44

1. 10 g. Weight.

2. 2 mL. Volume.

3. 6.3 kg. Weight.

4. 0.75 mg. Weight.

5. 100 mcg. Weight.

6. 0.02 L. Volume.

7. 4.2 mcg. Weight.

8. 4 L. Volume.

9. 1000 mL. Volume.

10. 3.7 kg. Weight.

11. 2 cm. Length.

12. 30 mL. Volume.

13. 3 m. Length.

14. 74 kg. Weight.

15. 4 mm. Length.

16. 3.5 L. Volume.

17. 25 m. Length.

18. 60 mcg. Weight.

19. 2.5 cm. Length.

20. 2 g. Weight.

Conversion of Metric Units, pp. 45-46

1. Larger to smaller, multiply by 1000 or move decimal point three places to the right: 1.7 L = 1700 mL.

2. Larger to smaller, multiply by 1000 or move decimal point three places to the right: 0.5 g = 500 mg.

3. mL is the abbreviation for milliters, so 0.5 mL.

4. Smaller to larger, divide by 1000 or move decimal point three places to the left: 100 mg = 0.1 g.

5. Smaller to larger, divide by 1000 or move decimal point three places to the left: 400 mcg = 0.4 mg.

6. Smaller to larger, divide by 1000 or move decimal point three places to the left: 100 mL = 0.1 L.

7. Larger to smaller, multiply by 1000 or move decimal point three places to the right: 0.5 mg = 500 mcg.

8. Larger to smaller, multiply by 1000 or move decimal point three places to the right: 1 mg = 1000 mcg.

9. mg to mcg is larger to smaller, so 0.4 mg = 400 mcg; both are per mL so they are equivalent.

10. g to mg is larger to smaller, so 0.04 g = 40 mg. You have more than enough.

International Units and Milliequivalent Measures, p. 47

1. 1,000,000 units

2. 20,000 units

3. 17 units

4. 7200 units

5. 500,000 units

6. 20 mEq or 20 milliequivalents

7. 30 mEq or 30 milliequivalents

8. 15 mEq or 15 milliequivalents

9. 40 mEq or 40 milliequivalents

10. 10 mEq or 10 milliequivalents

Chapter Review, pp. 47-48

1. 5 mL. Volume.

2. 1.5 mg. Weight.

3. 0.25 mg. Weight.

4. 2.5 mL. Volume.

5. 5 g. Weight.

6. Yes.

7. 5000 mg.

8. 0.05 mg.

9. Yes.

10. 2000 mg.

11. 0.06 L.

12. 2500 mL.

13. 0.125 g.

14. 0.12 L.

15. 30,000 mcg.

16. 500 mg.

17. 1 cm.

18. 2500 mcg.

19. 0.5 g.

20. 250 mcg.

21. 20 mEq.

22. 30 mEq.

23. 15 mEq.

24. 40 mEq.

25. 10 mEq.

Comprehensive Review
Chapter 1, pp. 49-51

1. c.

2. a.

3. a.

4. More.

5. More.

6. Exactly.

7. Less.

8. Less.

9. More.

10. Exactly.

11. 7.5. Human error check: less than 8.

12. 0.375. Human error check: less than 2.

13. 50.6 mg. Human error check: less than 51.

14. 0.6 mg. Human error check: less than 2.

15. 0.5 mg. Human error check: less than 3.

16. 10.45 mg. Human error check: less than 12.

17. 2.875 mg. Human error check: less than 4.

18. 15 mg. Human error check: less than 16.

19. 3.25 mg. Human error check: less than 5.

20. 2 g. Human error check: less than 5.

21. 2 mg. Human error check: 2.

22. 5 mg. Human error check: 5.

23. 2.5 mg. Human error check: less than 3.

24. 15 mg. Human error check: 15.

25. 6.5 mg. Human error check: less than 7.

26. 1.5 mg. Human error check: less than 2.

27. 2.25 gram. Human error check: less than 3.

28. 0.9 mg. Human error check: less than 2.

29. 4.5 mg. Human error check: less than 5.

30. 2.25 mg. Human error check: less than 3.

Chapter 2, pp. 51-54

1. 5.0

2. 0.250

3. 975

4. 1000

5. 17,350.0

6. 12.35

7. 0.100

8. 0.075

9. 188.76

10. 1646.0

11. Dividend 7.5, divisor 1.5, answer 5. Check: $5 \times 15 = 75$.

12. Dividend 1, divisor 0.25, answer 4. Check: $4 \times 2.5 = 1$.

13. No. Dividend 3, divisor 1.5, answer 2. Check: $2 \times 1.5 = 3$.

14. Dividend 62.5, divisor 25, answer 2.5. Check: $25 \times 2.5 = 62.5$.

15. Dividend 0.125, divisor 0.125, answer 1. Check: $0.125 \times 1 = 0.125$.

16. Dividend 0.5, divisor 0.2, answer 2.5. Check: $2.5 \times 0.2 = 0.5$.

17. Dividend 1.8, divisor 0.6, answer 3. Check: $3 \times 0.6 = 1.8$.

18. Dividend 7.5, divisor 2.5, answer 3. Check: $2.5 \times 3 = 7.5$.

19. Dividend 2.25, divisor 0.75, answer 3. Check: $3 \times 0.75 = 2.25$.

20. No. Two 2.5 tablets and one 1.25 tablet.

21. 1.2 mg.

22. 3.75 mg.

23. 0.5 mg.

24. 4.25 mg.

25. 5.65 mg.

26. 1.25 g.

27. 75 mcg.

28. 1.2 mg.

29. 0.075 mg.

30. 0.25 mg.

31. 2 tablets.

32. 2 capsules.

33. 4 tablets.

34. 1½ tablets.

35. 2½ tablets.

36. 3 capsules.

37. No. ½ tablet.

38. 2 tablets.

39. 2 tablets.

40. 3 tablets.

41. 36 ounces.

42. 37.5 ounces.

43. 5.5 L.

44. 4 L.

45. 1350 mL.

46. 600 mL.

47. 10.2 g.

48. 13.8 g.

49. 480 mL.

50. 270 mL.

Chapter 3, pp. 54-56

1. c

2. c

3. c

4. c

5. a

6. a

7. b

8. b

9. a

10. a

11. $\frac{3}{4}$

12. $\frac{1}{6}$

13. $\frac{1}{16}$, 0.1

14. $\frac{20}{1}$, 20

15. $\frac{3}{5}$, 0.6

16. $\frac{7}{6}$, 1.2

17. $\frac{3}{8}$, 0.4

18. $\frac{16}{1}$, 16

19. $\frac{4}{1}$, 4

20. $\frac{18}{35}$, 0.5

21. $\frac{7}{5}$, 1.4

22. $\frac{24}{5}$, 4.8

23. $\frac{1}{8}$, 0.1

24. $\frac{3}{8}$, 0.4

25. $\frac{9}{20}$, 0.5

26. $\frac{5}{4}$, 1.3

27. $\frac{4}{1}$, 4

28. $\frac{2}{5}$, 0.4

29. $\frac{15}{1}$, 15

30. $\frac{25}{6}$, 4.2

31. $\frac{4}{9}$, 0.4

32. $\frac{5}{28}$, 0.2

33. $\frac{12}{1}$, 12

34. $\frac{30}{1}$, 30

35. $\frac{3}{4}$, 0.8

36. 4 mL

37. 0.4

38. 1.1

39. 0.5

40. 18.2

41. 2.1

42. 7.1

43. 6

44. 0.4

45. 22.8

46. 2.8

47. 150 mL

48. 560 calories, 2240-calorie diet

49. 300 mL

50. 6 units

Chapter 4, p. 56

1. 4 g. Weight.

2. 5 mL. Volume.

3. 69.3 kg. Weight.

4. 0.25 mg. Weight.

5. 10 m. Length.

6. 0.05 L. Volume.

7. 160 mcg. Weight.

8. 3 L. Volume.

9. 31 cm. Length.

10. 13 mm. Length.

11. 1500 mL.

12. 400 mg.

13. 0.8 mL.

14. 0.2 g.

15. 0.6 mg.

16. 0.2 L.

17. 500 mcg.

18. 500 mcg.

19. Yes, they are equivalent.

20. Yes, you have more than enough.

CHAPTER 5
Conversion

Converting Within the Metric System, p. 59

1. 50 mcg (larger to smaller conversion factor 1000)

2. 0.0006 g (smaller to larger conversion factor 1000)

3. 2500 mg (larger to smaller conversion factor 1000)

4. 75,000 mcg (larger to smaller conversion factor 1000)

5. 0.000006 mg (smaller to larger conversion factor 1000)

6. 35,000 mg (larger to smaller conversion factor 1000)

7. 0.05 g (smaller to larger conversion factor 1000)

8. 0.013 mg (smaller to larger conversion factor 1000)

9. 55 mcg (larger to smaller conversion factor 1000)

10. 0.6 mcg (larger to smaller conversion factor 1000)

Converting Within the Metric System, p. 61

1. Smaller to larger—move decimal three places to the left or divide by 1000: 6000 mcg = 6 mg.

2. Larger to smaller—move decimal three places to the right or multiply by 1000: 0.4 L = 400 mL.

3. Larger to smaller—move decimal three places to the right or multiply by 1000: 0.6 g = 600 mg.

4. Smaller to larger—move decimal three places to the left or divide by 1000: 1 g = 0.001 kg.

5. Smaller to larger—move decimal three places to the left or divide by 1000: 500 mcg = 0.5 mg.

6. Larger to smaller—move decimal three places to the right or multiply by 1000: 0.5 g = 500 mg.

7. Larger to smaller—move decimal three places to the right or multiply by 1000: 1.25 mg = 1250 mcg.

8. Larger to smaller—move decimal three places to the right or multiply by 1000: 0.8 g = 800 mg.

9. Larger to smaller—move decimal three places to the right or multiply by 1000: 0.2 g = 200 mg.

10. Larger to smaller—move decimal three places to the right or multiply by 1000: 0.1 kg = 100 g.

Converting Between Systems of Measurement, p. 63-64

1. 1 tablet

2. 5 mL = 1 teaspoon; 20 mL/5 mL = 4 teaspoons

3. 0.4 in = 1 cm; 6 in/0.4 in = 15 cm; 8 in/0.4 in = 20 cm

4. 1 L = 1000 mL, so 2 L = 2000 mL; 1 ounce = 30 mL and 2000 mL/30 mL = 66.7 ounces

5. 1 kg = 2.2 lb; 156 lb/2.2 lb = 71 kg; 71 × 2 = 142 mg

6. gr 1 = 60 mg; gr 5 = 5 × 60 = 300 mg

7. 1 tsp = 5 mL; 2 tsp = 2 × 5 = 10 mL

8. 1 L = 1 qt; 1.5 L = 1.5 quarts

9. gr 1 = 60 mg; gr $\frac{1}{4}$ = $\frac{1}{4}$ × 60 = 15 mg; 1 tablet

10. gr 1 = 60 mg; gr 1/200 = 1/200 × 60/1 = 3/10 or 0.3, so 0.4 mg/1 mL = 0.3 mg/X mL and 0.4 X = 0.3; X = 3/4 = 0.75 mL

Chapter Review, pp. 64-66

1. 1.33 mL
2. 1 tablespoon
3. 22 inches
4. 1.2 inches; 1.6 inches
5. 6 ounces
6. 7.5 mL
7. 0.32 grams
8. 10 ounces
9. 3750 units
10. 6400 mL
11. 12½ (12.5) glasses
12. 600 mg = 2 capsules
13. 2 tablespoons
14. 8 grains
15. ½ tablet
16. 1.5 mL
17. 2 mL
18. 477 mg
19. 0.027 mg
20. 5 grains
21. 2 tablespoons
22. 1 tablespoon
23. 2.5 mL
24. 4 teaspoons
25. 120 mg

CHAPTER 6
Percentages

Percentages, pp. 69-70

1. 4/100 and 0.04.
2. 0.9/100 or 9/1000 and 0.009.
3. 0.45/100 or 45/10,000 and 0.0045.
4. 50/100 = 1/2 and 0.5.
5. 10/100 = 1/10 and 0.1.
6. 25/100 = 1/4 and 0.25.
7. 35/100 and 0.35.
8. 75/100 or 3/4 and 0.75.
9. 0.6/100 or 6/1000 and 0.006.
10. 43/100 and 0.43.
11. 3% = 0.03 for every unit. 0.03 × 4 = 0.12 or 12%.
12. 20% = 20/100 = 1/5; yes.

Percentages of Medications in Solutions, p. 71

1. 0.3% = 0.3/100 = 3/1000 or 0.003
   1000 × 3/1000 = 3 or 1000 × 0.003 = 3   Answer: 3 g.

2. 10% = 10/100 = 1/10 or 0.1
   1000 × 1/10 = 100 or 1000 × 0.1 = 100   Answer: 100 g.

3. 20% = 20/100 = 1/5 or 0.2
   500 × 1/5 = 100 or 500 × 0.2 = 100   Answer: 100 g.

4. 25% = 25/100 = $\frac{1}{4}$ or 0.25
   500 × $\frac{1}{4}$ = 125 or 500 × 0.25 = 125   Answer: 125 g.

5. 0.45% = 0.45/100 or 0.0045
   500 × 0.45 /100 = 2.25 or 500 × 0.0045 = 2.25
      Answer: 2.25 g.

6. 0.1% = 0.1/100 or 1/1000 or 0.001
   50 × 1/1000 = 0.05 or 50 × 0.001 = 0.05   Answer: 0.05 g.

7. 10% = 10/100 = 1/10 or 0.1
   300 × 1/10 = 30 or 300 × 0.1 = 30   Answer: 30 g.

8. 20% = 20/100 = 1/5 or 0.2
   250 × 1/5 = 50 or 250 × 0.2 = 50   Answer: 50 g.

9. 5% = 5/100 = 1/20 or 0.05
   100 × 1/20 = 5 or 100 × 0.05 = 5   Answer: 5 g.

10. 3% = 3/100 = 0.03
    750 × 3/100 = 22.5 or 750 × 0.03 = 22.5 Answer: 22.5 g.

Chapter Review, pp. 71-72

1. 15/100, 0.15
2. 40/100, 0.4
3. 0.1/100, 0.001
4. 1.25/100, 0.0125
5. 0.03/100, 0.0003
6. 8/100 and 0.08
7. 0.6/100 or 6/1000 and 0.006
8. 0.25/100 or 25/10,000 and 0.0025
9. 50/100 = 1/2 and 0.5
10. 10/100 = 1/10 and 0.1
11. 45/100 = 9/20 and 0.45
12. 33/100 and 0.33

13. 80/100 or 4/5 and 0.8

14. 0.7/100 or 7/1000 and 0.007

15. 42/100 and 0.42

16. 3% = 0.03 for every unit. 3 × 0.3 = 0.09 or 9%.

17. 20% = 20/100 = 1/5; No.

18. (c).

19. (c).

20. 90%.

21. 1 mL

22. 35

23. 70%

24. 10

25. 212

CHAPTER 7
Ratio-Proportion Method
Ratio, pp. 74-75

1. 40 mg/1 mL or 40 mg:1 mL

2. 125 mg/5 mL or 125 mg:5 mL reduces to 25 mg/1 mL or 25 mg:
   1 mL

3. 250 mg/1 tablet or 250 mg:
   1 tablet

4. 100 mg/10 mL or 100 mg:10 mL reduces to 10 mg/1 mL or 10 mg:
   1 mL

5. 0.05 mg/1 tablet or 0.05 mg:
   1 tablet

6. 325 mg/1 tablet or 325 mg:
   1 tablet

7. 200 mg/5 mL or 200 mg:5 mL or 40 mg:1 mL

8. 50 mg/5 mL or 50 mg:5 mL or 10 mg:1 mL

9. 60 mg/1 tablet or 60 mg:1 tablet

10. 250 mg/1 tablet or 250 mg:
    1 tablet

Ratio Measures, p. 76-77

1. a

2. c

3. a

4. b

5. c

6. b

7. c

8. b

9. a

10. c

11. c

12. a

Solving for an Unknown (X) in the Ratio-Proportion Method, pp. 78-79

1. $X = 900$
   $9X = 27 \times 300$
   $9X = 8100 \quad X = 8100/9$

   $$9\overline{)8100}$$
   $$\underline{81}$$

2. $X = 51$
   $2X = 34 \times 3 \quad 2X = 102$
   $X = 102/2$

   $$2\overline{)102}$$
   $$\underline{10}$$
   $$02$$
   $$\underline{\ 2}$$

3. $X = 46$
   $0.65X = 23 \times 1.3$
   $0.65X = 29.9 \quad X = 29.9/0.65$

   $$65\overline{)2990}$$
   $$\underline{260}$$
   $$390$$
   $$\underline{390}$$

4. $X = 2.76$
   $1000X = 1200 \times 2.3$
   $1000 X = 2760$
   $X = 2760/1000 = 2.76$

   $$1000\overline{)2760.00}$$
   $$\underline{2000}$$
   $$7600$$
   $$\underline{7000}$$
   $$6000$$
   $$\underline{6000}$$

5. $X = 160$
   $1/8X = 2 \times 10$
   $1/8X = 20$

   $$X = \frac{20}{1/8}$$

   $20 \times 8/1 = 160$

6. $X = 0.4$
   $75X = 30$
   $X = 30/75$

   $$75\overline{)30.0}$$
   $$\underline{300}$$

7. $X = 1.32$
   $3000X = 2.2 \times 1800$
   $3000X = 3960$
   $X = 3960/3000$

   $$3000\overline{)3960.00}$$
   $$\underline{3000}$$
   $$9600$$
   $$\underline{9000}$$
   $$6000$$
   $$\underline{6000}$$

8. X = 6
   81X = 9 × 54
   81X = 486   X = 486/81

   $$\begin{array}{r} 6 \\ 81\overline{)486} \\ \underline{486} \end{array}$$

9. X = 1.5

   $$2X = \frac{1}{3} \times \frac{9}{1}$$

   $$2X = \frac{9}{3} = \frac{3}{1} \quad 2X = 3 \quad X = 3/2$$

   $$\begin{array}{r} 1.5 \\ 2\overline{)3.0} \\ \underline{20} \\ 10 \\ \underline{10} \end{array}$$

10. X = 750
    5X = 125 × 30   5X = 3750
    X = 3750/5 = 750

    $$\begin{array}{r} 750 \\ 5\overline{)3750} \\ \underline{35} \\ 25 \\ \underline{25} \end{array}$$

Calculating Medication Dosages, pp. 83-85

1. X = 7.5 mL

   $$\frac{40\ mEq}{15\ mL} = \frac{20\ mEq}{X\ mL}$$

   40X = 15 × 20   40X = 300
   X = 300/40

   $$\begin{array}{r} 7.5 \\ 40\overline{)300.0} \\ \underline{280} \\ 200 \\ \underline{200} \end{array}$$

2. X = 3 tablets

   $$\frac{2.5\ mg}{1\ tab} = \frac{7.5\ mg}{X\ tab}$$

   2.5X = 7.5   X = 7.5/2.5

   $$\begin{array}{r} 3 \\ 25\overline{)75} \\ \underline{75} \end{array}$$

3. X = 20 mL

   $$\frac{12.5\ mg}{5\ mL} = \frac{50\ mg}{X\ mL}$$

   12.5X = 5 × 50
   12.5X = 250   X = 250/12.5

   $$\begin{array}{r} 20 \\ 125\overline{)2500} \\ \underline{250} \end{array}$$

4. X = 10 mL

   $$\frac{15\ mg}{1\ mL} = \frac{150\ mg}{X\ mL}$$

   15X = 150   X = 150/15

   $$\begin{array}{r} 10 \\ 15\overline{)150} \\ \underline{15} \end{array}$$

5. X = 4 tablets

   $$\frac{0.5\ mg}{1\ tab} = \frac{2\ mg}{X\ tab}$$

   0.5X = 2   X = 2/0.5 = 20/5

   $$\begin{array}{r} 4 \\ 5\overline{)20} \\ \underline{20} \end{array}$$

6. X = 19.5 mL

   $$\frac{500\ mg}{15\ mL} = \frac{650\ mg}{X\ mL}$$

   500X = 15 × 650
   500X = 9750   X = 9750/500

   $$\begin{array}{r} 19.5 \\ 500\overline{)9750.0} \\ \underline{500} \\ 4750 \\ \underline{4500} \\ 2500 \\ \underline{2500} \end{array}$$

7. X = 8 tablets

   $$\frac{0.25\ mg}{1\ tab} = \frac{2\ mg}{X\ tab}$$

   0.25X = 2   X = 2/0.25

   $$\begin{array}{r} 8 \\ 25\overline{)200} \\ \underline{200} \end{array}$$

8. X = 4 tablets
   50 mcg = 0.05 mg

   $$\frac{0.05\ mg}{1\ tab} = \frac{0.2\ mg}{X\ tab}$$

   0.05X = 0.2   X = 0.2/0.05

   $$\begin{array}{r} 4 \\ 5\overline{)20} \\ \underline{20} \end{array}$$

9. X = 2 tablets

   $$\frac{0.125\ mg}{1\ tab} = \frac{0.25\ mg}{X\ tab}$$

   0.125X = 0.25   X = 0.25/0.125

   $$\begin{array}{r} 2 \\ 125\overline{)250} \\ \underline{250} \end{array}$$

10. X = 0.25 mL

    $$\frac{10,000\ Units}{1\ mL} = \frac{2500\ Units}{X\ mL}$$

    10,000X = 2500
    X = 2500/10,000

    $$\begin{array}{r} 0.25 \\ 10,000\overline{)2500.00} \\ \underline{20000} \\ 50000 \\ \underline{50000} \end{array}$$

Formula Method, pp. 89-92

1. larger, more, X = 6 mL
   D = 60
   H = 10
   V = 1

   $$\frac{60}{10} \times 1 = X$$

   $$\begin{array}{r} 6 \\ 10\overline{)60} \\ \underline{60} \end{array}$$

2. smaller, less, X = 0.75 mL
D = 15
H = 20
V = 1

$$\frac{15}{20} \times 1 = X$$

$$20\overline{)15.00}\ \ ^{0.75}$$
$$\underline{140}$$
$$100$$
$$\underline{100}$$

3. smaller, less, X = 0.5 mL
D = 0.2
H = 0.4
V = 1

$$\frac{0.2}{0.4} \times 1 = X$$

$$4\overline{)2.0}\ \ ^{0.5}$$
$$\underline{2.0}$$

4. smaller, less, X = 0.5 mL
D = 5
H = 10
V = 1

$$\frac{5}{10} \times 1 = X$$

$$10\overline{)5.0}\ \ ^{0.5}$$
$$\underline{50}$$
$$0$$

5. smaller, less, X = 0.5 mL
D = 12.5
H = 25
V = 1

$$\frac{12.5}{25} \times 1 = X$$

$$25\overline{)12.5}\ \ ^{0.5}$$
$$\underline{125}$$

6. larger, more, X = 2.1 mL
Must convert first: 0.63 mg × 1000 = 630 mcg.

$$\frac{630\ mcg}{300\ mcg} \times 1\ mL = X$$

$$300\overline{)630.0}\ \ ^{2.1}$$
$$\underline{600}$$
$$300$$
$$\underline{300}$$

7. larger, more, X = 1.25 mL
Must convert first: 0.25 mg × 1000 = 250 mcg.

$$\frac{250\ mcg}{200\ mcg} \times 1\ mL = X$$

$$200\overline{)250.00}\ \ ^{1.25}$$
$$\underline{200}$$
$$500$$
$$\underline{400}$$
$$1000$$
$$\underline{1000}$$

8. larger, more, X = 1.5 mL

$$\frac{600\ mcg}{400\ mcg} \times 1 = X$$

$$4\overline{)6}\ \ ^{1.5}$$
$$\underline{4}$$
$$20$$
$$\underline{20}$$

9. smaller, less, X = 4 mL
Must convert first: 400 mg ÷ 1000 = 0.4 g.

$$\frac{0.4\ g}{1\ g} \times 10\ mL = X$$

0.4 × 10 = 4

$$1\overline{)4}\ \ ^{4}$$

10. smaller, less, X = 0.25 mL
Must convert first: 0.05 mg × 1000 = 50 mcg.

$$\frac{50\ mcg}{200\ mcg} \times 1\ mL = X$$

$$200\overline{)50.00}\ \ ^{0.25}$$
$$\underline{400}$$
$$1000$$
$$\underline{1000}$$

Chapter Review, pp. 92-94

1. 1.5 or 1½ tablets

2. 1.25 mL

3. 2 capsules

4. 0.8 mL

5. 0.7 mL

6. 2 tablets

7. 1.6 mL

8. 2 tablets

9. 10 mg

10. 4 mL

11. 0.5 or ½ tablet

12. 2.5 mL

13. 1.5 or 1½ tablets

14. 1.6 mL

15. 1.6 mL

16. 2 tablets

17. 2 mL

18. 30 mL

19. 2 capsules

20. 12.5 mL

CHAPTER 8
Body Weight

Converting Pounds to Kilograms, pp. 95-96

1. 61.36

$$
22\overline{)1350.00} \\
\underline{132} \\
30 \\
\underline{22} \\
80 \\
\underline{66} \\
140 \\
\underline{132} \\
8
$$

2. 112.27

$$
22\overline{)2470.00} \\
\underline{22} \\
27 \\
\underline{22} \\
50 \\
\underline{44} \\
60 \\
\underline{44} \\
160 \\
\underline{154} \\
6
$$

3. 84.09

$$
22\overline{)1850.00} \\
\underline{176} \\
90 \\
\underline{88} \\
200 \\
\underline{198} \\
2
$$

4. 56.36

$$
22\overline{)1240.00} \\
\underline{110} \\
140 \\
\underline{132} \\
80 \\
\underline{66} \\
140 \\
\underline{132} \\
8
$$

5. 66.36

$$
22\overline{)1460.00} \\
\underline{132} \\
140 \\
\underline{132} \\
80 \\
\underline{66} \\
140 \\
\underline{132} \\
8
$$

6. 100.9

$$
22\overline{)2220.0} \\
\underline{22} \\
0200 \\
\underline{198} \\
2
$$

7. 91.36

$$
22\overline{)2010.00} \\
\underline{198} \\
30 \\
\underline{22} \\
80 \\
\underline{66} \\
140 \\
\underline{132} \\
8
$$

8. 79.54

$$
22\overline{)1750.00} \\
\underline{154} \\
210 \\
\underline{198} \\
120 \\
\underline{110} \\
100 \\
\underline{88} \\
12
$$

9. 70.9

$$
22\overline{)1560.00} \\
\underline{154} \\
200 \\
\underline{198} \\
2
$$

10. 76.36

$$
22\overline{)1680.00} \\
\underline{154} \\
140 \\
\underline{132} \\
80 \\
\underline{66} \\
140 \\
\underline{132} \\
8
$$

Calculating Body Weight, pp. 99-100
Keep answers to the tenth

1. 95.45 kg, 0.6 mg, 57 mg, 210/2.2 = 95.5 × 0.6 = 57.27 mg = 57.3 mg

2. 63.63 kg, 150 units, 9540 units, 140/2.2 = 63.63 × 150 = 9544.5 units

3. 100 kg, 15 mg, 1500 mg, 220/2.2 = 100 × 15 = 1500 mg

4. 60 kg, 0.8 mg, 48 mg, 132/2.2 = 60 × 0.8 = 48 mg

5. 73 kg, 10 mcg, 730 mcg, 73 × 10 = 730 mcg

6. 82 kg, 0.25 mg, 21 mg, 82 × 0.25 = 20.5 mg = 21 mg

7. 63.63 kg, 0.4 mg, 25 mg, 140/2.2 = 63.63 × 0.4 = 25.45 mg = 25.5 mg

8. 55.45 kg, 110.9 mg, 443.6 mg, 122/2.2 = 55.45 × 8 = 443.6 mg

9. 60 kg, 2.2 mg, 132 mg, 60 × 2.2 = 132 mg

10. 71.8 kg, 15 mg, 1077 mg, 158/2.2 = 71.8 × 15 = 1077.2 mg

Chapter Review, pp. 100-101

1. 46.2 mg

2. 8454.5 units

3. 754.6 mg

4. 32.2 mg

5. 820 mcg

6. 23.5 mg

7. 37.5 mg

8. 170.9 mg

9. 162.8 mg

10. 854.6 mg

11. 43.1 mg

12. 8454.6 units

13. 1159.1 mg

14. 37.1 mg

15. 365 mcg

16. 24 mg

17. 12.7 mg

18. 516.4 mg

19. 45 mg

20. 954.6 mg

CHAPTER 9
Using Syringes
Syringes, pp. 108-112

1. b

2. a

3. d

4. a

5. b

6. d

7. e

8. c

9. a or b

10. e

11. b

12. 12 mL

13. 0.3 mL

14. 0.25 mL

15. 16 mL

16. 2.7 mL

17. 2.3 mL

18. 8 mL

19. 0.3 mL

20. 1.2 mL

21. 1.6 mL

22.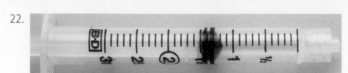

23.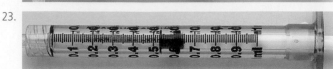

24.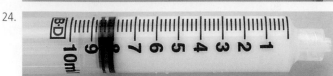

25.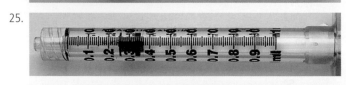

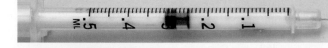

26.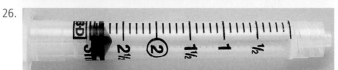

27.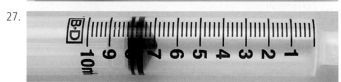

28.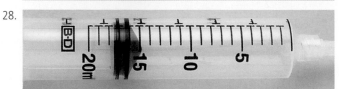

29.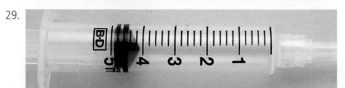

30.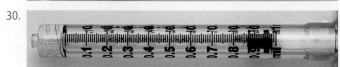

31.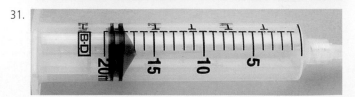

Prefilled Syringes, pp. 118-120

1. 0.1 mL, Yes, discard 0.1 mL.

$$\frac{5000 \text{ units}}{0.2 \text{ mL}} = \frac{2500 \text{ units}}{X \text{ mL}}$$

$$5000X = 500 \quad X = \frac{500}{5000} = \frac{1}{10}$$

$$10\overline{)1.0} \quad \frac{0.1 \text{ mL (administer)}}{}$$
0.1 mL discard

2. 0.5 mL, No, administer the entire syringe.
60 kg × 5 mcg = 300 mcg

3. 0.28 mL, Yes, discard 0.22 mL.

$$\frac{44 \text{ mcg}}{0.5 \text{ mL}} = \frac{25 \text{ mcg}}{X \text{ mL}} \quad 44X = 12.5$$

$$44\overline{)12.50} \quad \frac{0.28 \text{ mL (administer)}}{}$$
$$\underline{88}$$
$$370$$
$$\underline{352}$$

0.50 mL
$$\underline{-0.28 \text{ mL}}$$
0.22 mL discard

4. 0.8 mL, No discard. Administer the entire syringe.
0.04 g = 40 mg (move the decimal three places to the right)

5. 4 mL, No discard. Administer 4 syringes (4 mL).

$$\frac{600,000 \text{ units}}{1 \text{ mL}} = \frac{2,400,000 \text{ units}}{X \text{ mL}}$$

$$600,000X = 2,400,000$$

$$6\overline{)24} \quad \frac{4 \text{ mL (administer)}}{}$$

6. 0.5 mL, Yes, discard 0.5 mL.

$$\frac{50 \text{ mg}}{1 \text{ mL}} = \frac{25 \text{ mg}}{X \text{ mL}} \quad 50X = 25$$

$$50\overline{)25.0} \quad \frac{0.5 \text{ mL (administer)}}{}$$
$$\underline{250}$$

1.0 mL
$$\underline{-0.5 \text{ mL}}$$
0.5 mL discard

7. 0.75 mL, Yes, discard 0.25 mL.

$$\frac{4 \text{ mg}}{1 \text{ mL}} = \frac{3 \text{ mg}}{X \text{ mL}} \quad 4X = 3$$

$$4\overline{)3.00} \quad \frac{0.75 \text{ mL (administer)}}{}$$
$$\underline{28}$$
$$20$$
$$\underline{20}$$

1.00 mL
$$\underline{-0.75 \text{ mL}}$$
0.25 mL discard

8. 1.2 mL, Administer one full syringe and, from a second syringe, administer 0.2 mL and discard 0.8 mL.

9 kg × 4 mg = 36 mg

$$\frac{30 \text{ mg}}{1 \text{ mL}} = \frac{36 \text{ mg}}{X \text{ mL}} \quad 30X = 36$$

$$30\overline{)36.0} \quad \frac{1.2 \text{ mL (administer)}}{}$$
$$\underline{30}$$
$$60$$
$$\underline{60}$$

1.0 mL
$$\underline{-0.2 \text{ mL}}$$
0.8 mL discard from second syringe

9. 0.6 mL, Yes, discard 0.4 mL

$$\frac{4 \text{ mg}}{1 \text{ mL}} = \frac{2.5 \text{ mg}}{X \text{ mL}} \quad 4X = 2.5$$

$$4\overline{)2.50} \quad \frac{0.62 \text{ mL} \quad (\text{administer } 0.6)}{}$$
$$\underline{24}$$
$$10$$
$$\underline{8}$$
$$2$$

1.00 mL
$$\underline{-0.63 \text{ mL}}$$
0.37 mL discard

10. 1 mL, No discard. Administer the entire syringe.

20,000 mcg (move decimal point three spaces to the left) = 20 mg

$$\frac{20 \text{ mg}}{1 \text{ mL}} = \frac{20 \text{ mg}}{X \text{ mL}}$$

20X = 20

X = 1 mL   No discard required

About 0.5-mL and 1-mL Syringes and Insulin Syringes, pp. 121-124

1. 5 units

2. 0.65 mL

3. 0.35 mL

4. 0.29 mL

5. 0.47 mL

6. 10 units

7. 78 units

8. 0.2 mL

9. 66 units

10. 0.22 mL

11.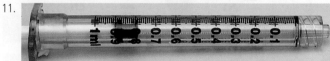

12.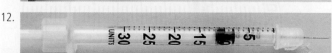

13.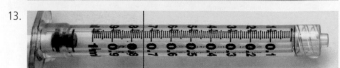

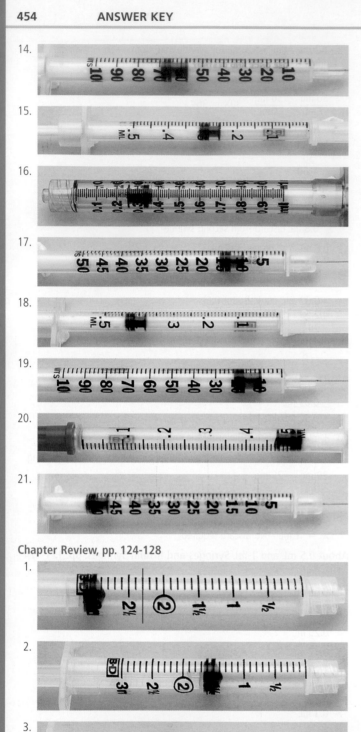

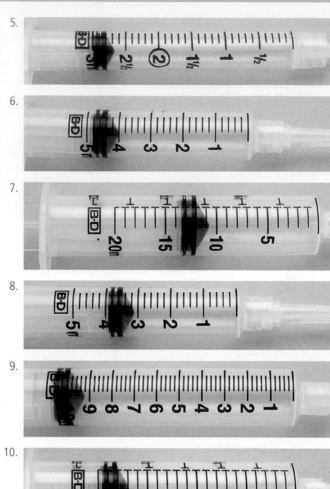

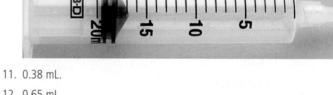

11. 0.38 mL.

12. 0.65 mL.

13. 0.87 mL.

14. 0.75 mL.

15. 27 units.

16. 0.3 mL.

17. 0.6 mL.

18. 0.1 mL.

19. 13 units.

20. 0.8 mL.

CHAPTER 10

Oral Medications

Medication Labels, pp. 137-141

1. Dilaudid; hydromorphone HCl; 2 mg; metric.

2. Acetaminophen; Tylenol; 160 mg/5 mL, 80 mg per ½ teaspoon; metric and household; suspension liquid.

3. Mycophenolate; CellCept; 250 mg; metric; Roche; 09/2014; capsule; store at 25° C (77° F).

4. Tylenol; acetaminophen; 500 mg; metric; caplets; McNeil.

5. Prilosec OTC; omeprazole; 20 mg; metric; 03/14; delayed-release tablets.

6. Tylenol; acetaminophen; 325 mg; caplets; metric.

7. Zofran; ondansetron hydrochloride; 8 mg; metric; tablets; GlaxoSmithKline.

8. Mucinex; guaifenesin; 600 mg; metric; 11/2014; extended-release tablets; Adams.

9. Vibramycin; doxycycline monohydrate; 25 mg per 5 mL or each teaspoon; metric and household; 1 Jul/14; oral suspension; Pfizer Labs.

10. Difulcan; fluconazole; 10 mg/mL; metric; 1 Jun 14; oral suspension; Roerig.

Calculating Solid Medication Dosages, pp. 144-148

1. Yes, acetaminophen, yes, yes, larger, 2 caplets.

   Ratio-proportion method:

   $$\frac{325 \text{ mg}}{1 \text{ caplet}} = \frac{650 \text{ mg}}{X \text{ caplet(s)}} \quad 325X = 650$$

   $$325)\overline{650} \quad \begin{array}{c} 2 \text{ caplets} \\ \underline{650} \end{array}$$

   Formula method:

   $$\frac{650 \text{ mg}}{325 \text{ mg}} \times 1 = 2 \text{ caplets}$$

2. Yes, Glucophage, yes, same, 1 tablet.

3. Yes, captopril, yes, same, 1 tablet.

4. Yes, furosemide, yes, yes, larger, 3 tablets.

   Ratio-proportion method:

   $$\frac{40 \text{ mg}}{1 \text{ tablet}} = \frac{120 \text{ mg}}{X \text{ tablet(s)}} \quad 40X = 120$$

   $$40)\overline{120} \quad \begin{array}{c} 3 \text{ tablets} \\ \underline{120} \end{array}$$

   Formula method:

   $$\frac{120 \text{ mg}}{40 \text{ mg}} \times 1 = 3 \text{ tablets}$$

5. Yes, Detrol, yes, same, 1 tablet.

6. Yes, digoxin, yes, no, same, 1 tablet.
   250 mcg = 0.25 mg

7. Yes, lorazepam, yes, same larger, 2 tablets.

   Ratio-proportion method:

   $$\frac{1 \text{ mg}}{1 \text{ tablet}} = \frac{2 \text{ mg}}{X \text{ tablet(s)}} \quad X = 2 \text{ tablets}$$

   Formula method:

   $$\frac{2 \text{ mg}}{1 \text{ mg}} \times 1 = 2 \text{ tablets}$$

8. 0.8 mg

   Ratio-proportion method:

   $$\frac{0.4 \text{ mg}}{1 \text{ tablet}} = \frac{X}{2 \text{ tablets}} = X = 0.4 \times 2 \quad X = 0.8 \text{ mg}$$

   Formula method:

   $$\frac{X \text{ mg}}{0.4 \text{ mg}} \times 2 \text{ tablets} \quad X = 0.8 \text{ mg}$$

9. Yes, metoprolol tartrate, yes, yes, larger, 2 tablets.

   Ratio-proportion method:

   $$\frac{50 \text{ mg}}{1 \text{ tablet}} = \frac{100 \text{ mg}}{X \text{ tablet(s)}} \quad 50X = 100$$

   $$50)\overline{100} \quad \begin{array}{c} 2 \text{ tablets} \\ \underline{100} \end{array}$$

   Formula method:

   $$\frac{100 \text{ mg}}{50 \text{ mg}} \times 1 = 2 \text{ tablets}$$

10. Yes, levothyroxine, yes, yes, same, 1 tablet.
    50 mcg = 0.05 mg

Calculating Liquid Medication Dosages, pp. 154-159

1. 20 mg/5 mL, 25 mL

   Ratio-proportion method:

   $$\frac{20 \text{ mg}}{5 \text{ mL}} = \frac{100 \text{ mg}}{X \text{ mL}} \quad 20X = 500$$

   $$20)\overline{500} \quad \begin{array}{c} 25 \text{ mL (administer)} \end{array}$$

   Formula method:

   100 mg/20 mg × 5 mL = 25 mL

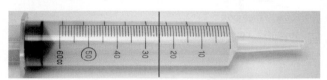

2. Penicillin VK, 125 mg/5 mL, 20 mL

   Ratio-proportion method:

   $$\frac{125 \text{ mg}}{5 \text{ mL}} = \frac{500 \text{ mg}}{X \text{ mL}}$$

   Reduce: $\frac{25}{1} = \frac{500}{X}$

   $$25X = 500 \quad X = 20 \text{ mL}$$

   $$25)\overline{500} \quad \begin{array}{c} 20 \text{ mL (administer)} \end{array}$$

   Formula method:

   500 mg/125 mg × 5 mL = 20 mL

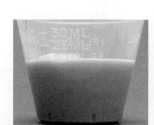

3. Zantac, 15 mg/mL, 20 mL

   Ratio-proportion method:

   $$\frac{15 \text{ mg}}{1 \text{ mL}} = \frac{300 \text{ mg}}{X \text{ mL}} \quad 15X = 300$$

   $$15)\overline{300} \quad \begin{array}{c} 20 \text{ mL (administer)} \\ \underline{300} \end{array}$$

   Formula method:

   300 mg/15 mg × 1 mL = 20 mL

4. Mellaril, 30 mg/1 mL, 10 mL

   Ratio-proportion method:

   $$\frac{30 \text{ mg}}{1 \text{ mL}} = \frac{300 \text{ mg}}{X \text{ mL}} \quad 30X = 300$$

   $$30)\overline{300.00} \quad \begin{array}{c} 10 \text{ mL (administer)} \end{array}$$

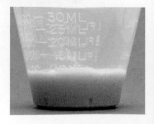

Formula method:

300 mg/30 mg × 1 mL = 10 mL

5. Kaon CL, 40 mEq/15 mL, 30 mL

Ratio-proportion method:

$$\frac{40\ mEq}{15\ mL} = \frac{80\ mEq}{X\ mL} \quad 40X = 1200$$

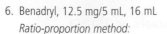

$$40\overline{)1200} \quad \frac{30\ mL\ (administer)}{}$$

Formula method:

80 mEq/40 mEq × 15 mL = 30 mL

6. Benadryl, 12.5 mg/5 mL, 16 mL

Ratio-proportion method:

$$\frac{12.5\ mg}{5\ mL} = \frac{40\ mg}{X\ mL} \quad 12.5X = 200$$

Remember to move decimal point in both the dividend and the divisor to the right.

$$125\overline{)2000} \quad \frac{16\ mL\ (administer)}{}$$
$$\underline{125}$$
$$750$$
$$\underline{750}$$

Formula method:

40 mg/12.5 mg × 5 mL = 16 mL

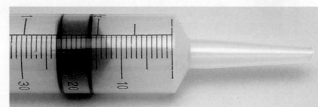

7. Cleocin Pediatric, 75 mg/5 mL, 3.3 mL

Ratio-proportion method:

$$\frac{75\ mg}{5\ mL} = \frac{50\ mg}{X\ mL} \quad 75X = 250$$

$$75\overline{)250.00} \quad \frac{3.33\ mL\ (round\ to\ nearest\ tenth)}{}$$
$$\underline{225}$$
$$250$$
$$\underline{225}$$
$$250$$
$$\underline{225}$$

Formula method:

50 mg/75 mg × 5 mL = 3.3 mL

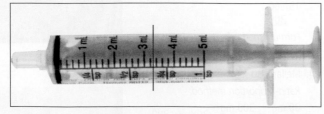

8. Cefixime, 100 mg/5 mL, 10 mL

Ratio-proportion method:

$$\frac{100\ mg}{5\ mL} = \frac{200\ mg}{X\ mL}$$

Reduce: $\dfrac{20}{1} = \dfrac{200}{X}$

20X = 200 mL   X = 10 mL

Formula method:

$$\frac{200\ mg}{100\ mg} \times 5\ mL = 10\ mL$$

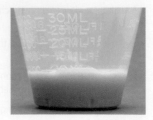

9. Lanoxin, 0.05 mg/mL, 3 mL

Ratio-proportion method:

150 mcg = 0.15 mg

$$\frac{0.05\ mg}{1\ mL} = \frac{0.15\ mg}{X\ mL} \quad 0.05X = 0.15$$

$$5\overline{)15} \quad \frac{3\ mL}{}$$
$$\underline{15}$$

Formula method:

$$\frac{0.15\ mg}{0.05\ mg} \times 1\ mL = 3\ mL$$

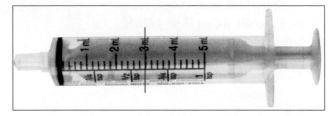

10. Amoxil, 125 mg/5 mL, 10 mL

0.25 g = 250 mg

Ratio-proportion method:

$$\frac{125\ mg}{5\ mL} = \frac{250\ mg}{X\ mL}$$

Reduce: $\dfrac{1}{5} = \dfrac{2}{X}$ X = 10 mL

Formula method:

$$\frac{250\ mg}{125\ mg} \times 5\ mL = 10\ mL$$

Chapter Review, pp. 160-172

1. Yes, no, larger, 2 tablets.

2. Yes, yes, yes, larger, 2 tablets.

3. Yes, yes, larger, 2 tablets.

4. Yes, yes, larger, 2 tablets.

5. Yes, yes, 10 mL.

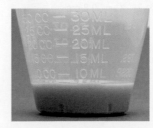

6. Yes, yes, 10 mL.

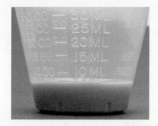

7. Yes, 3 capsules.

8. Yes, yes, larger, 2 tablets.

9. Yes, yes, larger, 2 tablets.

10. Yes, yes, yes, 10 mL.

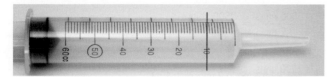

11. Yes, yes, 36 tablets.

12. Yes, yes, 3 tablets.

13. Yes, yes, larger, 4 tablets.

14. Yes, yes, yes, larger, 3 tablets.

15. Yes, yes, larger, 3 tablets.

16. Yes, no, 6 capsules.

17. Yes, yes, 10 mL.

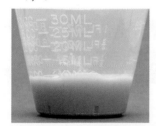

18. Yes, yes, larger, 10 mL.

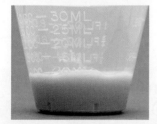

19. Yes, yes, yes, larger, 2 tablets.

20. Yes, no, larger, 2 tablets.

21. Yes, yes, larger, 4 tablets.

22. Yes, yes, same, 1 tablet.

23. Yes, yes, larger, 2 tablets.

24. Yes, yes, same, 1 tablet.

25. No, request appropriate medication and send wrong medication back to pharmacy.

26. Yes, yes, smaller, 2.5 mL.

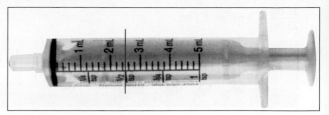

27. 1.2 mg.

CHAPTER 11
Parenteral Medications

Parenteral Medications, pp. 180-182

1. Ampicillin; ampicillin sodium; 500 mg; intramuscular or intravenous.

2. Ativan; lorazepam; 2 mg/mL; intramuscular; intravenous route requires dilution.

3. Demerol; meperidine hydrochloride; 100 mg/mL; yes; no.

4. Midazolam; 1 mg/mL; intramuscular or intravenous.

5. Diflucan; fluconazole; 2 mg/mL; intravenous injection; no; yes.

6. Magnesium sulfate; 1 g/2 mL; intravenous.

7. Diphenhydramine hydrochloride; 50 mg/mL; intramuscular or intravenous; no; yes.

8. Nitroglycerin; 5 mg/mL; intravenous infusion only; intravenous push; no; yes.

9. Neupogen; filgrastim; 300 mcg/mL; subcutaneous or intravenous; no; yes.

10. Concentrated sodium chloride; 234 mg/mL or 4 mEq/mL; intravenous or subcutaneous route after dilution.

Calculating Parenteral Dosages, pp. 187-191

1. Larger, 1.7 mL

Ratio-proportion method:

$$\frac{15 \text{ mg}}{1 \text{ mL}} = \frac{25 \text{ mg}}{X \text{ mL}} \quad 15X = 25$$

1.66 (round to nearest tenth)
15)25.0
15
100
90
10

Formula method:

$$\frac{25 \text{ mg}}{15 \text{ mg}} \times 1 \text{ mL} = 1.7 \text{ mL}$$

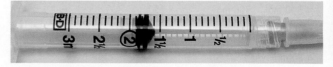

2. Larger, 1.2 mL

Ratio-proportion method:

$$\frac{25 \text{ mg}}{1 \text{ mL}} = \frac{30 \text{ mg}}{X \text{ mL}} \quad 25X = 30 \quad X = 1.2 \text{ mL}$$

1.2 mL
25)30.0
25
50
50

Formula method:

$$\frac{30 \text{ mg}}{25 \text{ mg}} \times 1 \text{ mL} = 1.2 \text{ mL}$$

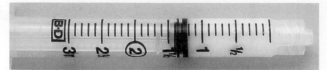

3. Larger, 1.6 mL

   Ratio-proportion method:

   $$\frac{100 \text{ mg}}{1 \text{ mL}} = \frac{160 \text{ mg}}{X \text{ mL}} \quad 100X = 160 \quad X = 1.6 \text{ mL}$$

$$\begin{array}{r} 1.6 \text{ mL} \\ 100\overline{)160.0} \\ \underline{100} \\ 600 \\ \underline{600} \end{array}$$

   Formula method:

   $$\frac{160 \text{ mg}}{100 \text{ mg}} \times 1 \text{ mL} = 1.6 \text{ mL}$$

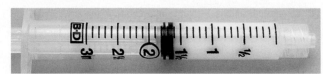

4. Larger, 4 mL, 2 mL/min

   Ratio-proportion method:

   $$\frac{10 \text{ mg}}{1 \text{ mL}} = \frac{40 \text{ mg}}{X \text{ mL}} \quad 10X = 40 \quad X = 4 \text{ mL}$$

$$\begin{array}{r} 4 \text{ mL} \\ 10\overline{)40} \end{array}$$

   Formula method:

   $$\frac{40 \text{ mg}}{10 \text{ mg}} \times 1 \text{ mL} = 4 \text{ mL}$$

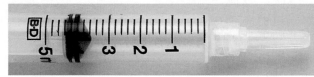

$$\frac{4 \text{ mL}}{2 \text{ min}} = 2 \text{ mL/min}$$

5. The same, 2 mL

   Ratio-proportion method:

   $$\frac{300 \text{ mg}}{2 \text{ mL}} = \frac{300 \text{ mg}}{X \text{ mL}} \quad \text{Reduce:} \quad \frac{150}{1} = \frac{300}{X}$$

   $$150X = 300 \quad X = 2 \text{ mL}$$

   Formula method:

   $$\frac{300 \text{ mg}}{300 \text{ mg}} \times 2 \text{ mL} = 2 \text{ mL}$$

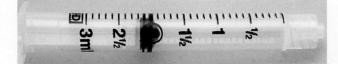

6. Larger, 1.5 mL

   Ratio-proportion method:

   $$\frac{5 \text{ mg}}{1 \text{ mL}} = \frac{7.5 \text{ mg}}{X \text{ mL}} \quad 5X = 7.5 \quad X = 1.5 \text{ mL}$$

   Formula method:

   $$\frac{7.5 \text{ mg}}{5 \text{ mg}} \times 1 \text{ mL} = 1.5 \text{ mL}$$

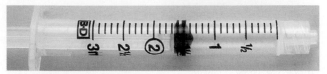

7. Smaller, 0.1 mL, 0.1 mL

   Ratio-proportion method:

   $$\frac{5000 \text{ units}}{0.2 \text{ mL}} = \frac{2500 \text{ units}}{X \text{ mL}} \quad 5000X = 500 \quad X = 0.1 \text{ mL}$$

   Formula method:

   $$\frac{2500 \text{ units}}{5000 \text{ units}} \times 0.2 \text{ mL} = 0.1 \text{ mL}$$

   Discard 0.1 mL.

8. Larger, 2 mL

   Ratio-proportion method:

   $$\frac{150 \text{ mg}}{1 \text{ mL}} = \frac{300 \text{ mg}}{X \text{ mL}} \quad 150X = 300 \quad X = 2 \text{ mL}$$

   Formula method:

   $$\frac{300 \text{ mg}}{150 \text{ mg}} \times 1 \text{ mL} = 2 \text{ mL}$$

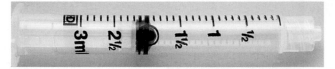

9. Smaller, 0.5 mL

   Ratio-proportion method:

   $$\frac{40 \text{ mg}}{1 \text{ mL}} = \frac{20}{X \text{ mL}} \quad 40X = 20 \quad X = 0.5 \text{ mL}$$

   Formula method:

   $$\frac{20 \text{ mg}}{40 \text{ mg}} \times 1 \text{ mL} = 0.5 \text{ mL}$$

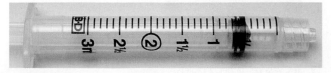

10. Larger, 2 mL

    Ratio-proportion method:

    $$\frac{25 \text{ mg}}{1 \text{ mL}} = \frac{50 \text{ mg}}{X \text{ mL}} \quad 25X = 50 \quad X = 2 \text{ mL}$$

    Formula method:

    $$\frac{50 \text{ mg}}{25 \text{ mg}} \times 1 \text{ mL} = 2 \text{ mL}$$

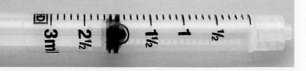

Chapter Review, pp. 191-199

1. 1.5 mL.

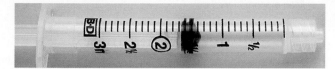

2. 0.87 mL.

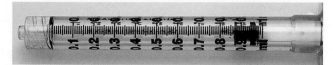

3. 3 mL.

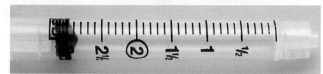

4. 0.35 mL.

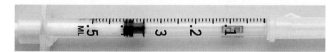

5. 1 mL, give 0.2 mL/min.

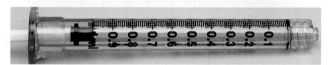

6. Add 10 mL to each liter.

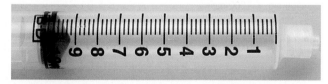

7. 3 mL; 3 mL over 1 minute.

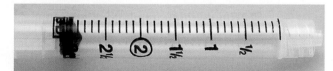

8. 1 mL.

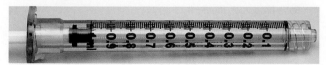

9. 0.5 mL.

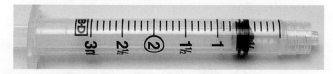

10. 0.5 mL.

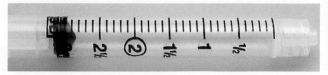

11. 3 mL, 1.5 mL/min.

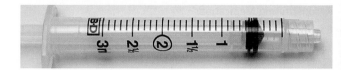

12. 0.4 mL.

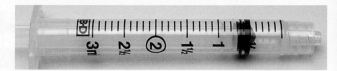

13. 1.5 mL.

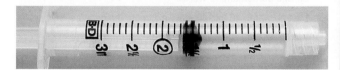

14. 3.8 mL, 1.5 minutes

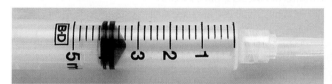

15. 0.67 mL.

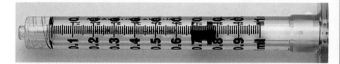

16. 1.5 mL and 23 seconds

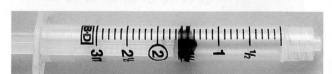

17. 1.6 mL.

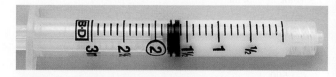

18. 600 mg/12 mL and 12 minutes.

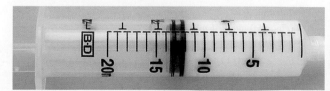

19. 0.5 mL.

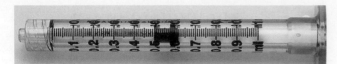

20. 1.2 mL.

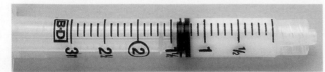

CHAPTER 12
Reconstituting Medications
Reading the Label, pp. 203-205

1. Water; 63 mL; 125 mg/5 mL; store dry powder and reconstituted suspension at 25° C (77° F); 10 days.

2. Distilled water; 24 mL; 10 mg/mL; between 41° F and 86° F. Discard unused portion after 2 weeks.

3. Purified water; 46 mL; 40 mg/5 mL; room temperature; 30 days.

4. Water; 47.6 mL; 25 mg/5 mL; see package insert; 2 weeks.

5. Water; 105 mL; 250 mg/5 mL; store below 30° C (86° F), protect from moisture; 14 days.

Parenteral Powders, pp. 214-219

1. 11.5 mL; 1,000,000 units/mL; 4 mL.

   Ratio-proportion method:

   $$\frac{1,000,000 \text{ units}}{1 \text{ mL}} = \frac{4,000,000 \text{ units}}{X \text{ mL}}$$

   Reduce by 1,000,000: $\frac{1}{1} = \frac{4}{X}$ X = 4 mL

   Formula method:

   $$\frac{4,000,000 \text{ units}}{1,000,000 \text{ units}} \times 1 \text{ mL} = 4 \text{ mL}$$

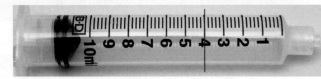

2. 1.8 mL; 500 mg/2 mL, 2 mL.

   Ratio-proportion method:

   $$\frac{250 \text{ mg}}{1 \text{ mL}} = \frac{500 \text{ mg}}{X \text{ mL}}$$

   250 X = 500
   X = 2 mL

   $$250\overline{)500} \atop \underline{500} \atop 0 \atop ^{\displaystyle 2}$$

   Formula method:

   500 mg/250 mg × 1 mL = 2 mL

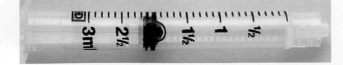

3. 9.8 mL; 5000 units/mL; 4.2 mL; 10,500 units; 2.1 mL.
   21 kg × 1000 units = 21,000 units/day

   Ratio-proportion method:

   $$\frac{5000 \text{ units}}{1 \text{ mL}} = \frac{21,000 \text{ units}}{X \text{ mL}}$$

   Reduce by 1000: $\frac{5}{1} = \frac{21}{X}$ 5X = 21 X = 4.2 (each dose is 2.1 mL)

   2.1 × 5000 = 10,500 units

   Formula method:

   21,000 units/5000 units × 1 mL = 4.2 mL per day
   (in two doses of 2.1 mL)

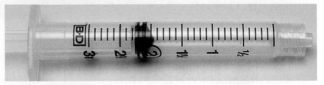

4. 95 mL; 100 mg/mL, 10 mL.

   Ratio-proportion method:

   $$\frac{100 \text{ mg}}{1 \text{ mL}} = \frac{1000 \text{ mg}}{X \text{ mL}}$$ Reduce by 100: $\frac{1}{1} = \frac{10}{X}$ X = 10

   Formula method:

   1000 mg/100 mg × 1 mL = 10 mL

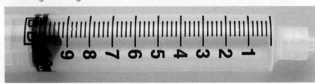

5. 9 mL; 400 mg/mL, 3.8 mL.

   Ratio-proportion method:

   $$\frac{400 \text{ mg}}{1 \text{ mL}} = \frac{1500 \text{ mg}}{X \text{ mL}}$$

   Reduce by 100: $\frac{4}{1} = \frac{15}{X}$ 4X = 15 X = 3.8

   Formula method:

   1500 mg/400 mg × 1 mL = 3.8 mL

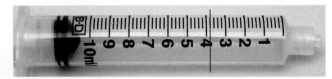

6. 3 mL; 300 mg/mL, 2.5 mL.

   Ratio-proportion method:

   $$\frac{300 \text{ mg}}{1 \text{ mL}} = \frac{750 \text{ mg}}{X \text{ mL}}$$

   Reduce by 30: $\frac{10}{1} = \frac{25}{X}$ 10X = 25 X = 2.5

   Formula method:

   750 mg/300 mg × 1 mL = 2.5 mL

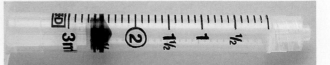

7. 3 mL; 280 mg/mL, 1.8 mL.

Ratio-proportion method:

$$\frac{280\ mg}{1\ mL} = \frac{500\ mg}{X\ mL}$$

Reduce by 10: $\frac{28}{1} = \frac{50}{X}$ $28X = 50$ $X = 1.8$

Formula method:

500 mg/280 mg × 1 mL = 1.8 mL

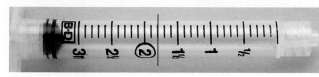

8. 6.6 mL; 250 mg/mL, 2 mL.

Ratio-proportion method:

$$\frac{250\ mg}{1\ mL} = \frac{500\ mg}{X\ mL}$$

Reduce by 250: $\frac{1}{1} = \frac{2}{X}$ $X = 2$

Formula method:

500 mg/250 mg × 1 mL = 2 mL

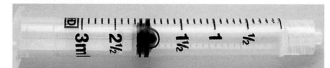

9. 11.5 mL; 250 mg/mL, 1.5 mL.

Ratio-proportion method:

$$\frac{250\ mg}{1.5\ mL} = \frac{250\ mg}{X\ mL}$$ $250\ X = 375$ $X = 1.5\ mL$

Formula method:

250 mg/250 mg × 1.5 mL = 1.5 mL

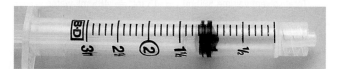

10. 2.5 mL; 330 mg/mL, 1.5 mL.

Ratio-proportion method:

$$\frac{330\ mg}{1\ mL} = \frac{500\ mg}{X\ mL}$$

Reduce by 10: $\frac{33}{1} = \frac{50}{X}$ $33X = 50$ $X = 1.5$

Formula method:

500 mg/330 mg × 1 mL = 1.5 mL

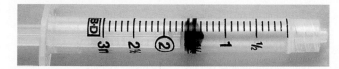

Oral Medications, pp. 224-230

1. 59 mL; 250 mg/5 mL, 10 mL.

Ratio-proportion method:

$$\frac{250\ mg}{5\ mL} = \frac{500\ mg}{X\ mL}$$

Reduce: $\frac{1}{5} = \frac{2}{X}$ $X = 10\ mL$

Formula method:

500 mg/250 mg × 5 mL = 10

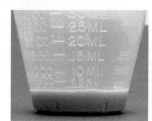

2. 100 mg; 5 mL; 15 mL, 10 mL.

Ratio-proportion method:

$$\frac{100\ mg}{5\ mL} = \frac{200\ mg}{X\ mL}$$

Reduce by 100: $\frac{1}{5} = \frac{2}{X}$ $X = 10$

Formula method:

For day 1: 200 mg/100 mg × 5 mL = 10 mL
For day 2-5: 100 mg/100 mg × 5 mL = 5 mL

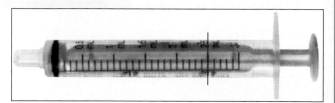

3. 46 mL; 40 mg/5 mL, 2.5 mL.

Ratio-proportion method:

$$\frac{40\ mg}{5\ mL} = \frac{20\ mg}{X\ mL}$$

Reduce by 20: $\frac{2}{5} = \frac{1}{X}$ $2X = 5$ $X = 2.5\ mL$

Formula method:

20 mg/40 mg × 5 mL = 2.5 mL

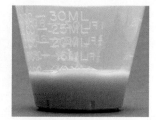

4. 47.6 mL; 25 mg/5 mL, 20 mL.

Ratio-proportion method:

$$\frac{25\ mg}{5\ mL} = \frac{100\ mg}{X\ mL}$$

Reduce by 25: $\frac{1}{5} = \frac{4}{X}$ $X = 20$

Formula method:

100 mg/25 mg × 5 mL = 20 ml

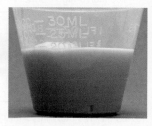

5. 24 mL; 10 mg/mL, 7.5 mL.
   Ratio-proportion method:

   $$\frac{10 \text{ mg}}{1 \text{ mL}} = \frac{75 \text{ mg}}{X \text{ mL}}$$

   Reduce by 10: $\frac{1}{1} = \frac{7.5}{X}$ X = 7.5

   Formula method:
   75 mg/10 mg × 1 mL = 7.5 mL

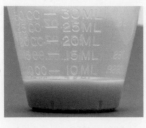

6. 78 mL; 125 mg/5 mL, 10 mL.
   Ratio-proportion method:

   $$\frac{125 \text{ mg}}{5 \text{ mL}} = \frac{250 \text{ mg}}{X \text{ mL}}$$

   Reduce by 125: $\frac{1}{5} = \frac{2}{X}$ X = 10

   Formula method:
   250 mg/125 mg × 5 mL = 10 mL

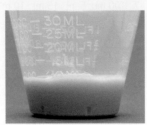

7. 69 mL; 100 mg/5 mL, 20 mL.
   Ratio-proportion method:

   $$\frac{100 \text{ mg}}{5 \text{ mL}} = \frac{400 \text{ mg}}{X \text{ mL}}$$

   Reduce by 100: $\frac{1}{5} = \frac{4}{X}$ X = 20

   Formula method:
   400 mg/100 mg × 5 mL = 20 mL

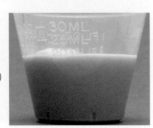

8. 45 mL; 200 mg/5 mL, 10 mL.
   Ratio-proportion method:

   $$\frac{200 \text{ mg}}{5 \text{ mL}} = \frac{400 \text{ mg}}{X \text{ mL}}$$

   Reduce by 200: $\frac{1}{5} = \frac{2}{X}$ X = 10

   Formula method:
   400 mg/200 mg × 5 mL = 10 mL

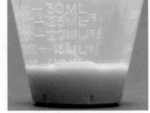

9. 75 mL; 75 mg/mL, 6.7 mL.
   Ratio-proportion method:

   $$\frac{75 \text{ mg}}{5 \text{ mL}} = \frac{100 \text{ mg}}{X \text{ mL}}$$ 75X = 500   X = 6.7

   Formula method:
   100 mg/75 mg × 5 mL = 6.7 mL

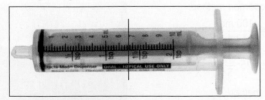

10. 63 mL; 125 mg/5 mL, 7 mL.

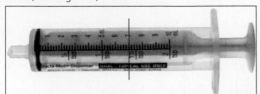

Ratio-proportion method:

$$\frac{125 \text{ mg}}{5 \text{ mL}} = \frac{175 \text{ mg}}{X \text{ mL}}$$

125X = 875   X = 7

Formula method:
175 mg/125 mg × 5 mL = 7 mL

Liquid Concentrates, pp. 233-235

1. $\frac{2}{5}$, 50 mL; 20 mL; 30 mL;

   40% = 40/100 (reduce fraction by 20)

   $$\frac{2}{5} = \frac{20 \text{ mL}}{X \text{ mL}}$$ 2X = 100   X = 50 mL

   Total solvent volume 50 mL − 20 mL = 30 mL water

2. $\frac{1}{10}$; 900 mL; 90 mL; 810 mL

   $$\frac{1}{10} = \frac{90 \text{ mL}}{X \text{ mL}}$$ X = 900 mL

   Total solvent volume 900 mL − 90 mL = 810 mL water

3. $\frac{1}{20}$; 250 mL; 5 mL or 1 tsp; 245 mL;

   2% = 2/100 (reduce fraction by 2)

   Convert teaspoons to mL = 5 mL

   $$\frac{1}{50} = \frac{5}{X}$$ X = 250 mL

   Total solvent volume 250 mL − 5 mL = 245 mL water

4. $\frac{1}{20}$; 1000 mL; 50 g; 950 mL; 5% is 5/100 (reduce fraction by 5)

   $$\frac{1}{20} = \frac{X}{1000}$$ 20X = 1000   X = 50 grams total solute

   Total solvent volume 1000 mL − 50 mL = 950 mL water

5. $\frac{3}{100}$; 500 mL; 15 mL or 3 tsp; 485 mL; 3% = 3/100

   $$\frac{3}{100} = \frac{X}{500}$$ 100X = 1500   X = 15 cc (3 tsp) total solute

   Total solvent volume 500 mL − 15 mL = 485 mL water

6. $\frac{3}{4}$; 200 mL; 150 mL; 50 mL

   $$\frac{3}{4} = \frac{X}{200}$$ 4X = 600   X = 150 mL

   Total solvent volume 200 mL − 150 mL = 50 mL water

7. $\frac{1}{4}$; 480 mL; 120 mL; 360 mL

   $$\frac{1}{4} = \frac{X}{480}$$ 4X = 480   X = 120 mL total solute

   Total solvent volume 480 mL − 120 mL = 360 mL water

8. $\frac{1}{5}$; 500 mL; 100 g; 20% = 20/100 (reduce fraction by 20)

   $$\frac{1}{5} = \frac{X}{500}$$ 5X = 500   X = 100 grams total solute

9. $\frac{3}{4}$; 100 mL; 75 mL; 25 mL; 75% = 75/100 (reduce fraction by 25)

   $$\frac{3}{4} = \frac{X}{100}$$ 4 X = 300   X = 75 mL total solute

   Total solvent volume 100 mL − 75 mL = 25 mL

10. $\frac{1}{4}$; 300 mL; 60 mL; 240 mL

    $$\frac{1}{4} = \frac{X}{240}$$ 4X = 240   X = 60 mL total solute

    Total solvent volume 300 mL − 60 mL = 240 mL water

ANSWER KEY

Chapter Review, pp. 235-244

1. 3 mL.

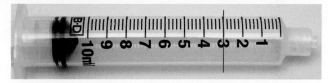

2. 13 mL.

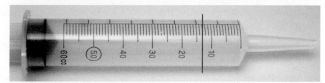

3. 5 mL.

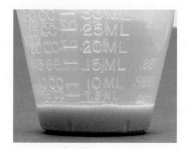

4. 7 mL.

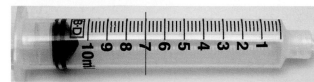

5. 20 mL.

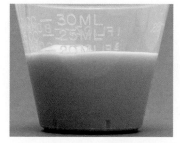

6. 2.3 mL.

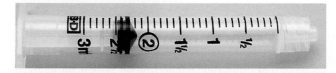

7. 1 mL.

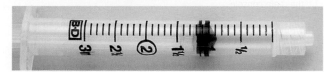

8. 16 mL.

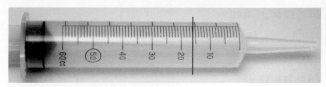

9. 10 mL.

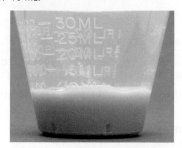

10. 2 mL.

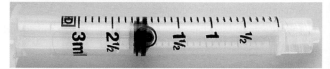

11. 1.3 mL.

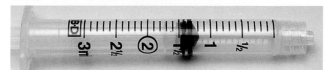

12. 0.5 mL.

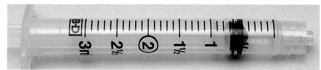

13. 11 mL.

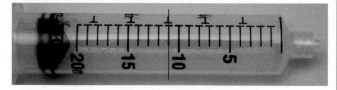

14. 1.5 mL.

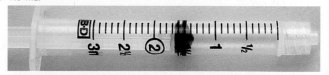

15. 1.8 mL.

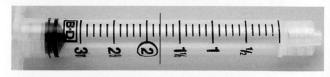

16. 2.4 mL.

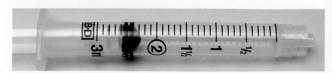

17. 120 mL; 60 mL.

18. 240 mL; 120 mL.

19. 66.7 mL; 16.7 mL.

20. 1 can.

CHAPTER 13
Unit Dose, Card System, and Computerized Medication Administration System

Unit Dose System, p. 248

1. False. The medications may also be kept in rolling carts.

2. False. The pharmacy staff will restock medications every 24 hours, but they also will deliver medications that are ordered throughout the day.

3. True. Nurses are not responsible for stocking the drawers in the unit dose system.

4. False. The nurse should perform a calculation to see if she can administer the ordered dose using the dose in the drawer.

5. True. This can result in a delayed or missed dose for the patient from whom the medication is borrowed.

6. False. Controlled substances are kept in a separate area and are locked up at all times.

7. 4 mL

   Ratio-proportion method:

   $$\frac{125 \text{ mg}}{5 \text{ mL}} = \frac{100 \text{ mg}}{X \text{ mL}}$$

   Reduce: $\frac{25 \text{ mg}}{1 \text{ mL}} = \frac{100 \text{ mg}}{X \text{ mL}}$ $25X = 100$ $X = 4 \text{ mL}$

   Formula method:

   $$\frac{100 \text{ mg}}{125 \text{ mg}} \times 5 \text{ mL} = 4 \text{ mL}$$

8. 0.5 tablet or ½ tablet.
   Convert mcg to mg by moving decimal point three places to the left.
   62.5 mcg = 0.0625 mg

   Ratio-proportion method:

   $$\frac{0.125 \text{ mg}}{1 \text{ tab}} = \frac{0.0625 \text{ mg}}{X \text{ tab}}$$ $0.125X = 0.0625$

   $$125\overline{)62.5}^{\;0.5}$$

   Formula method:

   $$\frac{0.0625 \text{ mg}}{0.125 \text{ mg}} \times 1 \text{ tab} = 0.5$$

9. 0.5 mL

   Ratio-proportion method:

   $$\frac{30 \text{ mg}}{1 \text{ mL}} = \frac{15 \text{ mg}}{X \text{ mL}}$$ $30X = 15$

   $$30\overline{)15.0}^{\;0.5}$$

   Formula method:

   $$\frac{15 \text{ mg}}{30 \text{ mg}} \times 1 \text{ mL} = 0.5$$

10. 1.5 mL

    Ratio-proportion method:

    $$\frac{30 \text{ mg}}{1 \text{ mL}} = \frac{45 \text{ mg}}{X \text{ mL}}$$ $30X = 45$

$$30\overline{)45.0}^{\;1.5}$$
$$\underline{30}$$
$$150$$
$$\underline{150}$$

Formula method:

$$\frac{45 \text{ mg}}{30 \text{ mg}} \times 1 \text{ mL} = 1.5 \text{ mL}$$

Card System, p. 251

1. True. Routine and as-needed medications are kept on individual cards for each patient.

2. True. This helps the nurse organize the medications according to the time they are to be given.

3. False. This information is printed onto the cards at the pharmacy each time they resupply medications.

4. False. The computerized MAR will be supplied by the pharmacy each time the medications are restocked.

5. True. Medications are usually changed with less frequency in settings that utilize the card system.

6. False. Each blister-pack will contain unwrapped pills, with no individual labels on each pill.

7. False. All doses of each controlled substance are kept on individual cards, with a separate inventory sheet for signing out each dose to the patient to whom it is administered.

8. $\frac{0.5 \text{ mg}}{1 \text{ tab}} = \frac{1.5 \text{ mg}}{X \text{ tab}}$ $0.5X = 1.5$

   $X = 3$ tablets

9. 0.5 tablet or ½ tablet
   Yes if tablet scored

   Ratio-proportion method:

   $$\frac{60 \text{ mg}}{1 \text{ tab}} = \frac{30 \text{ mg}}{X \text{ tab}}$$ $60X = 30$

   $$60\overline{)30.0}^{\;0.5}$$

   Formula method:

   $$\frac{30 \text{ mg}}{60 \text{ mg}} \times 1 \text{ tab} = 0.5 \text{ tablets}$$

10. 2 tablets
    1.6 mcg × 62.5 kg = 100 mcg

    Ratio-proportion method:

    $$\frac{50 \text{ mcg}}{1} = \frac{100 \text{ mcg}}{X \text{ tab}}$$ $50X = 100$ $X = 2$ tablets

    Formula method:

    $$\frac{100 \text{ mcg}}{50 \text{ mcg}} \times 1 \text{ tab} = 2 \text{ tablets}$$

Computerized Medication Administration System, pp. 255-256

1. False. The pharmacy enters individual patient medication orders into the main console.

2. False. Any medication prescribed for a patient can be stored in the station, even those requiring refrigeration if the station is equipped with the appropriate equipment.

3. True. This can serve as a check against the MAR and prevent a medication error involving administering a medication twice.

4. False. Any medication ordered on the patient can be profiled. The screen can be programmed to inform the nurse if the medication is stored somewhere other than within the station.

5. False. Documentation is done on the MAR after the medication is given but does not necessarily require the nurse to reenter the station.

6. False. The nurse may need to do a calculation to determine how much of the medication provided should be used to administer the ordered dose.

7. True. With this system, the medications are stored by name of the medication, not by individual patient, allowing the nurse to access a medication anytime it is stocked in the system by overriding the profiled medication screen.

8. Remove 1 cartridge; 0.6 mL
   Ratio-proportion method:

   $$\frac{10,000\ units}{1\ mL} = \frac{6000\ units}{X\ mL}$$

   $10,000X = 6000$

   $X = \dfrac{6000}{10,000}$ Reduce: $\dfrac{6}{10}$

   $X = 0.6\ mL$

   Formula method:

   $$\frac{6000\ units}{10,000\ units} \times 1\ mL = 0.6\ mL$$

9. Three 500-mg capsules and two 250-mg capsules
   Convert g to mg
   $2\ g = 2000\ mg$
   Determine the amount to give from the amount on hand.
   $500\ mg \times 3\ capsules = 1500\ mg$
   $2000\ mg - 1500\ mg = 500\ mg\ remaining$

   $$\frac{250\ mg}{1\ cap} = \frac{500}{X\ cap}$$

   $250X = 500$ $X = 2\ capsules$

10. 12.5 mL
    Ratio-proportion method:

    $$\frac{200\ mg}{5\ mL} = \frac{50\ mg}{X\ mL}$$ $20X = 250$

    $X = \dfrac{250}{20}$ Reduce: $\dfrac{25}{2}$

    $X = 12.5\ mL$

    Formula method:

    $$\frac{50\ mg}{20\ mL} \times 5\ mL = 12.5\ mL$$

Chapter Review, pp. 256-258

1. False.
2. False.
3. True.
4. False.
5. True.
6. False.
7. False.
8. True.
9. False.
10. True.
11. False.
12. False.

13. 1.5 tablets.
14. 4 tablets.
15. 2.5 tablets.
16. 5 tablets.
17. 8 mL.
18. 0.5 mL.
19. One 500 mg capsule plus two 250 mg capsules.
20. 7.5 mL.

CHAPTER 14
Medication Records
Preprinted Forms, p. 263

1. True.

2. False. Each form is used for a 7-day period.

3. True.

4. False. They can be documented as long as the nurse indicates that the patient took them himself or herself.

5. False. All intramuscular, subcutaneous, and intradermal medications administered should have the site documented.

6. True.

7. False. These forms can be individualized with times.

8. *Step 1:* Calculate the total dosage per day.
   $X = 3\ mg \times 2$
   $X = 6\ mg$

   Step 2: Calculate the dosage for the 2 days.
   $X = 6\ mg \times 2$
   $X = 12\ mg$

   The patient will receive 12 mg over the 2 days and 4 mg the first day for a total of 16 mg.

9. $\dfrac{0.75\ mg}{1\ tab} = \dfrac{3\ mg}{X\ tab}$ $0.75X = 3$

   $75\overline{)300}$ with quotient 4

   $X = 4\ tabs$

10. $\dfrac{25\ mg}{1\ tab} = \dfrac{37.5\ mg}{X\ tab}$ $25X = 37.5$

    $X = 1.5\ tablets$

Computerized MARs and Bar Codes, pp. 268-269

1. True. Information can be entered one time and then retrieved as needed and also updated when needed.

2. False. Patients are not reliable sources, because they can become confused or forget their dose. It is better to contact the nurse who was supposed to administer the medication to be certain.

3. True. The system can be set up to allow printing out the sheets if the policy dictates or the records can be maintained electronically with the nurses entering data as the medication is administered.

4. False. The patient receives one bracelet on admission, and this bracelet can be used throughout the patient's stay.

5. $X = \dfrac{100\ mg}{50\ mg/dose}$

   $X = 2\ doses$

   The patient can receive two doses.

6. $\dfrac{250 \text{ mg}}{10 \text{ mL}} = \dfrac{35 \text{ mg}}{X \text{ mL}}$ $250X = 350$

$X = \dfrac{350}{250}$

$X = 1.4 \text{ mL}$

The nurse will administer 1.4 mL.

7. $\dfrac{6 \text{ mg}}{1 \text{ kg}} = \dfrac{X \text{ mg}}{18 \text{ kg}}$ $X = 108$

$X = 108 \text{ mg}$

The patient will receive 108 mg in 24 hours.

8. $\dfrac{108 \text{ mg}}{3 \text{ dose}} = \dfrac{X \text{ mg}}{1 \text{ dose}}$ $3X = 108$

$X = \dfrac{108}{3}$

$X = 36 \text{ mg}$

Each dose will contain 36 mg.

9. $\dfrac{1 \text{ kg}}{2.5 \text{ mg}} = \dfrac{18 \text{ kg}}{X \text{ mg}}$ $X = \dfrac{18 \text{ kg} \times 2.5 \text{ mg}}{1 \text{ kg}}$

$X = 45 \text{ mg}$

The patient's dose of 36 mg does not exceed the recommended guideline.

10. The doses are not equal, so the nurse would receive an error message if she scanned the medication after scanning the patient's bracelet.

Chapter Review, pp. 269-272

1. 4 mL.

2. 4 mL.

3. 1.3 mL.

4. 3 tablets.

5. 2 mL.

6. 10 mL.

7. 4 doses. The patient can receive 4 doses.

8. 1 mL. The nurse will administer 1 mL.

9. 80 mg. The patient will receive 80 mg in 24 hours.

10. 80 mg. Each dose will contain 26.7 mg.

11. Yes.

12. 0.5 gram. The doses are not equal, so the nurse would receive an error message if she scanned the medication after scanning the patient's bracelet.

13. 2 mL.

14. 2 mL.

15. 1 mL.

16. 2 tablets.

17. 10 mL.

18. 20 mL.

19. 2.5 mL.

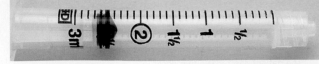

20. 3 tablets.

CHAPTER 15
Introduction to Intravenous Therapy
Calculating Large Volume Solution Hourly Infusion Rates, pp. 293-294

1. $\dfrac{2000 \text{ mL}}{24 \text{ hr}} = 83 \text{ mL/hr (83.3)}$

2. $\dfrac{500 \text{ mL}}{8 \text{ hr}} = 63 \text{ mL/hr (62.5)}$

3. $\dfrac{1000 \text{ mL}}{12 \text{ hr}} = 83 \text{ mL/hr (83.3)}$

4. $\dfrac{1500 \text{ mL}}{15 \text{ hr}} = 100 \text{ mL/hr}$

5. $\dfrac{500 \text{ mL}}{10 \text{ hr}} = 50 \text{ mL/hr}$

6. $\dfrac{250 \text{ mL}}{2 \text{ hr}} = 125 \text{ mL/hr}$

7. $\dfrac{1000 \text{ mL}}{10 \text{ hr}} = 100 \text{ mL/hr}$

8. $\dfrac{250 \text{ mL}}{6 \text{ hr}} = 42 \text{ mL/hr (41.7)}$

9. $\dfrac{240 \text{ mL}}{4 \text{ hr}} = 60 \text{ mL/hr}$

10. $\dfrac{3000 \text{ mL}}{14 \text{ hr}} = 214 \text{ mL/hr (214.3)}$

Calculating Small Volume Infusion Rates, p. 298

1. 60 minutes = 1 hour

$\dfrac{250 \text{ mL}}{1 \text{ hr}} = 250 \text{ mL/hr}$

2. 30 minutes = 0.5 hours

$\dfrac{250 \text{ mL}}{0.5 \text{ hr}} = 500 \text{ mL/hr}$

3. $\dfrac{60 \text{ min}}{1 \text{ hr}} = \dfrac{45 \text{ min}}{X \text{ hr}}$

$X = 0.75 \text{ hours}$

$\dfrac{180 \text{ mL}}{0.75 \text{ hr}} = 240 \text{ mL/hr}$

4. $\dfrac{60 \text{ min}}{1 \text{ hr}} = \dfrac{15 \text{ min}}{X \text{ hr}}$

$X = 0.25 \text{ hours}$

$\dfrac{100 \text{ mL}}{0.25 \text{ hr}} = 400 \text{ mL/hr}$

5. $\dfrac{50 \text{ mL}}{0.25 \text{ hr}} = 200 \text{ mL/hr}$

6. $\dfrac{60 \text{ min}}{1 \text{ hr}} = \dfrac{20 \text{ min}}{X \text{ hr}}$

$X = 0.33 \text{ hours}$

$\dfrac{100 \text{ mL}}{0.33 \text{ hr}} = 303 \text{ mL/hr}$

7. 30 minutes = 0.5 hours

$\dfrac{250 \text{ mL}}{0.5 \text{ hr}} = 500 \text{ mL/hr}$

8. $\dfrac{60 \text{ min}}{1 \text{ hr}} = \dfrac{10 \text{ min}}{X \text{ hr}}$

   $X = 0.17$ hours

   $\dfrac{50 \text{ mL}}{0.17 \text{ hr}} = 294.1$ mL/hr

9. 30 minutes $= 0.5$ hours

   $\dfrac{50 \text{ mL}}{0.5 \text{ hr}} = 100$ mL/hr

10. $\dfrac{100 \text{ mL}}{1.5 \text{ hr}} = 66.7$ mL/hr

Gravity Infusions: Calculating Drops/Minute (gtt/min), pp. 305-307

1. $\dfrac{125 \text{ mL}}{60 \text{ min}} = 2.08 = 2.1$ mL/min

   $\dfrac{15 \text{ gtt}}{1 \text{ mL}} = \dfrac{X \text{ gtt}}{2.1 \text{ mL}} = 31.5$ gtt/min $= 32$ gtt/min

2. 100 gtt/min (microdrip mL/min same as gtt/min)

3. 200 mL/60 min $= 3.33 = 3.3$ mL/min

   $\dfrac{10 \text{ gtt}}{1 \text{ mL}} = \dfrac{X \text{ gtt}}{3.3 \text{ mL}} = 33$ gtt/min

4. 2000 mL/20 hr $= 100$ mL/hr

   100 mL/60 min $= 1.66 = 1.7$ mL/min

   $\dfrac{20 \text{ gtt}}{1 \text{ mL}} = \dfrac{X \text{ gtt}}{1.7 \text{ mL}} = 34$ gtt/min

5. 83 mL/min 83 gtt/min

6. 150 mL/60 min $= 2.5$ mL/min

   $\dfrac{20 \text{ gtt}}{1 \text{ mL}} = \dfrac{X \text{ gtt}}{2.5 \text{ mL}} = 50$ gtt/min

7. 90 mL/hr/60 min $= 1.5$ mL/min

   $\dfrac{15 \text{ gtt}}{1 \text{ mL}} = \dfrac{X \text{ gtt}}{1.5 \text{ mL}} = 22.5$ gtt/min $= 23$ gtt/min

8. 120 mL/60 min $= 2$ mL/ min

   $\dfrac{10 \text{ gtt}}{1 \text{ mL}} = \dfrac{X \text{ gtt}}{2 \text{ mL}} = 20$ gtt/min

9. $\dfrac{50 \text{ mL}}{20 \text{ min}} = 2.5$ mL/min

   $\dfrac{10 \text{ gtt}}{1 \text{ mL}} = \dfrac{X \text{ gtt}}{2.5 \text{ mL}} = 25$ gtt/min

10. 100 mL/30 min $= 3.33 = 3.3$ mL/min

    $\dfrac{15 \text{ gtt}}{1 \text{ mL}} = \dfrac{X \text{ gtt}}{3.3 \text{ mL}} = 49.5$ gtt/min $= 50$ gtt/min

Calculating Total Infusion Times, p. 311

1. $\dfrac{125 \text{ mL}}{1 \text{ hr}} = \dfrac{1000 \text{ mL}}{X \text{ hr}}$ $125X = 1000$ $X = 8$ hr

   Completion time: 0315 hours (3:15 AM).

2. $\dfrac{50 \text{ mL}}{1 \text{ hr}} = \dfrac{1000 \text{ mL}}{X \text{ hr}}$

   $50X = 1000$ $X = 20$ hr

   Completion time: 0445 hours (4:45 AM).

3. $\dfrac{80 \text{ mL}}{1 \text{ hr}} = \dfrac{250 \text{ mL}}{X \text{ hr}} = 80X = 250X = 3.1$, or 3 hr

   Completion time: 1600 hours (4 PM).

4. $\dfrac{75 \text{ mL}}{1 \text{ hr}} = \dfrac{380 \text{ mL}}{X \text{ hr}}$

   $75X = 380$ $X = 5.1$, or 5 hr

   Completion time: 1215 hours (12:15 PM).

5. $\dfrac{75 \text{ mL}}{1 \text{ hr}} = \dfrac{500 \text{ mL}}{X \text{ hr}}$

   $75X = 500$ $X = 6.7$, or 7 hr

   Completion time: 2100 hours (9 PM).

6. $\dfrac{42 \text{ mL}}{1 \text{ hr}} = \dfrac{500 \text{ mL}}{X \text{ hr}}$ $42X = 500$ $X = 11.9$, or 12 hr

   Completion time: 2200 hours (10 PM).

7. $\dfrac{50 \text{ mL}}{1 \text{ hr}} = \dfrac{200 \text{ mL}}{X \text{ hr}}$ $50X = 200$ $X = 4$ hr

   Completion time: 1815 hours (6:15 PM).

8. $\dfrac{25 \text{ mL}}{1 \text{ hr}} = \dfrac{80 \text{ mL}}{X \text{ hr}}$ $25X = 80$

   $X = 3.2$, or 3 hr

   Completion time: 1400 hours (2 PM).

9. $\dfrac{200 \text{ mL}}{1 \text{ hr}} = \dfrac{100 \text{ mL}}{X \text{ hr}}$

   $200X = 100$ $X = 0.5$ hr

   0.5 hr $\times$ 60 minutes $= 30$ minutes

   Completion time: 1630 hours (4:30 PM).

10. $\dfrac{400 \text{ mL}}{1 \text{ hr}} = \dfrac{100 \text{ mL}}{X \text{ hr}}$ $400X = 100$ $X = 0.25$ hr

    0.25 hr $\times$ 60 minutes $= 15$ minutes

    Completion time: 1415 hours (2:15 PM).

Chapter Review, pp. 311-314

1. 125 mL/hr.
2. 83 mL/hr.
3. 100 mL/hr.
4. 50 mL/hr.
5. 133 mL/hr.
6. 2.1 mL/min; 32 gtt/min.
7. 2.5 mL/min; 150 gtt/min.
8. 1.7 mL/min; 17 gtt/min.
9. 2.5 mL/min; 50 gtt/min.
10. 1.25 mL/min; 75 gtt/min.
11. 4.2 mL/min; 84 gtt/min.
12. 1 mL/min; 60 gtt/min.
13. 5 mL/min; 100 gtt/min.
14. 2.5 mL/min; 25 gtt/min.
15. 8.3 gtt/min; 125 gtt/min.
16. 10 hr 1400 (2 PM).
17. 13 hr 0945 (9:45 AM).
18. 3.75 hr 1245 (12:45 PM).
19. 8 hr 0315 (3:15 AM).
20. 10 hr 0800 (8 AM).

CHAPTER 16
Calculating Intravenous Heparin Dosages

Calculating Infusion Rates Based on Heparin Units/Hour, pp. 320-321

1. $\dfrac{25{,}000\ units}{250\ mL} = \dfrac{600\ units}{X\ mL}$

   Reduce fraction: $\dfrac{25{,}000}{250} = \dfrac{100}{1}$

   $\dfrac{100\ units}{1\ mL} = \dfrac{600}{X\ mL}$ $100X = 600$ $X = 6\ mL/hr$

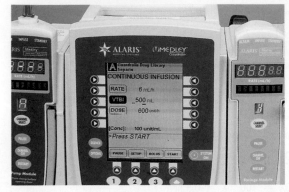

2. $25{,}000/250 = 1\ mL = 100\ units\ heparin;\ 700 \times 1/100 = 7\ mL/hr.$

   $\dfrac{25{,}000\ units}{250\ mL} = \dfrac{550\ units}{X\ mL}$

   Reduce fraction: $\dfrac{25{,}000}{250} = \dfrac{100}{1}$

   $\dfrac{100\ units}{1\ mL} = \dfrac{550}{X\ mL}$ $100X = 550$ $X = 5.5\ mL/hr$

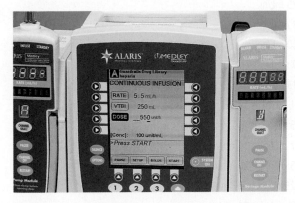

3. $\dfrac{50{,}000\ units}{250\ mL} = \dfrac{400\ units}{X\ mL}$

   Reduce fraction: $\dfrac{50{,}000}{250} = \dfrac{200}{1}$

   $\dfrac{200\ units}{1\ mL} = \dfrac{400}{X\ mL}$ $200X = 400$ $X = 2\ mL/hr$

4. $\dfrac{50{,}000\ units}{250\ mL} = \dfrac{600\ units}{X\ mL}$

   Reduce fraction: $\dfrac{50{,}000}{250} = \dfrac{200}{1}$

   $\dfrac{200\ units}{1\ mL} = \dfrac{600}{X\ mL}$ $200X = 600$ $X = 3\ mL/hr$

5. $\dfrac{25{,}000\ units}{500\ mL} = \dfrac{800\ units}{X\ mL}$

   Reduce fraction: $\dfrac{25{,}000}{500} = \dfrac{50}{1}$

   $\dfrac{50\ units}{1\ mL} = \dfrac{800}{X\ mL}$ $50X = 800$ $X = 16\ mL/hr$

6. $\dfrac{50{,}000\ units}{500\ mL} = \dfrac{1800\ units}{X\ mL}$

   Reduce fraction: $\dfrac{50{,}000}{500} = \dfrac{100}{1}$

   $\dfrac{100\ units}{1\ mL} = \dfrac{1800}{X\ mL}$ $100X = 1800$ $X = 18\ mL/hr$

7. $\dfrac{25{,}000\ units}{250\ mL} = \dfrac{2400\ units}{X\ mL}$

   Reduce fraction: $\dfrac{25{,}000}{250} = \dfrac{100}{1}$

   $\dfrac{100\ units}{1\ mL} = \dfrac{2400}{X\ mL}$ $100X = 2400$ $X = 24\ mL/hr$

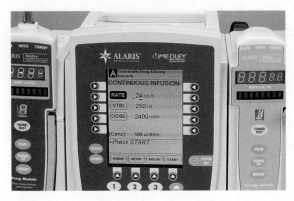

8. $\dfrac{25{,}000\ units}{250\ mL} = \dfrac{400\ units}{X\ mL}$

   Reduce fraction: $\dfrac{25{,}000}{250} = \dfrac{100}{1}$

   $\dfrac{100\ units}{1\ mL} = \dfrac{400}{X\ mL}$ $100X = 400$ $X = 4\ mL/hr$

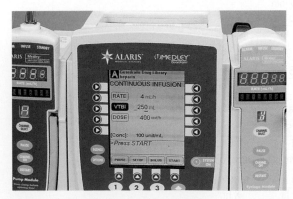

9. $\dfrac{25{,}000 \text{ units}}{250 \text{ mL}} = \dfrac{1700 \text{ units}}{X \text{ mL}}$

Reduce fraction: $\dfrac{25{,}000}{250} = \dfrac{100}{1}$

$\dfrac{100 \text{ units}}{1 \text{ mL}} = \dfrac{1700}{X \text{ mL}}$ $100X = 1700$ $X = 17 \text{ mL/hr}$

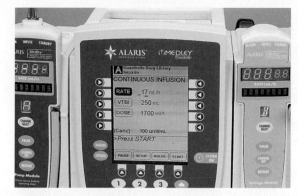

10. $\dfrac{50{,}000 \text{ units}}{500 \text{ mL}} = \dfrac{1200 \text{ units}}{X \text{ mL}}$

Reduce fraction: $\dfrac{50{,}000}{500} = \dfrac{100}{1}$

$\dfrac{100 \text{ units}}{1 \text{ mL}} = \dfrac{1200}{X \text{ mL}}$ $100X = 1200$ $X = 12 \text{ mL/hr}$

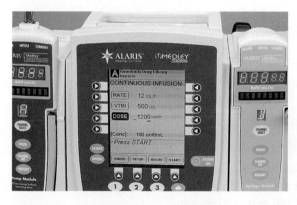

Calculating Infusion Rates Based on Heparin Units/Hour, p. 324

1. 2500 units/hr.

$\dfrac{25{,}000 \text{ units}}{250 \text{ mL}} = \dfrac{X \text{ units}}{25 \text{ mL}}$

Reduce fraction: $\dfrac{25{,}000}{250} = \dfrac{100}{1}$

$\dfrac{100 \text{ units}}{1 \text{ mL}} = \dfrac{X \text{ units}}{25 \text{ mL}}$ $1X = 2500$ $X = 2500$

2. 1200 units/hr.

$\dfrac{25{,}000 \text{ units}}{250 \text{ mL}} = \dfrac{X \text{ units}}{12 \text{ mL}}$

Reduce fraction: $\dfrac{25{,}000}{250} = \dfrac{100}{1}$

$\dfrac{100 \text{ units}}{1 \text{ mL}} = \dfrac{X}{12 \text{ mL}}$ $X = 1200$

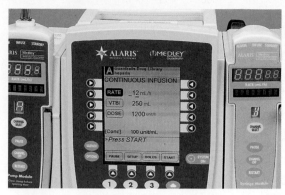

3. 1100 units/hr.

$\dfrac{50{,}000 \text{ units}}{1000 \text{ mL}} = \dfrac{X \text{ units}}{22 \text{ mL}}$

Reduce fraction: $\dfrac{50{,}000}{1000} = \dfrac{50}{1}$

$\dfrac{50 \text{ units}}{1 \text{ mL}} = \dfrac{X \text{ units}}{22 \text{ mL}}$ $X = 1100$

4. 2000 units/hr.

$\dfrac{25{,}000 \text{ units}}{250 \text{ mL}} = \dfrac{X \text{ units}}{20 \text{ mL}}$

Reduce fraction: $\dfrac{25{,}000}{250} = \dfrac{100}{1}$

$\dfrac{100 \text{ units}}{1 \text{ mL}} = \dfrac{X}{20 \text{ mL}}$ $X = 2000$

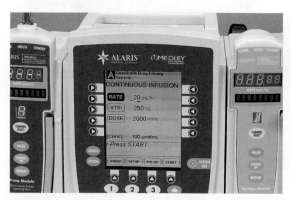

5. 2000 units/hr.

$\dfrac{50{,}000 \text{ units}}{1000 \text{ mL}} = \dfrac{X \text{ units}}{40 \text{ mL}}$

Reduce fraction: $\dfrac{50{,}000}{1000} = \dfrac{50}{1}$

$\dfrac{50 \text{ units}}{1 \text{ mL}} = \dfrac{X \text{ units}}{40 \text{ mL}}$ $X = 2000$

6. 2600 units/hr.

$$\frac{50,000 \text{ units}}{500 \text{ mL}} = \frac{X \text{ units}}{26 \text{ mL}}$$

Reduce fraction: $\frac{50,000}{500} = \frac{100}{1}$

$$\frac{100 \text{ units}}{1 \text{ mL}} = \frac{X \text{ units}}{26 \text{ mL}} \quad X = 2600$$

7. 3800 units/hr.

$$\frac{25,000 \text{ units}}{250 \text{ mL}} = \frac{X \text{ units}}{38 \text{ mL}}$$

Reduce fraction: $\frac{25,000}{250} = \frac{100}{1}$

$$\frac{100 \text{ units}}{1 \text{ mL}} = \frac{X \text{ units}}{38 \text{ mL}} \quad X = 3800$$

8. 1800 units/hr.

$$\frac{50,000 \text{ units}}{250 \text{ mL}} = \frac{X \text{ units}}{9 \text{ mL}}$$

Reduce fraction: $\frac{50,000}{250} = \frac{200}{1}$

$$\frac{200 \text{ units}}{1 \text{ mL}} = \frac{X \text{ units}}{9 \text{ mL}} \quad X = 1800$$

9. 1200 units/hr.

$$\frac{25,000 \text{ units}}{250 \text{ mL}} = \frac{X \text{ units}}{12 \text{ mL}}$$

Reduce fraction: $\frac{25,000}{250} = \frac{100}{1}$

$$\frac{100 \text{ units}}{1 \text{ mL}} = \frac{X \text{ units}}{12 \text{ mL}} \quad X = 1200$$

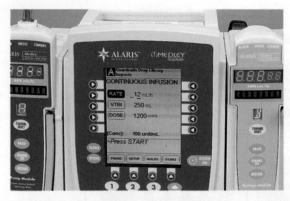

10. 2700 units/hr.

$$\frac{25,000 \text{ units}}{500 \text{ mL}} = \frac{X \text{ units}}{54 \text{ mL}}$$

Reduce fraction: $\frac{25,000}{500} = \frac{50}{1}$

$$\frac{50 \text{ units}}{1 \text{ mL}} = \frac{X \text{ units}}{54 \text{ mL}} \quad X = 2700$$

Heparin Based on Protocol and PTT Results, pp. 334-337

1. Give 4.9 mL bolus.

Bolus dose of heparin: 80 units × 61 kg = 4880 units.

$$\frac{1000 \text{ units}}{1 \text{ mL}} = \frac{4880 \text{ units}}{X \text{ mL}}$$

$1000X = 4880 \quad X = 4.9$

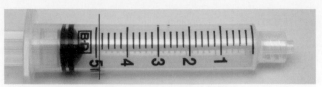

Initial intravenous infusion rate: 22 mL/hr

18 units × 61 kg = 1098 units/hour.

$$\frac{25,000 \text{ units}}{500 \text{ mL}} = \frac{1098 \text{ units}}{X \text{ mL}}$$

$$\frac{50}{1} = \frac{1098}{X} \quad 50X = 1098$$

X = 21.96 mL/hr (round to nearest tenth) 22 mL

Adjust the dose of heparin intravenous bolus based on partial thromboplastin time. Bolus: 4.9 mL.

(PTT) results: 80 units × 61 kg = 4880 units.

$$\frac{1000 \text{ units}}{1 \text{ mL}} = \frac{4880 \text{ units}}{X \text{ mL}}$$

$1000X = 4880 \quad X = 4.88$ (round to nearest tenth)

Adjust intravenous drip based on the PTT results: Increase infusion rate 4.9 mL/hr

4 units × 61 kg = 244 units/hour ↑.

$$\frac{50 \text{ units}}{1 \text{ mL}} = \frac{224 \text{ units}}{X \text{ mL}}$$

$50X = 244 \quad X = 4.88$ (round to nearest tenth)

2. Give 6.2 mL bolus.

80 units × 77 kg = 6160 units.

$$\frac{1000 \text{ units}}{1 \text{ mL}} = \frac{6160 \text{ units}}{X \text{ mL}}$$

$1000X = 6160 \quad X = 6.16$ mL (round to nearest tenth)

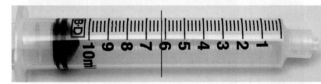

Initial intravenous infusion rate: 27.7 mL/hr.

18 units × 77 kg = 1386 units/hour.

$$\frac{25,000 \text{ units}}{500 \text{ mL}} = \frac{1386 \text{ units}}{X \text{ mL}}$$

$$\frac{50}{1} = \frac{1386 \text{ units}}{X \text{ mL}} \quad 50X = 1386 \quad X = 27.7 \text{ mL/hr}$$

Adjust the dose of heparin intravenous bolus based on PTT results: 80 units × 77 kg = 6160 units. Bolus 6.2 mL.

Adjust intravenous drip based on the PTT results: Increase infusion rate 6.2 mL/hr.

4 × 77 = 308 units/hour ↑.

$$\frac{50 \text{ units}}{1 \text{ mL}} = \frac{308 \text{ units}}{X \text{ mL}}$$

$50X = 308 \quad X = 6.16$ (round to nearest tenth)

3. Give 6.6 mL bolus dose of heparin.

80 units × 82 kg = 6560 units.

$$\frac{1000 \text{ units}}{1 \text{ mL}} = \frac{6560 \text{ units}}{X \text{ mL}}$$

$1000X = 6560 \quad X = 6.56$ (round to nearest tenth)

Initial intravenous infusion of heparin: 29.5 mL/hr.

18 units × 82 kg = 1476 units/hour.

$$\frac{25,000}{500} = \frac{1476 \text{ units}}{X \text{ mL}}$$

$$\frac{50}{1} = \frac{1476}{X} \quad 50X = 1476$$

X = 29.5 mL/hr

Adjust the dose of heparin intravenous bolus based on PTT results. Bolus with 6.6 mL.

80 units × 82 kg = 6560 units.

Adjust intravenous drip based on the PTT results: Increase infusion rate 6.6 mL/hr.

4 units × 82 kg = 328 units/hour ↑.

$$\frac{50 \text{ units}}{1 \text{ mL}} = \frac{328 \text{ units}}{X \text{ mL}}$$

50X = 328   X = 6.56 (round to nearest tenth)

4. Give 6 mL bolus dose of heparin.

80 units × 75 kg (165 pounds/2.2 kg) = 6000 units.

$$\frac{1000 \text{ units}}{1 \text{ mL}} = \frac{6000 \text{ units}}{X \text{ mL}}$$

1000X = 6000   X = 6

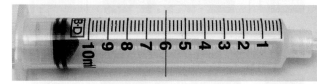

Initial intravenous infusion of heparin: 27 mL/hr.

18 units × 75 kg = 1350 units/hour.

$$\frac{25,000 \text{ units}}{500 \text{ mL}} = \frac{1350 \text{ units}}{X \text{ mL}}$$

$$\frac{50}{1} = \frac{1350}{X} \quad 50X = 1350 \quad X = 27 \text{ mL/hr}$$

Adjust the dose of heparin intravenous bolus based on PTT results: 80 units × 75 kg = 6000 units. Bolus is 6 mL.

Adjust intravenous drip based on the PTT results: Increase rate 6 mL/hr.

4 units × 75 kg = 300 units/hour ↑.

$$\frac{50 \text{ units}}{1 \text{ mL}} = \frac{300 \text{ units}}{X \text{ mL}}$$

50X = 300   X = 6

5. Give 7 mL bolus dose of heparin.

80 units × 88 kg = 7040 units.

$$\frac{1000 \text{ units}}{1 \text{ mL}} = \frac{7040 \text{ units}}{X \text{ mL}}$$

1000X = 7040   X = 7.04 (round to nearest tenth which is a whole number)

Initial intravenous infusion of heparin: 31.7 mL/hr.

18 units × 88 kg = 1584 units/hour.

$$\frac{25,000 \text{ units}}{500 \text{ mL}} = \frac{1584 \text{ units}}{X \text{ mL}}$$

$$\frac{50}{1} = \frac{1584}{X} \quad 50X = 1584$$

X = 31.7 mL/hr

Adjust the dose of heparin intravenous bolus based on PTT results: 80 units × 88 kg = 7040 units. Bolus is 7 mL.

Adjust intravenous drip based on the PTT results: Increase infusion rate 7 mL/hr.

4 units × 88 kg = 352 units/hour ↑.

$$\frac{50 \text{ units}}{1 \text{ mL}} = \frac{352 \text{ units}}{X \text{ mL}}$$

50X = 352   X = 7.04 (round to nearest tenth which is a whole number)

6. Give bolus with 7.7 mL.

80 units × 96 kg = 7680 units.

$$\frac{1000 \text{ units}}{1 \text{ mL}} = \frac{7680 \text{ units}}{X \text{ mL}}$$

1000X = 7680   X = 7.68 (round to nearest tenth)

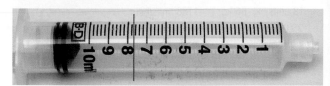

Initial intravenous infusion of heparin: 34.6 mL/hr.

18 units × 96 kg = 1728 units/hour.

$$\frac{25,000 \text{ units}}{500 \text{ mL}} = \frac{1728 \text{ units}}{X \text{ mL}}$$

$$\frac{50}{1} = \frac{1728}{X} \quad 50X = 1728 \quad X = 34.6 \text{ mL/hr}$$

Adjust the dose of heparin intravenous bolus based on PTT results: Give 3.8 mL bolus.

40 units × 96 kg = 3840 units.

$$\frac{1000 \text{ units}}{1 \text{ mL}} = \frac{3840 \text{ units}}{X \text{ mL}}$$

1000X = 3840   X = 3.84 (round to nearest tenth)

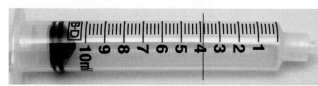

Adjust intravenous drip based on the PTT results: Increase infusion rate 3.8 mL/hr.

2 units × 96 kg = 192 units/hour ↑.

$$\frac{50 \text{ units}}{1 \text{ mL}} = \frac{192 \text{ units}}{X \text{ mL}}$$

50X = 192   X = 3.84 (round to nearest tenth)

7. Give 5.8 mL bolus dose of heparin.

80 units × 72 kg = 5760 units.

$$\frac{1000 \text{ units}}{1 \text{ mL}} = \frac{5760 \text{ units}}{X \text{ mL}}$$

1000X = 5760   X = 5.76 (round to nearest tenth)

Initial intravenous infusion of heparin: 25.9 mL/hr.

18 units × 72 kg = 1296 units/hour.

$$\frac{25,000 \text{ units}}{500 \text{ mL}} = \frac{1296 \text{ units}}{X \text{ mL}}$$

$$\frac{50}{1} = \frac{1296}{X} \quad 50X = 1296 \quad X = 25.9 \text{ mL/hr}$$

Adjust the dose of heparin intravenous bolus based on PTT results: Zero units.

Adjust intravenous drip based on the PTT results: Decrease rate 2.9 mL/hr.

2 units $\times$ 72 kg $=$ 144 units/hour $\downarrow$.

$$\frac{50 \text{ units}}{1 \text{ mL}} = \frac{144 \text{ units}}{X \text{ mL}}$$

50X $=$ 144   X $=$ 2.88 (round to nearest tenth) X $=$ 2.9

8. Give 5.3 mL bolus dose of heparin.

80 units $\times$ 66 kg $=$ 5280 units.

$$\frac{1000 \text{ units}}{1 \text{ mL}} = \frac{5280 \text{ units}}{X \text{ mL}}$$

1000X $=$ 5280   X $=$ 5.3

Initial intravenous infusion of heparin: 23.8 mL/hr.

18 units $\times$ 66 kg $=$ 1188 units/hour.

$$\frac{25,000 \text{ units}}{500 \text{ mL}} = \frac{1188 \text{ units}}{X \text{ mL}}$$

$$\frac{50}{1} = \frac{1188}{X} \quad 50X = 1188 \quad X = 23.8 \text{ mL/hr}$$

Adjust the dose of heparin intravenous bolus based on PTT results: Zero units, hold heparin for 1 hour.

Adjust intravenous drip based on the PTT results: Decrease rate 4 mL/hr.

3 units $\times$ 66 kg $=$ 198 units/hour $\downarrow$.

$$\frac{50 \text{ units}}{1 \text{ mL}} = \frac{198 \text{ units}}{X \text{ mL}}$$

50X $=$ 198   X $=$ 3.96 (round to nearest tenth which is a whole number) X $=$ 4.0

9. Give 6.2 mL bolus dose of heparin.

80 units $\times$ 77 kg (169.4 pounds/2.2 kg/pound) $=$ 6160 units.

$$\frac{1000 \text{ units}}{1 \text{ mL}} = \frac{6160 \text{ units}}{X \text{ mL}}$$

1000X $=$ 6160   X $=$ 6.16 (round to nearest tenth)

Initial intravenous infusion of heparin: 27.7 mL/hr.

18 units $\times$ 77 kg $=$ 1386 units/hour.

$$\frac{25,000 \text{ units}}{500 \text{ mL}} = \frac{1386 \text{ units}}{X \text{ mL}}$$

$$\frac{50}{1} = \frac{1386}{X} \quad 50X = 1386 \quad X = 27.7 \text{ mL/hr}$$

Adjust the dose of heparin intravenous bolus based on PTT results: Zero units.

Adjust intravenous drip based on the PTT results: Decrease rate by 3.1 mL/hr.

2 units $\times$ 77 kg $=$ 154 units/hour $\downarrow$.

$$\frac{50 \text{ units}}{1 \text{ mL}} = \frac{154 \text{ units}}{X \text{ mL}}$$

50X $=$ 154   X $=$ 3.08 (round to nearest tenth)

10. Give 6.6 mL bolus dose of heparin.

80 units $\times$ 82 kg $=$ 6560 units.

$$\frac{1000 \text{ units}}{1 \text{ mL}} = \frac{6560 \text{ units}}{X \text{ mL}}$$

1000X $=$ 6560   X $=$ 6.56 (round to nearest tenth)

Initial intravenous infusion of heparin: 29.5 mL/hr.

18 units $\times$ 82 kg $=$ 1476 units/hour.

$$\frac{25,000 \text{ units}}{500 \text{ mL}} = \frac{1476 \text{ units}}{X \text{ mL}}$$

$$\frac{50}{1} = \frac{1476}{X} \quad 50X = 1476 \quad X = 29.5 \text{ mL/hr}$$

Adjust the dose of heparin intravenous bolus based on PTT results: Zero units, hold heparin for 1 hour.

Adjust intravenous drip based on the PTT results. Decrease rate 4.9 mL/hr.

3 units $\times$ 82 kg $=$ 246 units/hour $\downarrow$.

$$\frac{50 \text{ units}}{1 \text{ mL}} = \frac{246 \text{ units}}{X \text{ mL}}$$

50X $=$ 246   X $=$ 4.92 (round to nearest tenth)

Chapter Review, pp. 337-340

1. 4 mL/hr.

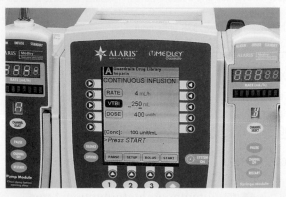

2. 6 mL/hr.

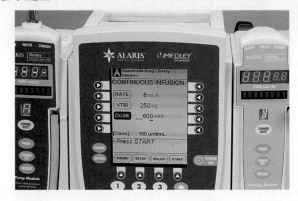

3. 3 mL/hr.

4. 2 mL/hr.

5. 12 mL/hr.

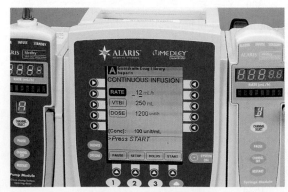

6. 12 mL/hr.

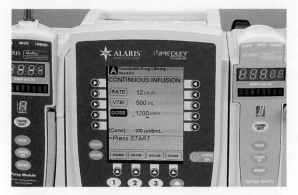

7. 11 mL/hr.

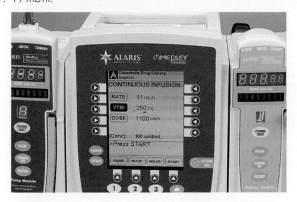

8. 5 mL/hr.

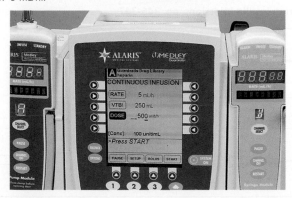

9. 15 mL/hr.

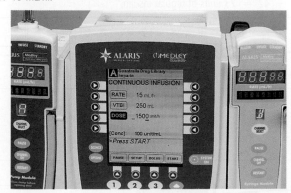

10. 10 mL/hr.

11. 2000 units/hr.

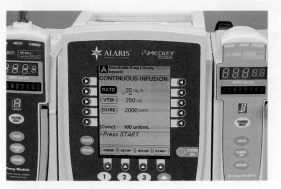

12. 1000 units/hr.

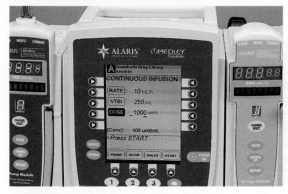

13. 850 units/hr.

14. 1100 units/hr.

15. 1750 units/hr.

16. 2400 units/hr.

17. 3400 units/hr.

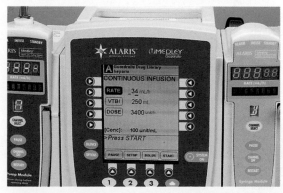

18. 2400 units/hr.

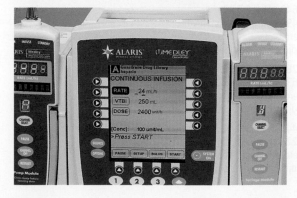

19. 700 units/hr.

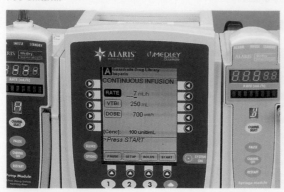

20. 2400 units/hr.

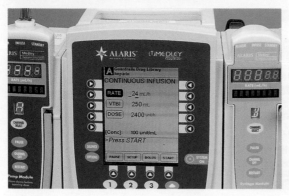

21. 5120 units; 5 mL.

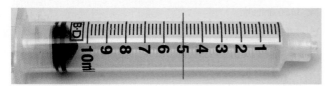

1152 units/hour; 23 mL/hr.
5120 units.
Adjust intravenous drip 256 units/hour ↑.

22. 5800 units; 5.8 mL bolus.

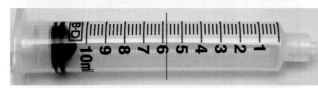

1305 units/hour; 26.1 mL/hr.
Zero units.
No change.

23. 6640 units; 6.6 mL.
1494 units/hour; 29.9 mL/hr
Zero units.
Adjust intravenous drip 166 units/hour ↓.

24. 7280 units; 7.3 mL.
1638 units/hour; 32.8 mL/hr.
Zero units.
Adjust intravenous drip 182 units/hour ↓.

25. 5440 units; 5.4 mL.
1224 units/hour; 24.5 mL/hr.
Zero units; hold heparin for 1 hour.
Adjust intravenous drip 204 units/hour ↓.

26. 5680 units; 5.7 mL.
1278 units/hour; 25.6 mL/hr.
Zero units.
No change.

27. 6000 units; 6 mL.

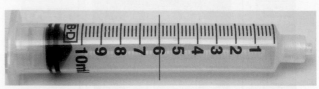

1350 units/hour; 27 mL/hr.
Zero units.
Adjust intravenous drip 150 units/hour ↓.

28. 6480 units; 6.5 mL.
1458 units/hour; 29.2 mL.
3240 units.
Adjust intravenous drip 162 units/hour ↑.

29. 6720 units; 6.7 mL.
1512 units/hour; 30.2 mL/hr.
6720 units.
Adjust intravenous drip 336 units/hour ↑.

30. 6320 units; 6.3 mL.
1422 units/hour; 28.4 mL/hr.
Zero units.
Adjust intravenous drip 158 units/hour ↓.

CHAPTER 17
Insulin
Preparing Insulin Injections, pp. 346-347

1.

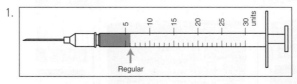

2.

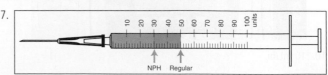

3. 65 − 42 = 23 units of regular insulin.

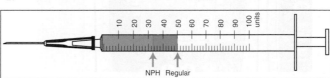

4. 47 − 35 = 12 units of regular insulin.

5. 65 − 30 = 35 units.

6. c.

7.

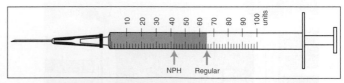

8. 100-unit syringe.

9.

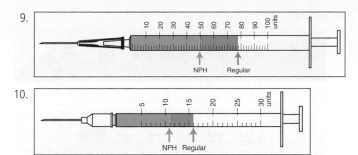

10.

Insulin Calculations Based on Blood Glucose Level and Food Intake, pp. 352-355

1. The patient does not need any insulin for his blood glucose level of 126 mg/dL. For lunch, the patient had a total of 75 grams of carbohydrate. To determine carbohydrate units, you must divide 75 by 15 for a total of 5 carbohydrate units. The patient should receive 0.8 units of insulin for every carbohydrate unit. You need to multiply 5 by 0.8, which is 4. Finally, you need to add the number of units to bring the blood glucose in to the target range with the amount of insulin needed to cover the meal. The patient needed zero units for blood glucose level adjustment and 4 units for the meal for a total of 4 units of insulin.

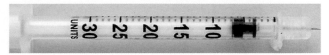

2. The patient is 25 mg/dL over the target blood glucose range (175 − 150 = 25). To determine the blood glucose units, divide 25 by 30, which is 0.83 units, and round up to 1 unit. The patient is to receive 1 unit of insulin for each blood glucose unit, or 1 unit (1 × 1). The patient consumed 128 grams of carbohydrate. To determine the number of carbohydrate units, you should divide 128 by 15, which is 8.53, and round to 9 carbohydrate units. The patient is to receive 0.8 units for every carbohydrate unit consumed. 9 carbohydrate units × 0.8 units of insulin is 7.2 units of insulin, which rounds to 7. To determine the total amount of insulin to be administered, add 7 units for the meal and 1 unit for the blood glucose level adjustment for a total of 8 units of insulin.

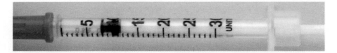

3. The patient's blood glucose level is below the target level of 150 mg/dL. Thus you do not need to administer any additional insulin. The patient is not eating at this time; thus you do not need to administer insulin for food consumption. The patient does not require any insulin at this time.

4. The patient is not over the target blood glucose range and does not need any additional insulin for the blood glucose. The patient will consume 98 grams of carbohydrate. To determine the number of carbohydrate units, you should divide 98 by 15, which is 6.53, and round to 7. The patient is to receive 0.8 units for every carbohydrate unit consumed. 7 carbohydrate units × 0.8 units of insulin is 5.6 units of insulin, which rounds to 6. To determine the total amount of insulin to be administered, add 6 units for the meal and 0 units for the blood glucose level adjustment for a total of 6 units of insulin.

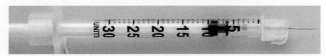

5. The patient is 98 mg/dL over the target blood glucose range (248 − 150 = 98). To determine the amount of insulin

needed for the increased blood glucose, divide 98 by 30, which is 3.27 units, and round to 3 units. The patient needs 1 unit of insulin for each blood glucose unit, or 3 units (3 × 1). The patient will consume 60 grams of carbohydrate. To determine the number of carbohydrate units, you should divide 60 by 15, which is 4. The patient is to receive 0.8 units for every carbohydrate unit consumed. 4 carbohydrate units × 0.8 units of insulin is 3.2 units of insulin, which rounds to 3. To determine the total amount of insulin to be administered, add 3 units for the meal and 3 units for the blood glucose level adjustment for a total of 6 units of insulin.

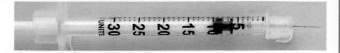

6. The patient is 8 mg/dL over the target blood glucose range (138 − 130 = 8). To determine the amount of insulin needed for the increased blood glucose, divide 8 by 30, which is 0.27 units, and round to 0 units. The patient does not need any insulin for the blood glucose level. The patient consumed 87 grams of carbohydrate. To determine the number of carbohydrate units, you should divide 87 by 8, which is 10.88, and round to 11 carbohydrate units. The patient is to receive 1 unit for every carbohydrate unit consumed. 11 carbohydrate units × 1 unit of insulin is 11 units of insulin. To determine the total amount of insulin to be administered, add 11 units for the meal and 0 units for the blood glucose level adjustment for a total of 11 units of insulin.

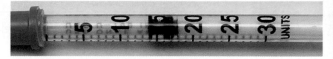

7. The patient is not over the target blood glucose range of 130 and does not need any additional insulin for blood glucose correction. The patient consumed 115 grams of carbohydrate. To determine the number of carbohydrate units, you should divide 115 by 8, which is 14.375, and round to 14 carbohydrate units. The patient is to receive 1 unit for every carbohydrate unit consumed. 14 carbohydrate units × 1 unit of insulin is 14 units of insulin. To determine the total amount of insulin to be administered, add 14 units for the meal and 0 units for the blood glucose level adjustment for a total of 14 units of insulin.

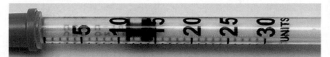

8. The patient is 19 mg/dL over the target blood glucose range (149 − 130 = 19). To determine the amount of insulin needed for the increased blood glucose, divide 19 by 30, which is 0.63 units, and round to 1 blood glucose unit. The patient should receive 1 unit of insulin for every unit of increased blood glucose or 1 unit (1 × 1 = 1). The patient consumed 124 grams of carbohydrate. To determine the number of carbohydrate units, you should divide 124 by 8, which is 15.5, and round to 16 carbohydrate units. The patient is to receive 1 unit for every carbohydrate unit consumed. 16 carbohydrate units × 1 unit of insulin is 16 units of insulin. To determine the total amount of insulin to be administered, add 16 units for the meal and 1 unit for the blood glucose level adjustment for a total of 17 units of insulin.

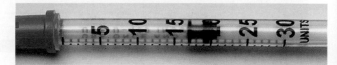

9. The patient is eating 48 grams of carbohydrates. To determine the number of carbohydrate units, you should divide 48 by 8, which is 6.

The patient needs to take 1 unit of insulin for every carbohydrate unit eaten. 6 × 1 = 6 units of insulin.

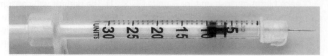

10. The patient's blood glucose is 78 mg/dL above the target range (198 − 120 = 78). To determine the amount of insulin needed for the increased blood glucose, divide 78 by 25, which is 3.12 units, and round to 3 units. The patient should receive one (1) unit of insulin for every unit increase in the blood glucose level. The patient should receive 3 units of insulin for the blood glucose adjustment.

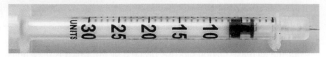

Chapter Review, pp. 355-360

1. 42 units.

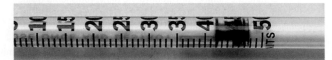

2. 34 units.

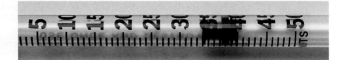

3. 30-unit syringe.

4. 100-unit syringe.

5. Regular insulin would be drawn up first.

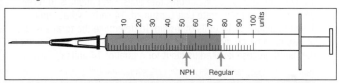

6. You should not give any regular insulin, since the blood glucose level is below 150 mg/dL.

7. 4 units.

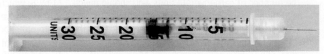

8. 13 units and contact physician.

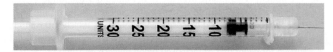

9. 11 units.

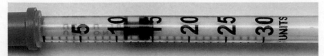

10. 14 units.

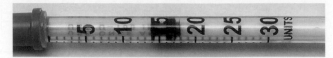

11. 3 units.

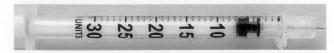

12. 5 units.

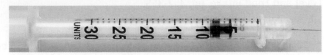

13. 3 units.

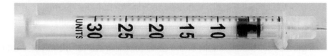

14. 8 units.

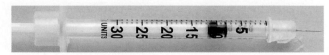

15. 4 units.

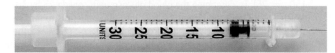

16. 2 units.

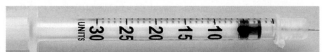

17. 2 units for blood glucose plus 3 units for carbohydrates = 5 units.

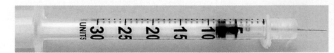

18. 2 units for glucose plus 2 units for carbohydrates = 4 units of insulin.

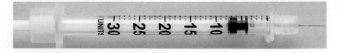

19. 7 units of insulin.

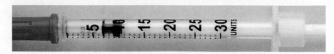

20. 2 units of insulin.

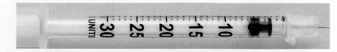

CHAPTER 18

Calculating Sliding-Scale Regular Insulin Dosages

Sliding Scale Prescription, pp. 364-366

1. You should not give any regular insulin, since the blood glucose level is below 150 mg/dL.

2. 4 units.

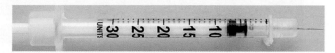

3. 13 units.

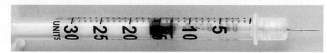

You should also call the physician on call to report this blood glucose.

4. 7 units.

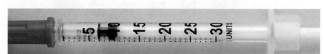

You should also recheck the patient's blood glucose in 2 hours.

5. 4 units.

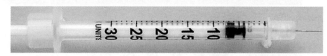

6. 4 units.

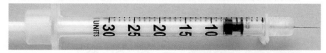

7. 4 units.

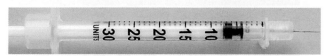

8. You should not give any regular insulin, since the blood glucose level is below 150 mg/dL.

9. 4 units.

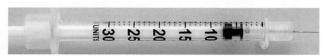

You should also recheck the patient's blood glucose level in 2 hours.

10. You should not give any regular insulin, since the blood glucose level is below 150 mg/dL.

Universal Formula, pp. 369-370

1. $160 - 100 = 60$ $60 \div 30 = 2$ units of regular insulin.

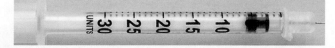

2. $223 - 100 = 123$ $123 \div 30 = 4.1$ units $= 4$ units of regular insulin.

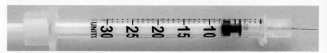

3. $302 - 100 = 202$ $202 \div 30 = 6.7$ units $= 7$ units of regular insulin.

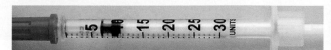

4. $254 - 100 = 154$ $154 \div 30 = 5.1$ units $= 5$ units of regular insulin.

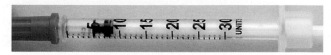

5. $273 - 100 = 173$ $173 \div 30 = 5.8$ units $= 6$ units of regular insulin.

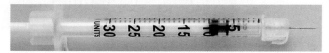

6. $494 - 100 = 394$ $394 \div 30 = 13.1$ units $= 13$ units of regular insulin.

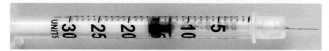

7. $184 - 100 = 84$ $84 \div 30 = 2.8$ units $= 3$ units of regular insulin.

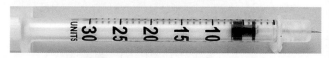

8. $389 - 100 = 289$ $289 \div 30 = 9.6$ units $= 10$ units of regular insulin.

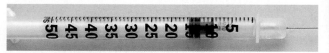

9. $214 - 100 = 114$ $114 \div 30 = 3.8$ units $= 4$ units of regular insulin.

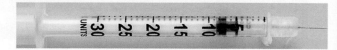

10. $246 - 100 = 146$ $146 \div 30 = 4.9$ units $= 5$ units of regular insulin.

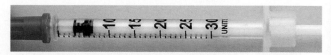

Chapter Review, pp. 370-374

1. 1 unit.

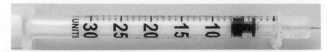

2. 3 units.

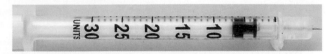

3. 0 units.

4. 3 units.

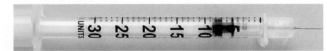

5. 5 units.

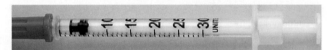

6. 2 units.

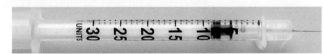

7. 5 units.

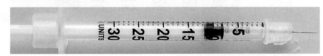

8. 8 units.

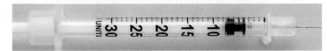

9. 4 units.

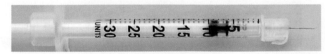

10. 6 units.

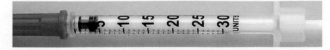

11. 1 unit.

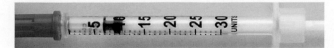

12. 7 units.

13. 5 units.

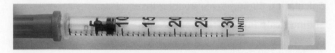

14. 6 units.

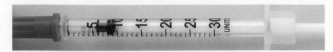

15. 3 units.

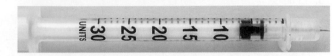

16. 3 units.

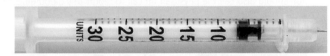

17. 6 units.

18. 5 units.

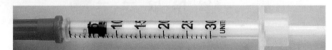

19. 7 units.

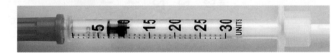

20. 9 units.

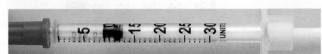

21. 3 units.

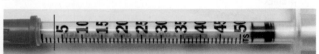

22. 0 units.

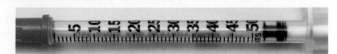

23. 5 units.

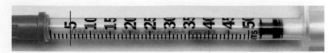

24. 2 units.

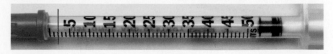

25. 6 units; contact physician immediately.

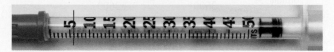

CHAPTER 19
Intake and Output

Output, p. 379

1. $\dfrac{100\ mL}{10\ mL} = \dfrac{1000\ mL}{X\ mL}$ Reduce: $\dfrac{10}{1} = \dfrac{1000}{X}$

   $10X = 1000$ $X = 100\ mL$

2. $\dfrac{200\ mL}{30\ mL} = \dfrac{1400\ mL}{X\ mL}$ Reduce: $\dfrac{20}{3} = \dfrac{1400}{X}$

   $20X = 4200$ $X = 210\ mL$

3. $\dfrac{100\ mL}{25\ mL} = \dfrac{600\ mL}{X\ mL}$ Reduce: $\dfrac{4}{1} = \dfrac{600}{X}$

   $4X = 600$ $X = 150\ mL$

4. $\dfrac{200\ mL}{40\ mL} = \dfrac{800\ mL}{X\ mL}$ Reduce: $\dfrac{5}{1} = \dfrac{800}{X}$

   $5X = 800$ $X = 160\ mL$

5. $\dfrac{200\ mL}{50\ mL} = \dfrac{500\ mL}{X\ mL}$ Reduce: $\dfrac{4}{1} = \dfrac{500}{X}$

   $4X = 500$ $X = 125\ mL$

6. $\dfrac{100\ mL}{40\ mL} = \dfrac{600\ mL}{X\ mL}$ Reduce: $\dfrac{5}{2} = \dfrac{600}{X}$

   $5X = 1200$ $X = 240\ mL$

7. $\dfrac{300\ mL}{25\ mL} = \dfrac{1200\ mL}{X\ mL}$ Reduce: $\dfrac{12}{1} = \dfrac{1200}{X}$

   $12X = 1200$ $X = 100\ mL$

8. $\dfrac{200\ mL}{30\ mL} = \dfrac{1000\ mL}{X\ mL}$ Reduce: $\dfrac{20}{3} = \dfrac{1000}{X}$

   $20X = 3000$ $X = 150\ mL$

9. $\dfrac{100\ mL}{30\ mL} = \dfrac{900\ mL}{X\ mL}$ Reduce: $\dfrac{10}{3} = \dfrac{900}{X}$

   $10X = 2700$ $X = 270\ mL$

10. $\dfrac{300\ mL}{50\ mL} = \dfrac{1500\ mL}{X\ mL}$ Reduce: $\dfrac{6}{1} = \dfrac{1500}{X}$

    $6X = 1500$ $X = 250\ mL$

Fluid Resuscitation for Burn Patients, pp. 383-384

1. A. $4 \times 90 \times 30 = 10,800\ mL$
   B. $10,800 \times 0.5 = 5400\ mL.$
   C. $5400/8 = 675\ mL/hr.$
   D. $10,800 \times 0.5 = 5400\ mL.$
   E. $5400/16 = 338\ mL/hr.$
   F. $1 \times 90 \times 30 = 2700\ mL/hr.$

2. A. $50\ lb/2.2 = 22.7\ kg$ as child's weight; $4 \times 22.7 \times 25 = 2270\ mL/24\ hr.$
   B. $2270 \times 0.5 = 1135\ mL.$
   C. $1135/8 = 142\ mL/hr.$
   D. $2270 \times 0.50 = 1135\ mL.$
   E. $1135/16 = 71\ mL/hr.$
   F. $1 \times 22.7 \times 25 = 567.5 = 568\ mL/hr.$

3. A. $73\ lb/2.2 = 33.2\ kg$ as weight; $4 \times 33.2 \times 35 = 4648\ mL/24\ hr.$
   B. $4648 \times 0.5 = 2324\ mL.$
   C. $2324/8 = 290.5 = 291\ mL/hr.$
   D. $4648 \times 0.5 = 2324\ mL.$
   E. $2324/16 = 145\ mL/hr.$
   F. $1 \times 33.2 \times 35 = 1162\ mL/hr.$

4. A. $106\ lb/2.2 = 48.2\ kg$ as weight; $4 \times 48.2 \times 20 = 3856\ mL/24\ hr.$
   B. $3856 \times 0.5 = 1928\ mL.$
   C. $1928/8 = 241\ mL/hr.$
   D. $3856 \times 0.5 = 1928\ mL.$
   E. $1928/16 = 121\ mL/hr.$
   F. $1 \times 48.2 \times 20 = 964\ mL/hr.$

5. A. $150\ lb/2.2 = 68.2\ kg$ as weight; $4 \times 68.2 \times 45 = 12,276\ mL/24\ hr.$
   B. $12,276 \times 0.5 = 6138\ mL.$
   C. $6138/8 = 767\ mL/hr.$
   D. $12,276 \times 0.5 = 6138\ mL.$
   E. $6138/16 = 384\ mL/hr.$
   F. $1 \times 68.2 \times 45 = 3069\ mL/hr.$

6. A. $80\ kg$ is the weight; $4 \times 80 \times 35 = 11,200\ mL/24\ hr.$
   B. $11,200 \times 0.5 = 5600\ mL.$
   C. $5600/8 = 700\ mL/hr.$
   D. $11,200 \times 0.5 = 5600\ mL.$
   E. $5600/16 = 350\ mL/hr.$
   F. $1 \times 80 \times 35 = 2800\ mL/hr.$

7. A. $96\ kg$ is the weight; $4 \times 96 \times 24 = 9216\ mL/24\ hr.$
   B. $9216 \times 0.5 = 4608\ mL.$
   C. $4608/8 = 576\ mL/hr.$
   D. $9216 \times 0.5 = 4608\ mL.$
   E. $4608/16 = 288\ mL/hr.$
   F. $1 \times 96 \times 24 = 2304\ mL/hr.$

8. A. $116\ kg$ is the weight; $4 \times 116 \times 70 = 32,480\ mL/24\ hr.$
   B. $32,480 \times 0.5 = 16,240\ mL.$
   C. $16,240/8 = 2030\ mL/hr.$
   D. $32,480 \times 0.5 = 16,240\ mL.$
   E. $16,240/16 = 1015\ mL/hr.$
   F. $1 \times 116 \times 70 = 8120\ mL/hr.$

9. A. $109\ kg$ is the weight; $4 \times 109 \times 36 = 15,696\ mL/24\ hr.$
   B. $15,696 \times 0.5 = 7848\ mL.$
   C. $7848/8 = 981\ mL/hr.$
   D. $15,696 \times 0.5 = 7848\ mL.$
   E. $7848/16 = 491\ mL/hr.$
   F. $1 \times 109 \times 36 = 3924\ mL/hr.$

10. A. $86\ kg$ is the weight; $4 \times 86 \times 60 = 20,640\ mL/24\ hr.$
    B. $20,640 \times 0.5 = 10,320\ mL.$
    C. $10,320/8 = 1290\ mL/hr.$
    D. $20,640 \times 0.5 = 10,320\ mL.$
    E. $10,320/16 = 645\ mL/hr.$
    F. $1 \times 86 \times 60 = 5160\ mL/hr.$

Chapter Review, pp. 384-386

1. 300 mL.

2. 80 mL.

3. 263 mL.

4. 200 mL.

5. 120 mL.

6. 150 mL.

7. 120 mL.

8. No; 1960 mL intake.

9. No; 120 mL minimum output.

10. No; 2300 mL intake.

11. A. 3683 mL/24 hr.
    B. 1842 mL.
    C. 230 mL/hr.
    D. 1842 mL.
    E. 115 mL/hr.
    F. 921 mL/hr.

12. A. 11,347 mL/24 hr.
    B. 5674 mL.
    C. 709 mL/hr.
    D. 5674 mL.
    E. 355 mL/hr.
    F. 2837 mL/hr.

13. A. 26,202 mL/24 hr.
    B. 13,101 mL.
    C. 1638 mL/hr.
    D. 13,101 mL.
    E. 819 mL/hr.
    F. 6551 mL/hr.

14. A. 17,600 mL/24 hr.
    B. 8800 mL.
    C. 1100 mL/hr.
    D. 8800 mL.
    E. 550 mL/hr.
    F. 4400 mL/hr.

15. A. 7280 mL/24 hr.
    B. 3640 mL.
    C. 455 mL/hr.
    D. 3640 mL.
    E. 228 mL/hr.
    F. 1820 mL/hr.

CHAPTER 20

Oncology

Formula Method, pp. 397-398

NOTE: The answers will be close but not exact between the two methods—nomogram and formula. Also note that the formula method in problems 1 through 10 all use the same formula, as follows:

$$\sqrt{Ht(cm) \times Wt(kg)}$$

1. Nomogram $= 2 \text{ m}^2 \times 1.2 \text{ mg/m}^2 = 2.4 \text{ mg}$

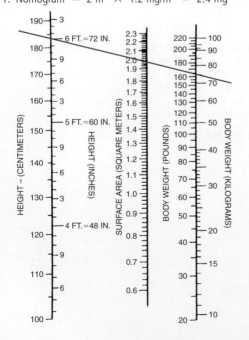

$$\text{Formula} = \frac{(72 \times 2.54) \times 75}{3600} = \frac{182.88 \times 75}{3600}$$

$$= \frac{13,716}{3600} = 3.81$$

$\sqrt{3.81} = 1.95$

$1.95 \text{ BSA} \times 1.2 = 2.3 \text{ mg}$

2. Nomogram $= 1.95 \text{ m}^2 \times 375 \text{ mg/m}^2 = 731 \text{ mg}$

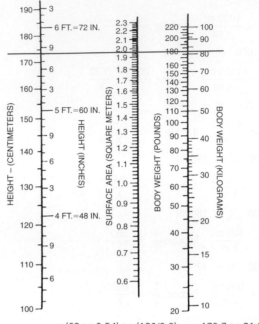

$$\text{Formula} = \frac{(68 \times 2.54) \times (180/2.2)}{3600} = \frac{172.7 \times 81.8}{3600}$$

$$= \frac{14,126.86}{3600} = 3.92$$

$\sqrt{3.92} = 1.98$

$1.98 \text{ BSA} \times 375 = 743 \text{ mg}$

3. Nomogram $= 2.54 \text{ m}^2 \times 125 \text{ mg/m}^2 = 318 \text{ mg}$
   BSA for 220 lb $= 2.3$
   BSA for 58 lb $= 1.3$
   BSA $2.3 + 1.3 = 3.6$

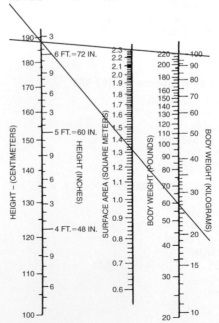

$$\text{Formula} = \frac{(74 \times 2.54) \times (278/2.2)}{3600} = \frac{187.9 \times 126.4}{3600}$$

$$= \frac{23,750.6}{3600} = 6.59$$

$$\sqrt{6.59} = 2.6$$

2.6 BSA × 125 = 325 mg

4. Nomogram = 1.95 m² × 135 mg/m² = 263 mg

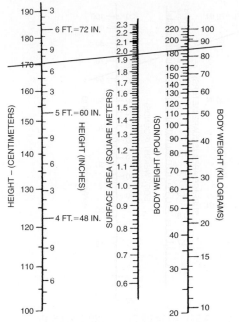

$$\text{Formula} = \frac{(67 \times 2.54) \times (185/2.2)}{3600} = \frac{170.2 \times 84.1}{3600}$$

$$= \frac{14,313.8}{3600} = 3.98$$

$$\sqrt{3.98} = 1.99$$

1.99 BSA × 135 = 269 mg

5. Nomogram = 1.8 m² × 20 mg/m² = 36 mg

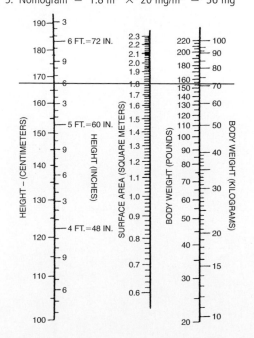

$$\text{Formula} = \frac{(66 \times 2.54) \times (72.72)}{3600} = \frac{167.6 \times 72.72}{3600}$$

$$= \frac{12,187.9}{3600} = 3.39$$

$$\sqrt{3.39} = 1.84$$

1.84 BSA × 20 = 36.8 mg

6. Nomogram = 1.91 m² × 100 mg/m² = 191 mg

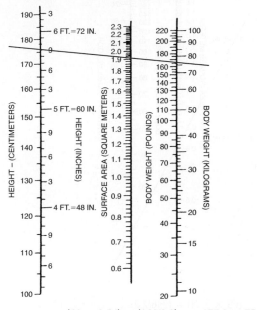

$$\text{Formula} = \frac{(69 \times 2.54) \times (166/2.2)}{3600} = \frac{175.3 \times 75.5}{3600}$$

$$= \frac{13,235.2}{3600} = 3.68$$

$$\sqrt{3.68} = 1.92$$

1.92 BSA × 100 = 192 mg

7. Nomogram $= 2.95 \text{ m}^2 \times 370 \text{ mg/m}^2 = 1092 \text{ mg}$
   BSA for 220 lb $= 2.15$
   BSA for 16 lb $= 0.8$
   BSA $2.15 + 0.8 = 2.95$

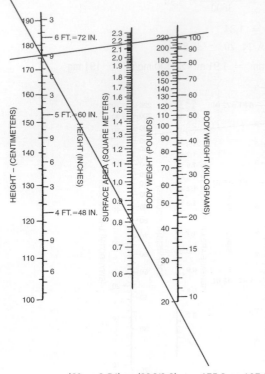

Formula $= \dfrac{(69 \times 2.54) \times (236/2.2)}{3600} = \dfrac{175.3 \times 107.3}{3600}$

$= \dfrac{18,809.7}{3600} = 5.22$

$\sqrt{5.22} = 2.28$

2.28 BSA $\times 370 = 844 \text{ mg}$

8. Nomogram $= 2.2 \text{ m}^2 \times 3.3 \text{ mg/m}^2 = 7.3 \text{ mg}$

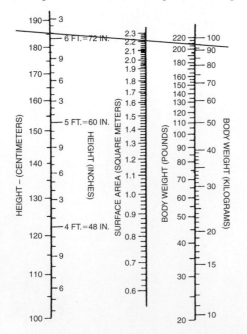

Formula $= \dfrac{(73 \times 2.54) \times (212/2.2)}{3600} = \dfrac{185.4 \times 96.4}{3600}$

$= \dfrac{17,872.6}{3600} = 4.96$

$\sqrt{4.96} = 2.23$

2.23 BSA $\times 3.3 = 7.36 \text{ mg}$

9. Nomogram $= 1.82 \text{ m}^2 \times 100 \text{ mg/m}^2 = 182 \text{ mg}$

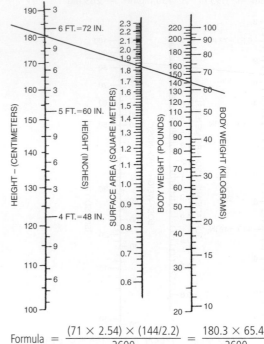

Formula $= \dfrac{(71 \times 2.54) \times (144/2.2)}{3600} = \dfrac{180.3 \times 65.45}{3600}$

$= \dfrac{118,010.6}{3600} = 3.28$

$\sqrt{3.28} = 1.81$

1.81 BSA $\times 100 = 181 \text{ mg}$

10. Nomogram = 3.6 m² × 500 mg/m² = 1800 mg
    BSA for 220 lb = 2.3
    BSA for 55 lb = 1.3
    BSA 2.3 + 1.3 = 3.6

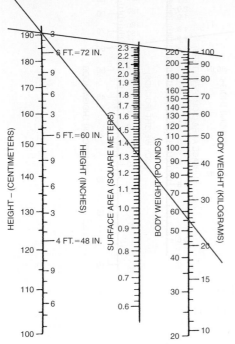

$$Formula = \frac{(75 \times 2.54) \times (275/2.2)}{3600} = \frac{190.5 \times 125}{3600}$$

$$= \frac{23,812.5}{3600} = 6.6$$

$\sqrt{6.6} = 2.57$

2.57 BSA × 500 = 1285 mg

Chapter Review, pp. 398-400

NOTE: The answers will be close but not exact between the two methods—nomogram and formula. Also note that the formula method in problems 1 through 10 all use the same formula, as follows:

$$\sqrt{\frac{Ht(cm) \times Wt(kg)}{}}$$

1. Nomogram = 2.56 mg

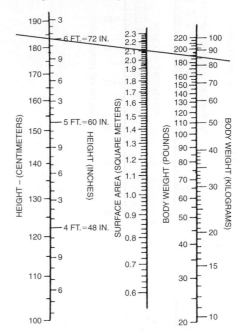

Formula = 2.5 mg

2. Nomogram = 653 mg

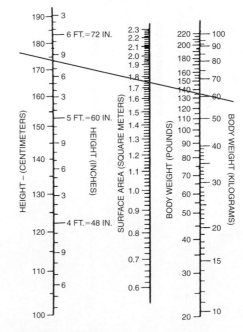

Formula = 645 mg

3. Nomogram = 225 mg

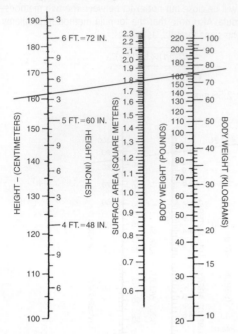

Formula = 229 mg

4. Nomogram = 230 mg

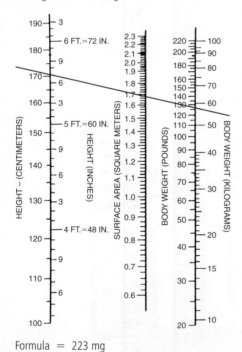

Formula = 223 mg

5. Nomogram = 34 mg

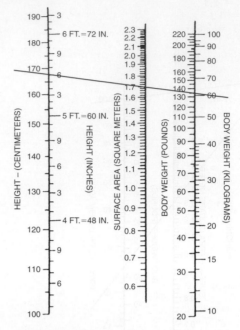

Formula = 34 mg

6. Nomogram = 180 mg

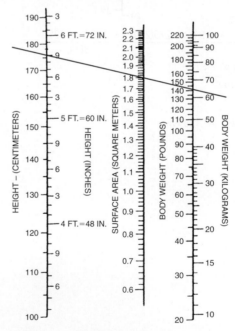

Formula = 177 mg

7. Nomogram = 674 mg

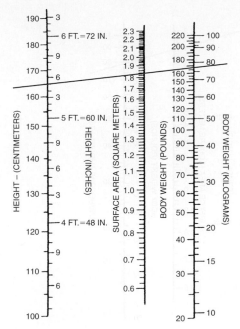

Formula = 692 mg

8. Nomogram = 6 mg

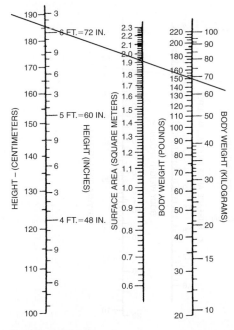

Formula = 6 mg

9. Nomogram = 172 mg

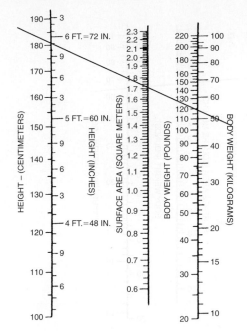

Formula = 162 mg

10. Nomogram = 1030 mg

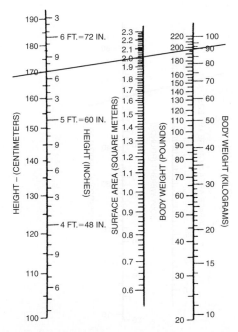

Formula = 1030 mg

11. Nomogram = 2 mg

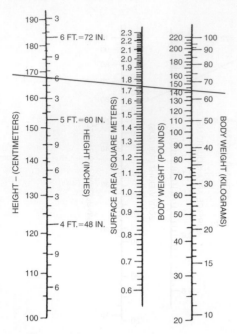

Formula = 2 mg

12. Nomogram = 653 mg

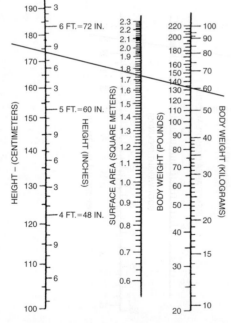

Formula = 641 mg

13. Nomogram = 263 mg

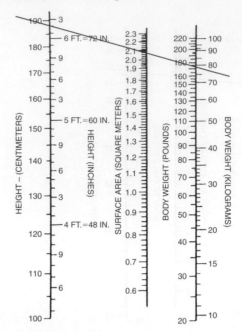

Formula = 254 mg

14. Nomogram = 243 mg

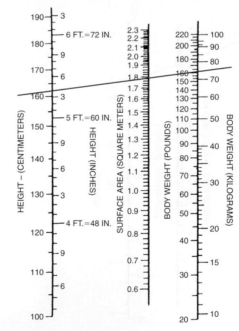

Formula = 247 mg

ANSWER KEY

15. Nomogram = 33 mg

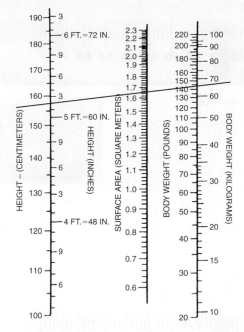

Formula = 34 mg

16. Nomogram = 180 mg

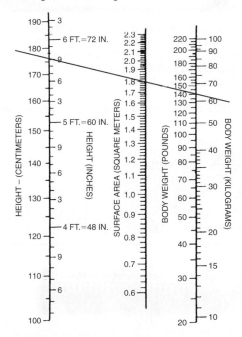

Formula = 179 mg

17. Nomogram = 577 mg

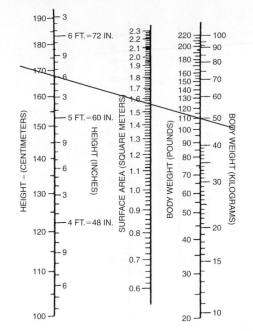

Formula = 570 mg

18. Nomogram = 6 mg

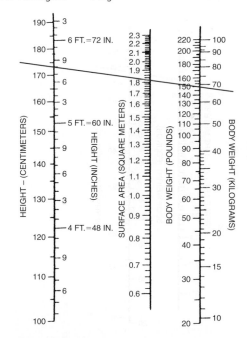

Formula = 6 mg

19. Nomogram = 210 mg

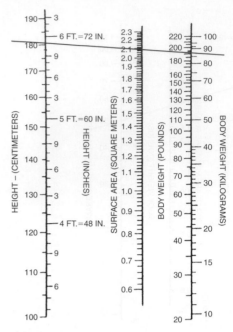

Formula = 209 mg

20. Nomogram = 900 mg

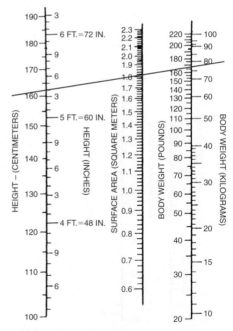

Formula = 930 mg

CHAPTER 21
Pediatrics
Medication Administration, pp. 411-417

1. A. 74 ÷ 2.2 = 33.6

33.6 − 31.4 kg = 2.2 kg

B. 1 g = 1000 mg

Ratio-proportion method:

$$\frac{1000 \text{ units}}{20 \text{ mL}} = \frac{400 \text{ mg}}{X \text{ mL}} \quad 1000X = 8000$$

X = 8 mL

Formula method:

400 mg/1000 mg × 20 mL = 8 mL

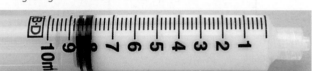

C. *Ratio-proportion method:*

$$\frac{15 \text{ mg}}{1 \text{ mL}} = \frac{75 \text{ mg}}{X \text{ mL}} \quad 15X = 75$$

X = 5 mL

Formula method:

75 mg/15 mg × 1 mL = 5 mL

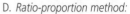

D. *Ratio-proportion method:*

$$\frac{2.5 \text{ g}}{10 \text{ mL}} = \frac{2 \text{ g}}{X \text{ mL}} \quad 2.5X = 20$$

X = 8 mL

Formula method:

2 g/2.5 g × 10 mL = 8 mL

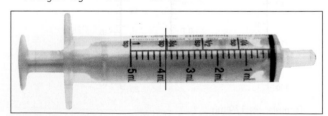

E. Merilee weighs 31.4 kg. The range of Pancrease 20 that she can receive is between 31.4 kg × 400 units = 12,560 units and 31.4 × 2500 units = 78,500 units. Merilee is receiving 3 capsules, each containing 20,000 units of lipase.
She receives 20,000 units × 3 at each meal or a total of 60,000 units of lipase.
Her dose of 60,000 units falls within the range of 12,560 units and 78,500 units.

2. A. *Ratio-proportion method:*

$$\frac{20 \text{ mg}}{1 \text{ mL}} = \frac{75 \text{ mg}}{X \text{ mL}} \quad 20X = 75$$

X = 3.8 mL

Formula method:

75 mg/20 mg × 1 mL = 3.8 mL

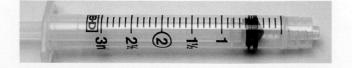

B. *Ratio-proportion method:*

$$\frac{150 \text{ mg}}{1 \text{ mL}} = \frac{60 \text{ mg}}{X \text{ mL}} \quad 150X = 60$$

X = 0.4 mL

Formula method:

60 mg/150 mg × 1 mL = 0.4 mL

C. *Ratio-proportion method:*

$$\frac{80 \text{ mg}}{2 \text{ mL}} = \frac{15 \text{ mg}}{X \text{ mL}} \quad 80X = 30$$

X = 0.375 (round to the nearest hundredth) = 0.38 mL.

Formula method:

15 mg/80 mg × 2 mL = 0.375 mL (round to the nearest hundredth) = 0.38 mL.

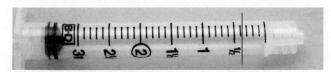

D. *Ratio-proportion method:*

$$\frac{40 \text{ mg}}{1 \text{ mL}} = \frac{60 \text{ mg}}{X \text{ mL}} \quad 40X = 60$$

X = 1.5 mL

Formula method:

60 mg/40 mg × 1 mL = 1.5 mL

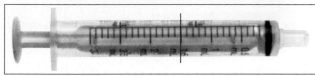

E. *Ratio-proportion method:*

$$\frac{100 \text{ mg}}{1 \text{ mL}} = \frac{90 \text{ mg}}{X \text{ mL}} \quad 100X = 90$$

X = 0.9 mL

Formula method:

90 mg/100 mg × 1 mL = 0.9 mL

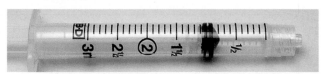

Zachary weighs 6 kg. His dose is 90 mg. To find the amount of mg/kg, divide the dose by his weight: 90/6 = 15 mg/kg.

3. A. 1g = 1000 mg

Ratio-proportion method:

$$\frac{1000 \text{ mg}}{20 \text{ mL}} = \frac{440 \text{ mg}}{X \text{ mL}} \quad 1000X = 8800$$

X = 8.8 mL

Formula method:

430 mg/1000 mg × 20 mL = 8.8 mL

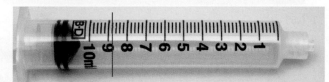

B. *Ratio-proportion method:*

$$\frac{40 \text{ mg}}{1 \text{ mL}} = \frac{35 \text{ mg}}{X \text{ mL}} \quad 40X = 35$$

X = 0.88 mL

Formula method:

35 mg/40 mg × 1 mL = 0.88 mL

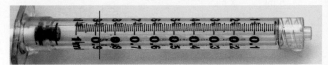

C. *Ratio-proportion method:*

$$\frac{50 \text{ mg}}{1 \text{ tab}} = \frac{75 \text{ mg}}{X \text{ tab}} \quad 50X = 75$$

X = 1.5 tablets

Formula method:

75 mg/50 mg × 1 tab = 1.5 tablets

D. *Ratio-proportion method:*

$$\frac{8 \text{ mg}}{1 \text{ tab}} = \frac{4 \text{ mg}}{X \text{ tab}} \quad 8X = 4$$

X = 0.5 tablet

Formula method:

4 mg/8 mg × 1 tab = ½ tablet

E. 10 hours at 40 mL/hour = 400 mL; 14 hours at 35 mL/hour = 490 mL; total number infused = 890 mL/24 hours.

4. A. Betony's BSA is 0.57 m².
   B. Her dose of Retrovir is 120 mg. To calculate the amount of medication per m², divide the dose by her m²: 120/0.57 = 210.5 mgm. This dose falls within the appropriate range of 180-240 mg/m².

   Ratio-proportion method:

$$\frac{10 \text{ mg}}{1 \text{ mL}} = \frac{120 \text{ mg}}{X \text{ mL}} \quad 10X = 120$$

X = 12 mL

Formula method:

120 mg/10 mg × 1 mL = 12 mL

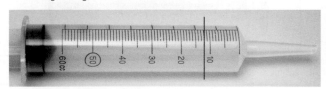

C. Her dose of Videx is 70 mg. To calculate the amount of medication per m², divide the dose by her m²: 70/0.57 = 122.8 mg. This dose falls within the appropriate range of 90-150 mg/m².

Ratio-proportion method:

$$\frac{10 \text{ mg}}{1 \text{ mL}} = \frac{70 \text{ mg}}{X \text{ mL}} \quad 10X = 70$$

X = 7 mL

Formula method:

70 mg/10 mg × 1 mL = 7 mL

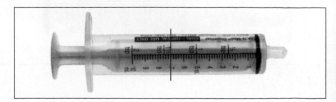

D. *Ratio-proportion method:*

$$\frac{50 \text{ mg}}{5 \text{ mL}} = \frac{65}{X \text{ mL}} \quad 50X = 325$$

X = 6.5 mL

Formula method:

65 mg/50 mg × 5 mL = 6.5 mL

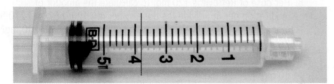

E. Betony receives 2 mL of Kaletra. She is receiving 2 × 80 mg = 160 mg of lopinavir and 2 × 20 mg = 40 mg of ritonavir.

Chapter Review, pp. 417-423

1. 0.29 mL

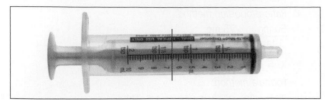

2. 3.75 mL round to 3.8 mL

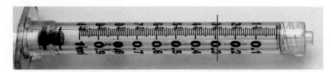

3. 7.5 mL

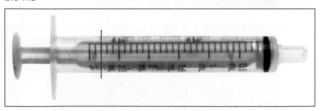

4. 2.8 mL

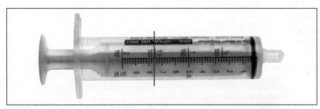

5. 4.3 mL

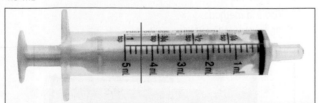

6. 7.4 mL

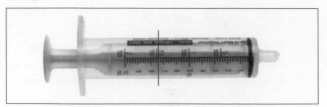

7. 7.4 mL

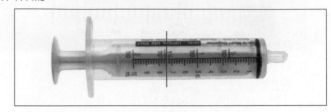

8. 16 mL

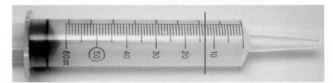

9. 2 capsules

10. 4 mL

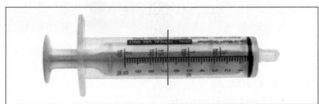

11. 6.6 mL

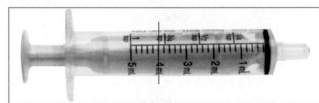

12. 0.45 mL

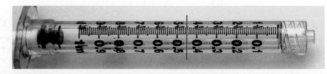

13. 0.65 mL

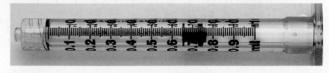

14. 0.84 mL

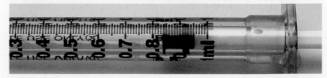

15. 4.8 mL

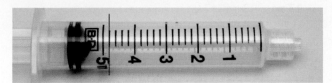

16. 0.9 mL

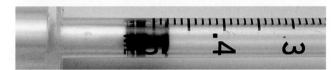

17. 0.48 mL

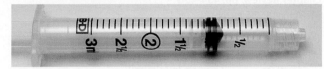

18. 0.68 mL

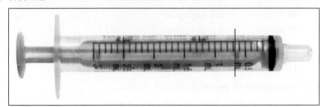

19. 2.7 mL

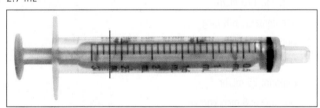

20. 7.5 mL

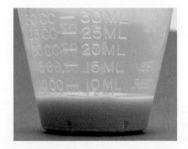

CHAPTER 22
Intensive Care Unit
Titration, pp. 433-434

1. Bumex: Give 1 mg as dose.

$$\frac{0.5\ mg}{1\ hr} = \frac{X\ mg}{2\ hr} \quad 1X = 0.5 \times 2 \quad X = 1\ mg$$

2. Propranolol: For initial dose of 1 mg/hr:

$$\frac{15\ mg}{500\ mL} = \frac{1\ mg}{X\ mL} \quad 15X = 500 \quad X = 33.3\ mL/hr$$

For maximum dose of 3 mg/hr:

$$\frac{15\ mg}{500\ mL} = \frac{3\ mg}{X\ mL} \quad 15X = 1500 \quad X = 100\ mL/hr$$

3. NTG: 10 mcg/min = 600 mcg/hr or 0.6 mg/hr

$$\frac{100\ mg}{250\ mL} = \frac{0.6\ mg}{X\ mL} \quad 100X = 150 \quad X = 1.5\ mL/hr$$

Titration table:

IV RATE	DOSE
1.5 mL/hr	10 mcg/min **(minimum)**
3 mL/hr	20 mcg/min
4.5 mL/hr	30 mcg/min
6 mL/hr	40 mcg/min
7.5 mL/hr	50 mcg/min
9 mL/hr	60 mcg/min **(maximum)**

20 mcg/min = 1200 mcg/hr or 1.2 mg/hr

$$\frac{100\ mg}{250\ mL} = \frac{1.2\ mg}{X\ mL} \quad 100X = 300 \quad X = 3\ mL/hr$$

30 mcg/min = 1800 mcg/hr or 1.8 mg/hr

$$\frac{100\ mg}{250\ mL} = \frac{1.8\ mg}{X\ mL} \quad 100X = 450 \quad X = 4.5\ mL/hr$$

40 mcg/min = 2400 mcg/hr or 2.4 mg/hr

$$\frac{100\ mg}{250\ mL} = \frac{2.4\ mg}{X\ mL} \quad 100X = 600 \quad X = 6\ mL/hr$$

50 mcg/min = 3000 mcg/hr or 3 mg/hr

$$\frac{100\ mg}{250\ mL} = \frac{3\ mg}{X\ mL} \quad 100X = 750 \quad X = 7.5\ mL/hr$$

60 mcg/min = 3600 mcg/hr or 3.6 mg/hr

$$\frac{100\ mg}{250\ mL} = \frac{3.6\ mg}{X\ mL} \quad 100X = 900 \quad X = 9\ mL/hr$$

4. Titration table:

IV RATE	DOSE
5 mcg/min	1.5 mL/hr
15 mcg/min	4.5 mL/hr
25 mcg/min	7.5 mL/hr
35 mcg/min	10.5 mL/hr
50 mcg/min	15 mL/hr

5 mcg/min = 300 mcg/hr or 0.3 mg/hr

$$\frac{100\ mg}{500\ mL} = \frac{0.3\ mg}{X\ mL} \quad 100X = 150 \quad X = 1.5\ mL/hr$$

15 mcg/min = 900 mcg/hr or 0.9 mg/hr

$$\frac{100\ mg}{500\ mL} = \frac{0.9\ mg}{X\ mL} \quad 100X = 450 \quad X = 4.5\ mL/hr$$

25 mcg/min = 1500 mcg/hr or 1.5 mg/hr

$$\frac{100\ mg}{500\ mL} = \frac{1.5\ mg}{X\ mL} \quad 100X = 750 \quad X = 7.5\ mL/hr$$

35 mcg/min = 2100 mcg/hr or 2.1 mg/hr

$$\frac{100\ mg}{500\ mL} = \frac{2.1\ mg}{X\ mL} \quad 100X = 1050 \quad X = 10.5\ mL/hr$$

50 mcg/min = 3000 mcg/hr or 3 mg/hr

$$\frac{100\ mg}{500\ mL} = \frac{3\ mg}{X\ mL} \quad 100X = 1500 \quad X = 15\ mL/hr$$

Formula:

$$\frac{500\ mL}{100\ mg} \times \frac{2\ mcg}{min} \times \frac{60\ min}{1\ hr} \times \frac{1\ mg}{1000\ mcg} =$$

$$\frac{150,000}{100,000} = 1.5\ mL/hr$$

5. Pronestyl: 30 mL/hr

2 mg/min = 120 mg/hr

$$\frac{2000 \text{ mg}}{500 \text{ mL}} = \frac{4}{1}$$

$$\frac{4 \text{ mg}}{1 \text{ mL}} = \frac{120 \text{ mg}}{X \text{ mL}} \quad 4X = 120 \quad X = 30 \text{ mL/hr}$$

Formula:

$$\frac{500 \text{ mL}}{2000 \text{ mg}} \times \frac{2 \text{ mg}}{\text{min}} \times \frac{60 \text{ min}}{1 \text{ hr}} = \frac{30,000}{500} = 30 \text{ mL/hr}$$

6. Pronestyl: 60 mL/hr

4 mg/min = 240 mg/hr

$$\frac{1000 \text{ mg}}{250 \text{ mL}} = \frac{4}{1}$$

$$\frac{4 \text{ mg}}{1 \text{ mL}} = \frac{240 \text{ mg}}{X \text{ mL}} \quad 4X = 240 \quad X = 60 \text{ mL/hr}$$

Formula:

$$\frac{250 \text{ mL}}{1000 \text{ mg}} \times \frac{4 \text{ mg}}{\text{min}} \times \frac{60 \text{ min}}{1 \text{ hr}} = \frac{60,000}{1000} = 60 \text{ mL/hr}$$

7. Lidocaine: 30 mL/hr

2 mg/min = 120 mg/hr

$$\frac{1000 \text{ mg}}{250 \text{ mL}} = \frac{4}{1}$$

$$\frac{4 \text{ mg}}{1 \text{ mL}} = \frac{120 \text{ mg}}{X \text{ mL}} \quad 4X = 120 \quad X = 30 \text{ mL/hr}$$

Formula:

$$\frac{250 \text{ mL}}{1000 \text{ mg}} \times \frac{2 \text{ mg}}{\text{min}} \times \frac{60 \text{ min}}{1 \text{ hr}} = \frac{3000}{1000} = 30 \text{ mL/hr}$$

8. Morphine sulfate: 62.5 mL/hr

$$\frac{100 \text{ mg}}{250 \text{ mL}} = \frac{25 \text{ mg}}{X \text{ mL}}$$

$$100X = 6250 \quad X = 62.5 \text{ mL/hr}$$

Formula:

$$\frac{250 \text{ mL}}{100 \text{ mg}} \times \frac{25 \text{ mg}}{\text{hr}} = \frac{6250}{100} = 62.5 \text{ mL/hr}$$

9. Morphine sulfate: 100 mL/hr

$$\frac{250 \text{ mL}}{100 \text{ mg}} \times \frac{40 \text{ mg}}{1 \text{ hr}} = \frac{10,000}{100} = 100 \text{ mL/hr}$$

$$\frac{100 \text{ mg}}{250 \text{ mL}} = \frac{40 \text{ mg}}{X \text{ mL}}$$

$$100X = 10,000 \quad X = 100 \text{ mL/hr}$$

Titration table:

IV RATE	DOSE
100 mL/hr	40 mg/hr **(minimum)**
200 mL/hr	80 mg/hr
300 mL/hr	120 mg/hr **(maximum)**

$$\frac{100 \text{ mg}}{250 \text{ mL}} = \frac{80 \text{ mg}}{X \text{ mL}}$$

$$100X = 20,000 \quad X = 200 \text{ mL/hr}$$

$$\frac{100 \text{ mg}}{250 \text{ mL}} = \frac{120 \text{ mg}}{X \text{ mL}}$$

$$100X = 30,000 \quad X = 300 \text{ mL/hr}$$

10. Atropine: 10 mL/hr

$$\frac{0.3 \text{ mg}}{1 \text{ mL}} = \frac{3 \text{ mg}}{X \text{ mL}}$$

$$0.3X = 3 \quad X = 10 \text{ mL/hr}$$

Formula:

$$\frac{1 \text{ mL}}{0.3 \text{ mg}} \times \frac{3 \text{ mg}}{1 \text{ hr}} = \frac{3}{0.3} = 10 \text{ mL/hr}$$

Chapter Review, pp. 434-436

1. Atropine: 2.5 mL/hr

2. Procainamide hydrochloride: 15 mL/hr

IV RATE	DOSE
15 mL/hr	2 mg/min **(minimum)**
30 mL/hr	4 mg/min **(usual maximum dose)**
45 mL/hr	6 mg/min

3. Cerebyx: 178 mL/hr

4. Morphine sulfate: 23 mL/hr

IV RATE	DOSE
23 mL/hr	0.2 mg/kg/hr **(minimum)**
46 mL/hr	0.4 mg/kg/hr
70 mL/hr	0.6 mg/kg/hr
93 mL/hr	0.8 mg/kg/hr
116 mL/hr	1.0 mg/kg/hr **(maximum)**

5. Theophylline ethylenediamine: 25 mL/hr

6. Dexmedetomidine hydrochloride: 45 mL/hr

7. Esmolol: 110 mL/hr

8. Remifentanil: 6.8 mcg

9. Dobutamine hydrochloride (Dobutrex): 20 mL/hr

10. NTG: 93.3 mcg/min

11. Heparin: 25 mL/hr

12. Dopamine: 8 mcg/kg/min

13. Dobutrex: 20 mg/hr

14. Dopamine: 16.8 mL/hr

15. Esmolol (Brevibloc): 186 mL/hr

16. Dopamine: 7.8 mcg/min

17. NTG: 66.7 mcg/min

18.
IV RATE	DOSE
30 mL/hr	4 mcg/min
45 mL/hr	6 mcg/min
60 mL/hr	8 mcg/min
75 mL/hr	10 mcg/min
90 mL/hr	12 mcg/min

19. Midazolam (Versed): 560 mcg

20. 6 mL/hr

IV RATE	DOSE
6 mL/hr	40 mcg/min
9 mL/hr	60 mcg/min
12 mL/hr	80 mcg/min
15 mL/hr	100 mcg/min
18 mL/hr	120 mcg/min

Index

Page numbers followed by *f*, *t*, and *b* indicate figures, tables, and boxes, respectively.